AF544839

Common Problems in Obstetric Anesthesia

Second Edition

Sanjay Datta, M.D., F.F.A.R.C.S. (Eng.)
Director of Obstetric Anesthesia
Brigham and Women's Hospital
Professor of Anaesthesia
Harvard Medical School
Boston, Massachusetts

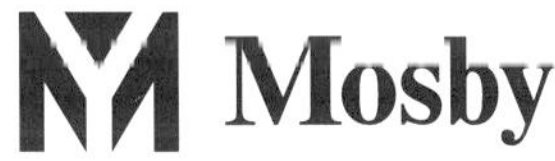

St. Louis Baltimore Berlin Boston Carlsbad Chicago London Madrid
Naples New York Philadelphia Sydney Tokyo Toronto

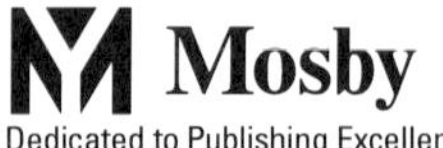

Dedicated to Publishing Excellence

Executive Editor: Susan M. Gay

Developmental Editor: Sandra Clark Brown

Project Manager: Linda Clarke

Project Supervisor: Victoria Hoenigke

Manufacturing Manager: Theresa Fuchs

Book Designer: Nancy McDonald

SECOND EDITION

Printed in the United States of America
Composition by the Clarinda Company
Printing/binding by Maple Vail-York

Mosby–Year Book, Inc.
11830 Westline Industrial Drive
St. Louis, MO 63146

Library of Congress Cataloging-in-Publication Data

Common problems in obstetric anesthesia / [edited by] Sanjay Datta.--
2nd ed.
p. cm.
Includes bibliographical references and index.
ISBN 0-8151-2348-5
1. Anesthesia in obstetrics. I. Datta, Sanjay.
RG732.C66 1995
617.9′682--dc20 94-34612
CIP

Contributors

Amr E. Abouleish, M.D.
Assistant Professor of Anesthesiology
The University of Texas Medical Branch
Galveston, Texas

Ezzat I. Abouleish, M.B., Ch.B., D.A., M.D.
Director of Obstetric Anesthesia
Professor of Anesthesiology
University of Texas Medical School
Department of Anesthesia
Houston, Texas

Angela M. Bader, M.D.
Director of Obstetric Anesthesia Research
Brigham and Women's Hospital
Assistant Professor of Anaesthesia
Harvard Medical School
Boston, Massachusetts

Deborah M. Barron, M.D.
Staff Anesthesiologist
Brigham and Women's Hospital
Clinical Instructor in Anesthesiology
Harvard Medical School
Boston, Massachusetts

David J. Birnbach, M.D.
Director of Obstetric Anesthesiology
St. Luke's-Roosevelt Hospital Center
Assistant Professor of Anesthesiology, Obstetrics and Gynecology
Columbia University College of Physicians and Surgeons
New York, New York

Norman H. Blass, M.D.
Distinguished Professor of Anesthesiology, Obstetrics and Gynecology
Department of Anesthesiology
The University of Texas Medical Branch
Galveston, Texas

George Blike, M.D.
Assistant Professor of Anesthesiology
Director of Obstetric Anesthesiology
Dartmouth-Hitchcock Medical Center
Lebanon, New Hampshire

Stuart Bramwell, M.D.
Director of Obstetric Anesthesia
Grady Memorial Hospital
Associate Professor of Anesthesiology and Obstetrics and Gynecology
Department of Anesthesia
Emory University
Atlanta, Georgia

Glen Z. Brooks, M.D.
Division Chief of Obstetric Anesthesia
North Shore University Hospital
Assistant Professor of Anesthesiology and Obstetrics and Gynecology
Cornell University Medical College
Manhasset, New York

Gerald A. Burger, M.D.
Captain
Medical Corps, U.S. Navy
Chairman
Department of Anesthesiology
Naval Medical Center
San Diego, California

William Camann, M.D.
Director of Obstetric Anesthesia Education
Brigham and Women's Hospital
Assistant Professor of Anaesthesia
Harvard Medical School
Boston, Massachusetts

Harvey Carp, Ph.D., M.D.
Director of Obstetric Anesthesia
Department of Anesthesia
Associate Professor of Anesthesiology and Obstetrics and Gynecology
University of Oregon Health Sciences Center
Portland, Oregon

Barry C. Corke, M.D., Ch.B., F.F.A.R.C.S.
Director of Obstetric Anesthesia
Medical Center of Delaware
Christiana Hospital
Jefferson Medical College
Newark, Delaware

Stephen B. Corn, M.D.
Staff Anesthesiologist
Brigham and Women's Hospital
Boston Children's Hospital
Instructor in Anaesthesia
Harvard Medical School
Boston, Massachusetts

John G. D'Alessio, M.D.
Assistant Professor of Anesthesiology
University of Tennessee College of Medicine at Memphis
Memphis, Tennessee

Sanjay Datta, M.D., F.F.A.R.C.S. (Eng.)
Director of Obstetric Anesthesia
Brigham and Women's Hospital
Professor of Anaesthesia
Harvard Medical School
Boston, Massachusetts

Carter Dodge, M.D.
Associate Professor of Anesthesiology and Pediatrics
Director of Pediatric Anesthesia
Dartmouth-Hitchcock Medical Center
Lebanon, New Hampshire

Hal S. Feldman, D.Sc.
Associate Director of Research
Brigham and Women's Hospital
Assistant Professor of Anaesthesia
Harvard Medical School
Boston, Massachusetts

Stephen P. Gatt, L.R.C.P., M.R.C.S., M.D., F.F.A.R.C.S., F.F.I.C.A.N.Z.C.A., (Intnsv. Cr.)
Senior Lecturer in Anaesthesia
University of New South Wales
Kensington, New South Wales, Australia
Director of Anaesthesia
Royal Hospital for Women
Paddington, New South Wales, Australia

Kenneth W. Gerard, M.D., Ph.D.
Director of Orthopedic Anesthesia
Medical Center of Delaware
Christiana Hospital
Clinical Assistant Professor of Anesthesiology
Jefferson Medical College
Newark, Delaware

Charles P. Gibbs, M.D.
Professor and Chairman
Department of Anesthesiology
University of Colorado School of Medicine
Denver, Colorado

Lesley I. Gilberton, M.D.
Staff Anesthesiologist
Brigham and Women's Hospital
Instructor in Anesthesia
Harvard Medical School
Boston, Massachusetts

Raymond Glassenberg, M.D.
Chief of Obstetric Anesthesia
Northwestern Memorial Hospital
Assistant Professor of Anesthesia
Northwestern University Medical School
Chicago, Illinois

Samuel Glassenberg
Director of Computer Graphics
CompuGraph
Wilmette, Illinois

Andrew P. Harris, M.D.
Director of Obstetric and Nelson 2 (TeLinde) O.R. Anesthesia
The Johns Hopkins Hospital
Associate Professor of Anesthesiology, Critical Care Medicine, and Gynecology and Obstetrics
The Johns Hopkins University School of Medicine
Baltimore, Maryland

Philip M. Hartigan, M.D.
Staff Anesthesiologist
Brigham and Women's Hospital
Instructor in Anaesthesia
Harvard Medical School
Boston, Massachusetts

Martha A. Hauch, M.D.
Staff Anesthesiologist
Brigham and Women's Hospital
Instructor in Anaesthesia
Harvard Medical School
Boston, Massachusetts

Ronald J. Hurley, M.D.
Associate Director of Obstetric Anesthesia
Brigham and Women's Hospital
Assistant Professor of Anaesthesia
Harvard Medical School
Boston, Massachusetts

Thomas H. Joyce, III, M.D.
Professor of Anesthesiology
University of Cincinnati College of Medicine
Cincinnati, Ohio

Nancy B. Kenepp, M.D.
Associate Professor of Anesthesia
Temple University Hospital
Temple University Medical School
Philadelphia, Pennsylvania

Brian King, M.D., Ph.D.
Fellow in Obstetrical Anesthesia
Department of Anesthesia
Brigham & Women's Hospital
Harvard Medical School
Boston, Massachusetts

Betty Lou Koffel, M.D.
Assistant Professor of Anesthesiology
University of Maryland School of Medicine
Baltimore, Maryland

Catherine K. Lineberger, M.D.
Assistant Professor of Anesthesiology
Department of Anesthesiology
Duke University Medical Center
Durham, North Carolina

Steven A. Lussos, M.D.
Staff Anesthesiologist
Fairfax Anesthesiology Associates
Fairfax Hospital
Falls Church, Virginia

Joseph S. Mallon, M.D., F.R.C.P.C.
Assistant Professor
Faculty of Medicine
Department of Anaesthesia
University of Toronto
Mount Sinai Hospital
Toronto, Ontario, Canada

Gordon L. Mandell, M.D.
Associate Chief of Anesthesiology
Magee-Women's Hospital
Assistant Professor of Anesthesiology
University of Pittsburgh School of Medicine
Pittsburgh, Pennsylvania

Ramon Martin, M.D., Ph.D.
Staff Anesthesiologist
Brigham and Women's Hospital
Assistant Professor of Anaesthesia
Harvard Medical School
Boston, Massachusetts

Graham H. McMorland, M.B., Ch.B., F.R.C.P.C.
Professor Emeritus
Department of Anaesthesia
University of British Columbia
Vancouver, British Columbia

J. Stephen Naulty, M.D.
Chairman
Department of Anesthesiology
Pennsylvania Hospital
Clinical Professor of Anesthesia and Obstetrics and Gynecology
University of Pennsylvania School of Medicine
Philadelphia, Pennsylvania

Nancy E. Oriol, M.D.
Director of Obstetric Anesthesia
Beth Israel Hospital
Assistant Professor of Anaesthesia
Harvard Medical School
Boston, Massachusetts

Marcia A. Procopio, M.D.
Assistant Professor of Anesthesiology
Dartmouth-Hitchcock Medical Center
Lebanon, New Hampshire

Jaya Ramanathan, M.D.
Director of Obstetric Anesthesia
Professor of Anesthesiology
University of Tennessee College of Medicine at Memphis
Memphis, Tennessee

Sivam Ramanathan, M.D.
Chief of Anesthesiology
Professor of Anesthesiology/Critical Care Medicine
Magee-Women's Hospital
University of Pittsburgh School of Medicine
Pittsburgh, Pennsylvania

Ram S. Ravindran, M.D.
Associate Professor of Anesthesiology
Department of Anesthesiology
Indiana University Medical Center
Indianapolis, Indiana

Kenneth L. Rodino, M.D.
Associate Professor
Department of Anesthesia
Northwestern Memorial Hospital
Northwestern University Medical School
Chicago, Illinois

Stephen H. Rolbin, M.D., F.R.C.P.C.
Assistant Professor
Faculty of Medicine
Department of Anaesthesia
University of Toronto
Mount Sinai Hospital
Toronto, Ontario, Canada

Francis A. Rosinia, M.D.
Director of Obstetric Anesthesia
Department of Anesthesia
Department of Obstetrics and Gynecology
Ochsner Medical Foundation
New Orleans, Louisiana

Mukesh C. Sarna, M.D., F.R.C.A., F.F.A.R.C.S.
Assistant Director of Obstetric Anesthesia
Beth Israel Hospital
Instructor in Anaesthesia
Harvard Medical School
Boston, Massachusetts

Markus C. Schneider, M.D.
Staff Anesthesiologist
Assistant Professor of Anaesthesiology
University Hospital-Kantonsspital
Basel, Switzerland

Ferne B. Sevarino, M.D.
Associate Director of Acute Pain Service
Associate Director of Obstetric Anesthesia
Associate Professor of Anesthesiology
Yale University School of Medicine
New Haven, Connecticut

Jonathan H. Skerman, B.D.Sc., M.Sc.D., D.Sc.
Vice Chairman for Administration and Research
Department of Anesthesiology
Professor of Anesthesiology
Professor of Obstetrics and Gynecology
Louisiana State University Medical Center
Shreveport, Louisiana

Christopher R. Swayze, M.D.
Clinical Assistant Professor of Anesthesiology
Department of Anesthesiology
Louisiana State University Medical Center
Shreveport, Louisiana

Katsuo Terui, M.D.
Staff Anesthesiologist
Teikyo University Ishihara Hospital
Ishihara
Chiba
Japan

Naomi Vaisrub, Ph.D.
Statistical Editor
Journal of the American Medical Association
Chicago, Illinois

Dana A. Vildus, M.D.
Staff Anesthesiologist
Brigham and Women's Hospital
Instructor in Anaesthesia
Harvard Medical School
Boston, Massachusetts

Donald H. Wallace, M.D.
Department of Anesthesiology and Pain Management
University of Texas
Southwestern Medical Center at Dallas
Dallas, Texas

Lisa Wollman, M.D.
Staff Anesthesiologist
Massachusetts General Hospital
Instructor in Anaesthesia
Harvard Medical School
Boston, Massachusetts

Preface

The first edition of *Common Problems in Obstetric Anesthesia* was published with twenty-nine chapters and contributions from sixty-six authors. Because of its interesting format, it served the clinicians interested in obstetric anesthesia in a very practical manner.

Obstetric anesthesia has advanced rapidly in recent years, hence necessitating the updating of the old chapters and the addition of a few new chapters.

The present edition now includes forty-six chapters with contributions from sixty-six authors. I hope the second edition will become more valuable because of its better clarity and addition of new information.

I wish to express my gratitude to all of the national, as well as international, contributors for their time and effort expended. It should also be noted that the authors generally expressed their own opinions and recommendations, which may not always reflect my own opinion.

Finally, I wish to thank Ms. Nancy F. Jeffery for her valuable help in completing this venture.

Contents

1

Cardiovascular and Respiratory Changes in Late Pregnancy

A 23-year-old primigravida at 39 weeks' gestation presents for preanesthetic evaluation and consultation. How will she differ from a nonpregnant woman with regard to her cardiovascular and respiratory systems?

Recommendations by Graham H. McMorland, M.D.

This is a healthy, young woman and any changes in her physiologic functions are likely to be those normally associated with pregnancy. However, because she is almost at term, the intensity and anesthetic implications of these changes will be maximal. One should note that the physiologic changes that occur during pregnancy are of such significance that they would cause concern to anesthesiologists if they were encountered in nonpregnant patients.

Cardiocirculatory System

A progressive increase in *blood volume* occurs during the second and third trimesters of pregnancy.[1] This increase is rapid in the second and early third trimesters, with little (or no) further rise in volume during the last few weeks of pregnancy. At term the total volume will have increased by 30% to 35% (1200 to 1500 ml). The increase in plasma volume (30% to 40%) will be relatively greater than that of the red cell mass (20% to 30%), resulting in hemodilution. This causes a fall in the hematocrit level (the so-called physiologic anemia of pregnancy) and a decrease in blood viscosity of 12% to 20%.

At term about half of the increased blood volume is in the enlarged uterus and placenta. Consequently, the effect of the normal blood loss (up to 500 ml during vaginal delivery and about 1000 ml at cesarean section) is minimized by an autotransfusion of 500 to 800 ml of blood from the contracting uterus.

The enlarged breasts, as well as the increased vasculature of the kidneys, skeletal muscles, and skin, provide additional reservoirs for the increased blood volume; and there is no evidence of circulatory overload in the normal gravida at term.

Cardiac output is markedly augmented during pregnancy. This is initially observed in the first trimester, rapidly rises until the thirtieth to the thirty-fourth week of gestation, and then maintains the level of augmentation until labor commences. At term the cardiac output has increased by 35% to 40%.[2] This elevation is due largely to an increase in stroke volume and, to a lesser degree, to an increased heart rate. During the first stage of labor, cardiac output will increase by a further 15% to 30% (in response to catecholamine secretion associated with pain and stress), and by 35% to 45% during the expulsive period. In the third stage of labor, the cardiac output will peak at 80% above prelabor values. This is followed by an initial rapid decline in cardiac output during the first postpartum hour and further gradual reduction, to reach normal, nonpregnant levels about 2 weeks after delivery.

Older data, which suggested that both blood volume and cardiac output decreased in the third trimester of pregnancy, were obtained with the patient in the supine position. Among others, Ueland and associates[2] were able to demonstrate that these observations were due primarily to compression of the vena cava and that when the patient is in a lateral or sitting position, this decrease is not noticed. When the patient is turned from the lateral to the supine position, the cardiac output will decrease by 14% to 20%, with a further fall of 17% in the lithotomy position, and 18% in a steep Trendelenburg tilt.

The clinical importance of this *aortocaval compression* is now well recognized.[3] Compression of the vena cava causes a decrease in venous return to the heart, resulting in reduced maternal cardiac output and hypotension. Partial compensation for this phenomenon occurs by peripheral vasoconstriction and collateral venous return via the epidural and azygos veins. Compression of the abdominal aorta gives rise to few maternal symptoms, but causes a significant decrease in blood flow to the lower extremities and reduction in uteroplacental perfusion. The latter effect, if uncorrected, will result in fetal hypoxia and acidosis. One should note that the gravid patient lying on her back, a "normal" blood pressure measured in an arm does not indicate adequate perfusion of the uterus, placenta, or lower limbs. A gravida in late pregnancy should never be allowed to lie supine, but should always adopt a lateral or sitting position, or at least have her pelvis tilted by means of a wedge under a hip.

Blood coagulation is markedly increased during pregnancy,[4] a hypercoagulable state that affords some protection against blood loss during parturition, but also renders the parturient particularly susceptible to thromboembolic phenomena. A significant increase occurs in total body and plasma levels of fibrinogen, as well as in levels of factors VII, VIII, and X.

Baroreceptor sensitivity has been demonstrated in studies using phenylephrine infusions.[5] With the patient in the left lateral position, the decrease in heart rate was noted as the blood pressure rose with incremental doses of phenylephrine. The heart rate will decrease by 0.9 beats/min for each 1 mm Hg increase in blood pressure compared with a decrease of 0.5 beats/min per 1 mm Hg in nonpregnant patients.

Vascular responsiveness to vasoconstrictor drugs, such as phenylephrine, epinephrine, and norepinephrine, is decreased in pregnancy.[6] Uterine vessels are less responsive to ephedrine (a mixed α-

and β-agonist) than to pure α-agonists, such as metaraminol, suggesting that ephedrine is the drug of choice for treating hypotension in pregnant patients. Ephedrine also increases fetal oxygen pressure (PaO_2) when used for treatment of hypotension.

However, recent studies have indicated that α agonists in small doses do not have significant adverse effects in pregnant patients and probably are safe to use for rapid treatment of severe hypotension.[7,8]

Anesthetic Considerations

Blood loss at delivery is well tolerated because of the increased blood volume during pregnancy and the autotransfusion (500 to 800 ml) from the contracting uterus. Blood transfusion, with its attendant risks, is rarely indicated in obstetric patients with uncomplicated deliveries.

Regional anesthesia, mostly because of the associated sympathetic block, will interfere with the ability of the parturient to compensate for vena caval compression by vasoconstriction. Patients receiving epidural or subarachnoid blocks should never be permitted to lie supine. When a lateral position is not practical (e.g., during cesarean section), the uterus must always be displaced laterally by means of a wedge under a hip (usually the left side) or by tilting the operating table laterally. An adequate intravenous preload with a dextrose-free crystalloid solution will aid in reducing the effect of vasodilatation and prevention of hypotension.

The distended epidural veins are easily punctured during insertion of an epidural needle or catheter, with increased risk of intravascular injection of toxic doses of local anesthetic drugs. For this reason, these drugs must always be administered in incremental small boluses. The distended veins also contribute to the decrease in capacity of the epidural space, reducing the volume of local anesthetic required.

Another consideration is that regional anesthesia can diminish, but not completely abolish, the increase in cardiac output during labor.

Hypotension must be rapidly treated, especially in the presence of sympathetic block produced by regional analgesia or anesthesia. Ephedrine, in intravenous increments of 5 to 10 mg, probably is the drug of choice. However, recent studies suggest that phenylephrine in small doses may be used safely when rapid restoration of blood pressure is required in the presence of severe hypotension.[7,8]

Respiratory System

Capillary engorgement of the respiratory mucosa may cause marked swelling of the upper airway. This will be aggravated by respiratory tract infections or the edema associated with preeclampsia. As a result of this engorgement, trauma and bleeding are easily produced and brisk epistaxis may follow attempts at nasotracheal intubation or suctioning.

Elevation of the diaphragm at term does not result in much (if any) decrease in total lung capacity, because of an associated increase in both transverse and anteroposterior diameters of the thorax.[9] Vital capacity is unchanged in the absence of pulmonary or cardiovascular disease, but the *functional residual capacity* (FRC) is reduced.[10] This latter effect, which is of clinical importance, is due largely to an increase in tidal volume (with an associated decrease in expiratory reserve volume). About one third of all parturients are likely to develop airway closure during normal tidal ventilation when in the supine position.[11,12]

Oxygen consumption is increased in pregnancy by 10% to 23% and is further increased by as much as 100% during labor.[13] *Minute ventilation* increases early in pregnancy and rises at term to 50% to 65% above that of the prepregnant state. This is related primarily to the increase in tidal volume and probably occurs in response to hormonal influences. Progesterone and possibly estrogen will sensitize the response of the respiratory center to carbon dioxide (CO_2).

Hyperventilation results in reduction of maternal arterial CO_2 pressure ($Pa{CO_2}$), at term, to about 32 mm Hg, but little maternal alkalosis occurs because of a compensatory rise in level of serum bicarbonate. During labor, hyperventilation will increase markedly as pain becomes more severe, and also as a result of popular psychoprophylactic analgesic techniques that concentrate on breathing patterns. The marked hyperventilation that occurs during painful uterine contractions often is followed by periods of decreased ventilation and maternal hypoxia.

Hyperventilation (especially iatrogenic, during general anesthesia) may result in progressive fetal acidosis.[14] There are a number of possible reasons for this. Hypocapnic uterine vasoconstriction may contribute, but decreased venous return associated with positive pressure ventilation probably is more important. Additionally, respiratory alkalosis will shift the maternal oxyhemoglobin dissociation curve to the left, thus reducing oxygen transfer to fetal hemoglobin.

Anesthetic Considerations

Manipulations such as laryngoscopy, intubation, and suctioning may readily cause trauma and bleeding from the congested, swollen mucosa. Generally it is advisable to use an endotracheal tube slightly smaller than one that would be selected for a nonpregnant patient to ensure rapid, smooth, and atraumatic intubation. In most patients this means a 7.5- or 7.0-mm internal diameter tube. In rare instances of severe mucosal swelling, even smaller tubes may be required. The intubation difficulties will be compounded by obesity with the associated short neck and large breasts. A selection of endotracheal tubes should always be readily available. The *polio* blade, or a short-handled laryngoscope, may be useful for morbidly obese patients.

The increase in oxygen consumption and reduced functional residual capacity will cause alarmingly rapid development of hypoxia and hypercapnia after even a short period of apnea, airway obstruction, or inhalation of a hypoxic gas mixture.[15] Endotracheal intubation must be performed rapidly and smoothly to reduce the apneic period to a minimum. However, even after conscientious preoxygenation, intubation will be associated with a precipitous fall of arterial oxygen pressure ($Pa{O_2}$).

Inhalation anesthesia is rapidly induced in pregnant women, mostly because hyperventilation (especially during labor) results in delivery of more of the anesthetic gas to the lung alveoli, and also because the decreased FRC permits less dilution of gases and hence higher alveolar concentrations. Animal studies indicate that at term, minimum alveolar concentration (MAC) for volatile gases is reduced by 25% to 40%,[16] probably due to increased levels of circulating endorphins and also, possibly, the sedative effect of progesterone.

One must remember that low concentrations of inhalation anesthetic agents being administered for analgesia during labor may unexpectedly produce anesthesia with loss of protective pharyngeal and laryngeal reflexes.

Epidural analgesia during labor will reduce the hyperventilation caused by pain, with consequent reduction in minute volume and oxygen consumption.[17] The associated hypocarbia and alkalemia are reduced, with resultant improvement in fetal acid-base status.

Summary

Pregnancy causes profound physiologic changes that affect both mother and fetus. These changes, especially those affecting the cardiovascular and respiratory systems, have significant implications for the management of analgesia and anesthesia.

1. Both blood volume and cardiac output increase markedly during pregnancy. During

labor, cardiac output will increase further and will peak during the third stage of labor at about 80% above prelabor values.

2. The clinical importance of *aortocaval compression* now is well recognized. In late pregnancy and during labor, the gravida should never assume a supine position. Sitting or lateral positions, or tilting the pelvis with a wedge will reduce the risk of this complication.
3. Ephedrine is the vasopressor of choice in parturients. However, recent studies have indicated that α-agonists in small doses may not have significant adverse effects in pregnant patients as was formerly taught.[7,8]
4. Respiratory changes include reduced FRC, capillary engorgement of respiratory mucosa, and increased minute volume and oxygen consumption. The latter effect, along with the reduced FRC, will cause alarmingly rapid development of hypoxia and hypercapnia during short periods of apnea (such as during endotracheal intubation).
5. Regional analgesia or anesthesia will reduce the increase in cardiac output during labor as well as the minute volume and oxygen uptake. However, the associated sympathetic block will inhibit the ability to compensate for vena cava compression by vasoconstriction.

The MAC for volatile anesthetic agents is reduced during pregnancy. Along with the hyperventilation, during labor, this will result in rapid induction of inhalation anesthesia.

References

1. Ueland K: *Cardiorespiratory physiology of pregnancy.* In Sciarra JJ, Droegemueller W, editors: *Gynecology and obstetrics,* vol 3, Hagerstown, 1979, Harper and Row.
2. Ueland K, Novy MJ, Peterson EN, et al: Maternal cardiovascular dynamics IV: the influence of gestational age on the natural cardiovascular response to posture and exercise, *Am J Obstet Gynecol* 1969; 104:856.
3. Marx GF: Aortocaval compression: Incidence and prevention, *Bull NY Acad Med* 1974; 50:443.
4. Hellgren M, Blomback M: Studies on blood coagulation and fibrinolysis in pregnancy during delivery and in the puerperium, *Gynecol Obstet Invest* 1981; 12:141.
5. Leduc L, Wasserstrum N, Spillman T, et al: Baroflex function in normal pregnancy, *Am J Obstet Gynecol* 1991; 165:1605.
6. Weiner CP, Martinez E, Chestnut DH, et al: Effect of pregnancy on uterine and carotid artery response to norepinephrine, epinephrine and phenylephrine in vessels with documented endothelium, *Am J Obstet Gynecol* 1989; 161:1605.
7. Ramanathan S, Grant GJ: Vasopressor therapy for hypotension due to epidural anesthesia for cesarean section, *Acta Anaesthesiol Scand* 1988; 32:559.
8. Wright PM, Iftikhar M, Fitzpatrick KT, et al: Vasopressor therapy for hypotension during epidural anesthesia for cesarean section: effects on maternal and fetal flow velocity ratios, *Anesth Analg* 1992; 75:56.
9. Alaily AB, Carrol KB: Pulmonary ventilation in pregnancy, *Br J Obstet Gynaecol* 1978; 85:518.
10. Prowse CM, Gaensler EA: Respiratory and acid-base changes during pregnancy, *Anesthesiology* 1965; 26:381.
11. Russell IF, Chambers WA: Closing volume in normal pregnancy, *Br J Anaesth* 1981; 53:1043.
12. Bevan DR, Holdcroft A, Loh LH, et al: Closing volume and pregnancy, *Br Med J* 1974; 1:13.
13. Eliasson AH, Phillips YU, Stajduhan KC, et al: Oxygen consumption and ventilation during normal labor, *Chest* 1992; 102:467.
14. Levinson G, Shnider SM, de Lorimer AA, et al: Effects of maternal hyperventilation on uterine blood flow and fetal oxygenation and acid base status, *Anesthesiology* 1974; 40:310.
15. Archer GW, Marx GF: Arterial oxygen tension during apnoea in parturient women, *Br J Anaesth* 1974; 46:358.
16. Palahniuk RJ, Shnider SM, Eger EI II: Pregnancy decreases the requirements for inhaled anesthetic agents, *Anesthesiology* 1974; 41:82.
17. Hagerdal M, Morgan CW, Sumner AE, et al: Minute ventilation and oxygen consumption during labor with epidural analgesia, *Anesthesiology* 1983; 59:425.

2

Pregnancy and Epidural Dose Requirements

A 33-year-old multipara, gravida 3, para 2 at term is scheduled for an elective repeat cesarean delivery. What are the considerations regarding the dose of the local anesthetic compared with the dose used for a nonpregnant individual?

Recommendations by Glen Z. Brooks, M.D.

Historically, determination of effective epidural dose requirements for full-term parturients has been made, for the most part, empirically. It has been realized for decades that epidural dose requirements are altered during pregnancy. One has also grown to appreciate the significance of the anatomic and physiologic changes that accompany the pregnant state. What has remained less clear are the specific aberrations of normal pregnancy that are responsible for the observed alterations in dose requirements, and to what extent each is important.

In addition, maternal physical characteristics, positioning during epidural injection, and injection techniques variably affect the distribution of drugs within the epidural space. These factors have not been as important in determining effective epidural doses as the effects of the anatomic and physiologic changes associated with pregnancy per se, but they also need to be considered.

Epidural analgesia has been an increasingly popular technique of pain relief for vaginal and abdominal deliveries for nearly five decades. Since caudal analgesia was used more commonly in the 1940s and 1950s, it is not surprising that perhaps the earliest reported observation of exaggerated epidural spread during labor was noted by Crawford and Chester in pregnant patients receiving caudal epidural analgesia.[1] In 1962, Bromage demonstrated that Crawford's and Chester's original observation also was true with lumbar epidural analgesia.[2] Other investigations supportive of this hypothesis followed.[3,4] Now it is generally agreed that during pregnancy, the injection of a given dose of local anesthetic agent into the epidural space results in a 30% to 35% greater segmental spread of analgesia than that observed in the nonpregnant state.

The phenomenon of exaggerated spread is not restricted to patients at term. Fagraeus and associates found that the extent of the analgesic segmental spread of 2% lidocaine was significantly increased even during the first trimester.[5] Increased sensitivity has been shown to extend into the early postpartum period as well.[6]

Proposed Causes for Change in Dose Requirements

Several causes for pregnancy-related changes in epidural dose requirements have been suggested.

Decreased Volume of Epidural Space

As the uterus enlarges during gestation, it produces a mechanical obstruction to blood flow through the inferior vena cava. This obstruction is the most dramatic when the patient is supine. In the presence of significant vena caval compression, blood must return to the heart through alternate routes: the azygous system and the intervertebral venous plexus. A marked increase in blood flow through the latter results in epidural venous engorgement and an effective decrease in the potential volume of the epidural space.[7] In theory, if the epidural space becomes a relatively smaller semirigid cylinder, any injected solution might be expected to spread further.[8] This logic was the basis for one of the first explanations for the exaggerated spread of epidurally administered anesthetic agents during pregnancy. Although support remains for this theory among some clinicians and investigators, probably it is not the only explanation and perhaps not even the most significant.

Altered Acid-Base Balance of Cerebrospinal Fluid

A second explanation for the augmented and more rapid segmental spread of epidural analgesia during pregnancy concerns well-known changes in acid-base balance.[9] These changes result from a progesterone-induced increase in alveolar ventilation during pregnancy with resultant hypocarbia $Paco_2$ 30 to 34 mm Hg. The metabolic compensation for this process is incomplete, and a slight increase in tissue and cerebrospinal fluid (CSF) pH can be expected. It has been suggested that even a small increase in pH will significantly narrow the gap between CSF pH and the pKa of a local anesthetic agent. Thus, the percentage of drug in the un-ionized form would increase, encouraging transneuronal diffusion of drug into neuroaxis cells.

Neurophysiologic Changes during Pregnancy

A better understanding of the neurophysiologic changes associated with pregnancy gives more important insight into the phenomenon of altered sensitivity to local anesthetic agents injected into the epidural space of gravid patients. Some early work in this area was done by Datta and associates studying rabbit vagus nerves.[10] When the isolated nerves from pregnant and nonpregnant rabbits were exposed to bupivacaine, the onset of conduction blockade was significantly more rapid in the nerve fibers of pregnant rabbits when compared with those of nonpregnant rabbits. At least in this mammalian species, pregnancy is associated with important neurophysiologic changes. The more rapid onset of conduction blockade probably indicates that the transneuronal diffusion of local anesthetic molecules is enhanced during pregnancy. Interestingly, Fagraeus and co-workers noted that even in early pregnancy, when the uterus is small and vena caval compression minimal, a significant increase occurs in the speed of onset of conduction blockade and the extent of segmental spread after injection of local anesthetics into the epidural space.[5] These observations support the concept of increased neuronal sensitivity to local anesthetic agents during pregnancy, rather than merely a change in the volume of the epidural space as an explanation for exaggerated spread.

Dramatic physiologic changes occur in the cardiovasculature and respiratory system of the pregnant woman that approach a nadir by the end of the first trimester. It is difficult to explain these physiologic responses in terms of uterine size, or even teleologically as compensation for the metabolic requirements of a growing fetus. Clearly, an altered hormonal state is the best explanation for these changes.

Progesterone is the hormone responsible for the increased ventilatory drive during pregnancy. Mounting evidence exists that progesterone also may be the hormone responsible for mammalian neurophysiologic changes noted during pregnancy. Studying pregnant, nonpregnant, and immediately postpartum women, Datta et al. found that the rise in CSF levels of progesterone in pregnant patients at term mirrored the dramatic rise in serum progesterone levels associated with pregnancy.[6] While these CSF levels began to rapidly fall in the postpartum period, both pregnant and early postpartum patients required significantly less lidocaine for comparable segmental levels of spinal anesthesia than did nonpregnant patients.

Increased neuronal sensitivity to anesthetic agents after chronic exogenous progesterone exposure has been demonstrated in other studies. Rabbits that had undergone oophorectomy and were treated for 8 days with injections of progesterone in peanut oil had significantly lower halothane minimum alveolar concentration levels than intact controls or animals that had undergone oophorectomy and were injected with peanut oil alone.[11] Using a similar model of a rabbit after oophorectomy, Moller and associates studied the relationship between chronic progesterone exposure and the electrophysiologic effects of lidocaine and bupivacaine on isolated Purkinje's fibers and ventricular muscle fibers.[12] Bupivacaine decreased the maximal rate of depolarization of both Purkinje's fibers and ventricular muscle to a significantly greater extent in progesterone-treated animals than in controls. The enhanced depressant effect of bupivacaine observed in progesterone-treated rabbits could not be demonstrated with lidocaine, nor does pregnancy per se alter the threshold for lidocaine-induced seizures in the rat.[13] Although these studies support the concept of an apparent increase in bupivacaine toxicity during pregnancy when compared with other local anesthetic agents, explanations of why pregnancy and chronic progesterone exposure selectively increase bupivicaine toxicity remain unclear.

Immediate pretreatment with progesterone has no effect on bupivacaine-induced conduction blockade in isolated rabbit vagus nerve.[14] Therefore, the progesterone molecule itself probably is not responsible for increased neuronal sensitivity to anesthetic agents. Rather, progesterone, or progesterone metabolites, may effect the synthesis of proteins responsible for the transneuronal penetration of anesthetic agents or the bioavailability of important neurotransmitters.

Whereas progesterone is one important hormone affecting the neurophysiologic factors of pregnancy, other hormones need to be considered and investigated as well, such a estrogen, catecholamines, serotonin, and prostaglandins.

Considerations when Determining Dose

The reason(s) for the observed increase in the extent and the rate of segmental spread of epidural analgesia associated with pregnancy may be singular or a combination of the above factors, or a yet undiscovered mechanism. However, decreased requirements must be considered when determining an appropriate dose of a local anesthetic agent to be administered epidurally to the pregnant patient.

Within a population of pregnant women, additional considerations exist when trying to predict the appropriate dose of a local anesthetic agent for a particular patient and task.

Physical Characteristics

Hodgkinson and Hussain found obesity to be a significant variable in the determination of the segmental spread of local anesthetics in the lumbar epidural space in patients undergoing cesarean section.[15] When injected in the lateral decubitus, obese patients were shown to experience a higher segmental level of analgesia than nonobese patients receiving the same epidural dose. However, the same authors in a later study found a decreased cephalad spread in obese versus nonobese parturients after administration of epidural anesthesia to patients in the sitting position.[16] This reduced spread became dramatic as body mass index rose.

In contrast to these studies involving pregnant patients, Duggen et al. were not able to establish a correlation between obesity per se and the extent of spread of epidural bupivacaine injected in the lateral position in either male or nonpregnant female patients for varicose vein surgery.[17] However, some correlation existed between segmental spread and body mass index with higher injectate volumes. But patient height and age had little effect on spread.

Within a population of pregnant women, except at extremes, height again seems to be of little significance in determining the extent of conduction blockade after the injection of a given dose of local anesthetic into the epidural space. Age, within the span of normal pregnancy, also appears to be of no significance.

Maternal Positioning

Differences exist between pregnant and nonpregnant patients with regard to the influence of positioning on the distribution of epidural anesthetic agents. The ultimate cephalad spread of epidural analgesia has been shown to be gravity dependent in nonpregnant patients. For example, when nonpregnant patients were kept in the lateral decubitus position during the period of injection only,[18] or during injection and for 15 minutes thereafter,[19] the cephalad spread of analgesia was statistically significantly greater on the dependent side.

Studying 35 term patients for elective cesarean section, Norris et al. randomly placed patients either on their left or right sides for epidural catheter placement and for 20 minutes after drug injection.[20] All patients then were placed in the supine position with left uterine displacement. In contrast to the findings noted above in nonpregnant patients, the authors found no significant difference in the spread of epidural blockade between dependent and nondependent sides in either group.

Pitkanen and co-workers studied 40 patients having elective cesarean section.[21] After injection of 0.5% bupivacaine (95 to 135 mg) with patients in the right lateral decubitus position, half of the patients were kept on their right sides and the other half were immediately turned to the left lateral decubitus position. After 30 minutes, all patients were turned to the supine position with left uterine displacement. Subsequent levels of the blocks on the right and left sides of each patient were determined, and the groups were compared. The authors did observe a two- to six-segment difference between the sides in some patients in each group. When this occurred, the block was always higher on the right side, the dependent side, at the time of injection. This suggested that if the spread of the bupivacaine was gravity dependent in pregnant patients at term, it was so only during injection and not in the period after injection. However, the number of patients who experienced any difference in the level of their blocks from right to left sides was not large enough to affect the outcome of the study. When both groups, and sides within each group, were compared, no significant differences occurred in the observed spread. It appears that, at least when injecting large volumes of local anesthetic agents of high concentration for cesarean section, changing maternal posture after injection does not significantly affect the ultimate bilateral level of the block.

In a nonobese population of pregnant women, administration of epidural anesthetics either in the lateral or in the sitting positions ultimately results in equal cephalad spreads. However, the onset of blockage of higher dermatomal segments has been reported to be delayed, and the quality of the block is inferior in patients injected while in the sitting position.[22] The effect of the lateral versus the sitting position at the time of injection on the spread of epidural anesthetics in obese patients has been discussed earlier in this section.

Lower volumes and concentrations of local anesthetics generally are employed during the administration of continuous epidural analgesics for labor. It has been my experience that in this clinical setting, positioning is important. With time, the continuous infusion of smaller masses of drugs leads to a unilateral block of the dependent side. This situation is best avoided by frequently turning the patient from side to side during pump infusion.

Injection Techniques

In nonobstetric patients, Omote and associates found equivalent dermatomal spread after slow injection (0.24 ml/sec) of a total of 14 ml of 2% lidocaine with epinephrine through a multiport epidural catheter when compared with more rapid injection (1.2 ml/sec) via a Tuohy needle.[23] Interestingly, the spread after needle injection at 0.24 ml/sec resulted in significantly less analgesic spread than injection via a multiport catheter at the same rate.

Crochetière et al. compared bolus with incremental injection techniques in patients who underwent cesarean section.[24] A T-4 dermatomal level was achieved after administration of similar doses of 2% lidocaine with epinephrine either as a bolus over 2 minutes via a Tuohy needle or incrementally over 10 minutes using an epidural catheter. However, patients receiving bolus injections had a significantly higher incidence of hypotension (52.2%) than patients who had received incremental injections (13.6%). They also noted that in spite of equal dermatomal levels of analgesics before incision, patients receiving slower injection experienced superior surgical analgesia.

In one study using small volumes of 0.5% bupivacaine, rapid injection over 5 seconds via an epidural catheter led to a faster onset of blockade than did slow injection over 40 seconds.[25] However, after 30 minutes, the extent of dermatomal spread was similar in both groups. This study may be of scientific interest when considering the effect of the speed of injection on the spread of drug in the epidural space. However, it should not be considered as an endorsement of rapid injection to achieve a faster onset of blockade. The dangers of rapid injection into either an unrecognized epidural vein or the subarachnoid space outweigh any possible benefits.

Comments and Recommendations

When performing a de novo epidural injection of anesthetic for cesarean section, I use a technique which has become a compilation of my own clinical experience, the published and unpublished observations of others, and an overwhelming concern for safety. The lateral decubitus position seems to be associated with less hypotension and superior surgical anesthesia than that achieved after injection of the same dose of local anesthetic in the sitting position. Also, most pregnant patients at term find the lateral decubitus position more comfortable than the sitting position. I also agree that greater safety and improved quality of the block are achieved by slow incremental injection rather than rapid bolus injection. Rapid injection forces the drug to spread more rapidly within the epidural space. The result is an epidural block with a dermatomal spread similar to that achieved with slow injection, but with a more rapid onset and, thus, a higher incidence of hypotension. Higher pressures created by rapid injection undoubtedly force more drug out of the epidural space through the intervertebral foramen. In spite of an apparently adequate level of the block based upon pinprick testing, it tends to be of poorer quality, especially once the peritoneum is reached. A possible explanation is that less drug remains available within the epidural space for adequate nerve root and cord penetration.

Slow injection does not require the placement of an epidural catheter. I prefer injecting all drugs directly through the epidural needle. Epidural catheters represent an additional opportunity for aberrant placement and serious complications, even if the epidural needle has been perfectly placed. After giving test doses, the selected local anesthetic agent is administered by slow incremental needle injection over 4 to 5 minutes while maintaining constant dialogue with the patient and monitoring vital signs. A block of predictable bilateral spread, quality, and duration can be established with great safety when 0.5% bupivacaine or 2% lidocaine with epinephrine is used.

Because of 2-chloroprocaine's short duration of action, single-needle injection for cesarean section is not practical and catheter placement is necessary for expected reinforcement. Likewise, if it is anticipated that the cesarean section will last longer than 2 hours, epidural catheter placement seems appropriate regardless of the local anesthetic chosen. Catheter placement also seems practical if the epidural catheter will be used for postoperative analgesia.

In instances where catheter placement is elected, it is best to use the catheter for all initial injections. This assures proper placement from the beginning of treatment and increases the likelihood that reinforcing doses will be safe and effective.

The epidural doses recommended for cesarean section are found in Table 2-1. These recommended doses are for nonobese patients with epidural anesthesia established when in the lateral decubitus position.

Because ropivacaine, a new local anesthetic agent, is not yet available for general use, I have not included it in the table. Current reports sug-

TABLE 2-1

Recommended Doses of Commonly Used Local Anesthetic Agents for Epidural Block for Cesarean Section

	Dosage*,†			
	Initial		Top-Up	
Anesthetic Agent	(ml)	(mg)	(ml)	(mg)
Bupivacaine 0.5%	22-26	110-130	10-12	50-60
2-Chloroprocaine 3.0%	18-22	540-660	8-10	240-300
Lidocaine‡ 2.0%	18-22	360-440	8-10	160-200

*Recommended dose ranges for nonobese patients of average height, 62 to 68 in (158 to 172 cm) in the lateral decubitus position. For extremes of height or if the patient is obese, these doses may be modified up to 20%.

†Initial and top-up doses include appropriate test dose(s).

‡With epinephrine 1:200,000.

gest that when used in concentrations and total doses similar to bupivacaine for cesarean section, a comparable quality of sensory analgesia is achieved. Ropivacaine also is associated with less motor block and decreased potential for cardiac toxicity when compared with bupivacaine.

After the initial epidural administration of any of the drugs listed in Table 2-1 at the level of the L2-3 interspace, a T-4 level of analgesia generally is attained. By placing the patient in a semisitting position for the first 5 minutes after injection, sacral analgesia seems to be more rapidly and effectively produced, reducing discomfort during bladder manipulation.

After chemical sympathectomy, the effect of vena caval compression by the uterus on blood pressure and cardiac output becomes more dramatic. At all times, patients must be positioned so that the uterus is adequately displaced from the vena cava to promote unobstructed blood return to the right side of the heart. This is attained most often by placing a wedge or blanket roll under the right hip. Volume loading with 1000 to 1500 ml of dextrose-free crystalloid before the onset of chemical sympathectomy also will help to attenuate dramatic maternal hemodynamic changes during cesarean section. (See Chapter 20.)

Summary

1. Epidural dose requirements for pregnant patients are significantly less (30% to 35%) than those required for nonpregnant patients of comparable age, height, and body habitus.
2. The decrease in epidural dose requirements begins in early pregnancy and continues until the early postpartum period.
3. Proposed mechanisms for the observed change in dose requirements include the following: a decrease in the effective volume of the epidural space, an increase in the availability of more diffusible un-ionized local anesthetic agent due to altered CSF acid-base balance, and hormonally influenced neurophysiologic changes.
4. Neurophysiologic changes associated with pregnancy seem to be the most influential factor. Nerves chronically exposed to progesterone experience an increase in the transneuronal diffusion of local anesthetic agents. As a result, a decreased dose of local anesthetic is necessary to achieve conduction blockage.
5. Obesity may further alter the expected spread of local anesthetic agents within the epidural space. When in the lateral decubitus during injection, obese patients experience greater cephalad spread compared with nonobese pregnant patients. However, after administration when patients are in the sitting position, decreased cephalad spread is observed.
6. Age and height, except at extremes, are not important variables in determining epidural dosage in a population of pregnant women.
7. When using large doses of local anesthetic agents in nonobese patients for cesarean section, positioning at the time of injection, and thereafter, has little effect on the ultimate cephalad or bilateral spread of the block.
8. Slow incremental injection via either an epidural needle or catheter is associated with equal to superior analgesia, less hypotension, and greater safety than is rapid bolus injection.

References

1. Crawford OB, Chester RV: Caudal anesthesia in obstetrics: a combined procaine-Pontocaine single injection technic, *Anesthesiology* 1949; 10:473.
2. Bromage PR: Spread of analgesic solutions in the epidural

space and their site of action: a statistical study, *Br J Anaesth* 1962; 24:161.

3. Hehre FW, Moyes AZ, Senfield RM, et al: Continuous lumbar peridural anesthesia in obstetrics II: Use of minimal amounts of local anesthetics during labor, *Anesth Analg* 1965; 44:89.
4. Kandel PF, Spoerel WE, Kinch RA: Continuous epidural analgesia for labour and delivery: review of 1000 cases, *Can Med Assoc J* 1966; 95:947.
5. Fagraeus L, Urban BJ, Bromage PR: Spread of epidural analgesia in early pregnancy, *Anesthesiology* 1983; 58:184.
6. Datta S, Hurley RJ, Naulty SJ, et al: Plasma and cerebrospinal fluid progesterone concentrations in pregnant and nonpregnant women, *Anesth Analg* 1986; 65:950.
7. Hipona FA, Yles R, Hehre FW: Venous encroachment on the spinal peridural space due to experimental IVC occlusion: possible clinical implications in late pregnancy, *Invest Radiol* 1966; 1:157.
8. Bromage PR: Continuous lumbar epidural analgesia for obstetrics, *Can Med Assoc J* 1961; 85:1136.
9. Sosis M, Bodner A: Further suggestions on epidural spread in pregnancy, *Anesthesiology* 1983; 59:600.
10. Datta S, Lambert DH, Gregus J, et al: Differential sensitivity of mammalian nerve fibers during pregnancy, *Anesth Analg* 1983; 62:1070.
11. Datta S, Migliozzi RP, Flanagan HL, et al: Chronically administered progesterone decreases halothane requirements in rabbits, *Anesth Analg* 1989; 68:46.
12. Moller RA, Datta S, Fox J, et al: Effects of progesterone on cardiac electrophysiologic action of bupivacaine and lidocaine, *Anesthesiology* 1992; 76:604.
13. Bucklin BA, Warner DS, Choi MM, et al: Pregnancy does not alter the threshold for lidocaine-induced seizures in the rat, *Anesth Analg* 1992; 74:57.
14. Bader AM, Datta S, Moller RA, et al: Acute progesterone treatment has no effect on bupivacaine-induced conduction blockade in the isolated rabbit vagus nerve, *Anesth Analg* 1990; 71:545.
15. Hodgkinson R, Hussain FJ: Obesity and the cephalad spread of analgesia following epidural administration of bupivacaine for cesarean section, *Anesth Analg* 1980; 59:89.
16. Hodgkinson R, Hussain FJ: Obesity, gravity and spread of epidural anesthesia, *Anesth Analg* 1981; 60:421.
17. Duggan J, Bowler GMR, McClure JH, et al: Extradural block with bupivacaine: influence of dose, volume, concentration and patient characteristics, *Br J Anaesthesiol* 1988; 61:324.
18. Seow LT, Lips RJ, Cousins JM: Effect of lateral posture on epidural blockade for surgery, *Anaesth Intensive Care* 1983; 11:97.
19. Grundy EM, Rao LN, Winnie AP: Epidural anesthesia and the lateral position, *Anesth Analg* 1978; 57:95.
20. Norris MC, Leighton BL, DeSimone CA, et al: Lateral position and epidural anesthesia for cesarean section, *Anesth Analg* 1988; 67:788.
21. Pitkanen MT, Paatero H, Rosenbery PH: The effect of maternal lateral position or position change on epidural anesthesia and plasma bupivacaine concentrations, *Reg Anesth* 1988; 13:157.
22. Reid JA, Thorburn J: Extradural bupivacaine or lignocaine anaesthesia for elective caesarean section: the role of maternal posture, *Br J Anaesth* 1988; 61:149.
23. Omote K, Namiki A, Iwasaki H: Epidural administration and analgesia spread: comparison of injection with catheters and needles, *J Anesthesia* 1992; 6:289.
24. Crochetière CT, Trépanier CA, Coté JJ: Epidural anaesthesia for caesarean section: comparison of two injection techniques, *Can J Anaesth* 1989; 36:133.
25. Griffiths RB, Horton WA, Jones IG, et al: Speed of injection and spread of bupivacaine in the epidural space, *Anaesthesia* 1987; 42:160.

3

Aspiration Risk in Parturients

A 26-year-old primigravida at term arrives at the hospital in active labor. Her obstetrician advised her to avoid eating after labor began. Why?

Recommendations by Charles P. Gibbs, M.D.

Because the cesarean section rate in the United States remains at about 25%,[1] the potential for this patient to require major anesthesia is not small. Aspiration and failure to be intubated are the two most common causes of maternal mortality at the time of general anesthesia for cesarean section.[2] In the United States, about 43% of patients receive general anesthesia for cesarean section.[3] As is discussed later in this chapter, aspiration of partially digested food produces severe lung damage. Thus, the recommendation not to eat once labor has begun is a very sound one. The more empty the stomach, the less risk exists for aspiration.

Incidence

A reliable incidence of aspiration during or surrounding the time of general anesthesia is difficult to determine because not all cases are diagnosed, and those that are diagnosed often are not reported. The report of Olsson and colleagues[4] of 185,000 cases of anesthesia found 83 cases of aspiration, producing an estimated incidence of 4.7 in 10,000 cases of anesthesia, or 1 in 2131. The incidence at the time of cesarean section was 1:661: almost a fourfold increase over the incidence of the general population. More recently, Warner and colleagues[5] reviewed 215,488 cases of general anesthesia and reported aspiration to have an incidence of 1 in 3216. For emergency operations, the incidence was 1 in 895 cases of anesthesia. Many cesarean sections are done as emergency operations.

Mortality and Morbidity

Mortality after aspiration of stomach contents ranges from 3% to 70%.[6-11] Five percent[4] and 4.6%[5] are the most recent figures and may be the most reliable. The difference in mortality rates is due, at least in part, to the different types of material aspirated and the therapy used, both of which are discussed in later sections of this chapter. Also, comorbid disease plays an important role.[5]

Morbidity is more difficult to define but consists of a multitude of serious complications, ranging from simple bronchospasm and mild hypoxia to pneumonitis and lung abscess to myocardial infarction and renal failure secondary to severe hypoxemia.[12-14] Olsson et al.[4] reported that 17% of patients who experienced aspiration required mechanical ventilation, and an additional 15% required a prolonged hospital stay. Warner et al.[5] reported that 19% of patients who experienced aspiration required mechanical ventilation.

The Pregnant Patient

As identified above, aspiration occurs more commonly in pregnant patients than in the general operating room (OR) population. Aspiration in pregnant patients is most likely to occur during a difficult intubation.[15] Failed and difficult intubations also occur more commonly in pregnant patients than in the general OR population.[16] Thus, the pregnant patient is at considerably more risk than others receiving general anesthesia. Why? Reasons can be divided into two categories: (1) those that are intrinsic to pregnancy; and (2) those that are iatrogenic.

Several factors are intrinsic to pregnancy. The enlarged uterus increases intraabdominal pressure and thus intragastric pressure.[17] However, the enlarged uterus is not necessary to produce the increased pressure, since the pressure is already elevated during the first trimester before the uterus rises out of the pelvis.[18] The production of gastrin, the hormone that increases both acidity and volume of gastric contents, is increased during pregnancy, particularly in the placenta, which is probably the site of production.[19] Motilin, a hormone that speeds gastric emptying, is depressed during pregnancy.[20] Gastric emptying is delayed during labor, and although the point is somewhat controversial, emptying time also may be delayed throughout pregnancy.[21,22] A recent study by Simpson and colleagues provides evidence that emptying time is delayed in the midtrimester.[23] Some professionals have suggested that the gastroesophageal angle is distorted by the encroaching uterus, making it less competent and perhaps explaining the high incidence of heartburn in pregnancy.[24,25] Although some have indicated that lower esophageal sphincter pressures are lower, sphincter pressures actually are normal during pregnancy, and the barrier pressure between the stomach and the esophagus is the same as in nonpregnant patients except for patients exhibiting heartburn.[26-28]

Iatrogenic factors that lead to increased risk of pulmonary aspiration of stomach contents in the pregnant patient include the use of narcotics and sedatives during labor. These agents retard gastric emptying even more than the delay caused by labor.[22] The lithotomy position increases intragastric pressure,[17] as does pushing on the uterus to aid delivery of the infant at the time of vaginal delivery. In the latter, if general anesthesia was electively used without an endotracheal tube, the stage would be set for an indefensible disaster.

"At Risk"

Any discussion of aspiration requires a discussion of the term "at risk." A patient is said to be at risk when there is more than 25 ml of gastric contents and the pH is less than 2.5.[8,29,30] Whereas considerable support exists regarding the significance of the pH value,[30,31] there is none to validate the significance of a volume value of 25 ml. Most authors and investigators now believe that the pH is the more critical determinant for degree of lung injury.[32-35] However, because the 25-ml value is so well entrenched in the literature and continues to be requoted despite newer data to the contrary, "at risk" to many clinicians will continue to mean pH less than 2.5 and volume greater than 25 ml.

Types of Gastric Aspirate

For this particular case, it is critically important to discuss types of gastric aspirate because it is the character of the aspirate that to a large extent determines the extent of lung injury, and it is partially digested food that causes the most severe injury. Historically, aspirates have been classified according to whether they were acid or nonacid liquids. More recently, investigators have described the histologic and physiologic effects of partially digested food particles. Aspiration of large particles or chunks of food produces airway obstruction and, if not relieved, death by asphyxia ensues. In these patients, all efforts are directed toward removing the food particle. Occasionally, bronchoscopy may be necessary. Nothing more will be said relating to this type of aspiration.

Acid Liquid

Acid liquid aspirate disperses throughout the lungs within 12 to 18 seconds and produces isolated areas of patchy atelectasis; within 3 minutes extensive areas of atelectasis occur.[36] Histologically, there are significant alveolar-capillary breakdown, intense capillary congestion, and interstitial edema and hemorrhage (Fig. 3-1).[37] However, necrosis usually does not occur and lung architecture remains intact. Physiologically, hypoxemia is the earliest, most dramatic, and most consistent response.[38-41] Because actual tissue destruction may not always be significant in the early hours after aspiration of acid, findings at this point are likely to reflect reflex responses, destruction of surfactant, alveolar edema, and atelectasis.[42] Later, the loss of fluid secondary to the pulmonary burn and resultant pulmonary edema may become so significant that hypotension and hypovolemia occur.[38] Pulmonary hypertension also occurs rapidly, mostly as a result of hypoxic vasoconstriction.

Nonacid Liquid

Nonacid liquid (pH greater than 2.5) aspirate produces few histologic abnormalities. There are occasional, widely scattered, discrete foci of inflammatory changes. Physiologically, nonacid liquid produces an immediate and significant decrease in arterial oxygen pressure ($Pa{O_2}$) and an increase in shunt Qsp/Qt.[8,38] However, shunt values usually return to baseline within 4 to 6 hours, as does $Pa{O_2}$ within 24 hours.[38] Notice that even with aspiration of liquids with a relatively neutral pH, a significant fall in $Pa{O_2}$ can result from reflex bronchospasm and destruction of lung surfactant, which may lead to atelectasis and pulmonary edema.[14]

Nonacid Food Particle

Nonacid food particles aspirate produces inflammation that is readily apparent in the bronchioles and lung tissues and varies from scattered to extensive, almost confluent areas. Edema and hemorrhage frequently are present. Later, the reaction changes more to a foreign body type of reaction. Lymphocytes and macrophages become prominent, and granuloma formation is evident around food particles in the aspirate. Physiologically, hypoxemia after aspiration of nonacid food particles is more severe than that after aspiration of acid liquid, and is nearly as severe as that after aspiration of acid food particles.[38]

Acid Food Particle

Acid food particle aspirate produces the most severe damage.[38] There are more extensive hemorrhagic pulmonary edema and multiple patches of actual alveolar septal necrosis, occasionally even obliterating the structure of the lung tissue (see Fig. 3-1). Hypoxemia in this category likewise is the most severe, as are hypercarbia and acidosis. Hypo

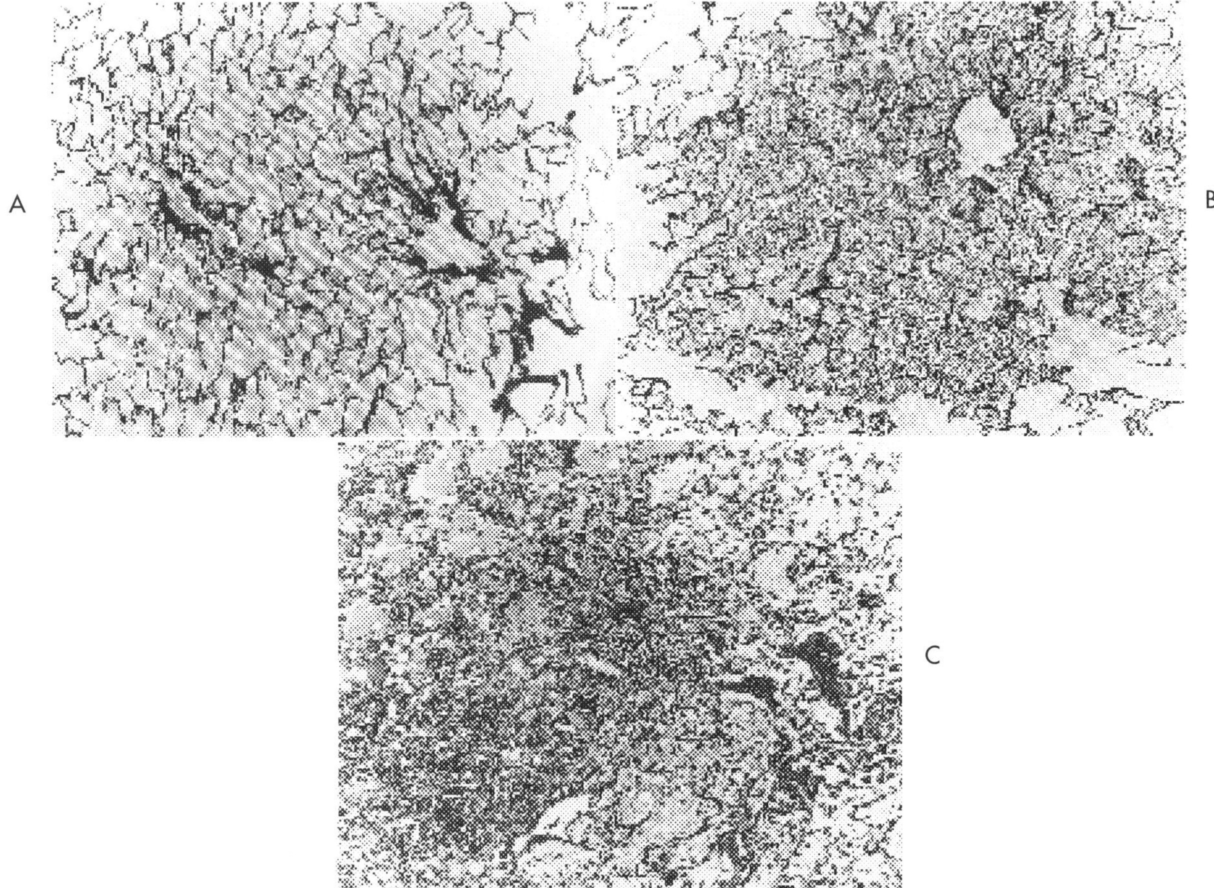

Fig. 3-1.
A, Lung after aspiration of normal saline. Essentially normal lung histologic findings. **B,** Lung after aspiration of liquid acid. Notice hemorrhage (red blood cells) and edema. Lung architecture has remained intact. **C,** Lung after aspiration of acid food particles at pH 1.8. Hemorrhage exudate is more extensive. Actual breakdown of alveolar walls and lung architecture also has occurred. *(From Gibbs CP, Modell JH: Management of aspiration pneumonitis. In Miller R, editor:* Anesthesia, *ed 3, New York, 1990, Churchill Livingstone, pp. 1293-1319.)*

tension is frequent and pulmonary hypertension is common. Most importantly, mortality is high and often occurs early. In one study of experimental animals who had acid food particle aspirate and who did not receive specific therapy, 50% died between 2 and 4 hours after the insult, and all animals died within 24 hours.[38] Table 3-1 provides blood gas values after various types of aspiration, and Fig. 3-1 depicts histologic changes. A review of Table 3-1 and Fig. 3-1 should convince even the most skeptical physician that consumption of food during labor is not human: it is dangerous.

TABLE 3-1

ARTERIAL BLOOD GAS TENSIONS AND pH OF DOGS 30 MINUTES AFTER ASPIRATION OF 2 ML/KG OF VARIOUS MATERIALS

Aspirate		Response		
Composition	pH	Pa_{O_2} (mm Hg)	Pa_{CO_2} (mm Hg)	pH
Saline	5.9	61	34	7.37
HCl acid	1.8	41	45	7.29
Food particles	5.9	34	51	7.19
Food particles	1.8	23	56	7.13

Pa_{O_2}, arterial oxygen pressure; Pa_{CO_2}, arterial carbon dioxide pressure.

From Gibbs CP, Modell JH: Management of aspiration pneumonitis. In Miller R, editor: *Anesthesia,* ed 3, New York, 1990, Churchill Livingstone, pp 1293-1319.

Signs, Symptoms, and Diagnosis

Aspiration of gastric contents can be dramatic with a full-blown picture that includes gastric contents in the oropharynx, wheezing, coughing, cyanosis, pulmonary edema, shock, hypoxemia, and roentgenographic findings. However, many (or indeed all) of these symptoms may be absent.[6,22] Often gastric contents are not seen in the oropharynx, particularly when the aspiration is a result of silent regurgitation rather than active vomiting. In this situation, unless stomach contents can be suctioned from the trachea, aspiration of stomach contents is only a presumption, and a positive diagnosis cannot be made.

Some clinicians measure pH of oral contents to get an indication as to whether aspiration has occurred. The maneuver is unreliable because the pH of gastric contents is rapidly altered by the more basic oral and tracheal secretions. Radiographic changes, when present, are extremely variable. Small irregular shadows constitute the most prominent and frequent finding initially. Landay et al.[13] found bilateral diffuse infiltrates in about 50% and no changes in 15% initially. Distribution usually is bilateral and favors perihilar or basal regions.

The *earliest* and *most reliable* sign of aspiration is hypoxemia, which follows aspiration of even the mildest and most benign aspirate. Even a saline aspirate causes a significant degree of hypoxemia.[38,39] Therefore, whenever there is any chance that aspiration has occurred, analysis of arterial oxygenation by pulse oximetry or measurement of oxygen tension in arterial blood is indicated. If hypoxemia is present, the patient should be treated.

Prevention

Regional anesthesia is the best way to avoid aspiration. However, when general anesthesia is required, the following preventive measures are helpful:

- Nothing by mouth
- Antacids
- Histamine-2 blocking agents
- Metoclopramide
- Head-up position
- Rapid sequence induction of anesthesia
- Cricoid pressure
- Endotracheal intubation
- Extubation awake

Nothing by Mouth

Some obstetricians, nurses, and nurse midwives have suggested that physicians should liberalize oral intake during labor.[40-43] Is nothing by mouth still appropriate? Studies have demonstrated that administration of clear liquids up to 2 hours before elective surgery does not increase gastric volume or acidity in nonpregnant patients, provided they do not also consume solid food.[44-55] Water, clear liquids, and tea—but not milk—are acceptable oral fluids before elective surgery in nonpregnant patients. However, several differences exist between laboring women and nonpregnant patients undergoing elective surgery, and these differences require a more cautious approach for the former type of patient. The interval between the last full meal and the onset of labor varies among patients. Indeed, some women are even advised to eat a full meal after the onset of labor and before they present to the labor and delivery unit. Second, many women receive opioids systemically or epidurally during labor. Opioids clearly result in delayed gastric emptying. Third, laboring women may require urgent cesarean section at any time. Thus the interval between the last oral intake and induction of anesthesia may be substantially less than 2 hours.

Guidelines for Perinatal Care, third edition,[56] published by the American College of Obstetricians and Gynecologists (ACOG) and the American Academy of Pediatrics, states the following:

> Patients should not ingest anything by mouth during labor except for small sips of water, ice chips, or preparations to moisten the mouth and lips. Hydration and nourishment during a long labor should be provided by means of the intravenous administration of fluids; this measure also minimizes acidemia and electrolyte imbalance.

Thus, it remains appropriate to restrict oral intake during labor. Even a policy that allows only ice chips may not guarantee low volumes of ingested fluid. In our institution, we have observed an oral fluid intake (in the form of ice chips) as low as 22 ml/hr and as high as 120 ml/hr during labor.[57] Thus we encourage judicious ingestion of ice chips and not unlimited consumption. We suggest that oral intake during labor should be limited to 60 ml/hr of water or another clear, nonparticulate liquid. This should represent a reasonable compromise between patient safety and comfort. Food should never be allowed. Not only does it cause severe lung damage if aspiration occurs, but it is also more slowly emptied from the stomach.[58] Time for gastric emptying of several different materials is shown in Fig. 3-2.

Antacids

An antacid will reduce the acidity of gastric fluid, but it will not reduce gastric volume. Thirty milliliters of nonparticulate antacid (e.g., 0.3 M sodium citrate: Bicitra, Alka-Seltzer Effervescent) is preferred.[59-61] Nonparticulate antacids are recommended over particulate antacids (e.g., magnesium trisilicate) because aspiration of a particulate antacid may cause pulmonary shunting and hypoxemia similar in magnitude to that caused by

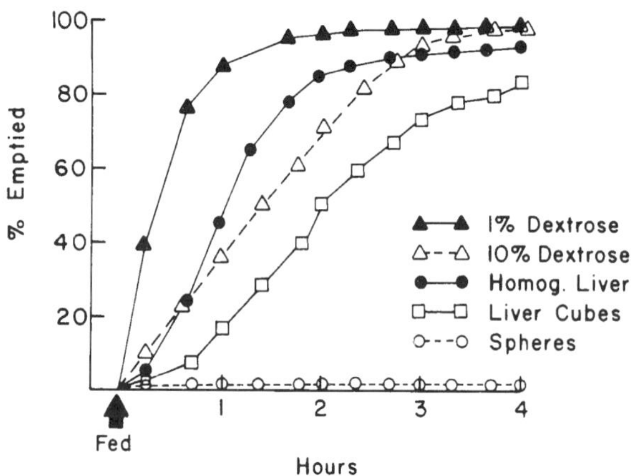

Fig. 3-2.
The rate of gastric emptying is influenced considerably by the makeup of any given meal. Notice the large difference in emptying times between 1% dextrose and cubes of liver. Solid plastic spheres pass very slowly if at all. Experiments performed in dogs. *(From Hinder RA, Kelly KA:* Am J Physiol *1977; 223:335.)*

acid aspiration and greater than that caused by saline.[62]

H_2 Antagonists

By blocking histamine receptors on the oxyntic cell, H_2 blockers significantly decrease gastric acid production and decrease volume. Cimetidine (given in doses of 200 to 400 mg intravenously, intramuscularly, or orally) reduces gastric acidity within 60 to 90 minutes. The usual regimen is 300 mg orally at bedtime and in the morning.[63-66] Intramuscular and intravenous use have few advantages over oral administration unless the patient cannot take anything by mouth. Oral preparations work nearly as fast and are considerably less expensive. The regimen for ranitidine is 150 mg orally at bedtime and in the morning. It is equally effective.[67-71]

Omeprazole inhibits the hydrogen ion pump on the gastric surface of the oxyntic cell.[72] The decrease in gastric acid production depends not on blood levels of the drug but on the binding of omeprazole to the hydrogen ion pump. Recently, some investigators have evaluated the prophylactic administration of omeprazole before cesarean section.[72-77] A two-dose regimen that includes oral administration of 40 mg at bedtime and on the morning of surgery consistently decreases gastric pH.[73] Orr et al.[76] concluded that a combination of omeprazole and metoclopramide is most effective in reducing both gastric acidity and gastric volume before elective cesarean section.

Metoclopramide

This agent is a procainamide derivative that is a cholinergic agonist peripherally and a dopamine receptor antagonist centrally. A 10-mg intravenous dose of metoclopramide increases lower esophageal sphincter tone and reduces gastric volume by increasing gastric peristalsis. Metoclopramide can have a significant effect on gastric volume in as little as 15 minutes.[78-80]

Head-Up Position

For patients subject to passive regurgitation of stomach contents, the head-up position decreases the incidence of actual regurgitation and thereby decreases the risk of pulmonary aspiration. Some clinicians argue in favor of the head-down position, claiming that it decreases the likelihood of pulmonary aspiration if the oropharynx fills with stomach contents. However, the head-up position decreases the likelihood of regurgitation itself.

Rapid-Sequence Induction

If the anesthesiologist is confident that endotracheal intubation will not present a problem, a rapid-sequence induction is indicated in patients considered at risk for aspiration. During general anesthesia the most dangerous time, in terms of aspiration of gastric contents, is the period from loss of consciousness to tracheal intubation with a cuffed endotracheal tube. A rapid-sequence induction permits completion of this process in the shortest possible time. The rapid-sequence induction is not itself without danger and risk. Failure to intubate the trachea once unconsciousness and paralysis are accomplished can result in hypoxia, asphyxia, aspiration, or all three. Results of a survey describing events surrounding 21 cases of aspiration revealed that 14 of 21 cases occurred during the process of a difficult intubation. In one instance, seven attempts had been made and in another instance four attempts had been made.[15] One should remember that the incidence of difficult intubation is 0.04% in all patients and 0.35% in obstetric patients.[16]

Cricoid Pressure

Sellick's maneuver is the simplest and most effective measure for minimizing the risk of aspiration.[81] However, the person applying cricoid pressure must know how to do so properly. Pressure is applied at the cricoid cartilage, not the thyroid cartilage or over the entire larynx. Pressure applied to the thyroid cartilage makes the intubation process more difficult, whereas pressure applied to the cricoid cartilage makes endotracheal intubation easier. Some prefer to place one hand behind the patient's neck while applying pressure at the cricoid cartilage. In addition to ensuring proper placement of pressure, the attendant must not release the pressure until the intubation is complete, the cuff is inflated, and correct placement is ensured.

Although it is not effective 100% of the time, when applied properly, cricoid pressure should prevent nearly all cases of aspiration. The maneuver will withstand an esophageal pressure head of at least 100 cm H_2O.[81] Thus, it should prevent aspiration of gastric contents after either regurgitation or vomiting. Some researchers have suggested that cricoid pressure should be released when vomiting occurs to prevent rupturing of the esophagus.[82] Such a consequence is mostly theoretical. Recently, Sellick[83] advocated that cricoid pressure not be released in these instances. When a trachea cannot be intubated and positive-pressure ventilation is required to prevent hypoxia, it is imperative that cricoid pressure be continued until the trachea is successfully intubated.

Endotracheal Intubation

Intubation of the trachea should be used in all patients at risk for aspiration, and obstetric patients are in the *at risk* category. If a difficult intubation is anticipated, the process should be accomplished before the administration of anesthesia. Although an awake intubation may be uncomfortable, the morbidity associated with aspiration is considerably more uncomfortable. Furthermore, when appropriate techniques are used, the process does not have to be brutal.

Awake Extubation

If intubation while the patient is awake or a rapid-sequence induction is indicated to prevent aspiration, then extubation while the patient is awake also is indicated. Extubation of an awake patient means that the patient is conscious, that is, awake, aware, and responding appropriately to commands. Gagging, coughing, bucking, and indiscriminately reaching for the endotracheal tube are not signs of consciousness; rather, they may be signs of stage 2 anesthesia, the excitement stage. If the endotracheal tube is removed during this stage, the patient may continue to be vulnerable to aspiration as well as laryngospasm.

Treatment

Although a thorough discussion of the treatment of aspiration is beyond the scope of this chapter, a few points need to be made. First, if a patient is hypoxic and if aspiration is suspected, some form of treatment should be instituted. The mainstay of treatment for most patients with aspiration will be mechanical ventilation with positive end expiratory pressure. Although most patients will require endotracheal intubation, some may be able to be managed with the application of continuous positive airway pressure via a mask. That decision will be determined by the physicians at the bedside. The amount of positive pressure and positive end expiratory pressure as well as the percentage of oxygen also will be determined at the bedside.

Although pulmonary lavage has been recommended by some physicians as routine treatment for pulmonary aspiration, this technique can decrease pulmonary compliance and Pa_{O_2} and increase intrapulmonary shunting. Because acidic aspirate reaches the periphery of the lung within 12 to 18 seconds,[84] lavage with bicarbonate solution is not helpful.

Corticosteroids first were recommended for treatment of patients with acid aspiration in 1961[85] and 1962.[85,86] Since that time, several studies of both animals and humans indicate that corticosteroid therapy provides some modification of the inflammatory response early after aspiration but does not alter the course of the disease.[87-89] However, it may interfere with normal healing mechanisms.[90] For these reasons, corticosteroids usually are not given.

Prophylactic antibiotics have been recommended by some investigators for patients who have had pulmonary aspiration of stomach contents.[89] However, they should not be used because they may alter the normal flora of the respiratory tract and thus may make the patient susceptible to secondary infection by more resistant organisms.[91] Antibiotics should be reserved for patients who show signs of clinical pulmonary infection, in which case the antibiotic most effective for the suspected offending organism, identified by Gram stains and cultures, should be used.

Recent animal reports suggest that instilling a surfactant replacement solution into the trachea after aspiration of acidic material may improve pulmonary function.[92] However, such therapy is still experimental.

Summary

Aspiration continues to be a serious threat to pregnant patients undergoing general anesthesia. If proper techniques and preventive measures are used, most cases can be prevented or the consequences ameliorated. Because aspiration of partially digested food causes the most severe physiologic and histologic derangements, patients should not eat once labor has begun except for small sips of water and ice chips.

References

1. Centers for Disease Control, *Morbid Mortal Weekly Rep* 1993; 42:15.
2. Hawkins J, Koonin L, Palmer S, et al: Anesthesia-related maternal deaths in the United States: a 12 year review 1979-1990, *Anesthesiology* 1993; 79:A982.
3. Gibbs CP, Krischer J, Peckham BM, et al: Obstetric anesthesia: a national survey, *Anesthesiology* 1986; 65:298.
4. Olsson GL, Hallen B, Hambracus-Jonzon K: Aspiration during anaesthesia: a computer-aided study of 185,358 anaesthetics, *Acta Anaesthesiol Scand* 1986; 30:84.
5. Warner MA, Warner ME, Weber JG: Clinical significance of pulmonary aspiration during the perioperative period, *Anesthesiology* 1993; 78:56.
6. Mendelson CL: The aspiration of stomach contents into the lungs during obstetric anesthesia, *Am J Obstet Gynecol* 1946; 52:191.
7. Arms RA, Dines DE, Tinstman TC: Aspiration pneumonia, *Chest* 1974; 65:136.
8. Awe WC, Fletcher WS, Jacob SW: The pathophysiology of aspiration pneumonitis, *Surgery* 1966; 60:232.
9. Cameron JL, Mitchell WH, Zuidema GD: Aspiration pneumonia: clinical outcome following documented aspiration, *Arch Surg* 1973; 106:49.
10. Dines DE, Titus JL, Sessler AD: Aspiration pneumonitis. *Mayo Clin Proc* 1970; 45:347.
11. Cameron JL, Caldini P, Toung J-K, et al: Aspiration pneumonia: physiologic data following experimental aspiration, *Surgery* 1972; 72:238.
12. LeFrock JL, Clark TS, Davies B, et al: Aspiration pneumonia: a 10-year review, *Am Surg* 1979; 45:305.
13. Landay ML, Christensen EE, Bynum LJ: Pulmonary manifestations of acute aspiration of gastric contents, *Am J Roentgenol* 1978; 131:587.
14. Wynne JW, Hood CI: Hypoxemia in the first hour after aspiration, *Chest* 1980; 78:546 (abstract).
15. Gibbs CP, Rolbin SH, Norman P: Cause and prevention of maternal aspiration, *Anesthesiology* 1984; 61:111 (letter to the editor).
16. Samsoon GLT, Young JRB: Difficult tracheal intubation: a retrospective study, *Anaesthesia* 1987; 42:487.
17. Spence AA, Mori DD, Finlay WEI: Observations on intragastric pressure, *Anaesthesia* 1967; 22:249.
18. Brock-Utne JG, Dow TGB, Dimopoulos GE, et al: Gastric and lower oesophageal sphincter (LOS) pressures in early pregnancy, *Br J Anaesthesiol* 1981; 53:381.
19. Attia RR, Ebeid AM, Fischer JE, et al: Maternal fetal and placental gastrin concentrations, *Anaesthesia* 1982; 37:18.

20. Christofides ND, Ghatei MA, Bloom SR, et al: Decreased plasma motilin concentrations in pregnancy, *Br Med J* 1982; 285:1453.
21. Davison JS, Davison MC, Hay DM: Gastric emptying time in late pregnancy and labour, *Br J Obstet Gynaecol* 1970; 77:37.
22. Holdsworth JD: Relationship between stomach contents and analgesia in labor, *Br J Anaesth* 1978; 50:1145.
23. Simpson KH, Stakes AF, Miller M: Pregnancy delays paracetamol absorption and gastric emptying in patients undergoing surgery, *Br J Anaesth* 1988; 60:24.
24. Greenan J: The cardio-oesophageal junction, *Br J Anaesth* 1961; 33:432.
25. Williams NH: Variable significance of heartburn, *Am J Obstet Gynecol* 1941; 42:814.
26. Brock-Utne JG, Dow TGB, Dimopoulos GE, et al: The effect of metoclopramide on the lower oesophageal sphincter in late pregnancy, *Anaesth Intensive Care* 1978; 6:26.
27. Dow TGB, Brock-Utne JG, Rubin J, et al: The effect of atropine on the lower esophageal sphincter in late pregnancy, *Obstet Gynecol* 1978; 51:426.
28. Lind JF, Smith AM, McIver DK, et al: Heartburn in pregnancy: a manometric study, *Can Med Assoc J* 1968; 98:571.
29. Roberts RB, Shirley MA: Reducing the risk of acid aspiration during cesarean section, *Anesth Analg* 1974; 53:859.
30. Teabeaut JR II: Aspiration of gastric contents: an experimental study, *Am J Pathol* 1952; 28:51.
31. Awe WC, Fletcher WS, Jacob SW: The pathophysiology of aspiration pneumonitis, *Surgery* 1966; 60:232.
32. James CF, Modell JH, Gibbs CP, et al: Pulmonary aspiration: effects of volume and pH in the rat, *Anesth Analg* 1984; 63:665.
33. Plourde G, Hardy JF: Aspiration pneumonia: assessing the risk of regurgitation in the cat, *Can Anaesth Soc J* 1986; 33:345.
34. Raidoo DM, Marszalek A, Brock-Utne JG: Acid aspiration in primates: a surprising experimental result, *Anaesth Intensive Care* 1988; 16:375.
35. Kennedy TP, Johnson KJ, Kunkel RG: Acute acid aspiration lung injury in the rat: biphasic pathogenesis, *Anesth Analg* 1989; 69:87.
36. Hamelberg W, Bosomworth PP: Aspiration pneumonitis: experimental studies and clinical observations, *Anesth Analg* 1964; 43:669.
37. Jones JG, Grossman RF, Berry M, et al: Alveolar capillary membrane permeability: correlation with functional, radiographic and postmortem changes after fluid aspiration, *Am Rev Respir Dis* 1979; 120:399.
38. Schwartz DJ, Wynne JW, Gibbs CP, et al: The pulmonary consequences of aspiration of gastric contents at pH values greater than 2.5, *Am Rev Respir Dis* 1980; 121:119.
39. Wynne JW, Hood CI: Hypoxemia in the first hour after aspiration, *Chest* 1980; 78:546 (abstract).
40. McKay S, Mahan C: How can aspiration of vomitus in obstetrics best be prevented? *Birth* 1988; 15:222.
41. Elkington KW: At the water's edge: where obstetrics and anesthesia meet, *Obstet Gynecol* 1991; 77:304.
42. Michael S, Reilly CS, Caunt JA: Policies for oral intake during labour: a survey of maternity units in England and Wales, *Anaesthesia* 1991; 46:1071.
43. Chestnut DH, Cohen SE: At the water's edge: where obstetrics and anesthesia meet, *Obstet Gynecol* 1991; 77:965 (letter in reply).
44. Agarwal A, Chari P, Singh H: Fluid deprivation before operation: the effect of a small drink, *Anaesthesia* 1989; 44: 632.
45. Goodwin AP, Rowe WL, Ogg TW, et al: Oral fluids prior to day surgery: the effect of shortening the preoperative fluid fast on postoperative morbidity, *Anaesthesia* 1991; 46: 1066.
46. Hutchinson A, Maltby JR, Reid CR: Gastric fluid volume and pH in elective inpatients I: coffee or orange juice versus overnight fast, *Can J Anaesth* 1988; 35:12.
47. Maltby JR, Sutherland AD, Sale JP, et al: Preoperative oral fluids: is a five-hour fast justified prior to elective surgery? *Anesth Analg* 1986; 65:1112.
48. Miller M, Wishart HY, Nimmo WS: Gastric contents at induction of anaesthesia: is a 4-hour fast necessary? *Br J Anaesth* 1983; 55:1185.
49. Scarr M, Maltby JR, Jani K, et al: Volume and acidity of residual gastric fluid after oral fluid ingestion before elective ambulatory surgery, *Can Med Assoc J* 1989; 141:1151.
50. Strunin L: How long should patients fast before surgery? Time for new guidelines, *Br J Anaesth* 1993; 70:1 (editorial).
51. Schreiner MS, Triebwasser A, Keon TP: Ingestion of liquids compared with preoperative fasting in pediatric outpatients, *Anesthesiology* 1990; 72:593.

52. Splinter WM, Schaefer JD: Ingestion of clear fluids is safe for adolescents up to 3 h before anaesthesia, *Br J Anaesth* 1991; 66:45.
53. Splinter WM, Schaefer JD: Unlimited clear fluid ingestion two hours before surgery in children does not affect volume or pH of stomach contents, *Anaesth Intensive Care* 1990; 18:522.
54. van der Walt JH, Carter JA: The effect of different preoperative feeding regimens on plasma glucose and gastric volume and pH in infancy, *Anaesth Intensive Care* 1986; 14:352.
55. van der Walt JH, Foate JA, Murrell D, et al: A study of preoperative fasting in infants aged less than three months, *Anaesth Intensive Care* 1990; 18:527.
56. Freeman RK, Poland RL: *Guidelines for perinatal care,* ed 3, 1992, American Academy of Pediatrics and American College of Obstetricians and Gynecologists.
57. Guyton TS, Gibbs CP: Ice chip consumption during labor, 1993 (unpublished data).
58. Hinder RA, Kelly KA: Canine gastric emptying of solids and liquids, *Am J Physiol* 1977; 233:335.
59. Gibbs CP, Spohr L, Schmidt D: The effectiveness of sodium citrate as an antacid, *Anesthesiology* 1982; 57:44.
60. Viegas OJ, Ravindran RS, Shumacker CA: Gastric fluid pH in patients receiving sodium citrate, *Anesth Analg* 1981; 60:521.
61. Chen CT, Toung TJ, Haupt HM, et al: Evaluation of the efficacy of Alka-Seltzer Effervescent in gastric acid neutralization, *Anesth Analg* 1984; 63:325.
62. Gibbs CP, Schwartz DJ, Wynne JW, et al: Antacid pulmonary aspiration in the dog, *Anesthesiology* 1979; 51:380.
63. Coombs DW, Hooper D, Colton T: Acid-aspiration prophylaxis by use of preoperative oral administration of cimetidine, *Anesthesiology* 1979; 51:352.
64. Johnston JR, McCaughey W, Moore J, et al: Cimetidine as an oral antacid before elective caesarean section, *Anaesthesia* 1982; 37:26.
65. Manchikanti L, Kraus JW, Edds SP: Cimetidine and related drugs in anesthesia, *Anesth Analg* 1982; 61:595.
66. Williams JG, Strunin L: Pre-operative intramuscular ranitidine and cimetidine: double blind comparative trial, effect on gastric pH and volume, *Anaesthesia* 1985; 40:242.
67. Dammann HG, Muller P, Simon B: Parenteral ranitidine: onset and duration of action, *Br J Anaesth* 1982; 54:1235.
68. Francis RN, Kwik RS: Oral ranitidine for prophylaxis against Mendelson's syndrome, *Anesth Analg* 1982; 61:130.
69. Maile CJ, Francis RN: Pre-operative ranitidine: effect of a single intravenous dose on pH and volume of gastric aspirate, *Anaesthesia* 1983; 38:324.
70. Brock-Utne JG, Downing JW, Humphrey D: Effect of ranitidine given before atropine sulphate on lower oesophageal sphincter tone, *Anaesth Intensive Care* 1984; 12:140.
71. Rout CC, Rock DA, Gouws E: Intravenous ranitidine reduces the risk of acid aspiration of gastric contents at emergency cesarean section, *Anesth Analg* 1993; 76:156.
72. Massoomi F, Savage J, Destache CJ: Omeprazole: a comprehensive review, *Pharmacotherapy* 1993; 13:46.
73. Yau G, Kan AF, Gin T, et al: A comparison of omeprazole and ranitidine for prophylaxis against aspiration pneumonitis in emergency caesarean section, *Anaesthesia* 1992; 47:101.
74. Moore J, Flynn RJ, Sampaio M, et al: Effect of single-dose omeprazole on intragastric acidity and volume during obstetric anaesthesia, *Anaesthesia* 1989; 44:559.
75. Ching MS, Morgan DJ, Mihaly GW, et al: Placental transfer of omeprazole in maternal and fetal sheep, *Dev Pharmacol Ther* 1986; 9:323.
76. Orr DA, Bill KM, Gillon KR, et al: Effects of omeprazole, with and without metoclopramide, in elective obstetric anaesthesia, *Anaesthesia* 1993; 48:114.
77. Ewart MC, Yau G, Gin T, et al: A comparison of the effects of omeprazole and ranitidine on gastric secretion in women undergoing elective caesarean section, *Anaesthesia* 1990; 45:527.
78. Wyner J, Cohen SE: Gastric volume in early pregnancy: effect of metoclopramide, *Anesthesiology* 1982; 57:209.
79. Olsson GL, Hallen B. Pharmacological evacuation of the stomach with metoclopramide, *Acta Anaesthesiol Scand* 1982, 26:417.
80. Brock-Utne JG, Dow TG, Welman S, et al: The effect of metoclopramide on the lower oesophageal sphincter in late pregnancy, *Anaesth Intensive Care* 1978; 6:26.
81. Sellick BA: Cricoid pressure to control regurgitation of stomach contents during induction of anesthesia, *Lancet* 1961; 2:404.
82. Notcutt WG: Rupture of the oesophagus following cricoid pressure? *Anaesthesia* 1981; 36:911.

83. Sellick BA: Rupture of the oesophagus following cricoid pressure? *Anaesthesia* 1982; 37:213.

84. Hamelberg W, Bosomworth PP: Aspiration pneumonitis: experimental studies and clinical observations, *Anesth Analg* 1964; 43:669.

85. Bannister WK, Sattilaro AJ, Otis RD: Therapeutic aspects of aspiration pneumonitis in experimental animals, *Anesthesiology* 1961; 22:440.

86. Bannister WK, Sattilaro AJ: Vomiting and aspiration during anesthesia, *Anesthesiology* 1962; 23:251.

87. Downs JB, Chapman RL Jr, Modell JH, et al: An evaluation of steroid therapy in aspiration pneumonitis, *Anesthesiology* 1974; 40:129.

88. Chapman RL Jr, Downs JB, Modell JH, et al: The ineffectiveness of steroid therapy in treating aspiration of hydrochloric acid, *Arch Surg* 1974; 108:858.

89. Chapman RL Jr, Modell JH, Ruiz BC, et al: Effect of continuous positive-pressure ventilation and steroids on aspiration of hydrochloric acid (pH 1.8) in dogs, *Anesth Analg* 1974; 53:556.

90. Wynne JW, Reynolds JC, Hood CI, et al: Steroid therapy for pneumonitis induced in rabbits by aspiration of foodstuff, *Anesthesiology* 1979; 51:11.

91. Wynne JW, Modell JH: Respiratory aspiration of stomach contents, *Ann Intern Med* 1977; 87:466.

92. Eijking EP, Gommers D, Vergear M, et al: Surfactant treatment of respiratory failure induced by hydrochloric acid aspiration in rats, *Anesthesiology* 1993; 78:1145.

4

Aspiration in Obstetrics

A 25 year-old multigravida was brought to the operating room for an emergency cesarean delivery for acute fetal distress. The anesthesiologist had some difficulty during induction of general anesthesia and intubation. The operation went well and resulted in the birth of a newborn with an Apgar score of 6 at 1 minute and 9 at 5 minutes. In the recovery room, the patient was dyspneic and cyanotic. X-ray film examination showed bilateral infiltrations, and the anesthesiologist made a diagnosis of acid aspiration. Discuss the treatment of this problem and the ways to prevent this complication.

Recommendations by Carter Dodge, M.D.
George Blike, M.D.

Epidemiology

Aspiration remains a distressingly common cause of maternal morbidity and mortality. Because the United States has no national maternal mortality survey, we rely on data from the United Kingdom where aspiration associated with failed or difficult endotracheal intubation represented the major cause of maternal mortality secondary to anesthesia. The causes of maternal death associated with anesthesia may be changing, however. During the time when rapid-sequence induction with cricoid pressure and tracheal intubation became common, the mortality associated with intubation has risen while mortality with aspiration has fallen.[1] In one British hospital over a 20-year period, the incidence of mortality from aspiration was 1 per 1500 general anesthetics administered for childbirth (Fig. 4-1).

To collect data in the United States, Gibbs and associates asked their colleagues in the Society for Obstetric Anesthesia and Perinatology to report all cases of maternal aspiration.[2] Seventy-nine physi-

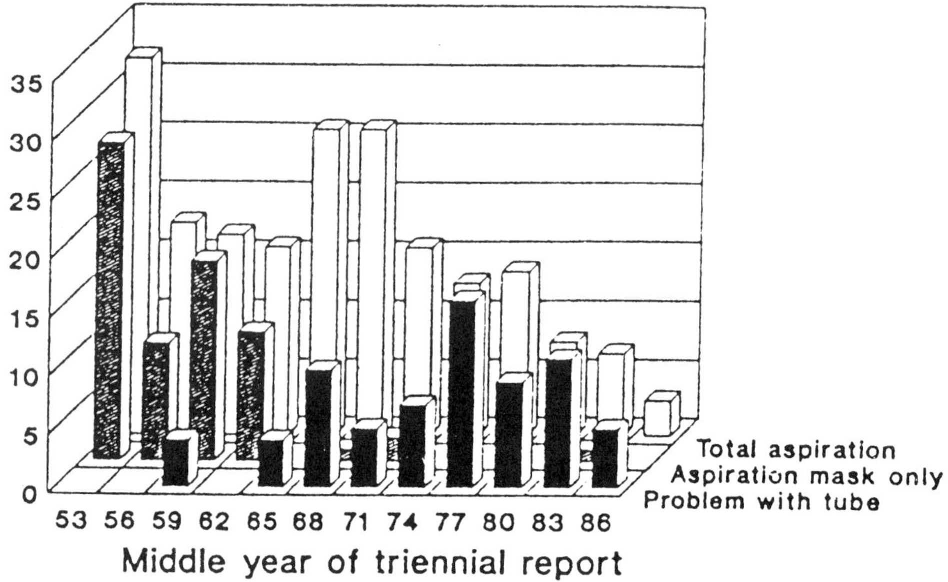

Fig. 4-1.

Maternal deaths associated with anesthesia from the 12 reports on confidential inquiries into maternal death in England and Wales (UK in last report) 1952 to 1987, Department of Health. London: HMSO. *Total aspiration* refers to deaths from aspiration pneumonitis. *Aspiration mask only* are those deaths from aspiration pneumonitis where tracheal intubation was not planned. *Problems with tube* include hypoxic deaths from esophageal intubation and failed intubation. *(From Vanner RG: Mechanisms of regurgitation and its prevention with cricoid pressure,* Int J Obstet Anesth *1993; 2:207.)*

cians reported 21 cases. All but two patients had been or were being intubated with cuffed oral endotracheal tubes. Their data remind us of the following:

1. General anesthesia for emergency cesarean section is particularly hazardous
2. A difficult or failed intubation increases the risk of aspiration
3. Even when accomplished with ease, endotracheal intubation per se does not prevent aspiration.

Diagnosis

Diagnosis of aspiration seldom is a problem, with clinical features unchanged since Mendelsen's description in 1946: ". . . progressive dyspnea, hypoxemia, wheezing, and patchy consolidation and collapse in the lungs. Usually in obstetrics, the clinical situation includes the discovery of a pharynx filled with gastric contents, difficulty with intubation, or regurgitation on emergence."

Several conditions cause diagnostic confusion. Amniotic fluid embolism presents with dyspnea, cyanosis, pulmonary edema, and chest pain. A predisposing factor is tumultuous labor with exceptionally strong contractions, either natural or stimulated with oxytocin. If the patient survives the initial shock-like episode, bleeding ensues with elevated fibrin split products, prolonged thrombin time, and decreased fibrinogen levels. An electrocardiogram may suggest strain on the right side of the heart, although time for confirmatory tests may be limited. The risk of pulmonary thromboembolism is increased fivefold during pregnancy so that it should be included in the differential diagnosis. Congestive heart failure becomes more likely if labor is inhibited with β-agonists like terbutaline or if the patient has preexisting heart disease.

Physiology

A great deal of uncertainty exists about the effects of pregnancy on upper gastrointestinal tract function. Whereas some early studies showed decreased gastric emptying times in parturients, the weight of evidence suggests that gastric emptying is normal in early labor. Acetaminophen is not absorbed from the stomach, but is rapidly absorbed from the small intestine. Blood levels correlate with gastric emptying. Normally, peak blood levels occur within 1 hour. With established labor and pain and after narcotic agents, peak levels of acetaminophen are delayed until 6 hours after ingestion.[3] Interestingly, epidural analgesia does not slow acetaminophen absorption to stress-free rates (Fig. 4-2).

Patients who have been in labor and who require an emergent cesarean section truly have full stomachs. In one report, gastric aspirates from patients coming for emergent cesarean section had a mean of 106 ml, with a maximum of 1000 ml, compared with aspirates from patients for elective sections who had a mean of 32 ml, with a maximum of 200 ml (Fig. 4-3).

In addition to increased gastric contents, parturients have altered lower esophageal sphincter function. Hey, a British anesthesiologist, obtained manometric measurements for pregnant women with heartburn, pregnant women without heartburn, and nonpregnant women as controls.[4] She found lower mean barrier pressures (gastric pressure minus maximum sphincter pressure) in pregnant women with heartburn than in a symptomatic preg-

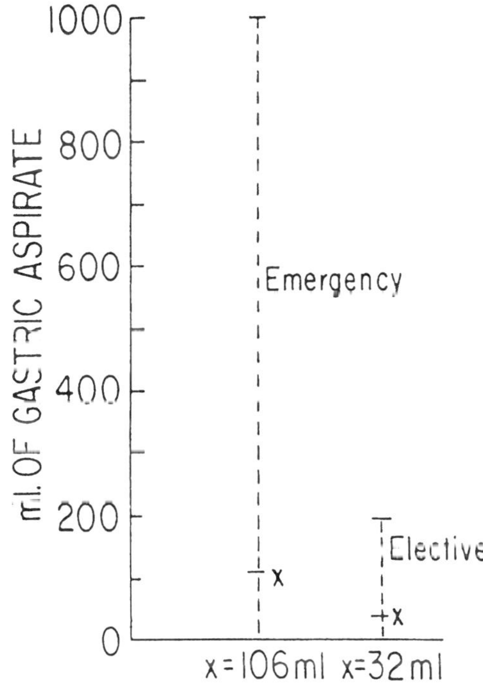

Fig. 4-2.
Plasma acetaminophen levels after 1.5 mg taken orally with 200 ml water. Notice that painful labor treated with meperidine reduces acetaminophen absorption. *(From Wilson J: Gastric emptying in labor: some recent findings and their clinical significance,* J Int Med Res *1978; 6(suppl 1):56.)*

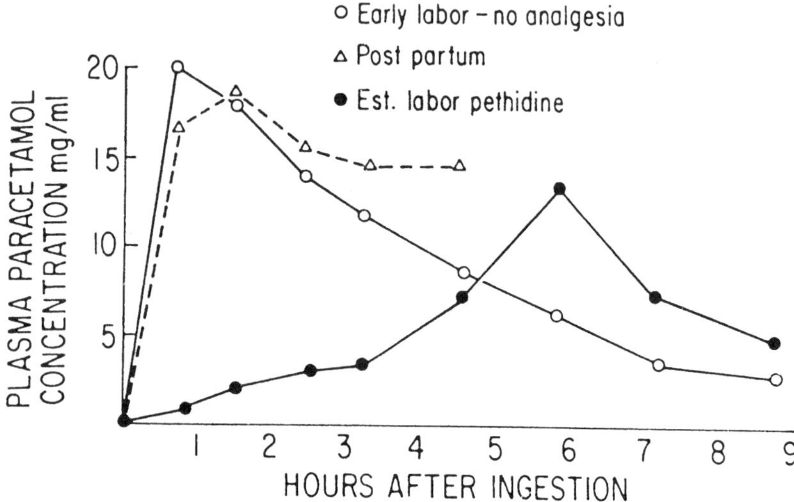

Fig. 4-3.

Volumes obtained from nasogastric aspiration after induction. Patients coming for emergent cesarean section may have large volumes of gastric contents. *(From Wilson J: Gastric emptying in labor: some recent findings and their clinical significance,* J Int Med Res *1978; 6(suppl 1):55.)*

nant women. A tremendous overlap occurred among the groups. Predicting any one individual's barrier pressure is impossible.

Unfortunately, it is difficult to wrap up this discussion of gastric function in pregnancy with a simple causal explanation. Levels of gastrin, which increases lower esophageal sphincter (LES) pressure, and progesterone, which decreases it, are unchanged in parturients with heartburn compared with asymptomatic pregnant women. Thus, hormonal explanations for altered gastrointestinal tract function are elusive.

Prevention

Pharmacologic

Because parturients with full stomachs frequently require anesthesia while in labor, a number of mechanical and pharmacologic approaches have been tried to minimize the danger of aspiration. Animal experiments suggest that a pH greater than 2.5 and a volume of aspirate less than 0.4 ml/kg usually result in minimal pulmonary damage.

During the 1970s, particulate antacids containing calcium, aluminum, and magnesium salts became the standard of care in some obstetric units, including our own. Problems included case reports of serious pulmonary complications when large amounts of gastric contents were aspirated, but the success of oral antacid regimens of 15 to 30 ml every 2 to 3 hours in raising the gastric pH was reassuring.

Gibbs and associates in 1979 demonstrated that dilute solutions of particulate antacids introduced into dog tracheas resulted in decreased arterial oxygenation and increased pulmonary shunting as profound as abnormalities caused by aspiration of hydrochloric acid at a pH of 1.8.[5] More worrisome, 1 month later when the lungs of surviving dogs were histologically normal, these dogs had an extensive intraalveolar cellular reaction. Furthermore, antacid particles were still present 1 month later.

One alternative to prophylaxis with particulate antacid suspensions is to use sodium citrate. This nonparticulate antacid is relatively harmless if aspiration occurs, producing only transient hypoxemia and minimal tissue changes. Gibbs and co-workers showed that the 30 ml of 0.3/M sodium citrate increased the gastric pH to greater than 2.5 in 98% of 52 samples tested from 26 patients undergoing elective cesarean sections.[5] Many studies, including this one, use historical controls in which 66% of patients undergoing elective cesarean sections had aspirates with a pH of less than 2.5.

Sodium citrate must be given frequently. Studies in healthy adults having elective surgery demonstrate pH elevation for 3 hours after 15 ml. However, in parturients shorter intervals are necessary. One study from Bowman-Gray School of Medicine found that 60 minutes after sodium citrate ingestion, gastric pH had dropped to less than 2.5 in 50% of parturients. Dose is also important. Some investigations have found a dose of 15 ml to be inadequate.

Sodium citrate's disadvantages include its unpleasant taste, which induces nausea in some patients, and a short duration of action. A further disadvantage is the drug's failure to lower gastric volumes. The main advantage of sodium citrate is its ability to raise gastric pH rapidly without causing pulmonary damage if aspiration occurs.

Cimetidine is an effective premedicant, especially in nonemergent obstetric anesthesia. After oral administration of 300 mg of cimetidine, peak levels are reached in 30 minutes. Higher peak levels are attained in 10 minutes after intramuscular (IM) administration. Single oral doses will suppress gastric acidity for longer than 8 hours in a normal man. It seems reasonable, therefore, to suppress nocturnal secretion by an oral dose of cimetidine in the evening before elective cesarean section and to give either oral or IM medication in the morning before elective operation.

A six-center study compared a regimen of 300 mg of cimetidine taken orally the evening before scheduled operation and 300 mg given IM between 1 and 3 hours preoperatively, with a regimen of two similarly timed doses of Mylanta II (Stuart Pharmaceuticals, Wilmington, DE)[6] The patients treated with cimetidine had lower fluid volumes in their stomachs, and fewer patients had gastric fluid pH of less than 2.5. This tendency toward reduced gastric volumes, in addition to higher pH, is a benefit associated with cimetidine that we often forget. A major objective of this study was to evaluate the possible effects of cimetidine treatment on the neonate. Cimetidine does cross the placenta readily. Umbilical vein levels were about 60% of maternal venous cimetidine levels. However, Apgar scores, Early Neonatal Neurobehavioral Scale scores, and neonatal gastric acidity were similar in the groups treated with cimetidine and with antacid.

Cimetidine is not as useful in emergency obstetric anesthesia. A single IM injection of cimetidine requires 60 minutes to be effective and fails to raise gastric pH above 2.5 in 10% of cases. Bolus intravenous cimetidine is not recommended because bradycardia, hypotension, and arrhythmias have resulted.

Unfortunately, cimetidine lacks Food and Drug Administration (FDA) approval for use in obstetrics. Regulatory approval was contingent on demonstration of the current incidence of obstetric aspiration and subsequent reduction of its morbidity by cimetidine, a Herculean task not likely to be undertaken.

Ranitidine, which does not inhibit the cytochrome P-450 system, has been promoted as a newer, presumably safer alternative to cimetidine. On a molar base it is 5 to 12 times more potent in inhibiting gastric secretions. Like cimetidine, it crosses the placenta and yields a fetal-maternal concentration ratio of 0.9. Given the difficulties that Smith Kline & French encountered winning FDA approval for cimetidine in obstetrics, we doubt that Glaxo, Inc. will mount the effort on behalf of ranitidine.

Omeprazole is a proton pump inhibitor which is activated to its effective form in the highly acidic environment of the stomach. Its noncompetitive inhibition of acid secretion is long lasting. It may be potentially useful in reducing gastric acidity in the pregnant patient undergoing either elective or emergency cesarean section. Orr and his group found that 40 mg taken orally the night before surgery and again at 6:00 A.M. the morning of surgery elevated gastric pH to 6.6.[7] Thirteen percent of patients were left with gastric pH values below 2.5. There are no known effects of omeprazole on the fetus, but umbilical vein concentrations are about 50% of those found in maternal plasma. Because omeprazole is between 5 and 10 times more expensive than cimetidine and ranitidine, we have not used it for antacid prophylaxis in our institution.

Metoclopramide initially was developed as an antiemetic, but subsequently was found to promote a rapid gastric clearance of solids and liquids through the stomach. In addition to its central antidopaminergic actions, the drug's action on the gut can be blocked with atropine, suggesting a postganglionic cholinergic site of action.

Metoclopramide does cross the blood-brain barrier and does cross the placenta. Fetal-maternal blood levels of 0.88 have been reported. Metoclopramide does inhibit serum cholinesterase and can lead to a 50% prolongation of succinylcholine induced neuromuscular blockade. The usual dose of metoclopramide is 10 mg IM or intravenously (IV) 1 hour, preferably longer, before induction of anesthesia.

The best evidence for the use of metoclopramide comes from a study in 1973. British parturients in this study also received meperidine in large doses, 150 mg, by current American standards. Gastric emptying was studied by giving a test meal of 750 ml of water containing phenol red as a marker through a nasogastric tube.[8] Interestingly, patients with a history of heartburn or dyspepsia, who might benefit most from treatment, were excluded from the study. Although the half-life of gastric emptying was reduced from 141 minutes in the placebo group to 51 minutes in the metoclopramide group, over 100 ml was still present in the stomach of the patients in the metoclopramide group after 2 hours. Metoclopramide does not suddenly and rapidly empty the stomach. Cohen and Barrier, in a study of patients having elective cesarean section, gave metoclopramide 10 mg an average of 12 minutes before the induction of general anesthesia and measured gastric contents by aspiration.[9] Not surprisingly, they found that gastric volume was unchanged in 30 patients compared with a similar number given placebo. The lesson is that metoclopramide may help empty the stomach if time is available, but it will not help us clinically in the setting of general anesthesia needed for an urgent or emergent cesarean section.

Identifying the Difficult Airway

Aspiration of gastric contents is sometimes a complication of management of the difficult airway. Prevention of aspiration might be possible if it were possible to identify in advance which patients are difficult intubations. The most promising currently available airway assessment is the modified Mallampati scoring system. Can this system help us manage the patient who needs a cesarean section for acute fetal distress?

A South African group in a hospital with 15,000 deliveries per year has prospectively evaluated this scoring system described by Mallampati and modified by Samsoon and Young.[10] The authors found a class IV airway in 6.6% of the mothers coming for cesarean section. A class IV airway means that the soft palate was not visible when the mother was asked to sit upright and open her mouth widely with her head in a neutral position and then asked to protrude her tongue maximally. They found that the relative risk of experiencing a difficult intubation compared with an uncomplicated class I airway was 11.3 for a class IV airway. If only class I and class IV airways are evaluated, the specificity of the test is 87%. This means the test is excellent at identifying the nondiseased. One might think that a test that can identify a large relative risk and has a good specificity might be an attractive test. Unfortunately, what anesthesiologists want to know is the positive predictive value. That is the probability of the condition (a difficult intubation) given a positive test (a class IV airway). Unfortunately, the predictive value of this screening is only 6.5%. This low predictive value means that the finding of a class IV airway is not helpful in managing the patient unless we are willing to do intubations of awake patients on the 93.5% of patients with the class IV anatomy in whom intubation will be easy. Although a short neck, receding mandible, and protruding maxillary incisors were independent risk factors associated with difficult intubations, there were not enough patients with multiple risk factors to determine the cumulative risk. Still lacking is a good preoperative predictor of failed intubation in the population coming for cesarean section.

Induction of General Anesthesia with Endotracheal Intubation

In many instances regional anesthesia for cesarean delivery is not feasible because of factors such as maternal hypovolemia, a coagulopathy, or the emergent need for cesarean section. In the case reported here, acute fetal distress precluded the use of regional anesthesia. Our patient developed aspiration pneumonitis, probably as a result of unrecognized aspiration that occurred during induction of general anesthesia. The risk of regurgitation and subsequent aspiration is greatest during the period when anesthesia is induced (i.e., when the upper esophageal sphincter is relaxed) until a cuffed endotracheal tracheal tube is placed. Preoxygenation followed by rapid sequence induction of anesthesia and endotracheal intubation while maintaining cricoid pressure has become widely accepted as the method of choice for preventing aspiration during this high-risk period. As previously noted in Fig. 4-1, deaths from aspiration dropped at the same time that use of this technique became widespread.

What Method of Preoxygenation Is Adequate?

Parturients are at increased risk for hypoxia after induction of general anesthesia because of a combination of increased oxygen consumption and diminished pulmonary reserve. During only 1 minute of apnea, parturients sustain an average 139 $\pm$ 13 mm Hg/min drop in arterial oxygen pressure (Pa_{O_2}) versus a 58 $\pm$ 8 mm Hg drop in nonpregnant women.[11] Standard preoxygenation for 3 to 5 minute delays hypoxia during apnea, allowing the anesthesiologist more time to safely secure the airway. However, 3 minutes of maternal preoxygenation during fetal distress carries the risk of increasing fetal morbidity and mortality. Four vital capacity breaths of 100% oxygen has been suggested to be as effective as 5 minutes of inhalation of 100% oxygen in increasing the Pa_{O_2} in nonpregnant patients.[12] Norris et al. confirmed that this 4 breaths/30-second technique is effective and safe in parturients undergoing elective cesarean delivery under general anesthesia.[13] In nonpregnant patients, although the time to desaturation (Sa_{O_2} of 90%) occurs more rapidly when the 4-breath preoxygenation method is used, it still took an average of 4 minutes to occur.[14] We use 4-breath preoxygenation in the setting of severe fetal distress to save time and to improve fetal outcome.

Cricoid Pressure

Although cricoid pressure is universally recommended for a rapid-sequence induction, the efficacy of the technique depends upon the induction drugs used, proper timing, good technique, and application of the correct amount of force.

Physiology of Regurgitation and Why Cricoid Pressure Is Effective

Normally regurgitation is prevented by the upper esophageal sphincter (UES). The UES consists of a 3-cm long sling of striated muscle attached to the cricoid cartilage. The pressure generated by the muscle of the UES is referred to as the upper esophageal sphincter pressure (UESP). When UESP is greater than gastric pressure, regurgitation of gastric contents does not occur. The UESP is controlled by the medulla. Consequently, UESP varies, ranging from about 40 mm Hg during wakefulness to 8 mm Hg during deep sleep. Because resting supine gastric pressures of 25 mm Hg are common in full-term parturients, reflux can easily occur. With some anesthetics and with muscle relaxants the UESP can decrease abruptly to about 10 mm Hg.[15] In the full-term parturient, gastric contents will regurgitate into the oropharynx under these conditions. The application of cricoid pressure attempts to replace the protective nature of the UES, which is lost as a result of UES relaxation at the induction of anesthesia. Cricoid pressure as described by Selleck consists of pressing the cricoid cartilage against the cervical vertebral body, trapping the esophagus in the process.

Anesthetic Effects on Upper Esophageal Sphincter Pressure

In a recent series of clinical studies in both live patients and cadavers, Vanner et al. may have answered some long-standing questions about cricoid pressure and the rapid-sequence induction of general anesthesia.[16-20] Using Dent sleeve manometry it was demonstrated that induction of anesthesia with thiopental, sedation with midazolam, and UES muscle relaxation with succinylcholine all reduce UESP to less than 10 mm Hg: a pressure low enough to allow the regurgitation of gastric contents into the pharynx. Interestingly, thiopental, 4 mg/kg, resulted in decreased UESP about 15 seconds before loss of consciousness as assessed by lid reflex. Not all anesthetics decrease UESP: halothane and ketamine have been shown to preserve UESP.[18,19]

How Much Cricoid Pressure Should Be Applied?

Cricoid pressure is a force and, therefore, is measured in newtons (9.81 N = 1 kg). Force is expressed in Newtons ($N = kg \cdot m \cdot sec^{-2}$), mass is expressed in kilograms, and 9.8 N equals the force of gravity on 1 kg. Several aspects of cricoid pressure have been investigated. In a cadaver study, 30 N of cricoid force prevented regurgitation of gastric saline infused at pressures up to 42 mm Hg.[20] In living patients, anesthetized and intubated, 40 N of cricoid force generated UEP ranging from 39 to 232 mm Hg (mean, 77).[16] Despite wide variation, 30 to 40 N of force can be expected to produce an UESP greater than 40 mm Hg, thus adequately replacing the function of the UES.

One can practice giving cricoid pressure using an infant scale commonly found in the obstetric suite. To simplify matters one can assume 10 N equals 1 kg on the scale. One can press on the scale as if giving cricoid pressure until the scale registers 3 to 4 kg to approximate the pressure one must apply clinically.

Does Head Position or Laryngoscopy Change the Efficacy of Cricoid Pressure?

Although head position and the amount of support behind the cervical spine have effects on the UESP, 30 to 40 N of cricoid force was effective in a study using an intubation pillow with integral neck support. In addition, laryngoscopy did not cause cricopharyngeal incompetence.[16]

How Do Awake Patients Tolerate Cricoid Pressure? What Should One Do if the Patient Retches?

Vanner studied 22 conscious volunteers and found that all subjects tolerated 20 N cricoid pressure for 20 seconds. However, with greater force, discomfort, nausea, and dyspnea were common.[7] Furthermore, Vanner's work with cadavers suggests that only pressures of 20 N or greater were associated with esophageal rupture.[10] Although a cadaver study may not model the clinical situation adequately, esophageal rupture is a catastrophic complication. Still, only one reported case exists of esophageal rupture and death associated with cricoid pressure. We maintain cricoid pressure during retching, but reduce the amount of force that is applied (Vanner suggests 20 N of force continue to be applied during retching).[20]

Can Cricoid Pressure Do Harm?

Unfortunately, even good therapies carry risks. The greatest risk associated with cricoid pressure is the potential for this technique to distort the anatomy of the larynx, resulting in airway obstruction and/or causing a failed intubation. We advocate decreasing cricoid force during laryngoscopy or mask ventilation as an early maneuver when difficulties are encountered. Difficult or failed intubation currently is a more common cause of maternal mortality than is aspiration.

Does a Cuffed Endotracheal Tube Protect Against Aspiration?

Some cases of aspiration are clinically significant, others are not. Whereas more than 70% of chronically intubated intensive-care patients aspirated methylene blue applied to the posterior pharynx, in no patient could the aspiration be proven to cause a pulmonary decompensation.[21] Although imperfect, a cuffed endotracheal tube does prevent large-volume aspiration despite evidence that subclinical aspiration still occurs.

At our institution, in the parturient described, a rapid-sequence induction of anesthesia would proceed as follows: (1) patient is placed on the OR table with left uterine displacement; (2) preoxygenation occurs by face mask 100% O_2 at 10-L flows with at least 4 vital-capacity breaths and additional breaths if time allows; (3) IV induction takes place with sodium thiopental followed by muscle relaxation with succinylcholine; (4) light cricoid pressure is applied before loss of lid reflex then force is increased as unconsciousness ensues; (5) ventilation is withheld and laryngoscopy is attempted after fasciculation's cease; (6) the trachea is intubated with a cuffed tube; (7) the tube position is confirmed by auscultation and an appropriate capnogram; and finally; (8) the obstetrician is advised to proceed with the surgical delivery.

Unfortunately, a rapid-sequence induction performed in the manner described does not guarantee against lethal aspiration. Two reported cases exist of patients who died from aspiration despite cricoid pressure and rapid-sequence induction of general anesthesia.[22]

Treatment of Aspiration

Aspiration can lead to morbidity and mortality immediately through asphyxiation, or in a delayed manner through adult respiratory distress syndrome (ARDS). Not all aspiration is clinically significant.

Hypoxia, as seen in our patient, occurs within minutes of aspiration and has multiple causes, including reflex airway closure, decreased surfactant activity, and interstitial and alveolar edema. All of these conditions contribute to large differences in alveolar arterial oxygen and a significant increase in venous admixture. Immediate therapy in our patient included administration of 100% oxygen by mask and rapid insertion of an endotracheal tube during cricoid pressure. Sedation can be added if hemodynamic conditions allow.

After aspiration, gastric acid is rapidly distributed throughout the lung, which causes damage immediately. Thus, attempts at lavaging with bicarbonate solutions are not helpful. Pathologic examination within the first few hours reveals epithelial degeneration, pulmonary edema, and hemorrhage with necrosis of type I alveolar cells. Large volume, low pH, and particulate matter all cause more severe forms of lung injury when aspiration occurs. It may be useful to obtain a specimen of the aspirate for pH analysis to estimate prognosis. Experimentally, as the pH of an aspirate decreases below 2.5, lung injury increases. As the pH decreases below 1.5, however, little additional damage to the lung occurs.

Treatment of aspiration pneumonitis or ARDS is directed toward maintaining oxygenation and cardiac output. Recent studies suggest that increased survival from severe ARDS can occur as a result of more appropriate ventilatory and cardiovascular support aimed at optimizing tissue oxygen delivery.[23] It is clear from computed tomographic studies that the lung injury associated with ARDS is diffuse and heterogeneous.[24] A two-compartment lung model has been developed which may justify the ventilatory strategies currently being used. One compartment is fluid filled, noncompliant, and underventilated; the other compartment is normal. Although positive end expiratory pressure (PEEP) has been used in the past to "recruit" abnormal alveolar units, over-distention of normal lung regions can damage lung directly. The newer ventilatory modes being used (pressure support, inverse ratio ventilation) all attempt to keep the alveoli as fully recruited as possible while avoiding iatrogenic damage to normal lung due to excessive airway pressures. Since only a portion of the lungs are being ventilated, lower tidal volumes have been recommended (6 to 8 ml/kg).

Despite its drawbacks, PEEP remains the primary method for recruiting nonventilated alveoli. PEEP is used to minimize the alveolar to arterial oxygenation gradient and maximize oxygen delivery. A simple, bedside method to find the optimal PEEP is to maximize pulmonary compliance. This can be done in several minutes using a volume ventilator by increasing the PEEP by 5-cm intervals from 0 to 20 cm of PEEP. The clinician observes the peak pressure generated in the sedated patient and adjusts the PEEP to minimize the difference between the peak inspiratory pressure reached and the PEEP setting. Success of this maneuver can be confirmed by blood gas analysis or by improvement of mixed venous oxygen saturation.

Our patient needs respiratory support because she is in respiratory failure. On the other hand, with the patient who is working hard to breathe but who is well oxygenated with supplemental oxygen, the decision to intubate and add PEEP may be more difficult. We tend to apply continuous positive airway pressure by face mask or PEEP by endotracheal tube early in the course of aspiration as some experiments with animals suggest this may reduce mortality. With severe aspirations, the PEEP necessary to improve oxygenation may depress cardiac output. In this situation, measurement of left ventricular filling pressures with a pulmonary artery catheter might be helpful.

Experimental evidence indicates that minimal, if any, benefits occur from using steroids in severe acid aspiration.[25] The clinician who uses steroids in the treatment must weigh their unproven benefits against possible complications. In addition, no well-controlled clinical studies exist on the use of antibiotics in acid aspiration.

Bronchoscopic examination may have value in one circumstance. The bronchoscopist can remove particulate matter that can cause airway obstruction. Overall, however, the need for bronchoscopy after aspiration is limited.

The prognosis for this patient depends upon the pH of the aspirate and the volume aspirated. In Mendelsen's original series of 66 patients, the mortality was zero.[26] But more recent clinical studies contradict this data, showing death rates of 35% to 60%. Thus, acid aspiration can be a potentially lethal disease.

The anesthesiologist's main goal is avoidance of the problem through maintaining a nonacid pH and, whenever possible, an empty stomach by pharmacologic and mechanical means. Since this is nearly impossible most of the time, a rapid induction of general anesthesia with cricoid pressure by a skilled practitioner will minimize, but not eliminate, this complication. When aspiration does occur, quick diagnosis and early institution of PEEP and mechanical ventilation may reduce the mortality associated with this potentially lethal complication.

Summary

Treatment of the case presented should include the following:

1. Endotracheal intubation
2. Maintenance of oxygenation and cardiac output
3. Pressure support where inverse ratio ventilation can be used to keep the alveoli as fully recruited as possible
4. PEEP still remains popular mode of therapy for these patients

References

1. Vanner RG: Mechanisms of regurgitation and its prevention with cricoid pressure, *Int J Obstet Anest* 1993; 2:207.
2. Gibbs CP, Rolbin SH, Norman P: Cause and prevention of maternal aspiration, *Anesthesiology* 1984; 61:111.
3. Wilson J: Gastric emptying in labor: some recent findings and their clinical significance, *J Int Med Res* 1978; 6(suppl 1):54.
4. Hey VMF: Gastro-oesophageal reflex in late pregnancy, *Anaesthesia* 1977; 32:372.
5. Gibbs CP, Spohr L, Schmidt D: The effectiveness of sodium citrate as an antacid, *Anesthesiology* 1982; 57:44.
6. Hodgkinson R, Glassenberg R, Joyce TH III, et al: Comparison of cimetidine (Tagamet) with antacid for safety and effectiveness in reducing gastric acidity before elective cesarean section, *Anesthesiology* 1983; 59:86.
7. Orr DA, Bill KM, Gillon KRW, et al: Effects of omeprazole, with and without metoclopramide, in elective obstetric anaesthesia, *Anaesthesia* 1993; 48:114.
8. Howard FA, Sharp DS: Effect of metoclopramide on gastric emptying during labour, *Br Med J* 1973; 1:446.
9. Cohen SE, Barrier G: Does metoclopramide decrease gastric volume in cesarean section patients? *Anesthesiology* 1983; 59:A403.
10. Rocke DA, Murray WB, Rout CC, et al: Relative risk analysis of factors associated with difficult intubation in obstetric anesthesia, *Anesthesiology* 1992; 77:67.
11. Archer GW, Marx GF: Arterial oxygen tension during apnoea in parturient women, *Br J Anaesth* 1974; 46:358.
12. Gold MI, Durate I, Muravchick S: Arterial oxygenation in conscious patients after 5 minutes and after 30 seconds of oxygen breathing, *Anesth Analg* 1981; 60:313.
13. Norris MC, Dewan DM: Preoxygenation for cesarean section: a comparison of two techniques, *Anesthesiology* 1985; 62:827.
14. Gambee AM, Hertzka RE, Fisher DM: Preoxygenation techniques: comparison of three minutes and four breaths, *Anesth Analg* 1987; 66:468.
15. Vanner RG: Mechanisms of regurgitation and its prevention with cricoid pressure, *Int J Obstet Anesth* 1993; 2:207.
16. Vanner RG, O'Dwyer JP, Pryle BJ, et al: Upper oesophageal sphincter pressure and the effect of cricoid pressure, *Anaesthesia* 1992, 47:95.
17. Vanner RG: Tolerance of cricoid pressure by conscious volunteers, *Int J Obstet Anesth* 1992; 1:195.
18. Vanner RG, Pryle BJ, O'Dwyer JP, et al: Upper oesophageal sphincter pressure and the intravenous induction of anaesthesia, *Anaesthesia* 1992; 47:371.
19. Vanner RG, Pryle BJ, O'Dwyer JP, et al: Upper oesophageal sphincter pressure during inhalational anaesthesia, *Anaesthesia* 1992; 47:950.
20. Vanner RG, Pryle BJ: Regurgitation and oesophageal rupture with cricoid pressure: a cadaver study, *Anaesthesia* 1992; 47:732.

21. Elpern EH, Jacobs ER, Bone RC: Incidence of aspiration in tracheally intubated adults, *Heart Lung* 1987; 16:527.
22. Whittington RM: Fatal aspiration (Mendelson's) syndrome despite antacids and cricoid pressure, *Lancet* 1979; 2:228.
23. Herbertson MJ, Cunningham K, Russell: The adult respiratory distress syndrome, *Curr Opin Anaesth* 1992; 5:218.
24. Gattinoni L, Pelosi P, Vitale G, et al: Body position changes redistribute lung computed-tomographic density in patients with acute respiratory failure, *Anesthesiology* 1991; 74:15.
25. Bone RC, Fisher CJ, Clemmer TP, et al: Early methylprednisolone treatment for septic syndrome and the adult respiratory distress syndrome, *Chest* 1987; 92:1032.
26. Mendelsen CL: Aspiration of stomach contents into lungs during obstetric anesthesia, *Am J Obstet Gynecol* 1946; 53:191.

5

Intravenous Fluid During Labor: Delivery by Cesarean Section

A 25-year-old primigravida is scheduled for an elective cesarean delivery for breech presentation. The patient selects spinal anesthesia. Discuss the choice of intravascular fluid for volume expansion before induction. What would you use in patients who are in labor?

Recommendations by Nancy B. Kenepp, M.D.

Overview of Anesthetic Management

Breech presentation, even with cesarean delivery, increases fetal and maternal risks. A history of accompanying infertility, multiple cesarean deliveries, grand multiparity, prematurity, or vaginal bleeding may forewarn the anesthesiologist of associated conditions such as uterine anatomic abnormalities, fibroid tumors, placenta previa, or abnormal placental implantation. These may complicate delivery of the fetus and uterine repair, and/or cause massive hemorrhage. Delivery of the aftercoming head may be complicated by fetal, bladder, or uterine injury, especially if the incision is transverse, the pregnancy is preterm, and the lower uterine segment has not been thinned out by labor. Although cesarean sections with breech presentations usually are uncomplicated, one should keep in mind the enumerated potentials.

Spinal Anesthesia in Obstetrics

For cesarean section, spinal anesthesia is efficient, reliable, and minimizes fetal drug exposure. However, in pregnancy, with increased abdominal girth and anesthetic sensitivity, the cephalad spread of the block is more difficult to predict. In addition, hypotension occurring with the onset of sympathetic blockade is more severe because the uterus obstructs venacaval and aortic outflow, and the parturient's cardiovascular and pulmonary reserves are decreased. If the patient has medical conditions exacerbating hypotension, epidural anesthesia, with slower onset of sympathetic block, facilitates avoiding maternal hypotension. Hypotension severe enough to compromise fetal well-being will occur, unless aggressive, preventive measures such as intravenous ephedrine and fluid administration, and left uterine displacement, are instituted. Expanding the blood volume by prehydration with intravenous fluid to alleviate the hypotensive effect of the sympathetic blockade is a major focus of this chapter.

Blood Availability

Since uterine atony may occur in patients who do not have any predisposing factors, all cesarean deliveries potentially require blood products. The fact that blood supplies are limited and that there is the risk of disease transmission has spurred recent investigation of and recommendations for blood transfusion associated with cesarean delivery. Several studies indicate poor predictability of need for blood products.[1,2] The majority of recipients lacked demonstrated risk factors such as anemia and antepartum bleeding. To preserve blood supplies, the availability of typed and crossmatched blood is recommended only for patients with placenta previa, abruption, and red blood cell antibodies. Other patients need a blood sample for type and screen sent to blood bank.

Autologous Blood Donation

With elective surgery, use of autologous blood to reduce the risk of infection associated with homologous blood transfusion has increased. Its application to elective cesarean section has been investigated. The safety of the blood donation procedure for mother and fetus has been established.[3,4] However, investigation has not revealed a population of parturients whose need for blood was a significant portion of that donated, or whose transfusion needs were confined to the volume they had predonated.[4-6] Even when narrowing the risk factors to preeclampsia, multiparity, multiple gestation, and elective cesarean section, and donating blood for three simultaneous factors (to increase transfusion probability maximally), it is estimated to cost at least $32,000 per case to prevent hepatitis, and $26,000,000 to prevent human immunovirus (HIV) transmission.[6] Predonation is cost effective only for patients with placenta previa. Unfortunately, this group also is unlikely to be able to donate a volume sufficient to preclude the need for homologous blood.

Preoperative Preparation

Preoperatively, the anesthesiologist should (1) establish proper preparation of the operating room and anesthesia equipment; (2) consider the advisability of sedative premedicants; (3) control gastric acidity and volume; and (4) consider the significant other's presence in the operating room. Personnel and equipment for monitoring and resuscitation of mother and fetus should be ready before administration of the spinal anesthetic. Although premedicants potentially depress the neonate, the fetus of an extremely anxious patient may benefit from maternal catecholamine suppression with a small dose of an appropriate sedative. Gastric volume and acidity should be reduced pharmacologically, as well as by prohibiting oral alimentation. Before administering the spinal anesthetic, one should plan the prevention and treatment of hypotension resulting from the rapidly developing sympathetic blockade.[7] Hypotension is prevented or attenuated by left uterine displacement; acute hydration with crystalloid or colloid intravenous fluids before administration of the spinal anesthetic; intravenous ephedrine or, if indicated, phenylephrine; and further intravenous fluid administration.

Preanesthetic Acute Hydration

Intravenous fluids used for acute hydration can be potentially harmful if not properly selected. Although they do not affect Apgar scores, all fluids have demonstrable effects on blood volume; hemoglobin concentration; and maternal and fetal pH, electrolyte, and metabolite concentrations. Blood volume and hemoglobin concentration changes alter maternal cardiac output and oxygen content. Metabolic changes compromise neonatal extrauterine adaptation by altering maternal and fetal carbohydrate metabolism immediately before birth, when maternal glucose supplies cease. To understand the consequences of acute hydration, it is necessary to consider maternal, fetal, and neonatal metabolism, and the content of various intravenous fluids.

Maternal Metabolism

Total glucose utilization increases in pregnancy. However, pregnancy-induced insulin resistance decreases maternal tissue glucose use. The relative amount of glucose available for fetal and placental tissues, which are not insulin resistant, thus increases. As in nonpregnant states, fasting reduces serum glucose, curtails glucose uptake, and induces the normal compensatory changes (i.e., increased glucagon and increased lipolysis, decreased insulin, and decreased cellular glucose uptake and utilization).

During labor, maternal serum glucose concentration does not correlate with duration of fasting; that is, serum glucose concentration does not decrease as labor progresses. Normal compensatory changes prevent hypoglycemia. Additionally, maternal catecholamine levels influence glucose metabolism and modify the effect of fasting on maternal serum glucose levels.

In adipose tissue, decreased glycerol availability causes release of free fatty acids. Free fatty acids are oxidized by liver mitochondria, producing acetyl coenzyme A, a ketone precursor and carbon source for gluconeogenesis. The liver also produces glucose from amino acids and glycogen.

Ketones and free fatty acids are the preferential muscle fuel. When energy needs exceed aerobic production capacity, glucose is the only source of pyruvate for anaerobic metabolism, which produces lactate. Thus, excessive muscle activity during labor may produce lactic acidosis and a precipitous fall in the blood glucose concentration as a result of anaerobic muscle metabolism.

Likewise, maternal hypotension, causing anaerobic metabolism, could cause maternal hypoglycemia. If such hypotension occurs when the parturient's serum glucose is already low from fasting, the available glucose could be depleted rapidly. Decreased glucose availability might secondarily sustain hypotension under these circumstances. Hypotension, which was difficult to reverse until intravenous glucose therapy was instituted, has been reported in two fasted parturients.[8]

Fetal and Placental Metabolism

Since small molecules diffuse across the placenta easily, fetal metabolite (and electrolyte) concentrations reflect those of the mother. Placental glucose utilization is independent of maternal serum glucose and insulin concentrations (as in red blood cells). On the other hand, fetal serum glucose correlates with maternal serum glucose and fetal glucose utilization appears integrated with maternal glucose utilization.[9]

Human fetal gluconeogenesis has not been demonstrated after a maternal overnight fast. However, in both sheep and dogs, fetal gluconeogenesis occurs after longer maternal fasts. Depressed glucose utilization and decreased glucose concentrations persist for 6 hours after birth in the neonates of fasted canines.

In humans, fetal hyperglycemia increases fetal glucose utilization. Insulin, pyruvate, and lactate production increase as glucose utilization increases.

Fivefold increases in fetal insulin can be demonstrated with as little as 10 to 20 g/hr of maternal intravenous dextrose (200 to 400 ml/hr of 5% dextrose).[10] Increased fetal glucose utilization can cause hypoxia, hypercarbia, and acidosis, probably by exceeding fetal aerobic capacity. Fetal catecholamines also increase lipolysis and gluconeogenesis, exacerbating the effects of hyperglycemia. Thus fetal hyperglycemia is especially dangerous if placental exchange is already compromised and fetal catecholamines are elevated.[11]

Neonatal Metabolism

The neonate's ability to maintain a normal blood glucose level depends upon the antepartum environment before the loss of maternally supplied glucose at birth. For example, when the rate of fetal anaerobic glycolysis exceeds glucose supply (as with hypoxia), clinical hypoglycemia is apparent at birth. On the other hand, increased fetal catecholamines activate fetal gluconeogenesis before birth, and thereby can deter the development of neonatal hypoglycemia. Conversely, fetal hyperglycemia (from maternal diabetes mellitus or iatrogenic origins) induces insulin release, increases glucose utilization, and secondarily depletes gluconeogenic enzymes. Thus fetal hyperglycemia provokes neonatal hypoglycemia by antenatally decreasing glucose forming capacity while accelerating its consumption.[12]

Passive fetal hypoglycemia (secondary to maternal fasting) might encourage neonatal hypoglycemia, but this appears not to be the situation. Maternal serum glucose concentration during labor does not correlate with neonatal glucose concentration or duration of maternal fasting.[13] Since maternal glucose concentration and utilization do correlate with that of the fetus, a lower maternal blood sugar decreases fetal glucose consumption, thereby deterring development of hypoglycemia in the neonate. It is also possible that maternal fasting induces fetal gluconeogenesis before birth.

Infusion of Dextrose Solutions

Maternal dextrose infusion previously was thought to improve the condition of the stressed fetus. Currently the evidence is overwhelming that dextrose infusion further compromises the fetus with impaired uteroplacental perfusion.[14,15] A number of studies have demonstrated undesirable metabolic changes in the normal fetus with excessive maternal dextrose administration. A significant rise in maternal lactate results from 10% dextrose infusion during labor.[16-18] Hydration before cesarean section with 1000 ml of 5% dextrose led to fetal hyperinsulinemia, acidosis, and raised serum lactate levels, as well as neonatal hypoglycemia and jaundice.[19-22]

On the other hand, very low maternal glucose concentrations have been observed after overnight fasts and in conjunction with crystalloid infusions during labor.[23,24] The amount of dextrose necessary to decrease protein catabolism and to increase insulin production in surgical patients has been established. In nonpregnant individuals, as little as 80 to 100 ml/hr (57 to 71 $mg \cdot kg^{-1} \cdot hr^{-1}$) of 5% dextrose halves urinary nitrogen excretion, and 120 ml/hr (85 $mg \cdot kg^{-1} \cdot hr^{-1}$) increases insulin production (indicating increased glucose use). It is likely that in resting parturients increased glucose consumption will occur with dextrose infusions of similar magnitude. Additional dextrose might increase fetal glucose utilization without providing further maternal protection.[19] Dextrose infusions of 400 ml/hr are associated with a significant increase in the incidence of neonatal hypoglycemia.[12] More than 200 ml/hr of 5% dextrose significantly increases fetal insulin concentrations.[10]

Infusion of Crystalloid Solutions

Crystalloid solutions containing sodium chloride, lactate, acetate, or gluconate also effect maternal and fetal well-being. The excessive chloride in normal saline is balanced in vivo by converting bicarbonate to lactic acid, thereby depleting the buffer base. Studies have reported decreases in maternal pH of up to 0.04 units with infusions of 1000 to 1200 ml of normal saline solution.[16,19,22] In the first of these studies, lactate and carbon dioxide concentrations were unchanged; in the last, lactate concentration increased.

Use of lactated Ringer's solution instead of sodium chloride eliminates bicarbonate depletion and increases maternal serum lactate concentration without raising serum pyruvate.[22] Increases in maternal and fetal serum lactate concentrations associated with sodium chloride and lactated Ringer's solutions do not reflect increases in anaerobic metabolism. Also, these crystalloids do not increase maternal pyruvate levels.

Infusion of gluconate solutions mirrors dextrose administration since in vivo conversion of gluconate to glucose increases serum glucose concentration. Acetate also is a metabolic substrate, and administering an acetate solution induces inhibition of glycolysis. Acetate administration also increases intracellular pyruvate, which in turn increases lactate concentration. Acetate and gluconate directly increase aerobic metabolism, which may be detrimental when fetal oxygenation is impaired. Acetate and gluconate, as substrates and intermediary products of carbohydrate metabolism, also have the potential to upset the fine tuning of fetal carbohydrate metabolism immediately before the baby's delivery, thereby disrupting neonatal metabolism.

Infusion of Free Water

Sodium-free solutions equilibrate rapidly within the entire body water space. They are ineffective in expanding maternal intravascular volume since only 15% of the volume infused remains in the intravascular compartment. Also, symptomatic dilutional hyponatremia occurs with concurrent Pitocin administration. Numerous studies relate significant decreases in fetal sodium to maternal infusions of more than 500 ml of dextrose in water during labor.[25-27] Neonatal hyponatremia, which may cause tachypnea,[28] occurs in 50% of neonates of mothers given 1000 ml of 5% dextrose in water before cesarean section.[29]

Infusion of Colloid Solutions

Hydroxyethyl starch, 5% albumin, and dextran all have been administered as alternatives to crystalloid infusion. Dextran 70, 7.5 ml/kg with 17.5 mg ephedrine, is superior to 15 mg/kg of dextran 70 in preventing maternal hypotension.[30] Unfortunately, dextran 40 has been associated with 32 cases of maternal anaphylaxis with associated fetal compromise.[31] Hydroxyethyl starch, 1000 ml, is not significantly different than 2000 ml of crystalloid solution.[32] Five percent albumin, 200 ml or 500 ml, with Ringer's lactate to total 1200 ml is similar in outcome to 1200 ml of Ringer's lactate. However, albumin concentrations and plasma oncotic pressure are better maintained with albumin solution.[33] When volumes of infusate are minimal, albumin is superior to Ringer's lactate in maintaining maternal blood pressure. Albumin is recommended for patients undergoing ritodrine or terbutaline treatment and for patients with severe preeclampsia or cardiac disease, in whom volume expansion is hazardous.[34] Otherwise, the additional expense of colloid solutions—and their lack of unequivocal superiority in preventing hypotension—does not justify their routine use.

Volume of Intravenous Fluid for Preload

Is it safe to rapidly administer intravenously as much as 30 ml/kg of crystalloid to parturients? Intravenous infusion of 500 to 2000 ml before administration of the spinal anesthetic has been recommended to prevent hypotension. Is this procedure effective? In a study of a preeclamptic parturient, 1500 ml of lactated Ringer's solution was administered, the endpoint being determined by a 30% increase in noninvasive Doppler cardiac output measurements. Hypotension during subsequent epidural anesthesia for cesarean section was avoided.[35] Other studies have demonstrated dubious effectiveness of prehydration in eliminating hypotension, especially with spinal anesthesia. Administration of 1000 ml Ringer's lactate increased cardiac output and prevented changes with epidural anesthesia. But with spinal anesthesia, the cardiac output decreased despite an initial elevation with volume expansion.[36] Increasing prehydration to 2000 ml of fluid before epidural anesthesia raised central venous pressure (CVP) but not dangerously, yet still permitted hypotension in 6.7% of patients.[37]

Increasing the rate of the infusion does not eliminate hypotension. Infusion of 20 ml/kg over 10 minutes increased CVP to 11.9 cm H_2O, but was no more effective than the same amount of fluid infused over 20 minutes in decreasing hypotension. More than 50% of patients receiving spinal anesthesia under these circumstances became hypotensive.[38]

Prehydration's contribution to preventing hypotension is relatively small. Hypotension develops in 82% to 92% of patients receiving spinal anesthesia for cesarean section without acute hydration or left uterine displacement.[39] With left uterine displacement, it occurs in 70% of patients receiving spinal anesthesia without a preload, and in 55% of those with a 20 ml/kg preload.[40] Thus prehydration with intravenous crystalloid appears to decrease the incidence of hypotension after administration of a spinal anesthetic by 15% to 20%.

Anesthetic Course

Recommendations for Dextrose Administration

Routine dextrose infusion before delivery is not recommended. Patients with prolonged fasting, malnutrition, or other reason for hypoglycemia need a blood sugar measurement. If the serum glucose is low, the patient should receive enough dextrose to prevent any further decrease before delivery. This can be accomplished by establishing a piggyback infusion of 5% dextrose at 50 to 85 $mg \cdot kg^{-1} \cdot hr^{-1}$ (80 to 120 ml/hr).

Recommendations for Acute Hydration

Routine prehydration is recommended for healthy parturients undergoing spinal anesthesia. Fluid volumes of up to 2000 ml or 20 ml/kg can be safely administered to healthy parturients before spinal anesthesia.[36,37] Prehydration with 30 ml/kg is too much volume for routine situations. An urgent procedure cannot be delayed for prehydration. Instead, the intravenous infusion is opened wide and other measures to prevent hypotension are instituted, such as intravenous infusion of ephedrine. In a group undergoing postpartum tubal ligations under spinal anesthesia, ephedrine infusion was superior to a crystalloid preload of 15 ml/kg in preventing hypotension.[41] Thus, use of prophylactic ephedrine infusion appears as effective in preventing hypotension as prehydration and is a reasonable alternative.

Rapidly administered fluids are warmed to reduce the incidence of shivering.[42] The first liter of fluid for acute hydration should be normal saline, since it primarily affects only pH. Subsequently Ringer's lactate is the fluid of choice. If the patient's condition warrants volume restriction, epidural anesthesia is a better choice. Prehydration is accomplished with hydroxyethyl starch or 5% albumin, with CVP monitoring as indicated.

Preventing Hypotension after Spinal Administration

After hydration, spinal anesthesia is induced using techniques and precautions appropriate for a cesarean section at term. The intravenous fluid should be running wide open immediately after the spinal anesthetic is administered. Hypotension is still expected in about 50% of parturients. Administration of prophylactic intravenous ephedrine has been repeatedly demonstrated to prevent hypotension under these circumstances, especially when the preload is reduced.[30,41] Laboring parturients undergoing cesarean section are less likely to experience hypotension, probably because uterine contractions provide an autotransfusion[39]; it might also be related to increased baseline catecholamine concentrations.

Additional measures to reduce the effect of the sympathetic blockade such as graduated compression stockings do not reduce the incidence of hypotension.[43] But providing an autotransfusion by elevating and wrapping the legs with an elastic bandage immediately after administering the spinal anesthesia does prevent hypotension.[44] This technique is cumbersome and requires extra personnel to accomplish, but it is a noninvasive, reversible means of rapidly increasing venous return after the sudden onset of sympathetic blockade.

Intravenous Fluid after Delivery

After delivery, the absence of the fetus permits less rigid control of intravenous dextrose and crystalloid administration. Intravenous therapy is determined by ongoing intraoperative maintenance and replacement fluid requirements, as in any other surgical procedure. In the event of significant hemorrhage, replacement of third-space and blood loss by conventional protocols for massive blood loss is required.[45] Blood loss estimates, adequacy of hemostasis, and hemoglobin concentration determine the need for red cell administration. Transfusion in conjunction with cesarean section has steadily decreased in recent years; in healthy parturients a hemoglobin less than 8 mg/dl usually prompts red cell therapy.[4,6,46]

Intravenous Fluids for Labor

Due to the reduced maternal morbidity from acid aspiration pneumonitis, permitting oral fluids during labor is a controversial issue.[47,48] Certainly patients receiving major conduction blocks cannot eat. If their labor is brief and without anesthetic intervention, intravenous fluids may be superfluous. Patients designated as *high risk* or who face a prolonged fast should receive intravenous dextrose and fluid supplementation to prevent dehydration and minimize ketone production.

Maternal Metabolism

Maternal glucose utilization during labor is determined by serum glucose concentration, catecholamine output, and the amount of muscular activity. Energy requirements may be increased in labor, but since muscle preferentially oxidizes ketones and free fatty acids, glucose requirements may be no greater than before labor unless muscular activity is excessive. Anaerobic glycolysis, occurring when muscle activity exceeds aerobic capacity, increases glucose utilization because glucose is the only source of pyruvate in the muscle. Vigorous muscle activity also produces heat that is dissipated as sweat. Thus strenuous labor may accelerate dehydration and produce a precipitous drop in the levels of maternal (and fetal) glucose.

Maternal Dextrose Requirements

How much glucose do laboring parturients need? Recently 5 g/hr has been recommended.[49] In fasting laboring parturients, maternal serum glucose concentration and the incidence of neonatal hypoglycemia are unrelated to the duration of fasting.[13] Maternal ketone concentrations during fasting labor increase minimally over a 2-hour period. A fivefold increase in umbilical cord insulin concentration occurs with infusion rates greater than 140 mg $\cdot$ kg^{-1} $\cdot$ hr^{-1} (200 ml/hr or 10 g/hr).[10] Thus an infusion of 5% dextrose at 200 ml/hr is excessive.

Decreases in maternal ketone concentrations during labor, indicating less dependence on gluconeogenesis for metabolic substrate, are more frequent with 5% dextrose infusions of 100 mg $\cdot$ kg^{-1} $\cdot$ hr^{-1} (140 ml/hr) than with infusions of 50 mg $\cdot$ kg^{-1} $\cdot$ hr^{-1}.[13] An infusion of 5% dextrose at 75 mg $\cdot$ kg^{-1} $\cdot$ hr^{-1} (about 80 to 100 ml/hr) limits maternal accumulation of ketones without increasing the likelihood of neonatal hypoglycemia.

Hydration during Labor

Maintenance and replacement fluid volumes for patients in labor should be calculated in the same manner as for those undergoing cesarean section. Maintenance fluid should be isotonic or 0.45% normal saline to prevent dilutional hyponatremia. Maintenance fluids can contain 5% dextrose since the infusion rate will fall within the guidelines for dextrose administration.

Replacement fluid, especially any infused before initiation of epidural analgesia, is administered as dextrose-free crystalloid solution, or if indicated, 5% albumin. Lactated Ringer's solution is preferable since the slow infusion rate for replacement fluids prevents significant increases in maternal serum lactate concentrations. A simple way of managing fluids is to use the crystalloid as the primary intravenous line, and piggyback 5% dextrose with an infusion pump. The combination of the two solutions approximates the infusion of 2.5% dextrose in a half-normal saline solution.

Hydration during Epidural Analgesia

Intravenous fluids should be prescribed for good reasons.[50] One should be aware of overhydrating by administering a bolus of fluid each time a local anesthetic is injected into the epidural catheter. Hypotension during the gradual onset of an epidural block from a small volume of dilute local anesthetic can be managed with the use of 500 ml to 1000 ml of intravenous fluid for prehydration. If the patient is redosed every 2 hours, the intravenous infusion should not be left wide open for 20 minutes while the block develops. A continuous epidural infusion avoids this problem. Fluid administration during prolonged labors can be adjusted with timely evaluation of intake and output, serum glucose and electrolytes, and urine ketones. One should limit dextrose to what is needed to prevent maternal accumulation of ketones. Volume should be replaced to maintain intravascular volume and urine output.

Summary

1. Hemorrhage from abnormal placentation or uterine injury is more common in breech than cephalic presentations.
2. Hypotension severe enough to compromise fetal well-being will occur with spinal anesthesia unless aggressive preventive measures are undertaken.
3. Autologous blood donation is not recommended. Typed and cross matched blood is necessary only for placenta previa, abruption, and RBC antibodies.
4. Fetal hyperglycemia increases fetal glucose use and causes hypoxia, hypercarbia, and acidosis.
5. Neonatal hypoglycemia is caused by maternal hyperglycemia, not by maternal fasting.
6. Parturients must receive less than 200 ml/hr of 5% dextrose intravenously. Free water, acetate and gluconate solutions, and dextran solutions are avoided.
7. Intravenous hydration before cesarean section with 20 ml/kg of normal saline or Ringer's lactate solution is safe; however, unless they are in labor, 50% of patients with spinal anesthesia will become hypotensive in spite of prehydration. Use of prophylactic ephedrine infusion will reduce the incidences of hypotension.

8. During labor use a combination of 5% dextrose at 80 to 100 ml/hr and lactated Ringer's solution limited to the volume necessary to maintain urine output and intravascular volume.

References

1. Dickason LA, Dinsmoor MJ: Red blood cell transfusion and cesarean section, *Am J Obstet Gynecol* 1992; 167:327.
2. Sherman SJ, Greenspoon JS, Nelson JM, et al: Identifying the obstetric patient at high risk of multiple-unit blood transfusions, *J Reprod Med* 1992; 37:649.
3. Droste S, Sorensen T, Price T, et al: Maternal and fetal hemodynamic effects of autologous blood donation during pregnancy, *Am J Obstet Gynecol* 1992; 167:89.
4. McVay PA, Hoag RW, Hoag MS, et al: Safety and use of autologous blood donation during the third trimester of pregnancy, *Am J Obstet Gynecol* 1989; 160:1479.
5. Andres RL, Piacquadio KM, Resnik R: A reappraisal of the need for autologous blood donation in the obstetric patient, *Am J Obstet Gynecol* 1990; 163:1551.
6. Combs CA, Murphy EL, Laros RK Jr: Cost-benefit analysis of autologous blood donation in obstetrics, *Obstet Gynecol* 1992; 80:621.
7. Wollman SB, Marx GF: Acute hydration for prevention of hypotension of spinal anesthesia in parturients, *Anesthesiology* 1968; 29:374.
8. Marx GF, Domurat MF, Costin M: Potential hazards of hypoglycaemia in the parturient, *Can J Anaesth* 1987; 34:400.
9. Patterson P, Philips L, Wood C: Relationship between maternal and fetal blood glucose during labor, *Am J Obstet Gynecol* 1967; 107:610.
10. Lucas A, Adrian TE, Aynsley-Greene A, et al: Iatrogenic hyperinsulinism at birth, *Lancet* 1980; 1:144.
11. Robillard JE, Sessions C, Kennedy RL, et al: Metabolic effects of constant hypertonic glucose infusion in well-oxygenated fetuses, *Am J Obstet Gynecol* 1978; 130:199.
12. Mendiola J, Grylack LJ, Scanlon JW: Effects of intrapartum glucose infusion on the normal fetus and newborn, *Anesth Analg* 1984; 61:32.
13. Kenepp NB, Cheek TC, Gabbe SG, et al: Intrapartum maternal intravenous dextrose administration, *Anesthesiology* 1985; 63:A436.
14. Mann LI, Pritchard JW, Symmes D: The effect of glucose loading on fetal response to hypoxia, *Am J Obstet Gynecol* 1970; 107:610.
15. Anderson GG, Codero L, Hon EH: Hypertonic glucose infusion during labor: effect on acid-base status, fetal heart rate and uterine contractions, *Obstet Gynecol* 1970; 36:405.
16. Lawrence GF, Brown VA, Parsons RJ: Feto-maternal consequences of high dose glucose infusion during labour, *Br J Obstet Gynecol* 1982; 89:27.
17. Morton KE, Jackson MC, Gilmar MDG: A comparison of the effects of four intravenous solutions for the treatment of ketonuria during labour, *Br J Obstet Gynecol* 1982; 89:27.
18. Evans SE, Crawford JS, Stevens ID, et al: Fluid therapy for induced labour under epidural analgesia: biochemical consequences for mother and infant, *Br J Obstet Gynaecol* 1986; 93:329.
19. Kenepp NB, Kumar S, Shelley WC, et al: Fetal and neonatal hazards of maternal hydration with 5% dextrose solutions prior to cesarean section, *Lancet* 1982; i:1150.
20. Datta S, Brown WU Jr: Acid-base status in diabetic mothers and their infants following general or spinal anesthesia for cesarean section, *Anesthesiology* 1977; 47:272.
21. Philipson EH, Kalhan SC, Riha MM, et al: Effects of maternal glucose infusion on fetal acid-base status in human pregnancy, *Am J Obstet Gynecol* 1987; 157:866.
22. Ramanathan S, Masih AK, Ashok U, et al: Concentrations of lactate and pyruvate in maternal and neonatal blood with different intravenous fluids used for prehydration before epidural anesthesia, *Anesth Analg* 1984; 63:69.
23. Jawalekar S, Marx GF: Effect of I.V. fluids on maternal and fetal blood glucose, *Anesthesiology* 1980; 53:A311.
24. Loong EP, Lao TT, Chin RK: Effects of intrapartum intravenous infusion of 5% dextrose or Hartmann's solution on maternal and cord blood glucose, *Acta Obstet Gynecol Scand* 1987; 66:211.
25. Tarno-Mordi WO, Shaw JCL, Liu D, et al: Iatrogenic hyponatremia of the newborn due to maternal fluid overload: a prospective study, *Br Med J* 1981; 283:639.
26. Dahlenburg GW, Burnell RH, Braybrook R: The relationship between cord serum sodium levels in newborn infants and maternal intravenous therapy during labour, *Br J Obstet Gynaecol* 1980; 87:519.
27. Morgan DB, Kirwan NA, Hancock KW, et al: Water intoxication and oxytocin infusion, *Br J Obstet Gynaecol* 1977; 84:6.

28. Singhi S, Chookang E, Hall J, et al: Iatrogenic neonatal and maternal hyponatremia following oxytocin and aqueous glucose infusion during labour, *Br J Obstet Gynaecol* 1982; 92:356.
29. Grylack LJ, Chu SS, Scanlon JW: Use of intravenous fluids before cesarean section: effects on perinatal glucose, insulin and sodium homeostasis, *Obstet Gynecol* 1984; 63:654.
30. Wennberg E, Frid I, Haljamae H, et al: Colloid (3% dextran 70) with or without ephedrine infusion for cardiovascular stability during extradural caesarean section, *Br J Anaesth* 1992; 69:13.
31. Barbier P, Jonville AP, Autret E, et al: Fetal risks with dextrans during delivery, *Drug Saf* 1992; 7:71.
32. Murray AM, Morgan M, Whitwam JG: Crystalloid versus colloid for circulatory preload for epidural caesarean section, *Anaesthesia* 1989; 44:463.
33. Ramanathan S, Masih A, Rock I, et al: Maternal and fetal effects of prophylactic hydration with crystalloids or colloids before epidural anesthesia, *Anesth Analg* 1983; 62:673.
34. Mathru M, Rao TL, Kartha RK, et al: Intravenous albumin administration for prevention of spinal hypotension during cesarean section, *Anesth Analg* 1980; 59:655.
35. Rozen EK, Preminger MK, Marx GF: Cardiac output measurements for guidance of perioperative intravenous hydration in an obstetric patient, *Int J Obstet Anesth* 1992; 1:114.
36. Robson SC, Boys RJ, Rodeck C, et al: Maternal and fetal haemodynamic effects of spinal and extradural anaesthesia for elective caesarean section, *Br J Anaesth* 1992; 68:54.
37. Lewis M, Thomas P, Wilkes RG: Hypotension during epidural analgesia for caesarean section: arterial and central venous pressure changes after acute intravenous loading with two litres of Hartmann's solution, *Anaesthesia* 1983; 38:250.
38. Rout CC, Akoojee SS, Rocke DA, et al: Rapid administration of crystalloid preload does not decrease the incidence of hypotension after spinal anaesthesia for elective caesarean section, *Br J Anaesth* 1992; 68:394.
39. Clark RB, Thompson DS, Thompson CH: Prevention of spinal hypotension associated with Cesarean section, *Anesthesiology* 1976; 45:670.
40. Rout CC, Rocke DA, Levin J, et al: A reevaluation of the role of crystalloid preload in the prevention of hypotension associated with spinal anesthesia for elective cesarean section, *Anesthesiology* 1993; 79:262.
41. Gajraj NM, Victory RA, Pace NA, et al: Comparison of an ephedrine infusion with crystalloid administration for prevention of hypotension during spinal anesthesia, *Anesth Analg* 1993; 76:1023.
42. Workhoven MN: Intravenous fluid temperature, shivering, and the parturient, *Anesth Analg* 1986; 65:496.
43. Lee A, McKeown D, Wilson J: Evaluation of the efficacy of elastic compression stockings in prevention of hypotension during epidural anaesthesia for elective caesarean section, *Acta Anaesthesiol Scand* 1987; 31:193.
44. Rout CC, Rocke DA, Gouws E: Leg elevation and wrapping in the prevention of hypotension following spinal anaesthesia for elective caesarean section, *Anaesthesia* 1993; 48:304.
45. Donaldson MDJ, Seaman MJ, Park GR: Massive blood transfusion, *Br J Anaesth* 1992; 69:621.
46. Camann WR, Datta S: Red cell use during cesarean delivery, *Transfusion* 1991; 31:12.
47. Elkington KW: At the water's edge: where obstetrics and anesthesia meet, *Obstet Gynecol* 1991; 77:304.
48. Abouleish E, Merriman T: In obstetrics: keep the water colorless and clear, *Anesth Analg* 1991; 73:674.
49. Benhamon D, Auroy Y: Fluid balance during labor: a French view, *Int J Obstet Anesth* 1993; 2:143.
50. Morton KE: Fluid management during labour: a British view, *Int J Obstet Anesth* 1993; 2:147.

6

Uteroplacental Circulation

A 23-year-old primigravida at term is admitted to the hospital in active labor. The fetal heart rate pattern is normal, and a uterine contraction occurs every 3 to 5 minutes with moderate intensity. One hour after her admission, the patient suddenly develops severe abdominal pain. The fetal heart rate is less than 100 beats per minute. After an appropriate examination, the obstetrician decides that the pain was due to a tetanic uterine contraction and the fetal bradycardia is the result of reduced uteroplacental perfusion. Explain the factors that affect uteroplacental blood flow. What therapeutic interventions can be used in such a situation?

Recommendations by Francis A. Rosinia, M.D.

A functional understanding of uteroplacental perfusion is essential for the safe practice of obstetric anesthesia. Uterine blood flow may be adversely affected by agents used to augment uterine activity and techniques used to relieve painful labor. Clinical appreciation of these factors is necessary because fetal hypoxia and acidosis result from impaired intervillous perfusion.

Uteroplacental Anatomy

The uterus benefits from the dual blood supply of the ovarian and uterine arteries. The ovarian artery, a long branch stemming directly from the aorta, enters the superior lateral aspect of the uterus through the broad ligament, where it forms an anastomosis with branches of the uterine artery. The ovarian artery's small contribution to uterine blood flow is in the upper one third of the uterus.[1] The uterine artery, a main branch of the internal iliac (hypogastric) artery, enters the lateral base of the uterus. The uterine arteries supply over 80% of the blood flow to the uterus. Uterine artery blood flow, in the myometrium, continues through the arcuate, radial, and spiral arteries to feed the intervillous space. Nutrient exchange in the intervillous space occurs across the semipermeable membrane of the fetal villi. This membrane consists of an outer layer of trophoblastic cells, a middle layer of connective tissue, and a fetal capillary wall. The thickness of this villous membrane separating fetal from maternal blood is about 2 to 3.5 μm. This is almost 10 times the length across which the pulmonary alveolar membranes exchange. Decidual veins drain the intervillous space into the uterine and ovarian veins to the central venous circulation.

Physiologic adaptation to pregnancy results in a dramatic increase in uterine blood flow. At term 10% of the maternal cardiac output is devoted to uterine perfusion, 80% to 90% of which feeds the placental intervillous space.[2] Greiss[3] investigated the pressure-flow relationship in the uterine vascular bed of the pregnant ewe. Regression analysis of uterine blood flow versus uterine blood pressure after complete aortic occlusion demonstrated a linear relationship ($r = .992$). This indicates that the uterine vascular bed during pregnancy operates at maximum hemodynamic efficiency, widely dilated, and without autoregulation.

Redistribution of pelvic blood flow in pregnancy has been documented by both angiographic and Doppler study of pregnant patients. Bieniarz and coworkers[4] performed pelvic arteriographs in nonpregnant and third-trimester pregnant women. Results showed dye flow in the internal iliac and dilated uterine artery system twice that in the external iliac arterial pathway. The exact opposite flow pattern was found in the nonpregnant women studied. The study also revealed an overgrowth of the uterine arcuate and spiral arteries that supplied the placenta. This did not occur in extraplacental uterine vessels. A recent Doppler flow study[5] of pregnant and nonpregnant women confirmed this redistribution of pelvic blood flow. In the nonpregnant versus the pregnant patients at 36 weeks of gestation, uterine blood flow increased from 9 to 353 milliliters per minute and uterine artery diameter increased from 1.4 to 3.4 mm.

These results show pregnancy causes a redistribution of the increased maternal cardiac output to a dilated, nonautoregulated uterine vascular bed for preferential placental perfusion.

Measurement of Uteroplacental Blood Flow

Direct measurement of uterine blood flow requires surgical placement of an electromagnetic flow probe on the uterine artery. Ethical considerations prohibit this invasive technique in pregnant women. Indirect measurement of uterine, intervillous, umbilical, and fetal blood flow can be studied in human subjects. An intravenous bolus injection of ^{133}Xe in saline distributes in the systemic circulation. The clearance of gamma radiation from the ^{133}Xe is measured for 10 to 15 minutes by scintillation detectors over the placenta and the uterine wall distant from the placenta. Intervillous and uterine myometrial blood flow then is estimated with a biexponential curve.[2] The ^{133}Xe method of blood flow measurement in pregnant women has been replaced by Doppler ultrasound assessment of blood flow. The Doppler effect occurs when an ultrasound wave is reflected from a target that is moving relative to the source of the ultrasound wave. The reflected wave undergoes a change in frequency relative to the transmitted wave. A moving column of blood cells will produce a change in frequency from the transmitted ultrasound wave. The difference in frequency is called the Doppler frequency shift. The velocity of moving blood cells is calculated from the Doppler frequency shift. Doppler ultrasound is used to measure blood flow in the uterine, umbilical, and fetal arteries. The pulsatility index (PI: peak systolic minus end-diastolic velocity divided by the mean flow velocity) and the systolic-diastolic (S/D) flow ratio are used as indices of downstream vascular resistance. Increased PI or

S/D ratio represents increased vascular resistance and decreased uteroplacental flow.[6]

Determinants of Uteroplacental Circulation

Uteroplacental circulation is determined by uterine blood flow (UBF). The following formula defines blood flow to the muscular uterus:

$$\text{UBF} = \frac{\text{uterine arterial pressure} - \text{uterine venous pressure}}{\text{uterine vascular resistance}}$$

Uterine arterial pressure is dependent on maternal arterial pressure and aortocaval compression. Uterine venous pressure varies only within a narrow range. Uterine artery vasodilatation is fixed, and unaffected by local factors. However, uterine artery vasoconstriction occurs with adrenergic stimulation, secretion of norepinephrine and epinephrine, local anesthetics, and vasopressors.[7] Uterine vascular resistance is determined by intrinsic vascular resistance and extrinsic pressure from uterine contractions. Management to optimize uteroplacental blood flow should be focused on maternal blood pressure and position, prevention of uterine artery vasoconstriction, and uterine muscular tone.

Uterine contractions result in a decrease of uterine blood flow through two mechanisms: (1) extrinsic compression of the distal aorta and iliac arteries and (2) compression of intramyometrial vessels. Uterine muscular contractions produce a firm uterus that assumes a larger anteroposterior diameter. A contracted uterus is more effective in compressing the aorta and inferior vena cava. This is strictly a local effect because brachial artery pressure may not show any change, but femoral artery pressure is diminished. Decreased uterine artery blood flow by extrinsic uterine compression is avoided by lateral uterine displacement.[8]

Fig. 6-1 illustrates a relaxed uterus with unimpaired intervillous perfusion. In this condition uterine perfusion pressure (mean arterial pressure minus venous pressure) normally is 70 to 80 mm Hg. Intramyometrial and amniotic fluid pressures, representing resistance to flow, are about 10 mm Hg. When the uterus contracts (Fig. 6-2) uterine vascular resistance increases. Increased uterine wall pressure first occludes venous drainage of the intervillous space by compression of uterine veins. Uterine venous pressure is increased, resulting in accumulation of blood in the intervillous space as diminished arterial perfusion continues. When uterine wall pressure exceeds mean arterial pressure, as illustrated in Fig. 6-2, blood flow through the intervillous space ceases. Fetal catabolites accumulate in the intervillous space without the normal replenishment that maternal blood provides. Hypox-

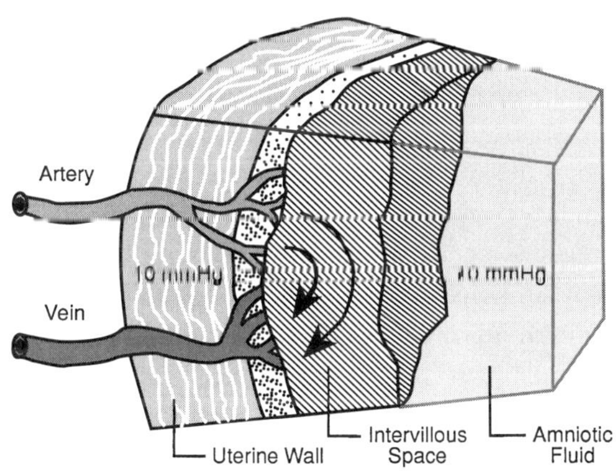

Fig. 6-1.
A relaxed uterine wall allows unimpeded intervillous space perfusion. *(From Poseiro JJ, Mendez-Bauer C, Pose SV, et al: Effect of uterine contractions on maternal blood flow through the placenta. In* Perinatal Factors Affecting Human Development, *Washington, D.C., 1969, Pan American Health Organization, Scientific Publication no 185.)*

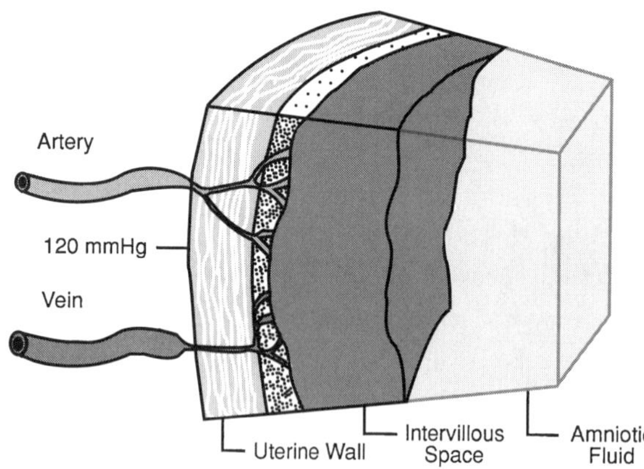

Fig. 6-2.
The contracted uterine wall interrupts arterial and venous blood flow. Intervillous space stasis results in hypoxia, hypercarbia, and acidosis. *(From Poseiro JJ, Mendez-Bauer C, Pose SV, et al: Effect of uterine contractions on maternal blood flow through the placenta. In* Perinatal Factors Affecting Human Development. *Washington, D.C., 1969, Pan American Health Organization, Scientific Publication no 185.)*

emia, hypercapnia, and acidosis may result in the intervillous space and the fetus.[8] Prolonged fetal decelerations are the clinical result.

Uterine contractions during labor should result in cervical dilatation, effacement, and fetal descent while allowing intervillous and fetal replenishment between contractions. Contractions during labor typically occur every 2 to 3 minutes, with a duration of 1 minute, an amplitude of 50 to 80 mm Hg, and adequate uterine relaxation between contractions. Increased frequency of contractions (tachysystole), increased uterine tone (uterine hypertonia) between contractions, or a tetanic uterine contraction may exceed uteroplacental reserve, resulting in fetal hypoxia and acidosis. Fetal bradycardia caused by increased uterine activity may be spontaneous or oxytocin-induced, or may result from breast hyperstimulation. Abruptio placentae will impair uteroplacental perfusion by two mechanisms: (1) uterine hypertonia and tetany and (2) separation of the placenta from the maternal blood supply. Cocaine use during pregnancy has been associated with an increased incidence of abruptio placentae.[9] Acute cocaine exposure to pregnant human myometrium results in an immediate increase in contractile activity.[10] Orgasmic coitus may also result in increased uterine activity and fetal bradycardia.[11]

Aortocaval compression will decrease uterine blood flow by decreasing uterine blood flow and increasing uterine venous pressure. Complete mechanical obstruction of the inferior vena cava by the gravid uterus at term with the patient in the supine position occurs uniformly.[12] However, Howard[13] found that only 11% of women at term had *supine hypotensive syndrome* when asked to lie on their backs. Variable routes of collateral pelvic venous return[4,12] account for the low incidence of postural hypotension in the term parturient. However, the supine position in the parturient at term will decrease intervillous blood flow[14,15] independent of maternal blood pressure and heart rate changes. Compression of the aorta and iliac arteries by the gravid uterus at term occurs with the patient in the supine position. This will reduce uterine arterial pressure without a change in brachial artery pressure. Lateral displacement of the uterus should be practiced with all parturients to maintain uterine blood flow.

Vasopressors used to increase maternal blood pressure may impair uterine blood flow by increasing uterine vascular resistance. Ephedrine is an indirect-acting vasopressor that stimulates both alpha and beta receptors. Ephedrine is the vasopressor of choice in the parturient because it will not diminish uterine blood flow when maternal hypotension is corrected. Methoxamine, metaraminol, and mephentermine will significantly reduce uterine blood flow, because of their predominantly alpha-mimetic effect.[16] Phenylephrine in small bolus doses when used to treat hypotension in healthy, pregnant patients at term having cesarean section under epidural[17] and spinal[18] anesthesia resulted in no significant difference in neonatal Apgar scores or acid-base values when compared with ephedrine. Doppler flow measurement of the maternal uterine artery; the placental arcuate artery; and the fetal umbilical, middle cerebral, and renal arteries was performed on healthy pregnant patients at term having cesarean section under spinal anesthesia.[19] Results showed a significant transient increase in maternal uterine and placental arcuate vascular resistance relative to baseline values in the group treated with phenylephrine prophylactic infusions and 100-μg boluses for hypotension. No significant differences occurred relative to baseline Doppler values in the ephedrine-treated group. Fetal Doppler results showed no increase in umbilical, middle cerebral, or renal artery vascular resistance relative to baseline in either group. Neonatal Apgar and acid-base values were within the normal range in both groups. Phenylephrine is a useful vasopressor in healthy pregnant women.

Local anesthetics when injected intravascularly will decrease uterine blood flow by an increase in uterine vascular resistance. This occurs as a result of uterine artery vasoconstriction and an increase in uterine muscular activity in pregnant patients. The vasoconstriction produced by local anesthetics appears to be through a direct mechanism, independent of alpha-adrenergic blockade.[20] This effect by local anesthetics becomes clinically significant during accidental intravascular injection with epidural anesthesia and after paracervical block.[21]

Epidural Anesthesia for Labor and Delivery and Uteroplacental Circulation

Epidural anesthesia complicated by hypotension will result in a reduction in uterine blood flow proportional to the decrease in maternal mean arterial pressure. Rapid crystalloid infusion is used before the initiation of epidural anesthesia to reduce the incidence and degree of hypotension from sympathetic blockade. A microsphere technique in pregnant ewes demonstrated a significant increase in maternal mean arterial pressure and uteroplacental blood flow after rapid crystalloid infusion.[22] The ewes that demonstrated postinfusion hemodilution (16.8% average decrease in hemoglobin concentration) showed a statistically significant increase "in both placental implantation-site blood flow and placental implantation-site oxygen delivery."[22]

The effect of epidural local anesthetic injection on uteroplacental blood flow has been measured in humans. Healthy pregnant women at term who were given intravenous bolus injection of ^{133}Xe before and after epidural blockade demonstrated a statistically significant increase in intervillous blood flow compared with the nonepidural group.[23] The increase in placental blood flow with epidural anesthesia for labor probably is due to reduced maternal circulating catecholamine levels.[24] The addition of epinephrine (5 μm/ml) to epidural local anesthetics for labor does not result in a decrease in intervillous blood flow.[25] Epidural anesthesia for labor conducted without significant maternal hypotension will not decrease uteroplacental blood flow.

Prolonged Fetal Heart Rate Deceleration

The normal range for fetal heart rate at term is 120 to 160 beats/min. Fetal bradycardia is defined as a baseline heart rate less than 120 beats/min. A baseline fetal heart rate is established after 15 minutes at that heart rate. A *prolonged deceleration* in fetal heart rate is defined as a deceleration of more than 30 beats/min that persists for more than 1 to 2 minutes.[26] This fetal heart rate pattern will occur as a result of fetal hypoxia or a fetal reflex. Decreased uterine blood flow, for any reason, leading to fetal hypoxia must be corrected for the fetus to recover. Reflex fetal heart rate decelerations can be associated with a vaginal examination, rapid descent of the fetus through the birth canal, and maternal voiding. The placenta, through intrauterine resuscitation, usually is the most effective therapy for fetal recovery when operative intervention is being considered.

Interventional Tocolysis for Fetal Distress

Interventional tocolysis is defined as maternal administration of a pharmacologic agent to decrease uterine muscular activity, allowing increased intervillous blood flow. Interventional tocolysis is a part of the management directed toward intrauterine resuscitation. The goal of intrauterine resuscitation is to increase uterine blood flow by optimization of maternal factors. These steps usually include discontinuation of oxytocin in augmented labor, correction of maternal hypotension by position change, rapid intravenous crystalloid infusion and ephedrine administration, and supplemental maternal oxygen administration. The next step should be interventional tocolysis when fetal decompensation has not been corrected and operative delivery appears imminent.[27] Clinical assessment of the cause of the fetal distress also is fundamental to the success of intrauterine resuscitation. The recent administration of a paracervical block, maternal supine position, or excessive uterine activity from oxytocin typically will respond well to intrauterine resuscitation without tocolysis. Severe abruptio placentae with concurrent fetal distress does not improve with intrauterine resuscitation, but requires immediate operative delivery and extrauterine neonatal management.

Prospective investigations of parturients that developed fetal distress, documented by fetal heart tracings and scalp pH less than 7.25, resulted in a significant decrease in uterine activity and improvement in fetal heart tracings and scalp pH in patients treated with 0.25 mg of terbutaline subcutaneously compared with controls.[28,29] Interventional tocolysis used in these patients after conservative therapy (maternal oxygen administration, lateral uterine displacement, and discontinuing oxytocin administration) showed no improvement in fetal heart tracings. Terbutaline is a predominantly beta-2-agonist that will increase maternal heart rate and pulse pressure. Administration of terbutaline for tocolysis is not appropriate in parturients with severe abruptio placentae, maternal cardiovascular disease, or other conditions worsened by beta-adrenergic stimulation. Intravenous administration of 0.25 mg of terbutaline is effective in the treatment of fetal distress,[30] resulting in an immediate decrease in uterine activity. Subcutaneous treatment with terbutaline will result in a delay of uterine response for a few minutes.[31] Magnesium sulfate (2 g intravenous bolus) also has been used for tocolysis in the management of fetal distress,[32] but when compared with terbutaline (0.25 mg of terbutaline given subcutaneously versus 4 g of magnesium by intravenous bolus) it was found to be less effective.[33]

Interventional tocolysis is effective in the management of acute intrapartum fetal distress when conventional methods of intrauterine resuscitation have failed. Intravenous terbutaline (0.25 mg) typically will improve a fetal heart tracing and scalp pH samples as a result of decreased uterine activity. Fig. 6-3 is an example of a patient with a fetal heart rate deceleration and uterine tetany effectively treated with interventional tocolysis. If fetal recovery does not improve after all methods of intrauterine resuscitation have been exhausted, the neonatal condition often is improved after operative delivery.[28] Effective use of intrauterine resuscitation may help avoid the "crash" cesarean section and make extrauterine neonatal management easier.

Summary

1. Patients should be evaluated for the potential causes of reduced uteroplacental perfusion.

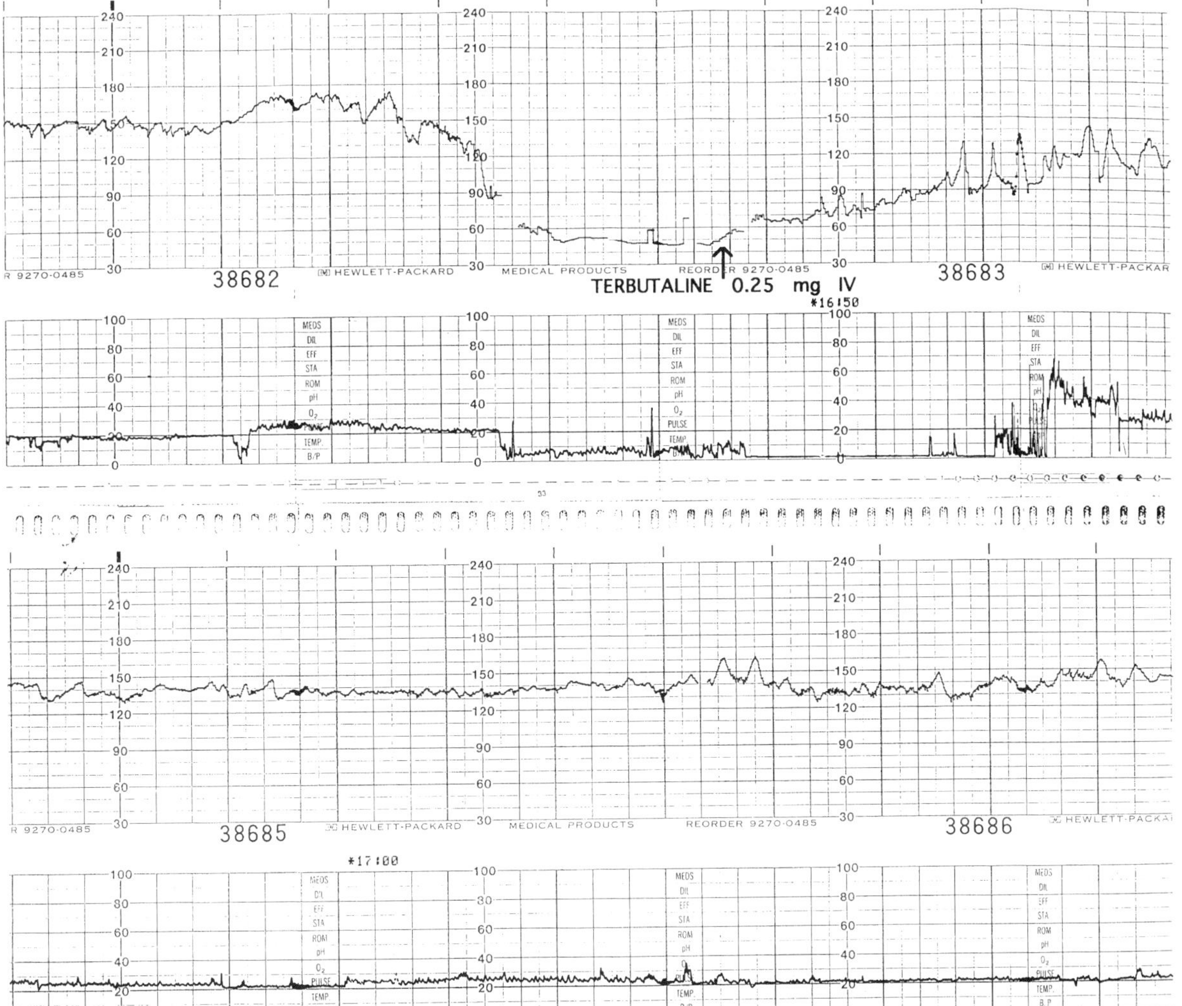

Fig. 6-3.

A healthy primigravida in spontaneous labor developed painful uterine tetany that was palpated at the bedside. Fetal bradycardia, refractory to maternal positioning and oxygen supplementation, was reversed with 0.25 mg of IV terbutaline. A vaginal delivery was accomplished 90 minutes later, with an Apgar score of 9/9 and an UA cord pH of 7.23.

2. One should begin intrauterine resuscitation with conservative methods: (a) discontinuation of oxytocin infusion, (b) optimization of maternal position, (c) correction of maternal hypotension with rapid intravenous crystalloid infusion and intravenous ephedrine, (d) administration of supplemental oxygen, and (e) monitoring of fetal heart tracing closely.
3. If conservative methods of intrauterine

resuscitation fail, one must consider administration of 0.25 mg of terbutaline intravenously and preparation for an operative delivery if fetal recovery does not occur.

References

1. Wehrenberg WB, Chaichareon DP, Dierschke DJ, et al: Vascular dynamics of the reproductive tract in the female rhesus monkey: relative contributions of the ovarian and uterine arteries, *Biol Reprod* 1977; 17:148.
2. Rekonen A, Luotola H, Pitkanen M: Measurement of intervillous and myometrial blood flow by an intravenous ^{133}Xe method, *Br J Obstet Gynaecol* 1976; 83:723.
3. Greiss FC: Pressure-flow relationship in the gravid uterine vascular bed, *Am J Obstet Gynecol* 1966; 96:41.
4. Bieniarz J, Julio W, Grainer L: Uteroplacental circulation: an angiographic study, Washington, D.C., 1969, Pan American Health Organization, Scientific Publication no 185.
5. Palmer SK, Zamudio S, Coffin C, et al: Quantitative estimation of human uterine artery blood flow and pelvic blood flow redistribution in pregnancy, *Obstet Gynecol* 1992; 80:1000.
6. Thompson RS, Trudinger BJ, Cook CM: Doppler ultrasound waveform indices: A/B ratio, pulsitality index and Pourcelot ratio, *Br J Obstet Gynecol* 1987; 95:581.
7. Greiss FC: A clinical concept of uterine blood flow during pregnancy, *Obstet Gynecol* 1967; 30:595.
8. Poserio JJ, Mendez-Bauer SV, Caldeyro-Barcia R: Effect of uterine contractions on maternal blood flow through the placenta, Washington, D.C., 1969, Pan American Health Organizations, Scientific Publication no 185.
9. Kain ZN, Rimar S, Barash P: Cocaine abuse in the parturient and effects on the fetus and neonate, *Anesth Analg* 1993; 77:835.
10. Monga M, Weisbrodt NW, Andres RL, et al: The acute effect of cocaine exposure on pregnant human myometrial contractile activity, *Am J Obstet Gynecol* 1993; 169:782.
11. Chayen B, Tejani N, Verma U, et al: Fetal heart rate changes and uterine activity during coitus, *Acta Obstet Gynecol Scand* 1986; 65:853.
12. Kerr MG, Scott DB, Samuel E: Studies of the inferior vena cava in late pregnancy, *Br Med J* 1964; 1:532.
13. Howard BK, Goodson JH, Mengert WF: Supine hypotension syndrome in late pregnancy, *Obstet Gynecol* 1953; 4:371.
14. Kauppila A, Koshinen M, Puolakka J, et al: Decreased intervillous and unchanged myometrial blood flow in supine recumbency, *Obstet Gynecol* 1980; 55:203.
15. Marx G, Patel S, Berman J, et al: Umbilical blood flow velocity waveforms in different maternal positions and with epidural analgesia, *Obstet Gynecol* 1986; 68:61.
16. Ralston DH, Shnider SM, deLorimier AA: Effects of equipotent ephedrine, metaraminol, mephentermine, and methoxamine on uterine blood flow in the pregnant ewe, *Anesthesiology* 1974; 40:354.
17. Ramanathan S, Grant GJ: Vasopressor therapy for hypotension due to epidural anesthesia for cesarean section, *Acta Anaesthesiol Scand* 1988; 32:559.
18. Moran DH, Perillo M, LaPorta RF, et al: Phenylephrine in the prevention of hypotension following spinal anesthesia for cesareasan delivery, *J Clin Anesth* 1991; 3:301.
19. Alahuhta S, Rasanen J, Jouppila P, et al: Ephedrine and phenylephrine for avoiding maternal hypotension due to spinal anesthesia for caesarean section: effects on uteroplacental and fetal haemodynamics, *Int J Obstet Anesth* 1992; 1:129.
20. Greiss FC, Still JG, Anderson SG: Effects of local anesthetic agents on the uterine vasculatures and myometrium, *Am J Obstet Gynecol* 1976; 124:889.
21. Asling JH, Shnider SM, Margolis AJ, et al: Paracervical block anesthesia in obstetrics, *Am J Obstet Gynecol* 1970; 107:626.
22. Crino JP, Harris AP, Parisi VM, et al: Effect of rapid intravenous crystalloid infusion on uteroplacental blood flow and placental implantation-site oxygen delivery in the pregnant ewe, *Am J Obstet Gynecol* 1993; 168:1603.
23. Hollmen AI, Jouppila R, Jouppila P, et al: Effect of extradural analgesia using bupivacaine and 2-chloroprocaine on intervillous blood flow during normal labor, *Br J Anaesth* 1982; 54:837.
24. Shnider SM, Abboud TK, Artal R, et al: Maternal catecholamines decrease during labor after lumbar epidural anesthesia, *Am J Obstet Gynecol* 1983; 147:13.
25. Albright GA, Jouppila R, Holmen A, et al: Epinephrine does not alter human intervillous blood flow during epidural anesthesia, *Anesthesiology* 1981; 54:131.
26. Gimovsky ML, Caritis SN: Diagnosis and management of hypoxic fetal heart rate patterns, *Clin Perinatol* 1982; 9:313.
27. Campbell WA, Vintzileos AM, Nochimson DJ: Intrauterine

versus extrauterine management/resuscitation of the fetus/neonate, *Clin Obstet Gynecol* 1986; 29:33.

28. Patriarco MS, Viechnicki BM, Hutchinson TA, et al: A study on intrauterine fetal resuscitation with terbutaline, *Am J Obstet Gynecol* 1987; 157:384.
29. Tajani NA, Verma UL, Chatterjee, et al: Terbutaline in the management of acute intrapartum fetal acidosis, *J Reprod Med* 1983; 28:857.
30. Shekarloo A, Mendez-Bauer C, Cook V, et al: Terbutaline (intravenous bolus) for the treatment of acute intrapartum fetal distress, *Am J Obstet Gynecol* 1989; 160:615.
31. Arias F: Intrauterine resuscitation with terbutaline: a method for the management of acute intrapartum fetal distress, *Am J Obstet Gynecol* 1978; 131:39.
32. Reece EA, Chervenak FA, Romero R, et al: Magnesium sulfate in the management of acute intrapartum fetal distress, *Am J Obstet Gynecol* 1984; 148:104.
33. Magann EF, Cleveland RS, Dockery JR, et al: Acute tocolysis for fetal distress: terbutaline versus magnesium sulfate, Abstracts, 41st Clinical Meeting ACOG, 1993.

7

Epidural Analgesia and the Progress of Labor

A 35-year-old parturient at term is admitted in active labor. On examination, the cervix is 4 cm dilated and 100% effaced. The patient wants epidural analgesia for pain relief; the obstetrician decides against it. The obstetrician's rationale is, apparently, epidural analgesia slows down the first and second stages of labor. Discuss the effect of epidural analgesia on the progress of labor.

Recommendations by Thomas H. Joyce III, M.D.

Why choose epidural analgesia for the laboring parturient? The late J. Selwyn Crawford, MD, said that pain usually subserves a protective function; however, the pain of uterine contractions subserves no useful function and, therefore, should be abolished.

Melzack has used the McGill Pain Questionnaire to compare the pain of labor with other painful conditions.[1] His studies suggest that the pain of uterine contractions is comparable with that associated with kidney stones, phantom limb syndrome, or an amputated digit. The physiologic consequences of pain are catecholamine release, anxiety, agitation, restless activity, and hyperventilation. Lederman and others have defined the parallel relationship between maternal anxiety, plasma catecholamines, and plasma cortisol as labor increases in intensity.[2] The elevation of maternal anxiety and plasma catecholamine has been shown to prolong the first stage of labor by the β-agonist effect on the myometrium.[3] Uncontrolled maternal hyperventilation can decrease fetal oxygenation and produce fetal acidosis. Maternal agitation, restlessness, and muscular activity will increase maternal metabolic oxygen usage. Analgesia—either parenteral or epidural—can decrease maternal catecholamine and cortisol levels.

Alternative methods of relieving anxiety and reducing maternal stress are the child birth education techniques and the Doula support method.[4,5] The Doula method uses a bedside female support person of the mother's background.

A U.S. study using support persons reported a decrease in medication usage (including oxytocin and epidural), forceps rate, and cesarean section rates. These human studies have been replicated in the animal (monkey) model showing that induced maternal stress results in fetal bradycardia, an increase catechol secretion, and a decrease in fetal pH and arterial oxygen pressure (PaO_2).[6] If maternal catecholamines alter myometrial contractility or produce multiple uterine pacemakers, a fundal dominate labor pattern may not occur, resulting in a prolongation of the first stage of labor. In these dysfunctional labors, the relief of maternal pain and anxiety frequently is followed by a rapid cervical dilatation when an otherwise lengthy labor would have been predicted. This phenomenon has been spoken of as *speeding up* labor.

In many obstetrical training programs, the clinical observation of a decrease in the amplitude of uterine contractions between 10 and 20 minutes after the epidural injection of a local anesthetic has been referred to as the *lidocaine effect*. This is commonly seen with all local anesthetic bolus injections at the height of absorption from the epidural space. Craft and co-workers reported this effect in 1972.[7] In their study they observed cervimetry in two 20-minute periods after injection of lidocaine or lidocaine with epinephrine. Cervical dilatation continued despite a decreased amplitude of the uterine contractions. Other reports noted this effect in their review of conduction and inhalation anesthesia on uterine contractions.[8,9] In a collaborative 11-university study of early amniotomy (<3 cm) versus spontaneous or artificial amniotomy (for scalp electrode), early amniotomy shortened the time of the first stage by 277 minutes versus 413 minutes in the conservatively managed group. The incidence of epidural analgesia and use of oxytocin were similar in both groups.[10]

A balance of sympathetic-parasympathetic tone influences the intensity and duration of the uterine contraction. Epidural analgesia for labor produces greater sympathetic block, thereby tending to increase the force and duration of uterine contractions. Whereas the alpha properties of norepinephrine can increase uterine contractions and decrease uterine blood flow, the β-agonist effects of epinephrine can diminish the frequency and duration of uterine contractions. Increased plasma epinephrine levels have been correlated with changes in the fetal heart rate, beat-to-beat variability, and variable decelerations.[11] Changes in uterine activity after injection of a local anesthetic in the epidural space have been thought to correlate with uterine blood flow. The article by Steiger and Nageotte shows a classic demonstration of high blood levels of a local anesthetic leading to uterine hypertonus and to fetal bradycardia requiring tocolytic therapy.[12]

Uterine blood flow is directly proportional to the mean maternal arterial pressure and inversely proportional to uterine vascular resistance. Local anesthetics produce no direct changes of the fetal heart rate.[13-15] If present in sufficient concentration, local anesthetics can produce uterine artery vasoconstriction and myometrial hypertonus.[16-18]

Recent technology has enabled investigators to study uterine and umbilical blood vessel flow in vivo.[19] The effect of different maternal positions on umbilical flow velocity waveforms detected little change from baseline other than a small, decreased systolic-diastolic (S/D) ratio with 2-chloroprocaine.[20] This change was considered insignificant. Morrow and co-workers demonstrated that the uteroplacental vessels are maximally dilated before labor in the healthy parturient.[21] The addition of epidural anesthesia did not negatively impact blood flow velocity in the mother or in the fetus. More recent work by Patton and colleagues. reported that although a fluid preload increased maternal heart rate, stroke volume, and cardiac output and decreased mean arterial pressure and systemic vascular resistance, the S/D ratios remained unchanged.[22] Whereas epidural analgesia returned cardiac output and stroke volume to baseline values, all other parameters were similar to those recorded after fluid loading. These authors likewise concluded that epidural anesthesia does not compromise uterine blood flow under normal circumstances. Fetal heart rate and S/D ratio studies in normal and hypertensive patients with epidural anesthesia detected no alteration of the fetal heart rate or umbilical S/D ratios.[23] These authors concluded that their findings demonstrated the beneficial effect of epidural block on maternal placental perfusion. Hughes et al. reported that whereas epidural block decreases maternal systolic and diastolic pressure and heart rate without treatable hypotension, no adverse changes were noticed in the velocimetry of umbilical or uterine arteries.[24] No significant differences were found before preload, after preload, or at the peak of the epidural block. Does epinephrine mixed with the local anesthetic affect umbilical artery velocity waveform ratios? Marx and colleagues found that when base flow was in the normal range, a fetus would tolerate epinephrine in the epidural solution.[25] However, when baseline flow indicated elevated vascular resistance, the presence of epinephrine produced vasoconstriction and diminished blood flow. The supine position long has been shown to modify uterine blood flow with potential disastrous effects on the fetus. In their study on uterine and umbilical flow velocity waveforms during the supine hypotensive syndrome, Pirkonen et al. reported that for women in the supine position, a 19% decrease in blood flow occurred, which was associated with a 26% rise in the uterine arterial S/D ratio.[26] This significant increase in resistance confirms that the lateral position with lateral displacement of the uterus is essential in late pregnancy. The reader is referred to a comprehensive review of obstetrics analgesia and anesthesia on uterine activity and uteroplacental blood flow by Conklin.[27] *Without maternal hypotension* or drug-induced uterine hypertonus, epidural analgesia has no negative impact on uterine or umbilical artery blood flow.

More than 100 papers in the medical literature state that epidural analgesia *is* or *is not* a causative factor in instrumental delivery.[28] I believe that in the 1980s a fairly good consensus existed in the anesthesia community that early and intense motor blockade of the perineal musculature would lengthen the second stage of labor an average of 30 minutes or longer, remove or modify the bearing-down reflex (which requires a good pushing coach), and might influence the fetal head not to rotate from transverse or posterior to the anterior presentation.

The decision by the obstetrician to shorten the second stage by vacuum extraction or forceps delivery for the benefit of the mother can be a factor. The American College of Obstetrics and Gynecology Committee on Forceps has published reports on the characteristics of normal labor.[29] For nulliparous women, the first stage of labor averaged 8.1 hours and for multiparous women it averaged 5.7 hours. The second stage of labor for nulliparous women averaged 54 minutes; for multiparous women it average 19 minutes. Their conclusions included a statement that conduction anesthesia lengthened the second stage of labor an average of 25 minutes, and that operative intervention after 2 hours in the second stage of labor must be modified to include fetal monitoring and clinical practice.

Over the last 50 years the clinical practice of anesthesia during labor has moved from caudal anesthesia to lumbar epidural anesthesia, high-concentration of local anesthetic, to analgesic agent with a low-concentration of local anesthetic, to low-concentration continuous-infusion epidural analgesia; to even lower doses of local anesthetic agent with the addition of epidural or intrathecal narcotic; to patient-controlled epidural analgesia with or without opioids; to intrathecal and epidural opioids given by single injection or continuous infusion (the walking epidural). See Chapter 16 for specific drugs and doses.

While reporting unpublished data from George Washington University (Washington, D.C.) Naulty noted a twofold to fivefold reduction in the use of outlet forceps, midforceps, and cesarean section in labor when anesthetic practice changed from the use of 1.5% lidocaine to bupivacaine 0.0625% with sufentanil.[30] Vertommen et al. reported that an epidural sufentanil-bupivacaine mixture reduced the incidence of instrumental deliveries from 36% to 24%.[31] In an classic report Chestnut and colleagues presented a randomized double-blind comparison of 0.0625% bupivacaine/0/0002% fentanyl versus 0.125% bupivacaine.[32] When saline replaced active solution, no change occurred in the length of the second stage of labor or the incidence of instrumental delivery. In two abstracts, Hawkins and coworkers presented data from a very large teaching hospital on the association of epidural analgesia and forceps delivery.[33,34] The power factors most likely to result in an instrumental delivery were (1) gestational age more than 41 weeks; (2) malpresentation of the fetal head; (3) previous cesarean section; (4) longer than 2 hours in the second stage of labor; and (5) epidural anesthesia. In this study multiparous patients were three times more likely than nulliparous patients to have a forceps delivery if epidural anesthesia was given. This study antedated the use of supplemental narcotics in low-dose continuous epidural analgesia. The changes that have occurred in clinical practice with the addition of supplemental opioid have minimized the occurrence and/or degree of perineal muscle relaxation. My clinical observation is that a lack of analgesia in the second stage of labor is more detrimental than analgesic perineum. Patients will be split 50:50 to push or not push effectively with perineal analgesia or absence of perineal analgesia.

Perhaps a short note should be made for the parturient presenting late in labor or the parturient who wishes to ambulate, to squat, or to assume the knee-chest position during labor. Epidural or intrathecal opioids will produce rapid analgesia for the first stage of labor with minimal side effects or pruritus, nausea, or urinary retention.[35,36] Opioids may not to minimally lengthen the first stage of labor. Analgesia is absent for pain or discomfort of the second and third stage of labor. Thus another technique such as pudendal block, local infiltration, inhalational analgesia, parenteral opioid, or spinal-epidural anesthesia is required if analgesia is requested.

Summary

1. Table 7-1 summarizes for the obstetrician in our case study the effects of epidural analgesia on mother and fetus during the first and second stage of labor.
2. Knowledge of these effects and skill, as well as good communication between the anesthesiologist and the obstetrician, are essential in maximizing the benefits of epidural analgesia while avoiding or minimizing the side effects of epidural analgesia.
3. Placing the mother in the supine position and the resultant maternal hypotension are to be avoided or corrected as rapidly as possible.

TABLE 7-1

Effects of Epidural Analgesia during First and Second Stages of Labor

Item	First Stage	Second Stage	Comment
Pain			
Primipara	++++	+++	Can lead to dysfunctional labor and change uterine and umbilical blood flow
Multipara	++	+++	
Maternal catecholamine	Lengthen	—	Can produce decreases in uterine blood flow and produce abnormal fetal heart rate patterns
Oxytocin	Shorten	Shorten	Can produce hypertonic uterus and fetal distress
Amide ester	—	—	Have potential to cause arterial constriction
Epidural block	Latent +/−	Lengthen, average 25 min	Second stage effects primarily related to perineal muscle relaxation
Epidural-intrathecal opioids	May not lengthen	—	Rapid onset of analgesia not effective for second-stage analgesia
Forceps delivery	—	+/−	Associated with epidural and other factors (see text)
New drugs	?	?	Alpha-2 agonists???
Obstetrician	Shorten by amniotomy and/or oxytocin	Shorten by oxytocin and/or instrumental delivery	Must know physiologic effects of epidural block on labor; latent-phase block becomes induction; communication is essential
Anesthesiologist	May shorten Meticulous technique	May relax or numb perineum	Must know fetal monitors; current knowledge and communication are essential

References

1. Melzack R: The myths of painless childbirth, *Pain* 1984; 19:321.
2. Lederman RP, Lederman G, Work BA, et al: The relationship of maternal anxiety, plasma catecholamine and plasma cortisol to progress in labor, *Am J Obstet Gynecol* 1978; 132:495.
3. Levinson G, Shnider SM: The effect of maternal fear and its treatment on uterine function and circulation, *Birth Fam J* 1979; 6:167.
4. Dick-Reed G: *Childbirth without fear,* New York, 1953, Harper and Row.
5. Kennell J, Klaus M, McGrath S, et al: Continuous emotional support during labor in a US hospital, *JAMA* 1991; 265:2197.

6. Morishma HO, Pederson H, Finster M: The influence of maternal physiological stress on the fetus, *Am J Obstet Gynecol* 1978; 131:286.
7. Craft JB, Epstein BS, Coakley CS: Effects of lidocaine with epinephrine versus lidocaine (plain) on induced labor, *Anesth Analg* 1972; 51:243.
8. Vasicka A, Kretchmer H: Effect of conduction and inhalation anesthesia on uterine contractions, *Am J Obstet Gynecol* 1961; 82:600.
9. Willdeck-Lund G: Effect of segmental epidural analgesia upon the uterine activity with specific reference to the use of different local anesthetic agents, *Acta Anaesth Scand* 1979; 23:519.
10. Fraser WD, Marcoux S, Montquin JM, et al: Effect of early amniotomy on the risk of dystocia in nulliparous women, *N Engl J Med* 1993; 328:1145.
11. Lederman RP, Lederman E, Work B, et al: Anxiety and epinephrine in nulliparous women in labor; relationship to duration of labor and fetal heart rate pattern, *Am J Obstet Gynecol* 1985; 53:870.
12. Steiger RM, Nageotte MD: Effect of uterine contractility and maternal hypotension on prolonged decelerations after bupivacaine epidural anesthesia, *Am J Obstet Gynecol* 1990; 163: 808.
13. Lavin JP, Samuels SV, Miodovnik M, et al: The effects of bupivacaine and chloroprocaine as local anesthetic for epidural anesthesia on fetal heart rate monitoring parameters, *Am J Obstet Gynecol* 1981; 141:717.
14. Hood DD, Parker RL, Meis PJ: Epidural bupivacaine does not effect fetal, heart rate tracings, *Soc Obstet Anesth Perinatology Abstr* 1993; 25:79.
15. Zilanti M, Salazar JR, Allen I, et al: Fetal heart rate and pH of fetal capillary blood during epidural analgesia in labor, *Obstet Gynecol* 1970; 36:881.
16. Fisburne JI, Greiss FC, Hopkinson R, et al: Response of the gravid uterine vasculature to arterial levels of local anesthetics, *Am J Obstet Gynecol* 1979; 133:753.
17. Greiss FC: Reactivities of the non gravid vasculature: effects of norepinephrine, *Am J Obstet Gynecol* 1978; 131:778.
18. Joyce TH, Aquino N, Kuckling A: The effect of local anesthetics on gravid human uterine artery strips in vitro, *ASA Abstr* 1976.
19. Fleischer A, Anyaegbunam AA, Schulman H, et al: Uterine and umbilical artery velocimetry during normal labor, *Am J Obstet Gynecol* 1987; 157:40.
20. Marx GF, Patel S, Berman JA, et al: Umbilical blood flow velocity waveforms in different maternal positions and with epidural analgesia, *Obstet Gynecol* 1986; 68:61.
21. Morrow RJ, Rolbin SH, Rictchie JWK, et al: Epidural anesthesia and blood flow velocity in mother and fetus, *J Can Anes Soc* 1989; 36:519.
22. Patton DE, Lee W, Miller J, et al: Maternal uteroplacental and fetoplacental hemodynamics and Doppler velocimetric changes during epidural anesthesia in normal labor, *Obstet Gynecol* 1991; 77:17.
23. Ramos-Santos E, Devoe LD, Wakefield ML, et al: The effects of epidural anesthesia on the Doppler velocimetry of umbilical and uterine arteries in normal and hypertensive patients during active term labor, *Obstet Gynecol* 1991; 77:20.
24. Hughes AB, Devoe LD, Wakefield ML, et al: The effects of epidural anesthesia on the Doppler velocimetry of umbilical and uterine arteries in normal term labor, *Obstet Gynecol* 1990; 75:809.
25. Marx GF, Edelstein ID, Schuss M, et al: Effects of epidural block with lignocaine and lignocaine-adrenaline on umbilical artery velocity wave ratios, *Br J Obstet Gynecol* 1990; 97: 517.
26. Pirkonen JP, Erkola RU: Uterine and umbilical flow velocity waveforms in the supine hypotensive syndrome, *Obstet Gynecol* 1990; 76:176.
27. Conklin KA: *Effects of obstetric analgesia on uterine activity and uteroplacental blood flow.* In Carsten ME, Miller JD, editors: *Uterine function,:Molecular and cellular aspects,* New York, Plenum, 1990.
28. Kilpatrick SJ, Laros RK Jr: Characteristics of normal labor, *Obstet Gynecol* 1989; 74:85.
29. Bailey PW, Howard FA: Epidural analgesia and forceps delivery; laying bogey, *Anaesthesia* 1983; 38:282.
30. Naulty JS: *Epidural analgesia for labor.* In Norris MC, editor: *Obstetric anesthesia,* Philadelphia, 1993, JB Lippincott.
31. Vertommen JD, Vandermeulen E, Van Aken H, et al: The effects of the addition of sufentanil to 0.125% bupivacaine on the quality of analgesia during labor and on the incidence of instrumental deliveries, *Anesthesiology* 1991; 74:809.
32. Chestnut DH, Laszewski LJ, Pollock KL, et al: Continuous epidural infusion of 0.0625% bupivacaine-0.0002% fentanyl during the second stage of labor, *Anesthesiology* 1990; 72:613.

33. Hawkins JL, Skjonsby BS, Joyce TH III, et al: The association of epidural analgesia and forceps delivery, *Anesth Analg* 1990; 70:S150.

34. Hawkins JL, Skjonsby BS, Kubicek M, et al: Is epidural analgesia the only variable associated with forceps delivery, *Anesth Analg* 1990; 70:S151.

35. Breen TW, Shapiro T, Glass G, et al: Epidural anesthesia in labor in an ambulatory patient, *Anesth Analg* 1993; 77: 919.

36. Grieco WM, Norris MC, Leighton BL, et al: Intrathecal sufentanil labor analgesia: the effects of adding morphine or epinephrine, *Anesth Analg* 1993; 77:1149.

8

Antenatal Monitoring of the High-Risk Fetus

A 27-year-old primigravida is admitted to the high-risk unit with severe hypertension. Discuss the antepartum evaluation of high-risk parturients.

Recommendations by Ramon Martin, M.D., Ph.D.

Anesthesia for the obstetric patient is an integral part of labor and delivery. For routine, normal deliveries this usually involves providing pain relief with an epidural technique. In pregnancies complicated by either maternal or fetal disease, the role of anesthesia is more central to patient care and can involve close monitoring with invasive lines during labor, fluid management, and discussion with the obstetricians about the timing and type of anesthesia. Equally important in the dialogue with the obstetricians is an understanding of the techniques used to assess the fetus, because this provides important information about how the fetus might tolerate labor and delivery. This chapter will review the causes of perinatal mortality, the techniques available to assess the fetus, and the clinical application to labor and delivery.

Perinatal Mortality

According to the National Center for Health Statistics,[1] the perinatal mortality rate (PMR) is defined as the number of late fetal deaths (after 28 weeks' gestation) plus early neonatal deaths (infants 0 to 6 days of age) divided by 1000 live births plus the fetal and neonatal deaths. In the United States, the PMR has declined by an average of 3% per year since 1965.[2] Over the last 6 years, fetal death rate alone has decreased 16% and neonatal mortality has fallen 21%. Of all fetal deaths, 22% occur between the thirty-sixth and fortieth weeks of gestation and another 10% occur beyond the forty-first week of gestation.

Congenital anomalies account for 25% of perinatal mortality and are the leading cause.[3] Premature labor and delivery was the most common event leading to death in this group. Overall, prematurity with associated respiratory distress syndrome (RDS) was the next most common cause of perinatal death. Intrauterine hypoxia and birth asphyxia account for 3% of the PMR, and placenta or cord complications accounted for 2% of the PMR. Several associated factors identified by Lammer et al.[4] were race (African-American), marital status (single), age (older than 34 and younger than 20 years of age), parity (>5) and lack of prenatal care. Multiple gestations were associated with 10% of all fetal deaths. This gives a PMR of 50/1000, which is seven times that of singleton pregnancies. More than half of all fetal deaths were associated with asphyxia or maternal causes, such as pregnancy-induced hypertension (PIH) or placental abruption.

If the first step to reducing the PMR further is recognizing the causes, then the next step is prevention. A study of perinatal mortality in the Mersey region of England showed that of 309 perinatal deaths, 182 (or 58.9%) were due to avoidable causes, primarily a delayed response to the following: abnormalities of the progress of labor or fetal heart rate tracing during labor and delivery, maternal weight loss with a resulting growth retarded fetus, and reductions in fetal movement.[5] Antepartum fetal monitoring is the means to decrease these fetal deaths. This is most useful when targeting specific groups of parturients who are at increased risk of perinatal mortality (Table 8-1).

TABLE 8-1
Parturients at Increased Risk of Perinatal Mortality

Maternal Disease	Fetal Disease
Postdates gestation	Neonatal asphyxia
Diabetes	Perinatal death
Previous stillbirth	Perinatal death
Pregnancy-induced hypertension	Fetal distress in labor
Maternal age older than 35 yr	Congenital anomalies
Maternal weight loss	IUGR
Premature labor	RDS

IUGR, intrauterine growth retardation; RDS, respiratory distress syndrome.

Techniques of Fetal Assessment

Maternal Assessment of Fetal Activity

Having a parturient count the fetal activity over a period of time is a simple and sensitive test of fetal well-being. It is based on the fact that from 28 weeks of gestation on, the fetus makes about 30 body movements each hour (about 10% of the total time), and the parturient is able to appreciate most of these.[6] Whereas fetal movement is reassuring, lack of movement can indicate either a quiet period, which usually can last 20 minutes (but can last as long as 75 minutes), or fetal compromise secondary to asphyxia. Factors that can decrease maternal appreciation of fetal activity are an anterior placenta, polyhydramnios, and obesity.[7]

Several studies have demonstrated that when patients reliably count fetal movements according to a set protocol, there is a significant reduction in fetal death.[8-10]

Amniocentesis

Performed before 15 weeks' gestation, early amniocentesis is an alternative to chorionic villus sampling to obtain fetal cells for diagnosis of genetic or morphologic abnormalities. Although the success of obtaining cells is the same as for chorionic villus sampling, the disadvantages are primarily due to the withdrawal of amniotic fluid. The volume of fluid removed is a much greater proportion of the total fluid volume, and this could increase fetal loss.

After 16 weeks' gestation, midtrimester amniocentesis with ultrasound guidance is safe, with a rate of fetal loss of 0.5% to 1.0%.[11,12] The amniotic fluid is used to grow fetal cells, which in turn, are used to scan for chromosomal aberrations. During the third trimester, amniocentesis is used to obtain fluid to assess fetal lung maturity.

Chorionic Villus Sampling

Performed between 9 to 12 weeks of gestation, chorionic villus sampling allows early determination of chromosomal abnormalities. Under ultrasound guidance, this technique is simply the aspiration of villi, through either the cervix or the abdomen. Because actual tissue is obtained, results from cells are available as early as 24 to 48 hours, and can also be analyzed for abnormalities in deoxyribonucleic acid or specific enzymatic reactions. Fetal loss was 2.3% to 2.5% in one randomized trial.[13] Limb reduction defects and oromandibular hypogenesis have been reported in a small number of infants after chorionic villus sampling,[14] but other studies[15,16] have not demonstrated any difference between the expected rates of appearance of these developmental aberrations.

Percutaneous Umbilical Blood Sampling

Starting at 18 weeks' gestation, fetal blood can be obtained transabdominally under ultrasound guidance by needle puncture of the umbilical cord. This is useful in diagnosing a range of problems:[17]

1. Hematologic abnormalities, such as hemoglobinopathies, isoimmunization, thrombocytopenia, and coagulation factor deficiencies
2. Inborn errors of metabolism
3. Infections by viruses, bacteria, or parasites
4. Chromosomal abnormalities, especially mosaicism

The risk to the fetus is greater than other tests, with an increase in fetal loss of 2%.[17] As a result, this test is usually reserved for situations where information cannot be obtained by other means.

Ultrasonography

Over the last two decades, ultrasound has become an important method of antepartum fetal assessment. Useful throughout gestation, it gives an accurate measurement of gestational age and provides an assessment of fetal growth as well as developmental abnormalities. It is also an important guide in the performance of amniocentesis, chorionic villus sampling, and cordocentesis. Real time ultrasound permits a dynamic assessment of fetal well-being by following, over time, fetal breathing activity, movements, and tone.

Despite its importance as a method of fetal assessment, controversy still exists about the routine use of ultrasound in pregnancy. In Helsinki, Finland, which like many other European countries advocates routine ultrasound screening, a randomized trial showed a significant decrease in perinatal mortality in the screened group compared with the control group.[18] This was due primarily to early detection of fetal malformations. A number of other studies have not found a benefit from routine ultrasound screening.[19,20] A recent large-scale study of 15,151 pregnant women demonstrated no difference in adverse perinatal outcome. Subgroups of women with postdates gestation, multiple pregnancies, or infants who are small for gestational age did not differ in perinatal outcome between the control and study populations.[21] This controversy is also fueled by the desire to contain medical costs by decreasing unnecessary testing.

During the first trimester, ultrasonography, particularly transvaginal sonography, can help determine whether a fetus is viable when there is vaginal bleeding, or determine the presence of other processes: ectopic pregnancy, uterine anomaly, or an adnexal mass. In addition, it can provide the first measurement of fetal crown-rump length as a measure of fetal age. During the second trimester, ultrasound assessment of biparietal diameter becomes an accurate measure of gestational age.[22] From 12 to 28 weeks of gestation, the relation between biparietal diameter and gestation is linear.[23] Ultrasonic assessment of fetal growth, when continued into the third trimester, is important in diagnosing deviations from normal growth such as growth retardation, macrosomia, or developmental anomalies. Diagnoses of oligohydramnios or polyhydramnios are made by ultrasound. As mentioned previously, real-time ultrasound measures variables that are the components of the biophysical profile (amniotic fluid volume, fetal breathing, limb movement, and tone). All of these measurements can have an effect on the course of labor and delivery.

Fetal Lung Maturity

Because fetal chronologic age does not necessarily correlate with functional maturity, particularly the pulmonary system, methods of assessing fetal maturity are important adjuncts in clinical decision making. The majority of perinatal morbidity and mortality results from complications of premature delivery. The most frequently seen complication is the RDS. This disorder is due to a particular deficiency of a surface-active agent (surfactant) that prevents alveolar collapse during expiration. Phospholipids, produced by fetal alveolar cells, are the major component of lung surfactant, and are produced in sufficient amounts by 36 weeks' gestation. The most commonly used technique measures the lecithin-sphingomyelin ratio (L/S). The concentration of lecithin, a component of surfactant, begins to rise in the amniotic fluid at 32 to 33 weeks' gestation and continues to rise until term. The concentration of sphingomyelin remains relatively constant, so that the ratio of the two provides an estimate of surfactant production that is not affected by variations in the volume of amniotic fluid. The risk of neonatal RDS when the L/S ratio is greater than 2 is less than 1%. If the ratio is less than 1.5, about 80% of neonates will develop RDS.

Disaturated phosphatidylcholine (SPC) is the major component of fetal pulmonary surfactant. The technique that separates SPC from lecithin in the amniotic fluid is complicated, and the results can be altered by abnormalities in amniotic fluid production and excretion (i.e., oligohydramnios or polyhydramnios). A value greater than 500 μg/dl amniotic fluid for SPC concentration is consistent with mature fetal lungs and a small risk of RDS.

The disadvantages in measuring the L/S ratio include the long turnaround time, the use of toxic chemicals, a lack of technical expertise, and the inability to standardize the test. As a result, few hospitals are able to perform the test. Another method, the TDx fetal lung maturity test, is automated and avoids the technical involvement in sample preparation and measurement. The test relies on the fluorescence polarization of a dye added to a solution of amniotic fluid that is then compared with values on a standard curve to determine the relative concentration of surfactant and albumin. The determined values are expressed in milligrams of surfactant per gram of albumin. With a cutoff of 50 mg/g for maturity, the TDx test was equal in sensitivity (0.96) and more specific (0.88 versus 0.83) when compared with the L/S ratio in one multicenter study.[24]

Biophysical Profile

The biophysical profile involves evaluation of immediate biophysical activities (fetal movement, tone, breathing movements, and heart rate activity) as well as semiquantitative assessment of amniotic fluid. The biophysical parameters reflect acute central nervous system (CNS) activity, and when present, correlate positively with the lack of depression (secondary to asphyxia) of the CNS. Amniotic fluid volume represents long-term or chronic fetal compromise.

Major indications for referral for biophysical profile include suspected intrauterine growth retardation, hypertension, postdates gestation, and diabetes.

The biophysical evaluation of the fetus is done by ultrasound with the sole purpose of detecting changes in fetal activity due to asphyxia. As has been mentioned previously, changes in fetal breathing movements, heart rate, and body movements are indicators of the state of fetal oxygenation. Superimposed on these factors are the nonrandom pattern of CNS output and the sleep state, with effects that might be mistaken for hypoxia. However, extending the period of observation to find a period of normal recovery for the latter conditions helps to differentiate asphyxia from normal variants.

The scoring of the fetal biophysical profile is an assessment of five variables (Table 8-2), four of which are monitored simultaneously by ultrasound. The variables are said to be normal or abnormal and are assigned a score of 2 for normal and 0 for abnormal. The nonstress test (NST) is monitored after the biophysical evaluation. When the test score is normal, conservative therapy is indicated, with some exceptions:

1. Postdate gestation with a favorable cervix
2. Growth-retarded fetus with mature pulmonary indices and a favorable cervix
3. Insulin-dependent diabetic woman at 37 weeks' gestation or more with mature pulmonary indices
4. Class A diabetic woman at term with a favorable cervix
5. Women with medical disorders (e.g., asthma, preeclampsia, PIH) that might pose a threat to maternal and fetal health.

Table 8-3 list recommendations for management of biophysical profile scores.

Several prospective studies, summarized in Table 8-4,[25-28] have shown that the majority of women studied (>97%) have normal test results and delivery outcome. Perinatal mortality varies inversely with the last score before delivery. In 1981 and

TABLE 8-2

Biophysical Profile Scoring

Variable	Score = 2	Score = 0
Fetal breathing movements	1 episode, 30-sec duration in 30 min	Absent
Gross body movements	3 discrete body/limb movements in 30 min	< 2 episodes in 30 min
Fetal tone	1 episode of extension/flexion of hand, limb, or trunk	Absent or slow movement
Fetal heart rate	2 episodes of acceleration with fetal movement in 30 min	< 2 episodes
Amniotic fluid vol	1 pocket, 1 × 1 cm	No amniotic fluid or a pocket < 1 × 1 cm

Vol, Volume.

TABLE 8-3

Interpretation and Management of Biophysical Profile Score

Score	Interpretation	Recommended Management
8-10	Normal infant	Repeat test in 1 wk*
6	Suspect asphyxia	Repeat test in 4-6 hr†
4	Suspect asphyxia	If > 36 wk, deliver If < 36 wk, repeat in 24 hr
0-2	Probable asphyxia	Deliver

*Repeat test twice a wk if mother is a diabetic or > 42 wk gestation.

†Deliver if oligohydramnios is present.

TABLE 8-4

Biophysical Profile and Perinatal Mortality

Study	No. Patients	No. Deaths	Perinatal Mortality
Manning et al.[25]	19,211	141	1.92
Baskett et al.[26]	5034	32	3.10
Platt et al.[27]	286	4	7.0
Schiffrin et al.[28]	158	7	12.6

1985, in large groups of patients, Manning et al.[29,30] found that the gross perinatal mortality rate decreased from 11.7 to 7.4 per 1000 and the corrected value decreased from 5 to 1.9 per 1000. In Manitoba, since the use of this testing, the stillbirth rate has decreased by 30%. A stillbirth occurring within a week of a normal test result is defined as a false-negative result. This ranges from 0.41 to 1.01 per 1000, with a mean of 0.64 per 1000.

The false-negative rate, although small, directly reflects the negative predictive accuracy of the test. Manning et al.[27] calculated from a study of 19,221 pregnancies a negative predictive accuracy of 99.224%, or the probability of fetal death after a normal test result as 0.726 per 1000 patients.

Because the ideal testing method would result in no false-negative deaths, the biophysical profile is not perfect. The cause of the imperfection is the probability of change in the fetal status from either a chronic condition or an acute variable. Whereas more frequent testing of all patients would decrease the false-negative rate, this has not been attempted because of the increased workload. The proper selection of patients requiring more vigilant monitoring (those judged to be at risk, e.g., women having an immature fetus with growth retardation, preeclampsia, or diabetes) would render this more feasible.

Nonstress Testing

Nonstress testing is the external detection of fetal heart rate and fetal movement in relation to uterine contractions, noting accelerations of fetal heart rate with fetal movement. These parameters are predictors of fetal outcome.

With the parturient recumbent in the semi-Fowler's position and left lateral tilt (to displace the uterus from the inferior vena cava and aorta), 20 minutes of consistent fetal heart rate tracing is followed, and a tocodynamometer is used to measure uterine contractions. Fetal movement is noted either by the mother by external palpation of the maternal abdomen or by spikes in the tocodynamometer tracing.

The test is usually interpreted as one of the following[31,32]:

1. *Reactive*—at least two fetal movements in 20 minutes with acceleration of the fetal heart rate to at least 15 beats/min, with long-term variability of at least 10 beats/min and a baseline rate within the normal range (Fig. 8-1)
2. *Nonreactive*—no fetal movement or acceleration of the fetal heart rate with movement, poor to no long-term variability, baseline fetal heart rate may be within or outside the normal range (Fig. 8-2)
3. *Uncertain reactivity*—fewer than two fetal movements in 20 minutes or acceleration to less than 15 beats/min, long-term variability amplitude less than 10 beats/min, baseline heart rate outside of normal limits.

Fetuses have sleep or inactive cycles that can last up to 80 minutes. The test administrator can either wait for a while or manually stimulate the infant.

A reactive test is associated with survival of the

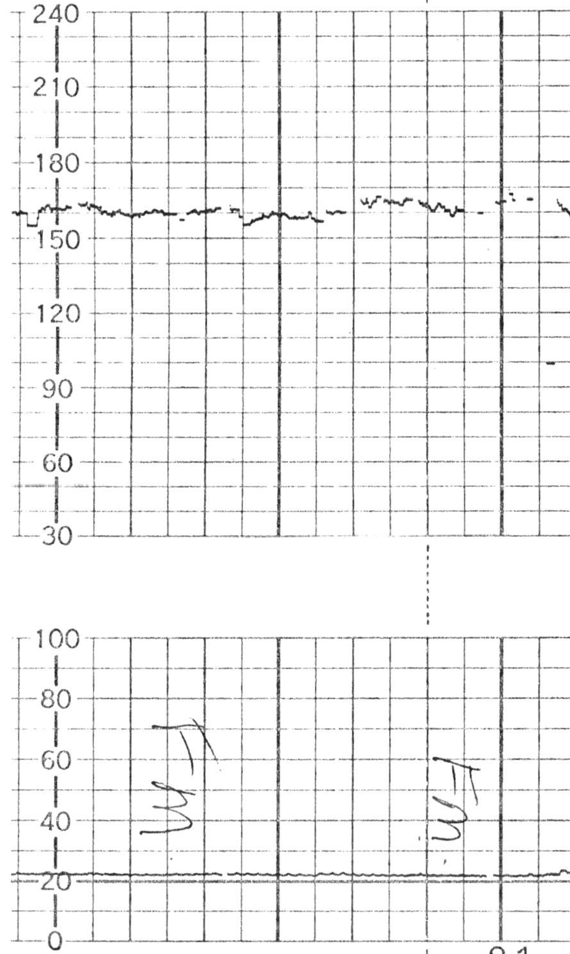

Fig. 8-1.

Reactive nonstress test, characterized by accelerations in the fetal heart rate with fetal movement (FM).

fetus for 1 or more weeks in more than 99% of cases.[31,33] A nonreactive test is associated with poor fetal outcome in 20% of cases.[34] Although the false-positive rate of this technique is high (80%), further evaluation needs to be done when a nonreactive result is obtained. The next step is usually a contraction stress test (CST). Similarly, an uncertain reactive pattern needs to be followed up with either another NST or a CST.

Contraction Stress Test

As its name implies, the CST assesses the fetal response (heart rate pattern) to regular uterine contractions. Using the same technique as the NST, the CST requires three adequate contractions within a 10-minute period, each with a duration of 1 minute. If there are not enough spontaneous contractions, augmentation with intravenous oxytocin is indicated. Beginning at a rate of 1.0 mU/min, the infusion is increased every 15 minutes until the requisite number of contractions are obtained. It is rarely necessary to exceed 10 mU/min.

Certain clinical situations present contraindications to CSTs: prior classic cesarean section, placenta previa, and women at risk of premature labor (premature rupture of membranes, multiple gestations, incompetent cervix, and women undergoing treatment for preterm labor).

The CSTs are interpreted as one of the following:

1. *Negative*—no late deceleration and normal baseline fetal heart rate
2. *Positive*—persistent late decelerations (even when the contractions are less frequent than three contractions within 10 minutes), possible absence of fetal heart rate variability
3. *Suspicious*—intermittent late deceleration or variable decelerations, abnormal baseline fetal heart rate
4. *Unsatisfactory*—poor quality recording or inability to achieve three contractions within 10 minutes
5. *Hyperstimulation*—excessive uterine activity (contractions closer than every 2 minutes or lasting longer than 90 seconds) resulting in late decelerations or bradycardia.

A negative result of a CST is associated with fetal survival for a week or more in 99% of cases,[31,32] whereas a positive result of a CST is associated with poor fetal outcome in 50% of cases.[34] Like the NST,

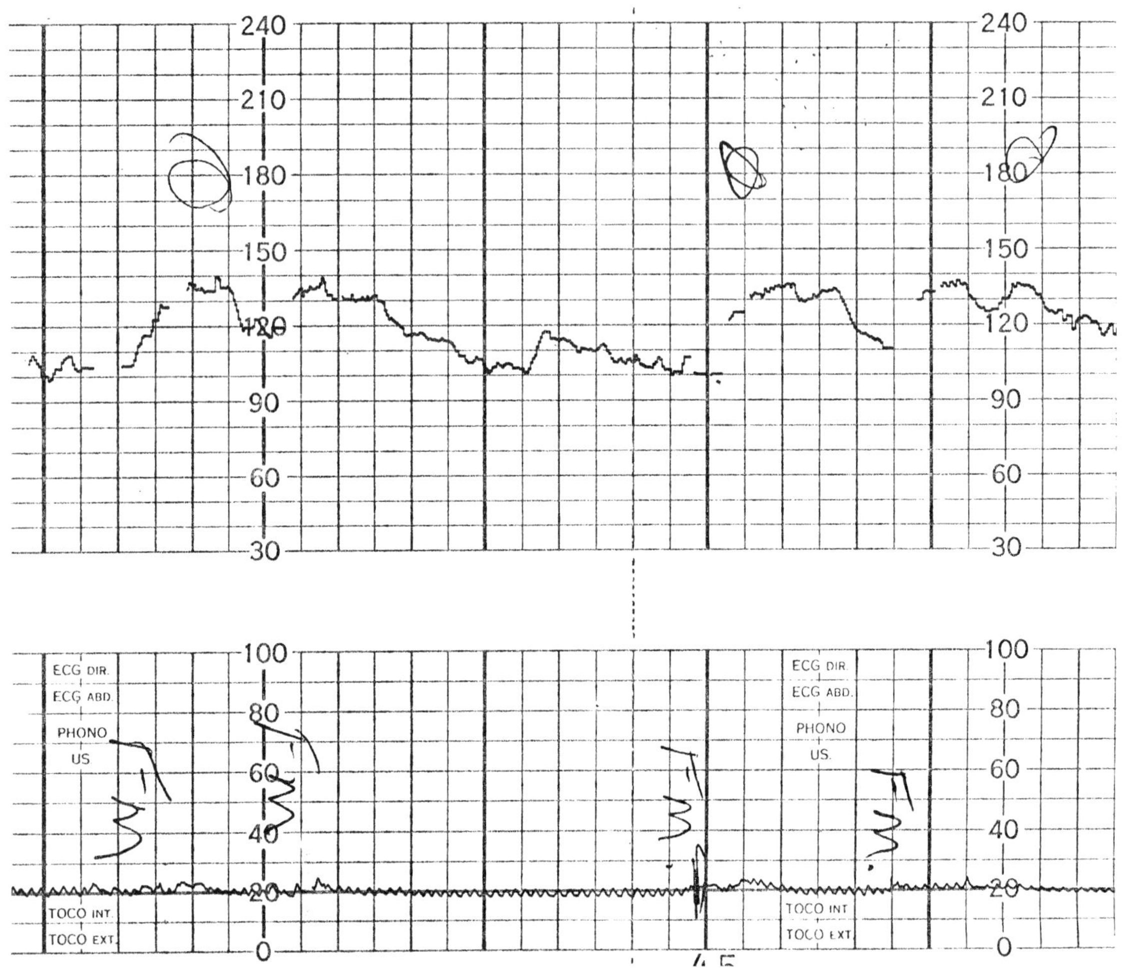

Fig. 8-2.
Nonreactive nonstress test, with no accelerations in fetal heart rate with fetal movement (FM).

the CST also has a high false-positive rate (50%), but the treatment, if delivery is indicated, can be a trial of induction of labor.

Fetal Scalp Sampling

Since first introduced by Saling and Schneider[35] in 1967, fetal blood sampling has become the final determinant in making a diagnosis of fetal hypoxia or asphyxia. The fetal blood sample is obtained from the presenting part (scalp or buttock) during labor. The instrumentation and technique of fetal blood collecting are described in many standard textbooks. In this brief discussion, mention is made of the indications for sampling as well as the prognostic significance of values obtained.

Although a full set of blood gas determinations (pH, carbon dioxide pressure [P_{CO_2}] and oxygen pressure [P_{O_2}]) can be done on as little as 0.25 ml of blood, most institutions obtain a minimal amount of blood for pH determination. Having the pH value alone does not allow differentiation between respiratory and metabolic acidosis. Treatment of the causes of acidosis is theoretically different. Metabolic acidosis requires immediate delivery, whereas respiratory acidosis should respond to standard resuscitation. In reality, the initial resuscitation measures (oxygen for the mother, uterine displacement, intravenous fluid bolus) generally are begun immediately with any severe deceleration. If a deceleration does not respond quickly to resuscitation, the clinical situation (stage of labor, presence of meconium, estimated fetal weight, gestation age, parity, etc.) will determine whether fetal scalp sampling is needed or if immediate delivery is necessary.

In human newborns, there is good correlation between the pH of scalp blood taken shortly before delivery and that of umbilical cord samples. Beard et al.,[36] correlating scalp blood pH and 2-minute Apgar scores, showed that a scalp pH above 7.25 was associated with an Apgar score greater than 7 in 92% of infants. When the scalp pH was less than 7.15, the Apgar score was less than 6 in 80% of cases. Fetal heart rate deceleration also has been found to correlate with pH values (Table 8-5).[37] This correlation is not always close, so fetal scalp sampling is used when any question exists about the fetal heart rate tracing.

TABLE 8-5

Correlation of Fetal Scalp pH and Fetal Heart Rate Pattern

Deceleration Pattern	Scalp pH
Early, mild variable	7.30 ± 0.04
Moderate variable	7.26 ± 0.04
Mild, moderate late	7.22 ± 0.06
Severe late, variable	7.14 ± 0.07

Data from Kubli FW, Hon EW, Khazin AF, et al: Observations on heart rate and pH in the human fetus during labor, *Am J Obstet Gynecol* 1969; 104:1190.

Other fetal heart rate patterns signal the need for fetal scalp sampling in addition to persistent late decelerations:

1. Absent or decreased short-term variability, which might be due to CNS depressants given to the mother
2. Variable deceleration when combined with reduced or absent short-term variability
3. Severe, persistent, variable decelerations.

The clinical situation provides indications for fetal scalp sampling, especially if there is decreased variability or severe deceleration.

Pulse Oximetry

Reflectance pulse oximetry is a refinement of conventional pulse oximetry, which requires transmitted light and provides a noninvasive method to assess fetal oxygenation. A study by Dildy et al.[38] demonstrated in healthy parturients in labor, when the sensor was placed between the cevix and the fetal presenting part, that a significant correlation existed between fetal oxygen saturation and umbilical vein saturation and pH, as well as umbilical artery pH. The relationship of umbilical artery pH and saturation to fetal oxygen saturation was not significant. The range of the values was large: for a fetal oximetry value of 60%, the umbilical vein saturation ranged from 30% to 70% and the pH from 7.25 to 7.38. Values for fetal pulse oximetry varied from 40% to 90% when, with delivery, the umbilical vein pH generally was greater than 7.24. Although there were statistical correlations, the wide range of values suggests a low specificity of the oximeter. In another study, fetal oxygen saturation was measured after giving a parturient supplemental oxygen and found a rise in fetal oxygen saturation; however, one third of the patients were excluded because of poor signal quality. Even more patients were excluded because of caput formation, fetal anemia, and meconium staining. Dildy et al.[38] studied 73 healthy parturients in labor and were unable to obtain a reliable signal 50% of the time. These preliminary studies suggest that there are still technical problems to be overcome, and as a result, the oximeter is not yet a useful clinical tool.

Summary

The reduction of perinatal morbidity and mortality is the sole purpose of fetal assessment, which spans the three trimesters of gestation. Chromosomal and developmental abnormalities are the focus of first- and early second-trimester studies. During the late and third trimesters, the emphasis shifts to causes of asphyxia and hypoxia. These problems tend to occur more frequently in parturients who have underlying diseases such as diabetes, PIH, drug addiction, malnutrition, and obesity. The important fetal assessments tests are as follows:

I. ANTEPARTUM
   A. NST
   B. Oxytocin challenge test
   C. Biophysical profile
   D. Fetal lung maturity test
II. INTRAPARTUM
   A. Fetal heart rate
   B. Scalp pH, P_{CO_2}, P_{O_2}

References

1. Friede A, Rochat R: Maternal mortality and perinatal mortality: definitions, data and epidemiology. In Sachs B, editor: *Clinical obstetrics,* Littleton, MA, 1985, PSG.
2. Vital Statistics of the United States, vol 2. Mortality, 1986. US Department of Health and Human Services, Public Health Services, Washington, DC, 1988.
3. Centers for Disease Control: Contribution of birth defects to infant mortality: United States, 1986, *MMWR* 1989; 38:633.
4. Lammer EJ, Brown LE, Anderka MT, Guyer B: Classification and analysis of fetal deaths in Massachusetts, *JAMA* 1989; 261:1757.
5. Mersey Region Working Party on Perinatal Mortality: Perinatal health. *Lancet* 1982; 1:491.
6. Patrick J, Campbell K, Carmichael L, et al: Patterns of gross fetal body movements over 24-hour observation intervals during the last 10 weeks of pregnancy, *Am J Obstet Gynecol* 1982; 142:363.
7. Sarokin Y, Dierker L: Fetal movement, *Clin Obstet Gynecol* 1982; 25:719.
8. Neldam S: Fetal movements as an indicator of fetal well being, *Lancet* 1980; 1:1222.
9. Rayburn W: Antepartum fetal assessment, *Clin Perinatol* 1982; 9:231.
10. Liston R, Cohen A, Mennui M, Gabbe S: Antepartum fetal evaluation by maternal perception of fetal movement, *Obstet Gynecol* 1982; 60:424.
11. Working Party on Amniocentesis: An assessment of the hazards of amniocentesis, *Br J Obstet Gynecol* 1978; 85(suppl):12.
12. Taber A, Philip J, Madsen M, et al: Randomised, controlled trial of genetic amniocentesis in 4606 low-risk women, *Lancet* 1986; 1:1287.
13. Jackson LG, Zachary JM, Fowler SE, et al: A randomized comparison of transcervical and transabdominal chorionic villus sampling, *N Engl J Med* 1992; 327:594.
14. Burton BK, Schulz CJ, Burd LI: Limb anomalies associated with chorionic villus sampling, *Obstet Gynecol* 1992; 79:726.
15. Manni G, Ibba RM, Lai R, et al: Limb-reduction defects and chorionic villus sampling, *Lancet* 1991; 337:1091.
16. Mahoney MJ: Limb abnormalities and chorionic villus sampling, *Lancet* 1991; 337:1422.
17. Shulman LP, Elias S: Percutaneous umbilical blood sampling, fetal skin sampling and fetal liver biopsy, *Semin Perinatol* 1990; 14:56.
18. Saari-Kemppainen A, Karjalainen O, Ylostalo P, et al: Ultrasound screening and perinatal mortality: controlled trial of systemic one-stage screening in pregnancy—the Helsinki Ultrasound Trial, *Lancet* 1990; 336:387.
19. Ewigman B, LeFevre M, Hesser J: A randomized trial of routine prenatal ultrasound, *Obstet Gynecol* 1990; 176:189.
20. Bekketeig LS, Eik-Nes SH, Jacobsen G, et al: Randomised controlled trial of ultrasonographic screening in pregnancy, *Lancet* 1984; 2:207.

21. Ewigman B, Crane JP, Frigoletto FD, et al: Effect of prenatal ultrasound screening on perinatal outcome, *N Engl J Med* 1993; 329:821.

22. Campbell S, Warsof S, Little D, et al: Routine ultrasound screening for the prediction of gestational age, *Obstet Gynecol* 1985; 65:613.

23. Kurtz A, Wapner R, Kurtz R, et al: Analysis of biparietal diameter as an accurate indicator of gestational age, *J Clin Ultrasound* 1980; 8:319.

24. Russell JC, Cooper CM, Ketchum CH, et al: Multicenter evaluation of TDx test for assessing fetal lung maturity, *Clin Chem* 1989; 35:1005.

25. Manning FA, Morrison I, Harmon CR, et al: Fetal assessment by fetal BPS: experience in 19,221 referred high-risk pregnancies II: the false negative rate by frequency and etiology, *Am J Obstet Gynecol* 1987; 157:880.

26. Baskett TF, Allen AC, Gray JH, et al: The biophysical profile score, *Obstet Gynecol* 1987; 70:357.

27. Platt LD, Eglington GS, Scorpios L, et al: Further experience with the fetal biophysical profile score, *Obstet Gynecol* 1983; 61:480.

28. Schiffrin BS, Guntes V, Gergely RC, et al: The role of real-time scanning in antenatal fetal surveillance, *Am J Obstet Gynecol* 1981; 140:525.

29. Manning FA, Baskett TF, Morrison I, et al: Fetal biophysical profile scoring: a prospective study in 1184 high-risk patients, *Am J Obstet Gynecol* 1981; 140:289.

30. Manning FA, Morrison I, Lange IR, et al: Fetal assessment based on fetal biophysical profile scoring: experience in 12,620 referred high-risk pregnancies I. Perinatal mortality by frequency and etiology, *Am J Obstet Gynecol* 1985; 151:343.

31. Schiffrin BS: The rationale for antepartum fetal heart rate monitoring, *J Reprod Med* 1979; 23:213.

32. Keegan KA, Paul RH: Antepartum fetal heart rate testing IV: The nonstress test as a primary approach, *Am J Obstet Gynecol* 1980; 136:75.

33. Evertson LR, Gauthier RJ, Collea JV: Fetal demise following negative contraction stress test, *Obstet Gynecol* 1978; 51:671.

34. Ott WJ: Antepartum biophysical evaluation of the fetus, *Perinatal Neonatal* 1978; 2:11.

35. Saling E, Schneider D: Biochemical supervision of the foetus during labor, *J Obstet Gynecol Br Common* 1967; 74:799.

36. Beard RW, Morris ED, Clayton SE: pH of fetal capillary blood as an indicator of the condition of the foetus, *J Obstet Gynecol Br Commonw* 1967; 74:812.

37. Kubli FW, Hon EW, Khazin AF, et al: Observations on heart rate and pH in the human fetus during labor, *Am J Obstet Gynecol* 1969; 104:1190.

38. Dildy GA, Clark SL, Loucks CA: Preliminary experience with intrapartum fetal pulse oximetry in humans, *Obstet Gynecol* 1993; 81:630.

9

Fetal Heart Rate Monitoring

A 28-year-old primigravida at term is admitted to the labor floor in active labor with a 5-cm dilation and 100% effacement of the cervix. Epidural analgesia is requested by her obstetrician to relieve her pain. What fetal heart pattern would be of concern to the anesthesiologist? Describe the different fetal heart rate patterns and their implications.

Recommendations by Ramon Martin, M.D., Ph.D.

In conjunction with fetal scalp sampling to measure acid-base balance, fetal heart rate (FHR) monitoring provides the main method of evaluating the fetus during the antepartum period as a part of nonstress testing, contraction stress testing, biophysical profile, and during labor and delivery. A review by Fenton and Steer[1] documents the historical use of FHR auscultation. First described by Marsac in 1650, a number of clinical studies have shown that perinatal morbidity and mortality are increased when the FHR is greater than 160 to 180 beats/min or less than 100 to 120 beats/min. Beginning in the 1940s, FHR was followed over a period of time as a more sensitive indicator of fetal well-being. This developed into continuous FHR monitoring, which charted beat-to-beat changes in the FHR.

Intermittent auscultation of the FHR is still a widely used means to monitor the fetus. In low-risk patients, this is done every 30 minutes, listening for 30 seconds during and after a contraction, when the parturient is in the first stage of labor and every 15 minutes during the second stage of labor. In high-risk patients, the frequency of listening is shortened to every 15 minutes during the first stage of labor and every 5 minutes during the second stage. Auscultation with a fetoscope or Doppler is able to detect changes in basal heart rate, variability, and decelerations in relation to uterine contractions. When abnormalities are noticed, either fetal scalp sampling and/or continuous FHR monitoring is indicated.

Continuous FHR monitoring entails measuring each fetal heart beat as well as the interval between two beats, calculating the FHR, and then plotting each successive rate. This can be done externally on the mother's abdomen with a Doppler ultrasound, a phonocardiographic monitor, or an electrocardiogram. An electrode, which is attached to the fetal scalp after rupture of the amniotic membranes, provides an internal or direct recording of FHR. Similarly, uterine contractions are measured either externally with a tocodynamometer or internally with a saline-filled catheter placed into the uterine cavity.

Fetal Heart Rate Patterns

The FHR pattern is characterized by its baseline between contractions and periodic changes in association with uterine contractions.[2] The baseline and periodic changes are further broken down into FHR and variability. This section considers the baseline FHR and its variants as well as variability.

Fetal heart rate is normal from 120 to 160 beats/min between contractions (Fig. 9-1). Rates greater than 160 beats/min are described as tachycardia

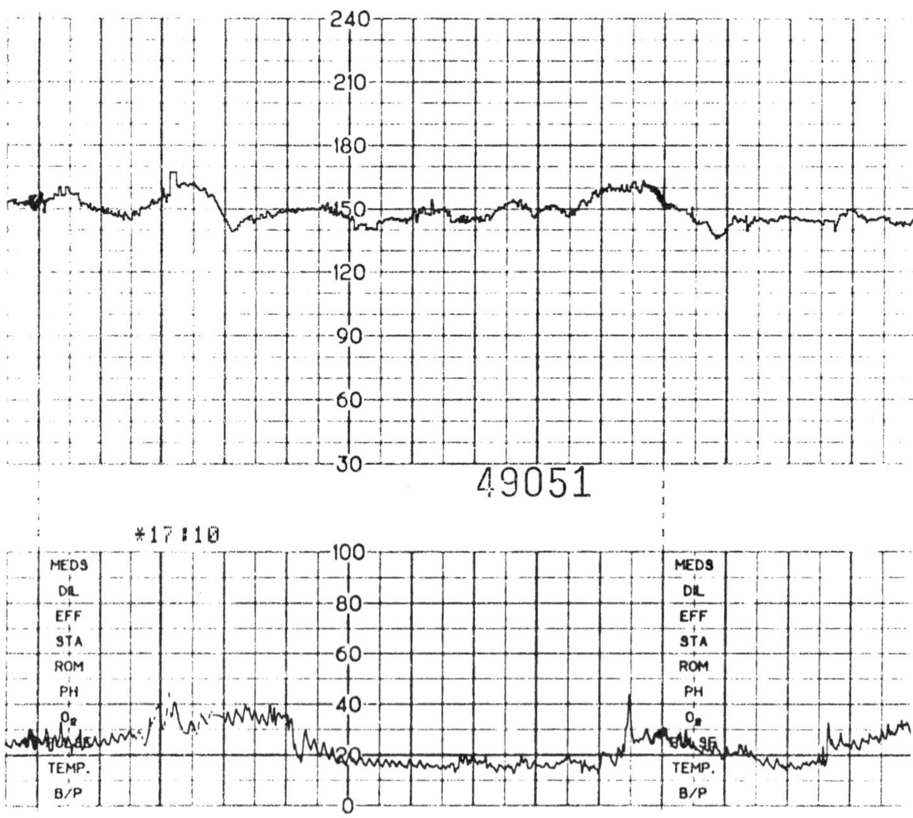

Fig. 9-1.
Normal heart rate pattern. The heart rate (140 beats/min) and short-term and long-term variability are normal. There are no periodic changes.

(Fig. 9-2) and those less than 120 beats/min as bradycardia. If the alteration in rate is less than 2 minutes in duration, it is called either an acceleration or a deceleration.

The usual, initial response of the normal fetus to acute hypoxia or asphyxia is bradycardia. A heart rate between 100 and 120 beats/min might signify either a compensated, mild hypoxic stress or may be idiopathic and benign. When the heart rate falls below 60 beats/min the fetus is in distress and requires either reversal of the cause of the bradycardia or emergency delivery. Other causes of bradycardia that are nonasphyxic in origin are bradyarrhythmias, maternal drug ingestion (especially β-blockers), and hypothermia. Tachycardia is occasionally seen with fetal asphyxia or with recovery from asphyxia, but is more likely seen secondary to the following:

- Maternal or fetal infection, especially chorioamnionitis
- Maternal ingestion of β-mimetic or parasympathetic blockers
- Tachyarrhythmias
- Prematurity
- Thyrotoxicosis

Variability in the FHR tracing describes the irregularity or the difference in interval from beat to beat. If the interval between heart beats were

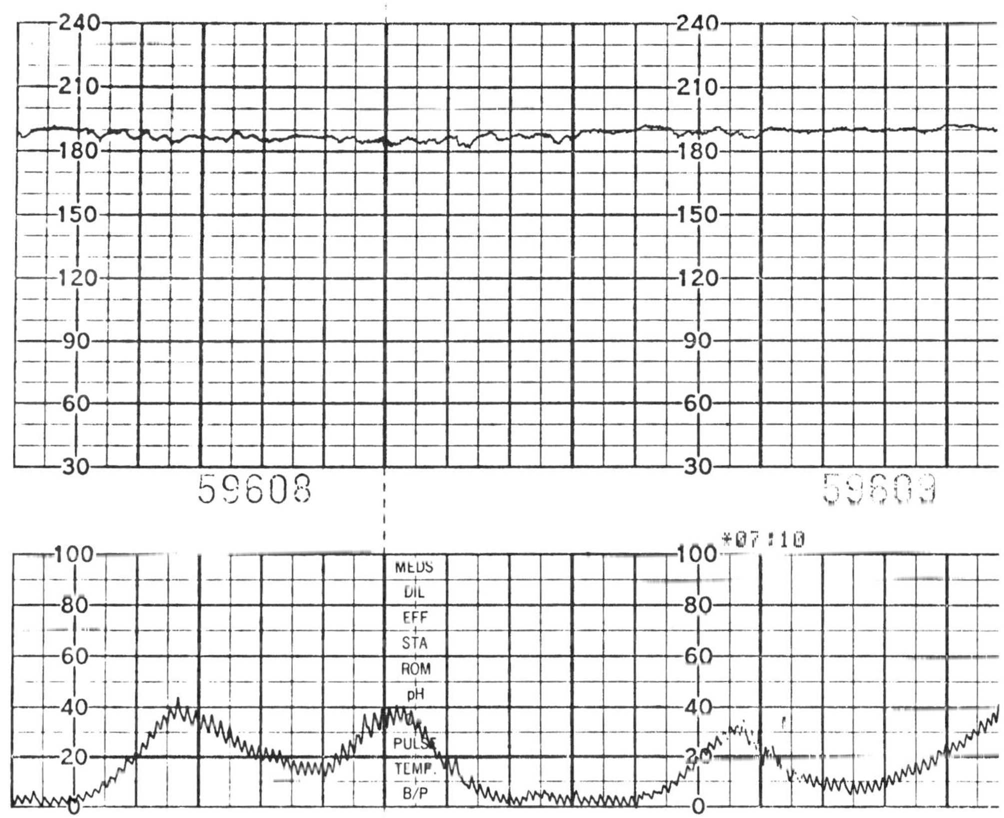

Fig. 9-2.

Tachycardia. In this case there was a maternal fever secondary to chorioamnionitis.

identical, then the tracing would be smooth (Fig. 9-3). In most healthy fetuses, one notes an irregular line. This is thought to be secondary to an intact nervous pathway through the cerebral cortex, midbrain, vagus nerve, and cardiac conduction system. It is thought that when asphyxia affects the cerebrum, there is decreased neural control of the variability. This is made worse by the failure of fetal hemodynamic compensatory mechanisms to maintain cerebral oxygenation. So with normal variability, irrespective of the FHR pattern, the fetus is not experiencing cerebral anoxia.

Variability is described as being either short term or long term. Short-term variability is the beat-to-beat difference, and it requires accurate detection of the heart rate. Because this can only be obtained with the fetal electrocardiogram, external monitors cannot be used to describe short-term variability, which is characterized as either present or absent. Long-term variability looks at a wider window of the FHR, between 3 and 6 minutes. It can be detected using either internal or external methods of FHR monitoring and is described by the approximate amplitude range in beats per minute as one of the following:

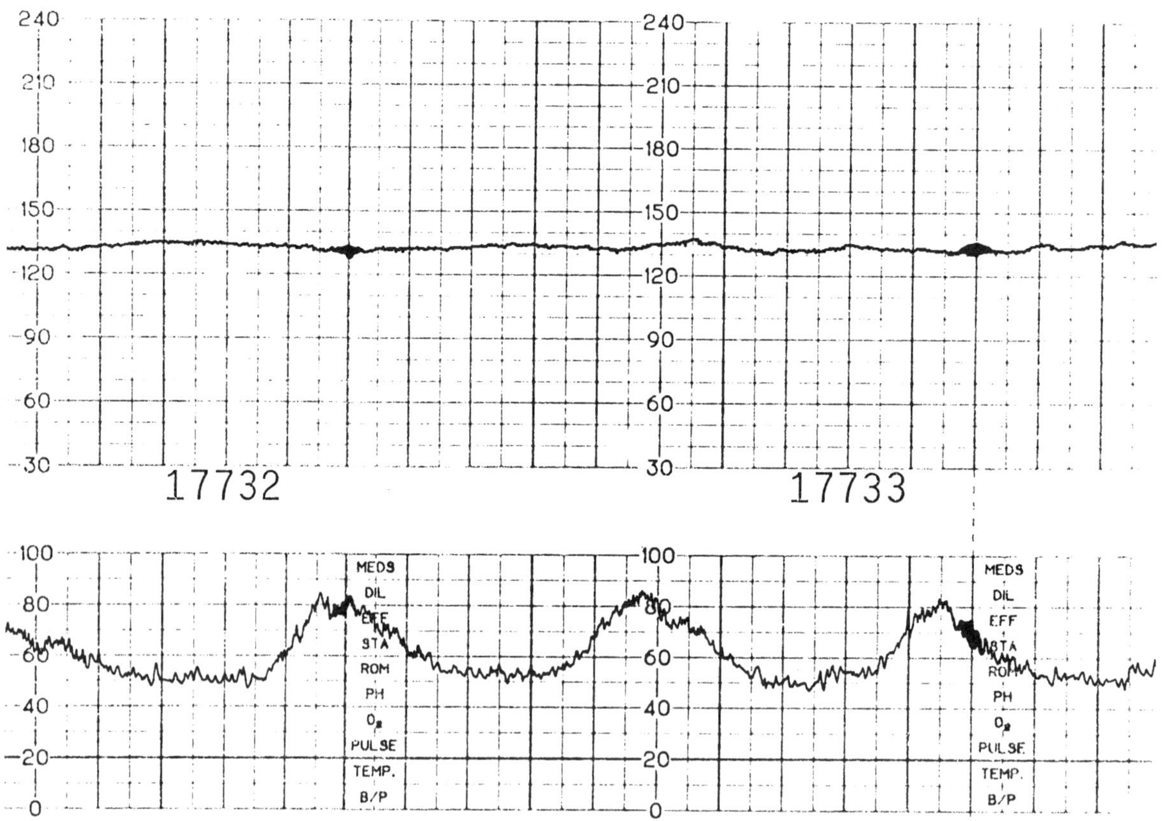

Fig. 9-3.
Decreased variability of the FHR.

1. *Normal*—the amplitude range is 6 beats/min or greater
2. *Decreased*—the amplitude range is between 2 and 6 beats/min
3. *Absent*—the amplitude range is less than 2 beats/min
4. *Saltatory*—the amplitude is greater than 25 beats/min. In addition to asphyxia, there are other causes of altered variability such as anencephaly, fetal drug effect (secondary to morphine, meperidine, diazepam, and magnesium sulfate), vagal blockade (due to atropine or scopolamine), and interventricular conduction delays (complete heart block).

Periodic changes in FHR occur in association with uterine contractions. Early accelerations occur concomitantly with a uterine contraction. They have a smooth contour and are a mirror image of the contraction (Fig. 9-4). The descent of the FHR is usually never more than 20 beats/min below the baseline. The cause is presumed to be due to a vagal reflex caused by a mild hypoxia, but is not associated with fetal compromise. Late decelerations also are smooth in contour and mirror the contrac-

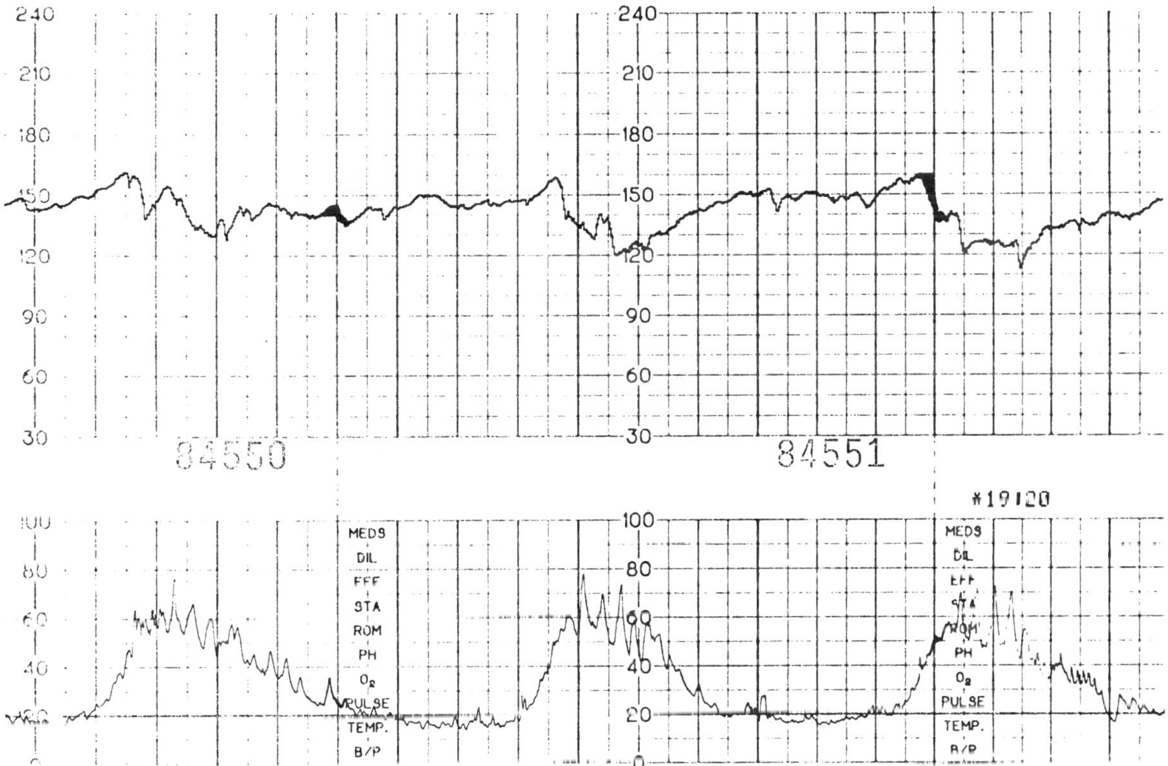

Fig. 9-4.
Early decelerations.

tion, but they begin 10 to 30 seconds after the onset of the contraction (Fig. 9-5). The depth of the decline is inversely related to the intensity of the contraction. Late decelerations have been classified as either reflex or nonreflex. Reflex late decelerations are due to maternal hypotension, which acutely decreases uterine perfusion to an otherwise healthy fetus. A uterine contraction on top of this insult further reduces oxygen flow, causing cerebral hypoxia, which then leads to the deceleration. In between contractions the FHR returns to baseline with good variability. The nonreflex late deceleration is due to prolonged hypoxia that leads to myocardial depression. Cerebral function also is depressed. This is seen with preeclampsia, intrauterine growth retardation, and prolonged repetitive late decelerations. Variability in FHR is either decreased or absent.

Variable decelerations differ in duration, shape, and decrease in FHR from contraction to contraction. The abrupt onset and cessation of the deceleration are thought to be due to increased vagal firing in response to compression of either the umbilical cord (during early labor) or dural stimulation with head compression (during the second stage of labor). The vagal activity causes bradycar-

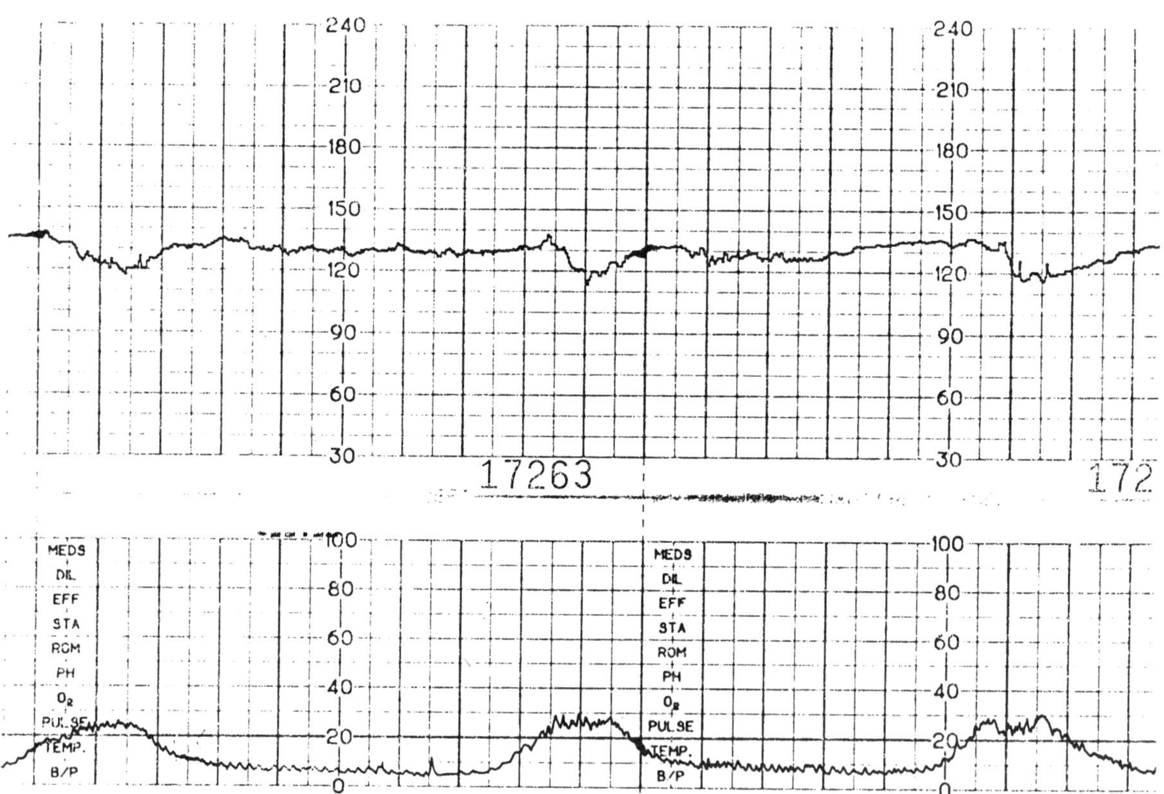

Fig. 9-5.
Late decelerations with decreased variability of the FHR between contractions.

dia, which decreases cardiac output as well as umbilical blood flow. Variable decelerations are described as severe when they (1) fall to 60 beats/min below the baseline FHR or (2) last longer than 60 seconds (Fig. 9-6). Otherwise they are classified as mild to moderate (Fig. 9-7). The normal fetus generally is able to tolerate mild-to-moderate variable decelerations for prolonged periods of time; however, severe variable decelerations eventually result in fetal compromise unless reversed.

Accelerations with uterine contractions represent the greater effect of sympathetic activity over the parasympathetic nervous system (Fig. 9-8). They indicate a reactive, healthy fetus and have a good prognostic significance.

The components of FHR described earlier comprise a normal pattern of a baseline rate of 120 to 160 beats/min, which has a variability of greater than 6 beats/min. One can see either no decelerations, early decelerations, or accelerations with contractions. This is associated with a good fetal outcome (i.e., Apgar score $>$ 7 at 5 minutes).[2,3] Depending on the severity and duration of the stress, other FHR patterns can be seen.

The acute stress pattern is a compensatory reac-

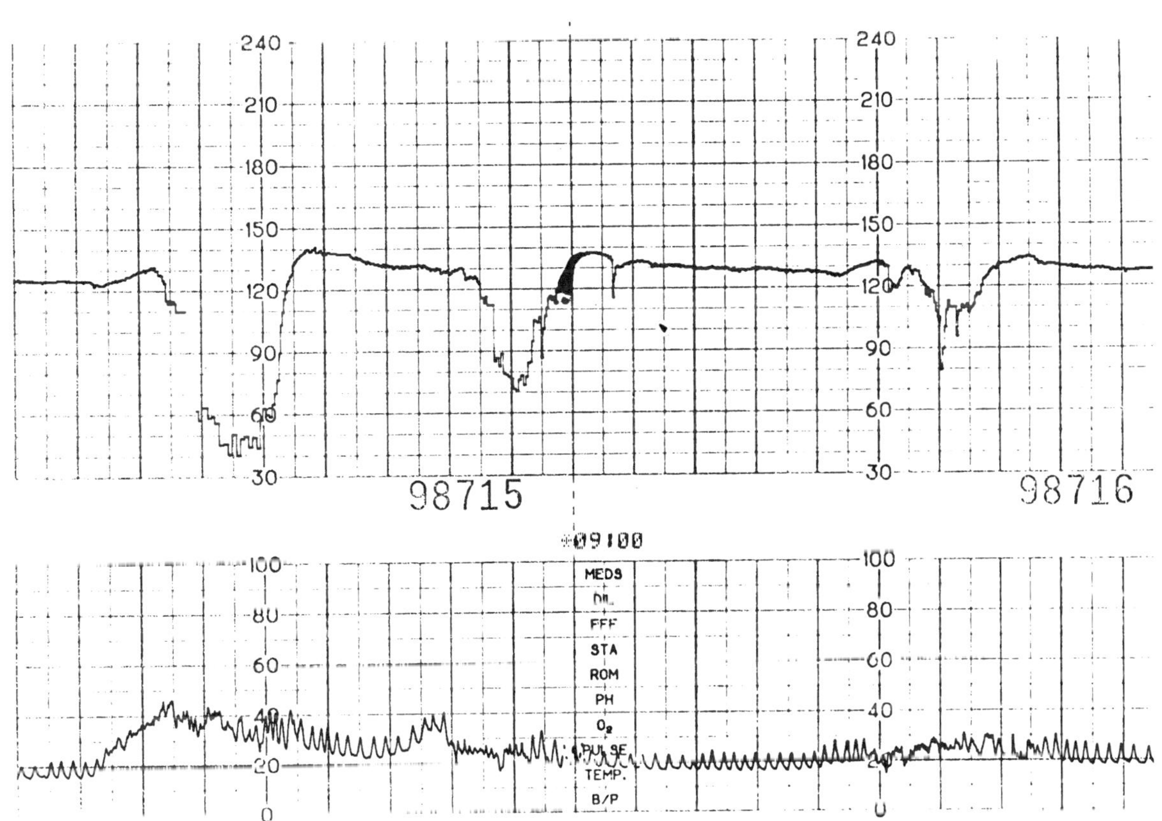

Fig. 9-6.
Severe, deep, variable decelerations with decreased variability of the FHR between contractions.

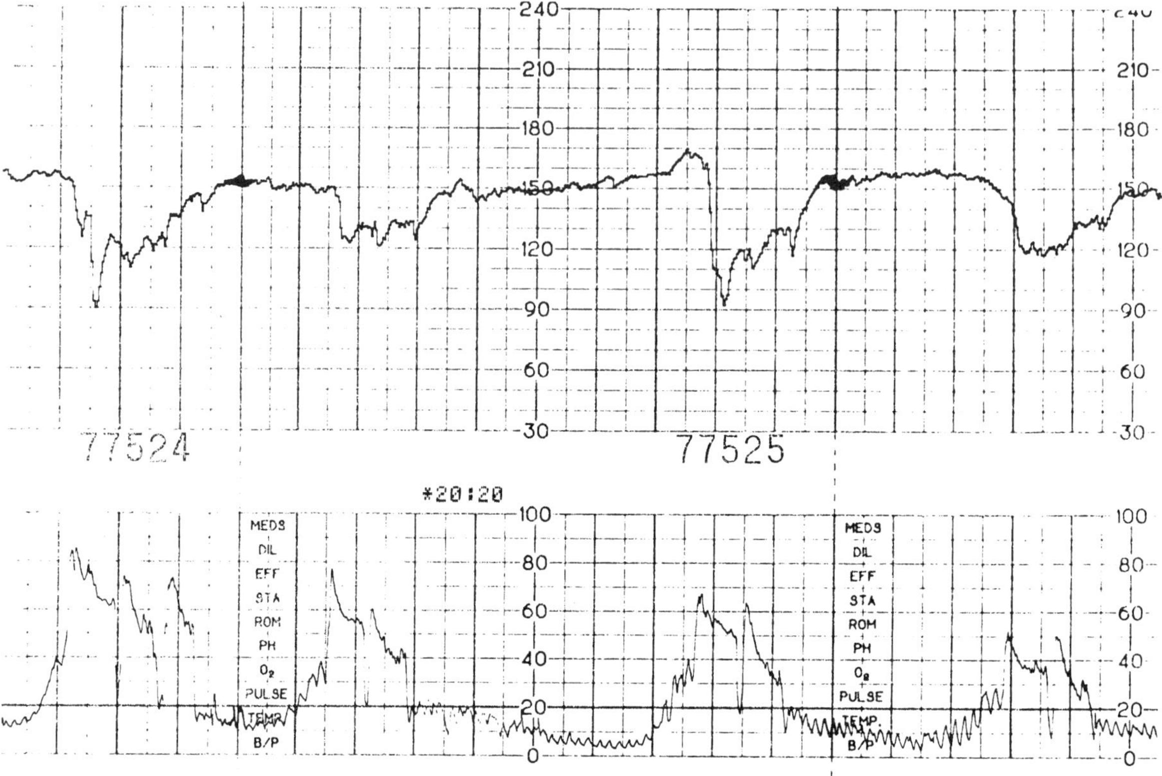

Fig. 9-7.
Mild-to-moderate variable decelerations with pushing during the second stage of labor.

tion in an otherwise healthy fetus to a short-lived period of asphyxia or hypoxia. The FHR usually demonstrates bradycardia, although tachycardia also is seen; however, the most important fact is that variability remains normal. There can be either late or variable decelerations. The fetal outcome is generally good[4] because the impact of the asphyxia is brief, with possible depression from carbon dioxide narcosis, which is rapidly reversible.

When the stress persists, bradycardia is more profound and is associated with decreased variability, as well as late and/or deep variable decelerations. This is a prolonged stress pattern that indicates mounting hypoxic damage to the heart and brain, resulting in the loss of compensatory mechanisms. Unless corrected, fetal death in utero can occur.

For a growth-retarded fetus, already compromised by a placenta with marginal function, persistent asphyxia results in a sinister pattern that is characterized by absent variability. The FHR displays severe variable or late decelerations, with a smooth rather than abrupt decrease and recovery in heart rate. Persistent bradycardia without variability also is called sinister.

Treatment of Fetal Heart Rate Patterns

The first step in treatment is to recognize and describe an abnormal FHR pattern. Then the cause

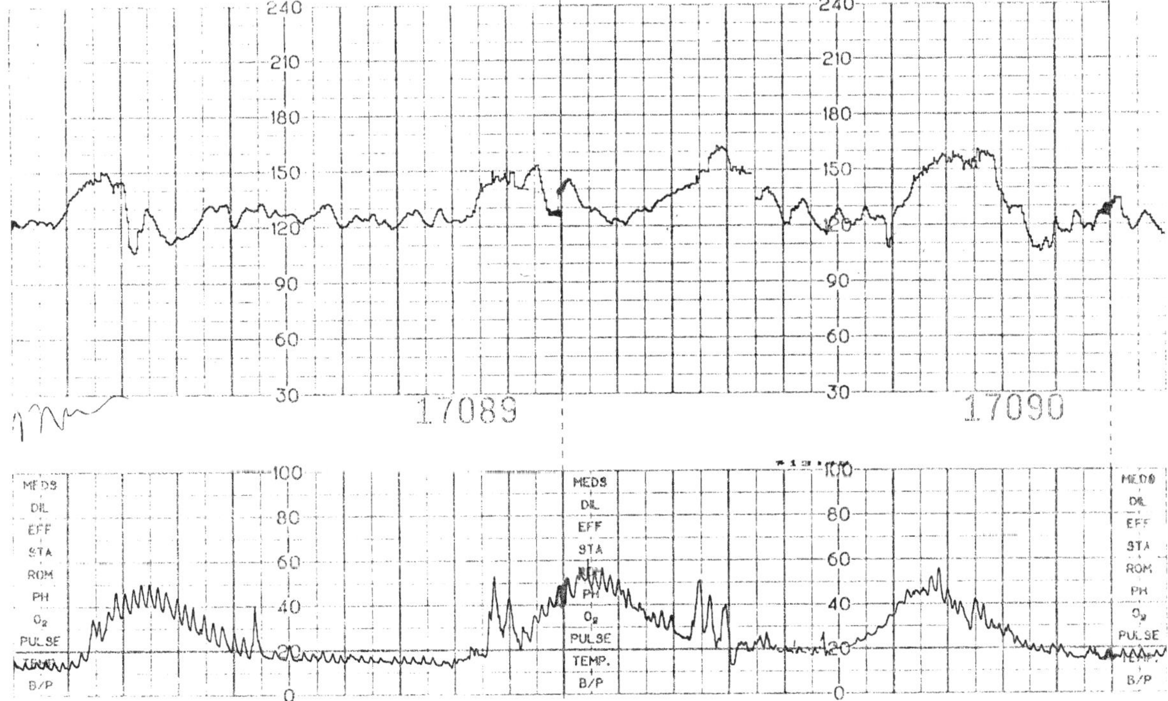

Fig. 9-8.

Accelerations with uterine contractions.

must be identified, and it should be corrected as quickly as possible. Causes and treatment of FHR patterns are presented in Table 9-1. If the pattern does not improve with these measures, then one needs to get more direct evidence of the fetal status (i.e., fetal scalp sampling) or deliver the fetus immediately.

Summary

Electronic FHR monitoring is now an important part of fetal assessment during the antepartum period. Its use to diagnose fetal distress, whether acute or chronic, has directly affected labor-and-delivery practice to decrease fetal morbidity and mortality. A review of the literature over the last 10 years, however, suggests that electronic monitoring has poor sensitivity in identifying morbidity and limited sensitivity in predicting its absence.[5] To determine if neonatal neurologic damage could be correlated with FHR tracing, this review looked at 10 studies and found the following:

1. There were several definitions of FHR patterns, making a comparison of data from various centers difficult.
2. FHR patterns had a poor predictive value on outcome.
3. A significant number of neonates with poor outcome had no monitoring abnormalities.
4. Monitoring FHR did not lead to effective treatment that had a significant impact on neonatal morbidity.

Although electronic FHR monitoring has been used for longer than 30 years, there is no standard

TABLE 9-1

TREATMENT OF FETAL HEART RATE PATTERNS

Pattern	Cause	Treatment
Bradycardia, late decelerations	Hypotension	IV fluids, ephedrine, change position
	Uterine hyperstimulation	Decrease oxytocin
Variable decelerations	Umbilical cord compression	Change position
	Head compression	Continue pushing if variability good
Late decelerations	Decreased uterine blood flow	Change position, O_2 for mother
Decrease in variability	Prolonged asphyxia	Change position, O_2 for mother

IV, Intravenous; O_2, oxygen.

associating brain damage with a specific FHR tracing. Currently no study has demonstrated that FHR monitoring either predicts or prevents neurologic morbidity. This does not deny the fact that electronic FHR monitoring is without merit. Rather, it needs to be further refined, standardized, and applied to particular clinical situations where physiologic correlations are possible.

The following are important aspects of fetal monitoring:

I. FHR
  A. Baseline
II. VARIABILITY
  A. Long term
  B. Short term
III. PERIODICITY IN RELATION TO UTERINE CONTRACTIONS
  A. Accelerations
  B. Decelerations

References

1. Fenton AN, Steer CM: Fetal distress, *Am J Obstet Gynecol* 1962; 83:354.
2. Hon EH, Quilligan EJ: The classification of fetal heart rate, *Conn Med* 1967; 31:779.
3. Schiffrin BS, Dame L: Fetal heart rate patterns: prediction of Apgar score, *JAMA* 1972; 219:1322.
4. Krebs HB, Petres RE, Dunn LJ, et al: Intrapartum fetal heart rate monitoring I: classification and prognosis of fetal heart rate patterns, *Am J Obstet Gynecol* 1979; 133:762.
5. Rosen MG, Diskensen JC: The paradox of electronic fetal monitoring: more data may not enable us to predict or prevent infant neurologic morbidity, *Am J Obstet Gynecol* 1993; 168:745.

10

Perinatal Pharmacology

The board examiner asks the candidate if the drugs used for obstetric pain relief cross the placenta to the fetus. The candidate answers, "Yes." The examiner responds, "Let us talk about placental transfer of drugs and disposition in the fetus and newborn."

Recommedations by Gerald A. Burger, M.D., Captain, Medical Corps, U.S. Navy

Placental Transfer: One Part of the Big Picture

The placental transfer of drugs is one facet of a much broader field of study: perinatal pharmacology. Perinatal pharmacology deals with the disposition and effects that chemical compounds (endogenous or exogenous) have on the mother and developing fetus from the time of conception until the end of the neonatal period (28 days of life). All anesthesiologists who care for pregnant women are practicing perinatal pharmacologists. Various foreign substances (drugs) are administered to the mother with a careful eye toward preventing fetal and subsequent neonatal complications. A basic understanding of the ways in which these drugs may affect mother and child becomes not only helpful, but necessary to practice safely.

**The views expressed in this article are those of the author and do not reflect the official policy or position of the Department of the Navy, Department of Defense, or the United States Government.*

Direct and Indirect Drug Effects

Drugs may produce (1) direct fetal effects (alterations in fetal and neonatal physiology or behavior) or (2) indirect fetal effects (alterations in the in utero environment leading to compromised oxygen transfer from mother to fetus). Direct fetal effects are assumed to be proportional to the quantity of the drug transferred across the placenta, whereas indirect effects are the result of compromised uteroplacental perfusion and fetal hypoxia. The interrelationship of mother and fetus is modeled as the maternal-placental-fetal unit.

The Maternal-Placental-Fetal Unit

Drug disposition and effects are studied in a multicompartmented model, the maternal-placental-fetal unit (Fig. 10-1). The model consists of three basic compartments, each with anatomic, physiologic, and pharmacologic characteristics very different from the others.

Maternal Compartment

Whereas all maternal systems are altered by pregnancy, those most important for this discussion are (1) changes in the cardiovascular physiology supporting the fetus in utero and (2) the alterations that occur in the maternal distribution and elimination of drugs.

Increases in maternal blood volume (25% to 40%) and cardiac output (30% to 50%) support the rapidly growing uteroplacental circulation, which at term receives 10% of the maternal cardiac output (500 to 700 ml/min). The uteroplacental circulation is connected to the maternal circulation in a parallel fashion. The major portion of blood flow to the uterus is conducted through uterine arteries, which arise from the internal iliac arteries well below the pelvic brim. The arteries subdivide to form an arcuate plexus within the uterine muscle, giving rise to the less muscular spiral arteries that penetrate placental decidual tissue and open on end to bathe fetal vessels in the placenta. Venous drainage from the placenta follows a course similar to

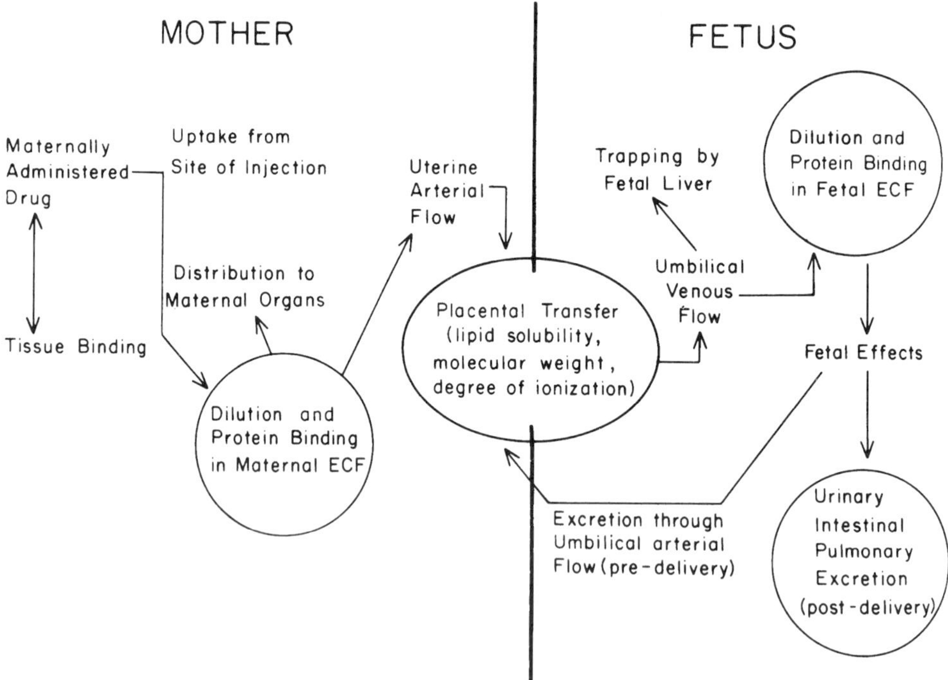

Fig. 10-1.

Perinatal drug transfer. *(From Ostheimer GW, editor:* Manual of obstetric anesthesia, *New York, 1984, Churchill-Livingstone.)*

the arteries emptying into the inferior vena cava. This complex supernumerary circulation is subject to many drug-induced alterations.

Increases in plasma volume of 40% to 50%, as well as an increase in total body water, lead to a relative decrease in the concentration of plasma proteins during pregnancy (decrease in milligrams per deciliter). While concentration of these proteins decreases, the total amount of protein during pregnancy actually increases (increase in total grams of serum protein). This absolute increase in serum protein causes an increase in the volume of distribution (V_d) for lipid-soluble drugs during pregnancy. Clearance for many drugs is increased during pregnancy (from increased renal blood flow and filtration), but not to as great an extent as V_d. The mismatch results in an increased half-life for many lipid-soluble drugs and leads to the persistence of the drug in the maternal tissues and increasing fetal exposure to the drug through availability for placental transfer. Unfortunately, many of the anesthetic drugs are very lipid soluble, falling within this category.

Placental Compartment

From a pharmacologist's point of view the placenta is a semipermeable membrane which drugs cross by simple diffusion, described by the Fick principle of diffusion. The placenta is considered pharmacologically inactive for anesthetic drugs.

Anatomically, the placenta is very complex. This disk-shaped intrauterine organ of gestation contains both maternal and fetal tissue functioning only to support the fetus. The maternal portion of the placenta forms the basal plate, which contains 180 to 320 spiral arteries as well as decidual tissue. The fetal portion forms the chorionic plate containing villi through which umbilical capillaries travel. The functional unit of the placenta is the *placentone,* which is defined as the intervillous space and chorionic villi perfused by a single spiral artery. The pattern of blood flow in the primate placenta is termed a villous-stream pattern, very different from other mammals. Maternal blood from the spiral arteries spurts into the intervillous space, bathing the chorionic villi that contain fetal umbilical capillaries. As with the maternal compartment, the physiologic character of the placental compartment is complex. Regulation of blood flow into the placenta from the mother and fetus is poorly understood. However, it is clear that only a portion of the placentones are functioning at one time. Notice that the human maternal and placental circulation is different from other species of mammals (including the sheep). For this reason, physiologic studies not done in humans or in primates may yield conclusions invalid in humans. Despite this limitation, much of what is preached as doctrine in obstetric anesthesia is the result of perinatal sheep research.

Fetal Compartment

The fetal compartment is very different physiologically and pharmacologically from the maternal side. The fetus must rely on the mother through the placenta for all of its support. Oxygenated blood from the placenta returns to the fetus by the single umbilical vein entering the body at the umbilicus. Fifty percent or more of this oxygenated blood is shunted through the ductus venosus directly into the inferior vena cava (IVC) while the remainder enters the portal circulation. From the IVC, blood flows into the right atrium (RA) where it mixes with poorly oxygenated blood returning from the upper torso and head. The majority of blood then passes into the left atrium via the foramen ovale into the left ventricle and into the aorta. Poorly oxygenated blood ultimately returns to the placenta via the paired umbilical arteries, which arise from the internal iliac arteries. Over 50% of the fetal cardiac output perfuses the placenta every minute.

The fetal circulatory pattern has a direct impact

on the fetal disposition of drugs transferred across the placenta. The pattern of fetal circulation in many instances actually minimizes the impact of a placentally transferred drug in the fetus through filtering and dilution.[1] Blood returning from the placenta that is shunted into the portal circulation is filtered by the fetal liver before perfusing other tissue. Whereas the fetus does not have a full complement of metabolizing enzymes, most (including the P-450 system) are present and will successfully inactivate foreign substances.[2] Additionally, blood entering the RA from the upper body tends to dilute any substances coming through the umbilical venous circulation. Some aspects of fetal drug uptake and distribution are not protective, however. Hepatic metabolism may be easily saturated in the fetus, leading to the accumulation of drugs in the fetus. Qualitative and quantitative differences in the tissue and serum protein binding affect V_d for most lipid soluble drugs, resulting in an increased plasma concentration of unbound or free drug in the fetus compared with the mother.[3] In addition, fetal tissue uptake follows a different pattern from maternal tissue uptake, allowing the fetus to concentrate drugs in sensitive systems such as the central nervous system and the cardiovascular system.[4] Renal function also may be immature, leading to decreased plasma clearance. Differences in the pH of fetal plasma compared with maternal plasma also may lead to *ion trapping* of drugs in the fetal circulation.[5,6]

Placental Transfer

For a drug to alter fetal physiologic makeup or neonatal behavior (direct effect), it must cross the placental membrane. This membrane separating maternal and fetal blood consists of three tissue layers: (1) trophoblastic epithelium on the surface of the chorionic villus, (2) connective tissue, and (3) fetal umbilical capillary endothelium. Compounds that are foreign to the body, like drugs, cross this lipid membrane by the process of simple diffusion. Important factors in the process of diffusion can be related by the Fick equation of simple diffusion:

$$Q/t = \frac{K \cdot A \cdot (C_{mat} - C_{fetal})}{D}$$

where

Q/t = Quantity transferred in a unit of time
K = Drug diffusion constant
A = Placental area for transfer
D = Diffusion distance across the membrane
$(C_{mat} - C_{fetal})$ = Concentration gradient of *free* drug across the placenta

The Fick equation assumes that only drug that is nonionized and not protein-bound (free drug) is transferred from mother to fetus. This assumption has been shown to be valid. The Fick equation also assumes that transfer across the placenta is ongoing and that equilibrium has not been achieved. For most anesthetic compounds with high lipid solubility and tissue binding (anesthetic gases not included), equilibrium is not attained during the course of drug administration. It is important to realize that *the Fick equation only describes the ease with which a drug is transferred, not the quantity transferred.*

Fick equation terms can be separated into three categories: the drug-diffusion constant, placental factors, and maternal-to-fetal gradient factors (Table 10-1).

The Drug-Diffusion Constant

Physicochemical properties of a drug greatly affect the ease of placental transfer. Substances with molecular weights greater than 500 daltons (da) cross the placenta with difficulty, and those with weights above 1000 Da do not cross. Most anesthetic drugs have molecular weights below 400 da and are subject to easy transfer. The dissociation constant (pKa) of a drug (pH at which 50% is ion-

TABLE 10-1
FICK EQUATION VARIABLES

Drug-Diffusion Constant (K)	Placental Factors (A and D)
Molecular weight	Placental area changes with disease
The pKa of drug	Diffuse distance changes with gestational age
Lipid solubility	

Maternal-Fetal Gradient (C_{mat} and C_{fetal})	
Maternal Free Drug Concentration	**Fetal Free Drug Concentration**
Dose administered	Concentration of drug in intervillous space
Site of administration	Alterations in fetal circulation due to asphyxia
Tissue distribution	Tissue distribution
Clearance of drug from body	Maternal transfer
Plasma pH	Clearance of drug from body
pKa, dissociation constant.	Plasma pH

Adapted from Ostheimer GW, editor: *Manual of obstetric anesthesia,* New York, 1984, Churchill-Livingstone.

ized and 50% nonionized) determines the fraction of a drug at plasma pH that is readily available for transfer across the placenta. For example, weak bases (local anesthetics) have pKa values close to the human body's pH, making a large proportion of drug available for transfer. The pKa is particularly important in placental transfer since pH differences frequently exist between maternal blood and fetal umbilical venous blood. Acidosis in the fetus can lead to accumulation of ionized drug in the fetus, a process known as *ion trapping.*[5]

Lipid solubility of a drug also is very important in determining the ease of placental transfer. Highly lipid-soluble compounds (thiopental or narcotics) are transferred very quickly despite unfavorable pKa values.[7] For lipid-soluble, low-molecular-weight, nonionized drugs (respiratory and anesthetic gases), (K) may approach infinity, making placental transfer limited only by placental perfusion. In that situation, uterine blood flow, not physical properties, is of greatest importance (see the following discussion).

Placental Factors

Placental factors are constant for any single maternal-placental-fetal unit. The area available for interface between maternal and fetal circulation averages 11 m^2 in the healthy parturient. Disease states of pregnancy (preeclampsia, diabetes, hypertension) can decrease this area, but the implications of these disease states on placental drug transfer remain unclear. However, we do know that these disease states reduce the area available for respiratory gas exchange, leading to a condition known as placental insufficiency. The distance that a drug must diffuse from the maternal to fetal circulations is 2 to 25 μ, depending upon gestational age. Early in gestation the distance is greater, leading to the assumption by some that the fetus may be protected in early gestation. Decreasing disease with maturity facilitates respiratory gas exchange and placental transfer of drugs, a mixed blessing to the fetus.

The Maternal-Fetal Gradient

One should recognize the striking pharmacokinetic and pharmacodynamic differences between maternal and fetal compartments. At the placental level, however, the pharmacokinetics are very simple. Only free drug (nonionized, nonprotein bound) will be transferred from mother to fetus. The free drug follows a concentration gradient. Factors that tend to change the amount of drug in the free state in both compartments may facilitate, retard, or reverse transfer of the drug to the fetus. The maternal-fetal gradient is a dynamic situation in which the mother initially may function as a drug donor and ultimately as a drug sink for the fetus, providing an efficient route of elimination for the drug. Interruption of fetal-to-maternal transfer of drug by birth leads to neonatal neurobehavioral drug effects.

Maternal free-drug concentration is dependent on the following:

- Dose of drug administered
- Site of administration (as seen with local anesthetic drugs in various tissue depots)
- Tissue distribution of the drug (tissue uptake will reduce circulating levels)
- Clearance of the drug from maternal plasma (metabolism and excretion of the drug will reduce free-drug levels since only free drug is available for clearance)

Fetal free-drug concentration is dependent on the following:

- Concentration of drug in the intervillous space (maternal free drug)
- The fraction of the umbilical venous flow entering the portal circulation. Normally 50% of umbilical venous flow is filtered through the portal circulation. Fetal hypoxemia decreases this percentage, leading to higher fetal blood levels
- The extent of dilution in the right atrium. Blood returning from the gut, upper torso, and head may dilute umbilical venous blood
- Tissue distribution since tissue uptake differs from that of mother in extent and site
- Maternal transfer (occurs when $C_{fetal} > C_{mat}$).
- Elimination through fetal renal clearance into the amniotic fluid.

Qualitative and quantitative differences in drug protein binding between mother and fetus allow the fetus to accumulate a quantity of active drug greater than that present in the mother. Fetal plasma protein binding is lower for many drugs (local anesthetics). If we measure the total plasma concentrations of a lipid-soluble drug like bupivacaine in the fetus and compare this value with maternal plasma concentration (fetal:maternal ratio) the ratio is 0.45. By this measurement this drug should be safer than a drug with a larger ratio (lidocaine ratio = 0.69) since transfer is less.[8] At equilibrium, however, whereas total plasma concentration may differ in the maternal artery, umbilical vein, and umbilical artery, free drug will be equal. Since free drug is the active form of the drug capable of causing an effect, protein binding appears to afford no margin of safety for one drug over another, as long as plasma binding sites are not saturated.

The factors that govern placental transfer of a drug, although important to discuss, remain difficult to study and nearly impossible to correlate clinically with fetal outcome. Direct drug effects on fetal-neonatal development caused by fetal tissue uptake are difficult to separate from the indirect effects that are discussed in the next section.

Drug Effects on Uteroplacental Circulation

In some situations a parenterally administered drug (ketamine) or an anesthetic technique (epidural analgesia or anesthesia) may create or contribute to fetal distress by altering uteroplacental perfusion. A decrease of uteroplacental perfusion reduces oxygen supply to the intervillous space and subsequently to the fetus. With little oxygen reserve (90 seconds in complete interruption of uteroplacental flow), it is not surprising that signs of fetal compromise (bradycardia) can follow a decrease in placental perfusion. In general, however, uteroplacental perfusion is luxuriant (50% more than needed) and fetal distress occurs because multiple factors have contributed to a substantial decrease in oxygen delivery.

Uteroplacental perfusion may be described by the equation:

$$\mathrm{UBF} = \frac{\mathrm{MAP} - \mathrm{UVP}}{\mathrm{UVR}}$$

where

UBF = Uteroplacental blood flow
MAP = Maternal mean arterial blood pressure

UVP = Uterine venous pressure

UVR = Uterine vascular resistance.

Many conditions (obstetric as well as anesthetic) can influence the terms of the above equation (Table 10-2). Common anesthetic alterations in uteroplacental blood flow include the following:

- Decreased MAP from sympathetic blockade in spinal or epidural anesthesia
- Decreased MAP and increased UVP from aortocaval compression during spinal or epidural anesthesia
- Increased UVR from high concentrations of local anesthetic (paracervical block)
- Increased UVR from intravenous ketamine (>2 mg/kg)

TABLE 10-2

FACTORS IN REDUCED UTEROPLACENTAL PERFUSION

Decreased Maternal Blood Pressure
Sympathetic blockade from spinal or epidural anesthesia
Aortocaval compression by the gravid uterus
Supine hypotensive syndrome
Increased Uterine Venous Pressure
Aortocaval compression by the gravid uterus
Uterine contractions (labor)
Hypertonic uterine contractions from
Abruptio placentae
Local anesthetic toxicity
Ketamine overdose
Oxytocin overdose
Increased Uterine Vascular Resistance
Chronic hypertension
Toxemia
Maternal hypoxemia
Maternal hypocarbia
Local anesthetic toxicity
Vasopressor agents

- Increased UVR from hypocarbia
- Increased UVR from hypoxemia

Whereas anesthetic drugs and techniques are responsible in some situations for aggravating fetal distress, maternal pathophysiologic characteristics and obstetric management more commonly are at fault. Among the factors listed in Table 10-2, aortocaval compression is the most common and the most preventable. All pregnant patients in the third trimester should be cared for in the left lateral decubitus position to ensure optimal uteroplacental perfusion. Maternal diseases certainly may reduce uteroplacental perfusion, making any additional decreases in placental flow from anesthetic drug or technique dangerous. This rationale frequently is used to defer elective obstetric anesthetic management. Although this reasoning cannot be faulted with our limited understanding of uteroplacental regulation, studies in Scandinavia (utilizing radioactive xenon washout techniques) have shown the placental perfusion in preeclampsia actually may be improved by cautious epidural analgesia.[9]

Regulation of uteroplacental perfusion is a very complex subject that is beyond the scope of this review. Our knowledge of this subject remains elementary due to difficulties in finding an animal model with placental structure similar to that of the human, and the ethical and legal issues involved in human study in the United States.

Assessing Direct Drug Effects in the Fetus and Neonate

Given a model as complex as the maternal-placental-fetal unit, it is not surprising that cause-and-effect relationships are difficult to demonstrate. Table 10-3 lists popular methods used to assess the direct effects that a drug may have on the fetus. Of the five methods listed, four are concerned with neonatal behavior and are termed *neurobehavioral assessments* (Apgar score, Brazelton Neonatal Behavioral Assessment score [NBAS], Early Neonatal Neurobehavioral Scale [ENNS], Neurologic and

TABLE 10-3
Assessment of Drug and Anesthetic Technique Effects in the Neonate

Apgar scores
Maternal-to-fetus ratio
Brazelton Neonatal Behavioral Assessment Score (NBAS)
Early Neonatal Neurobehavioral Scale (ENNS)
Neurologic and Adaptive Capacity Score (NACS)

Adaptive Capacity Score [NACS]). The fifth method (maternal-to-fetal ratio) is a pharmacologic determination of drug concentration in mother and fetus.

The fetal-to-maternal ratio is a frequently quoted value determined by the ratio of total fetal plasma drug concentration (usually an umbilical venous sample) divided by total maternal plasma concentration (usually a maternal venous sample) obtained at one point in the process of labor and delivery. Although popular, this technique does not give a valid determination of the quantity of drug transferred from mother to fetus unless equilibrium (umbilical venous concentration equals umbilical arterial concentration) has been obtained and free drug concentration, not total plasma concentration, is used as the measurement.[10] The Apgar score was developed by Virginia Apgar in the 1950s to focus attention in the delivery suite on the neonate. Its coarse physiologic measurements are designed to identify a neonate in need of resuscitation. Low Apgar scores suggest severe depression and intrauterine asphyxia rather than drug effect. The Apgar score is not sensitive enough to evaluate subtle drug effect on behavior.[11]

The NBAS was developed to assess the neonate's adjustment to the environment. It is a sensitive tool that can be used to assess subtle behavioral changes due to drug effect if other intrauterine variables have been controlled.[12] The NBAS is difficult to perform and tedious. Within the last 20 years, the ENNS and NACS have been developed to provide a simple, reproducible assessment of subtle drug effects.[13] So far none of these assessments has demonstrated a persistent effect of a properly used anesthetic drug in neonates.

Assessing Indirect Drug Effects in the Fetus and Neonate

Current techniques to assess uteroplacental perfusion include ^{133}Xe clearance; Doppler ultrasound flow velocity measurements of the umbilical and uterine arteries; and direct-flow probe measurement of uterine artery blood flow in the chronically instrumented, gravid ewe. Each of these techniques has significant drawbacks, making conclusions drawn from studies involving these techniques highly suspicious. Radioactive xenon clearance was developed by Reckonen et al. in Europe in the 1970s to measure uteroplacental perfusion.[14] Each determination involves a small but measurable dose of radiation. The fear of radiation exposure as well as cost has greatly limited the use of this technique.

Within the last 10 years analysis of Doppler ultrasound waveform velocities in uterine and umbilical vessels has been used to assess the impact of treatments and drugs on uteroplacental perfusion. The noninvasive technique involves the construction of Doppler flow systolic and diastolic waveforms for a vessel of interest. Changes in the waveforms with a treatment are said to reflect alterations in vascular resistance due to the treatment.[15] Doppler flow techniques provide only an indirect assessment of uteroplacental perfusion, require many assumptions, and are technically difficult to perform and reproduce.

Since the early 1970s, the laboratory preparation from the chronically instrumented pregnant ewe has provided most of the information we use clinically concerning drug effect on uteroplacental perfusion.[16] Its limitations include nonprimate placental structure, different physiologic response to many anesthetic drugs than would be seen in humans, and error induced by chronic instrumentation.

Despite our efforts in assessing uteroplacental perfusion, no practical method remains available for direct assessment in humans. We are forced to continue to rely on fetal heart rate changes, fetal pH changes, anecdotal reports, and the methods described earlier in this chapter to determine the potential for a drug or treatment to reduce uteroplacental perfusion in the pregnant human.

Effects of Anesthetic Drugs on the Fetus and Neonate

Our knowledge of the way in which a drug may affect the fetus or neonate is based on empiric observation rather than well-controlled study. Controlled studies are difficult to conduct in the gravid patient because of patient resistance, ethical considerations, legal concerns, wide variation in obstetric technique, and difficulty in the prepartum diagnosis of the fetus at risk for intrauterine asphyxia. For these reasons, we must realize that any information presented as fact concerning the way a specific drug interacts with the maternal-placental-fetal unit is subject to revision in the near future. Accepting this condition, we look at several classes of anesthetic drugs and consider their impact on the maternal-placental-fetal unit. It is helpful to organize thoughts about the impact of these drugs on the fetus by dividing their effects into direct effects (alterations in physiologic makeup and neurobehavior due to placental transfer) and indirect effects (alterations in fetal or neonatal physiologic makeup due to drug-induced fetal hypoxemia).

Anesthetic Induction Agents

The most commonly used induction agents in the United States are thiopental, ketamine, and recently, propofol.

Indirect Effects

Thiopental reduces uteroplacental perfusion about 20% by an undetermined mechanism at doses not affecting maternal blood pressure and cardiac output.[17] Most authors recommend a dose in the parturient of 4 mg/kg pregnant body weight to prevent significant changes in uteroplacental perfusion.

Ketamine is noted for its ability to maintain blood pressure, even in the face of hypovolemia. This salutary effect is the result of sympathetic nervous system support. Interestingly, ketamine has not been shown to decrease uteroplacental perfusion if intravenous doses are kept below 1.5 mg/kg. Doses in excess of this amount may trigger a tetanic uterine contraction, interrupting uteroplacental perfusion.[18]

Propofol does not appear to alter uteroplacental perfusion at doses of 2 mg/kg or less.

Direct Effects

Thiopental rapidly reaches peak concentrations in umbilical venous blood (within 1 minute). If the dose is kept at 4 mg/kg, Apgar scores are not affected. There is no advantage in delaying delivery to await maternal redistribution since the fetal brain receives very small amounts of the drug because of rapid hepatic clearance.[19]

Ketamine also rapidly crosses the placenta. In maternal doses less than 1 mg/kg, neurobehavioral scores appear better than those of infants delivered after a barbiturate induction. The better neurobehavioral score may be due to the neonatal central nervous system (CNS) stimulation. Increasing doses (more than 1 mg/kg) lead to neonatal neurobehavioral abnormalities.[20]

Propofol, although rapidly transferred across the placenta, appears to have little impact on neonatal neurobehavioral scores at moderate dosages.[21]

Inhalational Anesthetic Agents

Inhalational anesthetic agents may be used to produce complete analgesia or anesthesia. Most frequently the potent inhalational anesthetic drugs are used in analgesic concentrations to supplement a general anesthetic technique based on nitrous oxide. Direct and indirect effects depend on the amount of these agents administered. Potent agents (halothane, enflurane, and isoflurane) are considered separately from nitrous oxide.

Indirect Effects

Potent inhalational agents in analgesic concentrations have been shown to improve fetal oxygenation, presumably by decreasing uterine vascular resistance.[22] In anesthetic concentrations, decreases in maternal blood pressure and cardiac output lead to impaired uteroplacental perfusion that is proportional to the dose administered with a subsequent decrease in fetal oxygen tensions.

Nitrous oxide reduces oxygen delivery to the fetus by physically occupying space in the maternal alveolus. Concentrations of 50% or less are recommended in the parturient.

Direct Effects

Analgesic concentrations of the potent inhalational agents have been shown to have no neurobehavioral effect in the postdelivery period when used for cesarean section along with 50% nitrous oxide, even though their transfer is rapid across the placenta. Anesthetic concentrations of these agents reduce Apgar scores in proportion to length of administration.[23]

Nitrous oxide is rapidly transferred across the placenta, reaching equilibrium in the mother within 15 minutes. Maternal concentrations of 70% or more have been associated with low Apgar scores whereas concentrations of 50% of less are not.[24] Concerns about the teratogenicity of nitrous oxide have been raised from studies in animal embryos. Nitrous oxide exposure in the embryo appears to interfere with the function of the enzyme methionine synthetase leading to developmental abnormalities.[25] Currently the impact of this finding is unclear and is of little import to the developing human fetus exposed intermittently to nitrous oxide.

Muscle Relaxants

All muscle relaxants are quaternary ammonium compounds that are highly ionized at body pH and therefore slow to cross the placenta. Even so, some transfer occurs with detectable levels of both succinylcholine and the nondepolarizing agents present in fetal blood after cesarean delivery. Except in the case of overdose or congenital absence of pseudocholinesterase, direct fetal effects are not significant. In clinically useful doses, indirect effects of these drugs are insignificant. None of the muscle relaxants relax uterine muscle.

Narcotics

Narcotics are the most frequently used analgesic medications in obstetrics. Of the narcotics, meperidine is the most popular for labor analgesia. Narcotics may produce significant indirect and direct effects.[26]

Indirect Effects

Most prominent among narcotic side effects is respiratory depression, which may impair maternal oxygen-carrying capacity and compromise oxygen transfer to the fetus. Additionally, orthostatic hypotension is a side effect that may lead to decreased uteroplacental perfusion.

Direct Effects

Neonatal respiratory depression also is a common complication of maternal narcotic administration, leading to alterations in neurobehavioral and Apgar scores. Meperidine has been found to alter neurobehavioral scores for as long as 3 days after delivery due to its metabolism to two poorly metabolized, but CNS-active, compounds.[27] Narcotics also may alter fetal heart rate patterns in utero (meperidine decreases beat-to-beat variability).

Local Anesthetic Agents

Local anesthetic agents are widely used to provide both analgesia and surgical anesthesia in obstetrics. Their effects on uteroplacental blood flow and fetal neurobehavior remain controversial.

Indirect Effects

Local anesthetic agents may affect uteroplacental perfusion by virtue of their concentration in plasma, their local effect on blood vessel tone, or their ability to cause sympathetic blockade when used in spinal or epidural anesthesia. Systemic toxic reactions caused by high plasma levels of local anesthetic agent improperly administered lead to convulsions with concomitant maternal hypoxemia, acidosis, and hypercarbia. These conditions markedly reduce oxygen transfer to the fetus. Local anesthetic agents deposited in close proximity to the uterine arteries (as in paracervical block) may trigger vasospasm and uterine hypertonus, thus reducing placental perfusion. Spinal or epidural anesthesia may lead to maternal hypotension if poorly managed, thus decreasing uteroplacental perfusion. These unfortunate toxic effects can be avoided with careful use of these potentially lethal drugs.

Direct Effects

Local anesthetic agents cross the placenta easily after absorption from tissue depots. Equilibrium is slow to occur, making quantitative transfer difficult to measure. Controversy continues concerning the neurobehavioral consequences of local anesthetic transfer to the fetus. Controversial evidence exists regarding a small, evanescent (< 12 hours) local anesthetic effect on neonatal neurobehavior after epidural anesthesia using lidocaine and mepivacaine.[28] This has been refuted by other observers. Mepivacaine is no longer used for obstetric anesthesia because of its increased half-life in the fetus (9 hours) compared with that in the mother (3 hours).[29] Popular agents appear to be safe in concentrations transferred to the fetus from tissue depots.

Summary

1. Perinatal pharmacology is a complex, difficult, ever-evolving field of study.
2. A basic understanding of perinatal pharmacology is vitally important to the safe practice of obstetric anesthesia.

References

1. Finster M, Morishima HO, Boyes RN, et al: The placental transfer of lidocaine and its uptake by fetal tissues, *Anesthesiology* 1972; 36:159.
2. Dawkins MJ: Biochemical aspects of developing function in newborn mammalian liver, *Br Med Bull* 1966; 22:27.
3. Waddell WJ, Marlowe GC: *Disposition of drugs in the fetus.* In Mirkin BL, editor: *Perinatal pharmacology and therapeutics,* New York, 1976, Academic Press.
4. Mather LE, Long G, Thomas J: The binding of bupivacaine to maternal and fetal plasma proteins, *J Pharm Pharmacol* 1971; 23:359.
5. Brown WU Jr, Bell GC, Alper MH: Acidosis, local anesthetics and the newborn, *Obstet Gynecol* 1976; 48:27.
6. Morishima HO, Covino BG: Toxicity and distribution of lidocaine in non-asphyxiated and asphyxiated baboon fetuses, *Anesthesiology* 1981; 54:182.
7. Finster M, Morishima HO, Mark LC, et al: Tissue thiopental concentrations in the fetus and newborn, *Anesthesiology* 1972; 36:155.
8. Chantigian RC: *Pain relief and vaginal delivery.* In Ostheimer GW, editor: *Manual of obstetric anesthesia,* New York, 1992, Churchill Livingstone.
9. Jouppila P, Jouppila R, Hollmen A, et al: Lumbar epidural analgesia to improve intervillous flow during labor in severe pre-eclampsia, *Obstet Gynecol* 1982; 59:158.
10. Burger GA: *Obstetric anesthesia and uteroplacental blood flow.* In Ostheimer GW, editor: *Manual of obstetric anesthesia,* New York, 1992, Churchill-Livingstone.
11. Is the Apgar score outmoded? Lancet 1989; 1:591.

12. Brazelton TB: *Neonatal behavioral assessment scale*. In *Clinics in developmental medicine,* no. 50, London, 1973, Stastics Int Med Publ.
13. Amiel-Tison C, Barrier G, Shnider SM, et al: A new neurologic and adaptive capacity scoring system for evaluation of obstetric medications in full term newborns, *Anesthesiology* 1982; 56:340.
14. Rekonen A, Luotola H, Pitanen M, et al: Measurement of intervillous and myometrial blood flow by intravenous ^{133}Xe method, *Br J Obstet Gynaecol* 1976; 83:723.
15. Copel JA, Grannum PA, Hobbins JC, et al: *Doppler ultrasound in obstetrics.* In *Williams' obstetric,* suppl no. 16, Norwalk, CT, 1988, Appleton & Lange.
16. Ralston DH, Shnider SM, De Lorimar AA: Effect of equipotent ephedrine, metaraminol, mephentermine, and methoximine on uterine blood flow in the pregnant ewe, *Anesthesiology* 1974; 40:354.
17. Jouppila P, Kuika J, Hollmen A: Effect of induction of general anesthesia for cesarean section on intervillous blood flow, *Acta Obstet Gynaecol Scand* 1979; 58:249.
18. Marx GF, Hwang HS, Chandra P: Post partum uterine pressures with different doses of ketamine, *Anesthesiology* 1979; 50:163.
19. Morgan DJ, Blackman GL, Paull JD, et al: Pharmacokinetics and plasma binding of thiopental II. studies at cesarean section. *Anesthesiology* 1981; 54:474.
20. Janeczko GF, El-Etr AA, Younes S: Low-dose ketamine anesthesia for obstetrical delivery, *Anesth Analg* 1972; 51:41.
21. Dailland P, Cockshott ID, Lirzin JD, et al: Intravenous propofol during cesarean section: placental transfer, concentration in breast milk and neonatal effects: a preliminary study, *Anesthesiology* 1989; 71:827.
22. Palahniuk RJ, Shnider SM: Maternal and fetal cardiovascular and acid-base changes during halothane and isoflurane anesthesia in the pregnant ewe, *Anesthesiology* 1974; 41:462.
23. Warren TM, Datta S: Comparison of the maternal and neonatal effects of halothane, enflurane and isoflurane for cesarean delivery, *Anesth Analg* 1983; 62:516.
24. Datta S, Ostheimer GW, Weiss JB, et al: Neonatal effects of prolonged anesthetic induction for cesarean section, *Obstet Gynecol* 1981; 58:331.
25. Levinson G, Shnider SM: *Anesthesia for surgery during pregnancy.* In Shnider SM, Levinson G, editors: *Anesthesia for obstetrics,* Baltimore, 1993, Williams & Wilkins.
26. Chantigian RC: *Pain relief and vaginal delivery.* In Ostheimer GW, editor: *Manual of obstetric anesthesia,* New York, 1992, Churchill Livingstone.
27. Hodgkinson R, Hussain R: The duration of effect of maternally administered meperidine on neonatal behavior, *Anesthesiology* 1982; 56:51.
28. Brown WU Jr, Bell GC, Lurie AO, et al: Newborn blood levels of lidocaine and mepivacaine in the first post natal day following maternal epidural anesthesia, *Anesthesiology* 1975; 42:698.
29. Kuhnert BR: Effects of maternal epidural anesthesia on neonatal behavior, *Anesth Analg* 1984; 63:301.

11

Local Anesthetic Pharmacology

A 29-year-old primigravida at 39 weeks' gestation is referred to you by her obstetrician because she is "allergic to local anesthetic." Apparently, she had a dental procedure with a local anesthetic, during which time she experienced light-headedness and palpitations and "passed out." When she awoke in 90 seconds, the dentist said she had an allergic reaction. No swelling or difficulty in breathing was noticed. Discuss your evaluation of this patient and your choice of analgesia or anesthesia for labor, delivery, or cesarean section since she wishes to be awake for her delivery.

Recommendations by Jonathan Skerman, B.D.Sc., M.Sc.D., D.Sc.
Christopher Swayze, M.D.

Pharmacology of Local Anesthetics

In obstetric anesthesia practice, local anesthetics are the most popular agents for providing pain relief, both for labor and delivery and cesarean section. We indeed live in an era where there are various local anesthetics available to furnish our particular needs. Hence a thorough knowledge of these agents is important for the physician.

Pharmacologic Aspects

The structural characteristics of local anesthetics strongly influence their physicochemical properties and ultimately their clinical profile.[1,2] The molecular structure and physicochemical and pharmacologic properties of various local anesthetic agents are shown in Table 11-1.

Compounds showing local anesthetic activity commonly possess an amine and an aromatic component, linked by an intermediate chain. The clinically important local anesthetics usually are classed

TABLE 11-1
Chemical Structure and Physicochemical and Pharmacologic Properties of Some Commonly Used Local Anesthetics

	Chemical Configuration			Physicochemical Properties				Pharmacologic Properties		
Agent	Aromatic Lipophilic	Intermediate Chain	Amine Hydrophilic	Molecular Weight (base)	pKa (25° C)	Partition Coefficient	Protein Binding (%)	Onset	Relative Potency	Duration
Esters										
Procaine	$H-N(H)-C_6H_4-$	$COOCH_2CH_2-$	$N(C_2H_5)(C_2H_5)$	236	8.9	0.02	6	Slow	1	Short
Amethocaine	$H_9C_4N(H)-C_6H_4-$	$COOCH_2CH_2-$	$N(CH_3)(CH_3)$	264	8.5	4.1	76	Slow	8	Long
Chloroprocaine	$H_2N-C_6H_3(Cl)-$	$COOCH_2CH_2-$	$N(C_2H_5)(C_2H_5)$	271	8.7	0.14	—	Fast	1	Short
Amides										
Prilocaine	$C_6H_4(CH_3)-$	$NHCOCH(CH_3)-$	$N(H)(C_3H_7)$	220	7.9	0.9	55	Fast	2	Moderate
Lidocaine	$C_6H_3(CH_3)_2-$	$NHCOCH_2-$	$N(C_2H_5)(C_2H_5)$	234	7.9	2.9	64	Fast	2	Moderate
Mepivacaine	$C_6H_3(CH_3)_2-$	$NHCO$	piperidine $N-CH_3$	246	7.6	0.8	78	Fast	2	Moderate
Bupivacaine	$C_6H_3(CH_3)_2-$	$NHCO$	piperidine $N-C_4H_9$	288	8.1	27.5	96	Moderate	8	Long
Etidocaine	$C_6H_3(CH_3)_2-$	$NHCOCH(C_2H_5)-$	$N(C_2H_5)(C_3H_7)$	276	7.7	141	94	Fast	6	Long

Adapted from Finster M: *Toxicity of local anesthetics in the fetus and the newborn,* Bull N Y Acad Med 1976; 52:222.

into two groups based on the nature of their intermediate chain. Amino ester agents contain an ester linkage whereas amino amide compounds possess an amide intermediary. Essentially, the two groups differ in terms of stability, metabolism, and antigenic properties.

The pKa Constant

Each compound has a specific pKa value, the pH at which both the ionized and nonionized forms are in equilibrium. The pH at the site of administration affects the proportion of nonionized drug present. Agents with a low pKa relative to the pH at the injection site have a greater proportion of nonionized drug. Since this form diffuses most rapidly, these agents have a rapid speed of onset. This is reflected in the data in Table 11-1. Procaine, with a high pKa, has a slow onset of action at physiologic pH values whereas mepivacaine, with a relatively low pKa, has a fast onset.

However, one must remember that although the uncharged form is important for diffusion across the nerve membrane, the charged form will be ultimately responsible for binding with protein receptors. Hence both forms of the local anesthetic are important for neural blockade. The pKa also affects the placental transfer of the local anesthetic. Agents with low pKa values will transfer in larger amounts because of the greater amount of uncharged forms. The umbilical vein:maternal vein (UV:MV) concentration ratio of a local anesthetic is inversely proportional to the pKa of the local anesthetic; that is, mepivacaine with the lowest pKa (7.6) possesses the highest UV:MV ratio (0.8). Although a lower UV:MV ratio recently has been implicated in higher tissue binding of the local anesthetic to neonatal tissue,[3] the clinical importance of this factor is not clear.

Effect of Membrane Composition

The composition of the axonal membrane, which is about 90% lipid and 10% protein, can influence the profile of clinical agents. Drugs with high lipid solubility (defined by the partition coefficient) penetrate nerve membranes more easily and exhibit higher potency. Furthermore, agents showing high protein binding attach more strongly to nerve membrane proteins and show prolonged duration of action. In Table 11-1, a comparison between the properties of procaine and etidocaine demonstrates the impact of these phenomena.

Other Factors

There are known differences between bupivacaine and etidocaine in their capacity to induce motor block. This phenomenon, differential blockade, results from differences in the ability to penetrate *A* and *C* class fibers. The relatively high pKa of bupivacaine means it diffuses at a much slower rate across large, myelinated *A* fibers, involved in motor impulse conduction, than for *C* fibers, involved in pain conduction.

Localized blood flow at the site of administration affects the amount of drug undergoing vascular absorption and hence the amount remaining at the site of action. With the exception of cocaine, clinical concentrations of local anesthetic agents generally induce some degree of vasodilatation after administration.

The total dose of the agents ultimately will dictate the onset, quality, and duration of the block. With increased doses of local anesthetic, one can make the onset faster and the duration longer. In one study using epidural anesthesia for obstetric patients, it was shown that when the same volume is used, the onset, quality, and duration of the block improved by varying the concentration from 0.125% to 0.5%.[4] Another interesting observation was discovered when 600 mg of prilocaine was used epidurally: no difference in onset, adequacy, or duration of block was observed by administering either 30 ml of a 2% solution or 20 ml of a 3% solution.[5] However, one might observe a higher spread of the local anesthetic in the epidural space when a higher volume is used.

Pharmacokinetics of Local Anesthetics

The specific application of pharmacokinetic principles to local anesthetics offers the following potential advantages[6]

- Selection of a safe dose for single injection techniques, and safe rates of administration for continuous-conduction blockade techniques
- Selection of the best anesthetic for a specific procedure
- Proper awareness of events after accidental intravascular administration
- Identification of individuals most susceptible to the risks of toxic reactions.

Factors such as the rate of absorption (from the site of administration), tissue distribution, metabolism, and excretion all affect the blood concentration of a local anesthetic agent.[2]

Absorption

The dose, site of injection, and pharmacologic profile of the drug will influence absorption. The relationship between dose administered and the subsequent peak blood concentration tends to be linear. However, the site of injection can be particularly important, since a fixed dose of one specific drug may show potential toxicity in one site but not in others.[2]

Distribution

The pharmacokinetic characteristics of some amino amide agents reveal differences between the various compounds in terms of their rates of distribution and metabolism. For example, the potency and analgesic duration of lidocaine, mepivacaine, and prilocaine are very similar. However, prilocaine undergoes redistribution as well as metabolism at a much faster rate than the other two compounds, indicated by the value for the volume of distribution at steady state (VDSS).

Metabolism and Excretion

Differences also exist in the clearance rates of the amino amides, which undergo a more complex process of metabolism than the amino ester agents. The amino class of drugs is degraded primarily by the liver.

Plasma Binding of Local Anesthetics

The binding of local anesthetics to plasma proteins should be taken into account when making interpretations concerning the blood concentration of a specific agent.[5] In particular, pathologic conditions may exert a strong influence on the concentration of bound agent in plasma. For a fixed dose of lidocaine, the unbound fraction may show considerable variation, depending on the pathologic state of the patient.

Toxicity of Local Anesthetics

Under normal circumstances, the clinical administration of regional anesthesia is a relatively safe procedure with little risk of side effects. However, the initial concentrations at the specific site of action may be many thousand times greater than the systemic concentration.[8] Clinical signs of toxicity usually are associated with injection into the wrong site, such as accidental intravascular administration. This is not a toxicity problem by strict definition, but rather an overdose. Toxic side effects also can follow the injection of an excessive dose into the correct anatomic site.[9]

Toxicity of local anesthetics may be either local or systemic. In terms of systemic toxicity, local anesthetics primarily affect the central nervous system (CNS) and cardiovascular system, the former being the more susceptible.

Central Nervous System Toxicity

The main symptoms and signs associated with local anesthetic toxicity of the CNS are as follows: a biphasic response appears, ranging from initial excitation, then agitation, ultimately leading to seizures (convulsive activity) and then to terminal depression (coma, apnea).

The relative potency of an agent and hence its lipid solubility shows some correlation with its potential to cause CNS toxicity. Bupivacaine, for example, is about eight times more potent than procaine, and about seven times more toxic. Toxicity also is affected by the acid-base status of the subject; acidosis can lead to an increase in the relative toxicity of a local anesthetic.[10]

The early stages of CNS toxicity are easy to detect, provided that the anesthesia personnel maintain a constant rapport with the patient. Early recognition of toxicity and appropriate action may prevent not only development of the more serious stages of neurologic toxicity, but also may prevent progression to cardiovascular dysfunction.

Proper care when administering the drug may prevent the development of toxic sequelae. Proper care includes checking for accidental venipuncture (by slight aspiration of the syringe after insertion of the needle), ensuring that the recommended dose is not exceeded, and administering the drug slowly.

Cardiovascular Toxicity

The stages of cardiovascular toxicity that may develop from the effects of local anesthesia are as follows: initially, the concentration of a local anesthetic that induces convulsions in a patient will produce a marked rise in cardiac output and blood pressure; however, further increases in blood concentration will produce myocardial depression, hypotension, and ultimately a potentially irreversible cardiovascular collapse.

As observed with CNS toxicity, the cardiotoxicity of a local anesthetic agent is related to its anesthetic potency; bupivacaine, for example, is relatively more potent and more toxic than lidocaine. The development of CNS toxicity is unacceptable, but should it occur, consider that a greater margin of safety exists for lidocaine, compared with bupivacaine, in the relative risk of development of cardiovascular collapse.[9,11] Pregnancy also may influence the cardiotoxicity of some local anesthetic agents.[12]

Local Toxicity and Miscellaneous Effects

Toxicity effects on the CNS and cardiovascular systems are the main complications associated with the use of local anesthetics; regional neural toxicity usually is rare. However, incidents of prolonged sensorimotor defects have been reported after the use of chloroprocaine.[13] Studies have shown that this toxicity is due to the low pH and sodium bisulfite content of the solution.[14] Commercial reformulations of chloroprocaine without sodium bisulfite are now available; administration of clinical concentrations has not been shown to induce local neural damage.[2]

Allergic reactions can develop in a small proportion of patients treated with amino ester–based compounds due to the formation of the metabolite, para-aminobenzoic acid. Methemoglobinemia is a transient side effect occasionally seen after the administration of prilocaine as well as benzocaine.[9]

Adjuncts to Local Anesthetics

Addition of a vasoconstrictor agent such as epinephrine can enhance the performance of an agent by reducing the rate of absorption.[15] This means the agent remains in contact with the target nerve for a longer period of time, increasing duration of action and decreasing peak plasma levels. It is most effective at subcutaneous sites of administration. Local anesthetics supplemented with epinephrine are commercially available. Alternatively, the vasoconstrictor can be added just before use. It is not advisable to inject epinephrine near terminal arteries, since a risk exists of producing tissue necrosis and gangrene.[16]

The potential for combining two different agents has been studied to use the best features of each compound. Studies on combinations of agents possessing rapid onset (e.g., lidocaine or chloroprocaine) with the long-acting drug bupivacaine have failed to produce consistently favorable results, although a prilocaine-bupivacaine combination may show some promise.[17] Recently for labor, delivery, and postoperative pain relief, the combined use of opioids and local anesthetics has generated great interest. It has been hypothesized that combination of these two classes of compounds would produce synergistic effects, and because of the decreased doses of each compound used, a reduction would occur in the incidence and severity of side effects.[18]

Carbonation of agents has been studied to hasten the onset and increase the depth of anesthesia. Carbon dioxide diffuses into the axoplasm, decreasing intracellular pH. This not only favors the active, ionic form of the drug, but also helps to trap the ionized drug within the cell at its site of action.[3] Although it is difficult to demonstrate statistically significant differences between carbonated agents and their corresponding hydrochloride salts, improved action has been reported and, under certain conditions, this may be of clinical relevance.[17]

Alkalinization of local anesthetic solutions, to increase the amount of drug in the nonionic (diffusible) form available for penetration to the site of action, also has been examined. Some reports have claimed success with pH-adjusted 0.75% bupivacaine or mepivacaine, for example, although other studies failed to show a benefit in clinical trials. The potential increase in pH is limited by the solubility of free base in solution, and only minor increases may be possible with some agents before precipitation occurs.[17]

Warming the local anesthetic to a temperature of 100° F has been shown to reduce the time to onset of epidural anesthesia blockade. A decreased pKa due to increased temperature probably is the mechanism.[19]

Local Anesthetics for Regional Anesthesia

Lidocaine

Lidocaine, also known in Europe by its alternative generic name lignocaine, is the most versatile and commonly used agent because of its inherent potency, rapid onset, and moderate duration of action. It has been the agent of choice for the majority of outpatient procedures. Addition of vasoconstrictor agents greatly increases its duration.

It can be used for all forms of regional anesthesia with concentrations of 0.5% to 2% for injection. Because of its lower pKa (7.7 to 7.8) it has a faster onset of block, and addition of epinephrine will prolong its block.

Prilocaine

In terms of speed of onset and duration of effect, prilocaine has a similar clinical profile to lidocaine. However, its relatively lower vasodilatative activity allows it to be used without epinephrine, making it well suited for peripheral blockade. Its low toxicity provides a comparatively high margin of safety, particularly where large doses of agent are to be used. It is the agent of choice for intravenous regional anesthesia. Because of the possibility of maternal and neonatal methemoglobinemia, it is no longer used for obstetric patients.

Mepivacaine

Mepivacaine also has a similar clinical profile to lidocaine. It has less vasodilatative activity but also is less versatile. Its prolonged metabolism in the fetus and neonate has restricted its use in obstetric procedures.

It may be used for infiltration, peripheral nerve blockade, and extradural anesthesia in concentrations ranging from 0.5% to 2%. It is frequently used for central neural blockade when a compound with properties of profound motor blockade, and relatively short duration of action, is required. Because of its high UV : MV ratio (0.8) and prolonged half-life in neonates (8 hours), it is rarely used in parturients in the United States.

Bupivacaine

The major advantage of this agent is its long duration (3 to 10 hours on average), which makes it ideal for a number of indications where such a long duration is desirable. Concentrations ranging from 0.25% to 0.75% are available for various types of regional anesthesia. It also exhibits differential effects on sensory-motor blockade.

In low doses, 0.25% to 0.375%, it is currently the agent of choice for labor analgesia and postoperative analgesia. Higher concentrations (0.5% to 0.75%) are used for surgical procedures.

Due to its relatively high potential for cardiotoxicity, it is not recommended for intravenous regional anesthesia. Since 1983 the Food and Drug Administration has recommended against the use of 0.75% concentration of bupivacaine for epidural anesthesia in obstetrics in the United States.

Etidocaine

Etidocaine is characterized by a high lipid solubility, which results in a rapid onset and prolonged duration of action, with profound sensory and motor blockade. Although it is useful in surgical procedures where neuromuscular blockade is desired, its use is limited for extradural obstetric or postoperative analgesia.

Certain procedures (e.g., lower limb orthopedic surgery) may take advantage of both etidocaine and bupivacaine: an initial 1.5% dose of etidocaine can induce rapid and deep anesthesia and motor block, whereas subsequent administration of 0.5% bupivacaine provides excellent sensory anesthesia with minimal motor blockade. It is seldom used on obstetric patients because of the prolonged motor blockade as well as poor sensory anesthesia.

Chloroprocaine

Chloroprocaine is an amino ester compound with rapid onset, short duration of action, and low systemic toxicity (due to its rapid hydrolysis in plasma). These characteristics have dictated its use, primarily in epidural anesthesia for cesarean section, since the risks of systemic toxicity are minimal for both mother and fetus. However, because of its short duration of action, frequent reinforcement will be necessary (30 min). Despite the wide range of clinically effective local anesthetics that are currently available, the search continues for novel agents that demonstrate improvements in potency, duration of effect, and safety.[18]

Ropivacaine

A series of studies has been conducted on the amino amide–based compound ropivacaine, which is structurally intermediate between bupivacaine and mepivacaine. Pharmacologic, pharmacokinetic, and toxicologic data suggest that ropivacaine exhibits a duration of effect comparable with bupivacaine, but with less risk of inducing cardiotoxicity. Provided that current data can be extrapolated to regional anesthesia in men, ropivacaine offers considerable potential for future clinical use.[20-22]

Use of Ropivacaine in Obstetrics

Although ropivacaine offers more sensory-motor dissociation and also affords a greater margin of safety between cardiovascular system (CVS) toxicity and CNS toxicity, one must consider the effect of this agent on uterine blood flow to ensure its safety in the parturient. Santos and colleagues recently published their conclusions that neither ropivacaine nor bupivacaine, when infused intravenously as fast as 0.2 mg · kg · min and 0.1 mg · kg · min, respectively, led to any ill effects on uterine artery blood flow or fetal well-being.[23] This was important to determine, as it previously had been reported that ropivacaine, unlike its amino amide relatives, had vasoconstrictive properties when administered subcutaneously in animals.[24] Since pregnancy seems to enhance the cardiotoxicity of bupivacaine, the investigators also had looked at the systemic toxicity of ropivacaine during ovine pregnancy and concluded that ovine pregnancy does not enhance the systemic toxicity of ropivacaine.[25]

Currently, clinical trials of ropivacaine in obstetric patients are under way. It appears that ropivacaine is an exciting new agent offering greater motor and sensory dissociation than bupivacaine when administered epidurally while affording an increased margin of safety when comparing its cardiac and systemic toxicities. After further studies in humans are completed, it promises to offer greater patient satisfaction and comfort, particularly when used in the management of obstetric analgesia or anesthesia and postoperative pain control.

Allergic Effects

Reports of allergic reactions, hypersensitivity, or anaphylactic responses to local anesthetic agents appear periodically.[26,27] Unfortunately systemic toxic reactions to local anesthetic agents frequently are misdiagnosed as representing allergic- or hypersensitivity-type reactions.[28] The amino ester agents such as procaine have been shown to produce allergic-type reactions. Because these agents are derivatives of para-aminobenzoic acid, which is known to have an allergenic nature, it is not unusual that a certain percentage of the population will demonstrate allergic reactions to this class of local anesthetics. The advent of the amino amide local anesthetics, which are not derivatives of para-aminobenzoic acids, markedly changed the incidence of allergic-type reactions to local anesthetic drugs. Reactions of an allergic type to the amino amides are extremely rare, although several cases have been reported in the literature in recent years, which suggests that this class of agents can on rare occasions produce an allergic-type phenomenon.[26-28]

It should be remembered that solutions of amino amide agents from multiple-dose containers may contain a preservative, methylparaben, whose chemical structure is similar to that of para-aminobenzoic acid. A positive skin reaction has been shown in patients in whom methylparaben was administered intradermally.[29] Also, some patients are allergic to metabisulfite, which is present in epinephrine-containing local anesthetic solutions. Cross-sensitivity reactions are possible because many other drugs, foods, and beverages contain preservatives such as metabisulfite and hydroxybenzoate. Two patients suspected of having allergic reactions to local anesthetics were confirmed by challenge testing to have allergies to benzoate and metabisulfite.

Progressive challenge with dilute (1:1000) and then undiluted intradermal injection of local anesthetics has been successfully used to diagnose adverse responses to local anesthetics. It is important to use local anesthetic solutions without additives in such testing, and also for neural blockade in patients with a history of allergy to preservatives in foods and drugs.[28]

When epinephrine is used with local anesthetic solutions, it must be in a concentration and dose to produce the desired vasoconstriction without leading to epinephrine overdose. Although the optimal concentration has been controversial, most authorities now agree on a concentration of

1:200,000. More dilute solutions are of doubtful value; increasing the concentration does not achieve a correspondingly more effective vasoconstriction and increases the likelihood of toxicity. Even with a concentration of 1:200,000, a total dose of 200 μg should not be exceeded.

The principal side effects of epinephrine are hypertension, tachycardia or bradycardia, and cardiac arrhythmias. Such reactions are likely to occur if the local anesthetic solution is accidentally injected intravenously. It is wise to avoid the use of epinephrine in patients sensitive to catecholamines (patients with hypertension, thyrotoxicosis).

If the dentist responsible for the patient's treatment (discussed earlier in this chapter) is able to be contacted, it would be advisable to obtain as much information related to her untoward experience as possible. Specific attention should be paid to the local anesthetic used, the volume and concentration of same, whether or not epinephrine was part of the solution, and in what concentration. Many associated factors could be contributory; fear and apprehension could lead to fainting or a vasovagal attack; posture also could be implicated, along with an empty stomach. Some local anesthetic solutions used for dental procedures also contain concentrations of epinephrine 1:50,000,

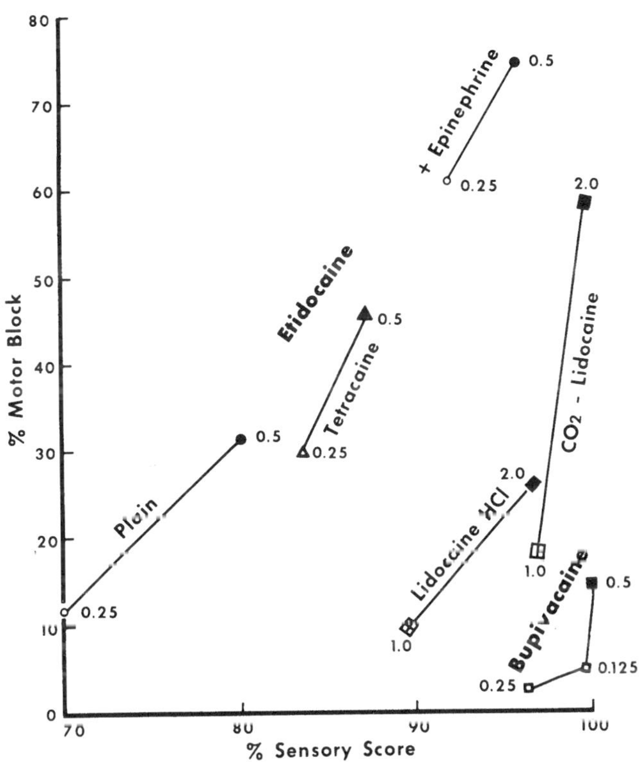

Fig. 11-1.

Epidural analgesia in labor. Quality of sensory and motor blockade with various analgesic solutions. Each point is the mean of 20 to 50 cases. ○, Etidocaine; △, tetracaine; ⊞, lidocaine; ■, bupivacaine. *(From Bromage PR, editor:* Epidural analgesia, *Philadelphia, 1978, WB Saunders.)*

and multiple ampules (usually 1.8 ml) may be used. The mucous membranes and alveolar bone of the oral cavity are extraordinarily vascular, and a direct intravascular injection of large amounts of epinephrine could have resulted in her light-headedness and palpitations. The presence of preservatives such as methylparaben in the epinephrine-containing local anesthetic might have been a contributing factor, but is unlikely.

In point of fact, although allergic reactions to the ester family of local anesthetics are known to occur, they are *not* common. Even more relevant in today's practice of infiltration and regional neural blockade using amide types of local anesthetics is the fact that clinically manifest allergic reactions in this group of drugs are *extremely rare*. Even though a variety of dilutional intradermal tests may be performed, skepticism still persists as to their effectiveness.[30]

As has been mentioned earlier in this chapter, an allergic reaction to amide local anesthetics is extremely rare, and if the skin test confirms this view, then the use of the agents will depend upon the procedure:

- For vaginal delivery, an ideal local anesthetic should be associated with good sensory analgesia with minimal motor blockade (Fig. 11-1). Bupivacaine 0.125% with opioids or bupivacaine 0.25% would be ideal for this situation.
- For cesarean section, the agents one can choose from include lidocaine 2%, with or without epinephrine (1 : 200,000), and bupivacaine 0.5%.

For elective cesarean section where there is no evidence of fetal distress or hypertension, lidocaine 2% with epinephrine can be used. If there is associated hypertension or if any other reason exists where maintenance of a stable cardiovascular system is necessary, bupivacaine 0.5% can be used if the patient is allergic to ester-type local anesthetic.

Summary

1. Use of a preservative-free local anesthetic is indicated.
2. An amino amide anesthetic agent would be the agent of choice in view of the fact that they are not derivatives of para-aminobenzoic acid.

References

1. Wildsmith JW: Peripheral nerve and local anaesthetic drugs, *Br J Anaesth* 1986; 58:692.
2. Covino BG: Pharmacology of local anesthetic agents, *Ration Drug Ther* 1987; 21:1.
3. Finster M: Toxicity of local anesthetics in the fetus and the newborn, *Bull N Y Acad Med* 1976; 52:222.
4. Littlewood DG, Buckley P, Covino BG, et al: Comparative study of various local anesthetic solutions in extradural block in labour, *Br J Anaesth* 1979; 51:47.
5. Tucker GT: Is plasma binding of local anesthetics important? *Acta Anaesthesiol Belg* 1988; 39:147.
6. Tucker GT: Pharmacokinetics of local anesthetics, *Br J Anaesth* 1986; 58:717.
7. Crawford OB: Comparative evaluation in peridural anesthesia of lidocaine, mepivacaine and L-67, a new local anesthetic agent, *Anesthesiology* 1964; 25:321.
8. Reynolds F: Adverse effects of local anaesthetics, *Br J Anaesth* 1987; 59:78.
9. Covino BG: Toxicity of local anesthetic agents, *Acta Anaesthesiol Belg* 1988; 39:159.
10. Englesson S: The influence of acid-base changes on central nervous system toxicity of local anaesthetic agents I: an experimental study in cats, *Acta Anaesthetic Scand* 1974; 18:79.
11. Morishima HO, Pedersen H, Finster M, et al: Bupivacaine toxicity in pregnant and non-pregnant ewes, *Anesthesiology* 1985; 63:134.
12. Santos AC, Pedersen H, Harmon TW, et al: Does pregnancy alter the systemic toxicity of local anesthetics? *Anesthesiology* 1989; 70:991.
13. Ravindran RS, Bond VK, Tasch MD, et al: Prolonged neural blockade following regional analgesia with 2-chloroprocaine injection, *Anesth Analg* 1980; 58:447.
14. Wang BC, Hillman DE, Spiedholz NI, et al: Chronic neurological deficits and Nesacaine-CE: an effect of the anesthetic,

2-chloroprocaine, or the antioxidant, sodium bisulfite? *Anesth Analg* 1984; 63:445.

15. Scott B: Adrenaline in local anesthetic solutions, *Acta Anaesthesiol Belg* 1988; 39:159.
16. Scott DB: *Techniques of regional anesthesia,* Fribourg: 1989, Med Globe SA.
17. Akerman B: Adjuncts to enhance the effectiveness of local anaesthetics, *Curr Opin Anaesth* 1989; 2:577.
18. Arthur GR, Covino BG: What's new in local anaesthetics? *Anaesthesiol Clin North Am* 1988; 6:357.
19. Mehta PM, Theriot E, Mehrotra D: A simple technique to make bupivacaine a rapid-acting epidural anesthetic, *Reg Anesth* 1987; 123:135.
20. Akerman B, Hellberg IB, Trossvik C: Primary evaluation of the local anaesthetic properties of the amino amide agent ropivacaine (LEA 103), *Acta Anaesthesiol Scand* 1988; 32:571.
21. Arthur GR, Feldman HS, Covino BG: Comparative pharmacokinetics of bupivacaine and ropivacaine, a new amide local anesthetic, *Anesth Analg* 1988; 67:1053.
22. Reiz S, Haggmark S, Johansson G, et al: Cardiotoxicity of ropivacaine: a new amide local anaesthetic agent. *Acta Anaesthesiol Scand* 1989; 33:93.
23. Santos AC, Arthur GR, Roberts DJ, et al: Effect of ropivacaine and bupivacaine on uterine blood flow in pregnant ewes, *Anesth Analg* 1992; 74:62.
24. Kopacz DJ, Carpenter RL, Mackey DC: Effect of ropivacaine on cutaneous capillary blood flow in pigs, *Anesthesiology* 1989; 721:69.
25. Santos AC, Arthur GR, Pedersen H, et al: Systemic toxicity of ropivacaine during ovine pregancy, *Anesthesiology* 1991; 75:137.
26. Brown DT, Beamish D, Wildsmith JAW: Allergic reaction to an amide local anesthetic, *Br J Anaesth* 1981; 53:435.
27. Reynolds F: Allergy reaction to an amide local anaesthetic, *Br J Anaesth* 1981; 53:901.
28. Fisher M McD, Graham R: Adverse responses to local anaesthetics, *Anaesth Intensive Care* 1984; 12:325.
29. Aldretti JA, Johnson DA: Evaluation of intracutaneous testing for investigation of allergy to local anesthetic agents, *Anesth Analg* 1970; 49:173.
30. Fisher M, Pennington JC: Allergy to local anaesthesia, *Br J Anaesth* 1982; 54:893.

12

Local Anesthetic Neurotoxicity

A 32-year-old primigravida at term is admitted for cesarean section for breech presentation. A continuous spinal with 5% hyperbaric lidocaine is used for the technique. During the next several days, the patient is unable to urinate or have a spontaneous bowel movement. Discuss the problem.

Recommendations by Ronald J. Hurley, M.D.
Hal S. Feldman, D.Sc.

Brief History of Local Anesthetics

The Incan civilization was essentially destroyed by the Spanish conquistadores under the command of Francisco Pizzaro in the midsixteenth century. The Incas chewed the leaves of the coca plant (Erythroxylon coca) as a stimulant. Additionally, there were reports of Incan surgeons allowing saliva containing coca to drip into the open incisions created during trephination to produce local anesthetic.[1] Very little scientific work was done with the coca plant until the leaves became available in Europe. In 1848 James Young Simpson published results of his studies of the topical application of various liquids in an attempt to produce local anesthesia. Although his efforts were unsuccessful, his insight was profound, ". . . if we would by any means induce a local anesthetic without that temporary absence of consciousness which is found in the state of general anesthesia, many would regard it as still a greater improvement in this branch of practice."[2] Others also experimented with various methods of producing local anesthesia, including James Moore's work on nerve compression and the spraying of ether on the skin studied by Benjamin Ward Richardson.

As the leaves of the coca plant became available for experimental use in Europe, researchers began to evaluate its properties. In 1857 Mantegazza described in some detail its systemic effects,[1] and in 1860 Niemann and Wohler isolated a purified substance from the leaf, which they termed *cocaine,* and reported that it caused numbness of the tongue.[2]

In 1868 Moreno y Maiz reported cocaine-induced seizures in animals.[3] An extensive evaluation of cocaine's pharmacologic properties was published by von Anrep in 1880. This report included its toxicity and ability to numb the skin if applied subcutaneously. Alexander Wood put forth the concept of blocking a nerve by the direct application of a drug in 1858.[2] Cocaine was destined to become an important drug in the development of local anesthesia.

Sigmund Freud became interested in cocaine and published his famous review, *Über Coca,* in 1884.[4] Together with his colleague, Karl Koller, work on the systemic effects of cocaine was begun. Koller, an intern in ophthalmology, wanted an agent which could be used as a local anesthetic in the eye. It did not take long for Koller to realize that cocaine was the agent he sought. On September 11, 1884, he performed an operation for glaucoma using cocaine as a topical anesthetic.[5] The news traveled quickly to the United States, and by November of that year the American medical literature had reported more than 150 successful cases of corneal and conjuctival anesthesia.[6] In the same year, Hall reported blocking of his own ulnar nerves and the removal of a small tumor after injecting cocaine into the supraorbital notch.[7] In 1885 J. Leonard Corning produced spinal anesthesia in the dog and in humans.[8]

In 1891 Quincke published his work concerning the injection of local anesthetic agents into the subdural space of the lumbar spinal cord.[9] Quincke realized that in humans, the spinal cord ended at the L_2 level, but the subarachnoid space extended to S_2. Therefore, injection by needle at the midlumbar region would avoid mechanical damage to the cord. Quincke developed the needle point design which bears his name for this purpose. Bier followed with his extensive work on cocaine spinal anesthesia and an early well-documented account of postdural puncture headache.[10]

Cocaine had been shown to be an effective local anesthetic agent. However, it was not without serious drawbacks. Many of the pioneer experimenters with cocaine had developed an addiction to the drug; this was a serious complication. As the drug became more widely used, its systemic toxicity became apparent. In 1891 Mattison published his study of the toxic actions of cocaine[11] outlining over 100 cases of toxicity including some deaths. Eggleston and Hatcher published data on cocaine acute toxicity in 1919.[12]

Cocaine's addiction liability and its potentially fatal toxicity prompted the search for a synthetic agent to replace it. A group of chemists under the direction of Einhorn produced procaine around 1905.[13] The search for additional synthetic agents continued, and in 1929 dibucaine was synthesized, and then in 1948 Löfgren reported his synthesis of lidocaine.[14]

Local Anesthetic Neurotoxicity

The use of local anesthetics in clinically available formulation for regional anesthesia has been shown to be generally safe. Large retrospective surveys reveal an incidence of persistent neurologic sequelae ranging from 0.01% to 0.03% for spinal anesthesia, from 0% to 0.09% for epidural anesthesia, and from 0% to 6% for brachial plexus block.[15-22] However, the last decade has been punctuated with alarming reports of possible neurotoxicity associated with commonly used local anesthetics. First came the reports of problems with chloroprocaine and then the recent report of continuous spinal anesthesia with microcatheters and 5% hyperbaric lidocaine. Cauda equina syndrome has been revisited with much speculation as to the etiology of this serious neurologic complication.

Cauda Equina Syndrome

The cauda equina begins at the third lumbar vertebra at birth and at the first lumbar vertebra in adults. The nerves lie in close proximity to each other and are especially vulnerable to toxic injury due to the lack of a dural sheath as they traverse a relatively long course before exiting at their respective foramina. Schneider et al.[21] point out that examination of anatomic preparations of the cauda equina in situ shows that the dorsal roots of the spinal nerves L-5 and S-1 are in the most dorsal position in the spinal canal. Therefore these sensory fibers represent the nerve roots which are most exposed to a hyperbaric local anesthetic solution pooling in that area.

Ferguson and Watkins[22] reported 14 patients who developed cauda equina syndrome after the administration of a spinal anesthetic and speculated as to the cause. Nicholson and Eversole[23] in 1946 described the symptoms in a review of the neurologic complication of spinal anesthesia:

> These cauda equina complications are generally brought to the anesthesiologist's attention because the patient fails to regain the use of his lower extremities at the usual time following spinal anesthesia. On examination, loss of motor and sensory function is generally found to involve the lumbosacral nerve distribution. Associated observations are urinary retention and incontinence of feces with the loss of anal sphincter tone. This loss of bowel and bladder function is the most ominous part of the entire clinical picture, and the return of function, when it occurs, is extremely slow. Impairment of sensation seems to be exceedingly variable. This loss of sensation may involve only the saddle area, one or both legs, or the entire body below the umbilicus.

Mechanisms of Neurologic Damage

Potential mechanisms of neurologic damage include trauma; ischemia; infection; and direct action of the local anesthetic, its diluent, or additives.

Trauma

Direct trauma to the peripheral nerve, spinal cord, or nerves of the cauda equina by catheter or needle is always possible. The mobility of the cauda equina protects these nerves from impalement, but the spinal cord and major peripheral nerve trunks are relatively fixed. Bromage[24] remarks on the ease with which a subarachnoid catheter can be passed into a dog's spinal cord. Intraneural injection of the cord was reported by Oswalt in 1989[25] in an attempted epidural on a patient under general anesthesia. However, usually penetration of the spinal cord or a peripheral nerve trunk is accompanied by a persistent paresthesia. Clinicians agree that injection in the face of a persistent paresthesia is contraindicated. However, evidence that spinal needles rarely cause neurologic injury themselves is provided by the follow-up of patients after diagnostic lumbar puncture. Reports of injury after these procedures are exceedingly rare.

Investigation of a nerve deficit should always include consideration of compression injury. Bony trauma, spinal neoplasm's herniated intervertebral discs, spinal stenosis, and expanding epidural hematomas and abscesses can mimic the rare complications of a regional anesthetic. Computer-assisted tomography (CT) and magnetic resonance imaging (MRI) can be invaluable in ruling out compression as a cause. A relatively rapid progression of neurologic symptoms can be an important clinical clue to the expanding mass lesion such as a hematoma or abscess. Intervention within hours is crucial in preserving neurologic function.

Ischemia

The blood supply to the spinal cord is segmentally derived from cervical, thoracic, lumbar, and sacral arteries by passage medially along the nerve roots to form anastomoses on the surface with the anterior and posterior spinal arteries. Interruption of this blood supply by trauma or surgical mishap can lead to paraplegia. Significant systemic hypotension (including that from spinal anesthesia) can produce similar ischemic damage. The cauda equina has no collateral blood flow. Branches of the iliac artery supply the lower part of the spinal cord and cauda equina. A cauda equina syndrome can be produced by a loss of blood supply from the iliac arteries.[26] Some patients may be especially prone to cord ischemia due to a deficiency in segmental anterior spinal artery supply.[27]

The effect of local anesthetics on neural microcirculation has been investigated in animals by several authors with variable results. Dohi et al.[28] used a microsphere technique in dogs and demonstrated no change after 10 to 50 mg of lidocaine in 7.5% dextrose. Mitchell et al.[29] used 5 ml of 2% lidocaine in the epidural space and showed a significant decrease in blood flow at 30 minutes. Since no systemic hypotension occurred, the authors speculated that either there was a decreased metabolic rate in the spinal cord or that there was a direct vasoconstrictive action of the lidocaine.

Epinephrine has been linked to the anterior spinal artery syndrome in a series of case reports.[30-32] Dohi and associates[28] showed that phenylephrine caused a dose-dependent reduction in neural blood flow.

Recently Schneider and associates[21] proposed that the lithotomy position may make patients more liable to ischemic changes. Placing the patient in the lithotomy position is linked to a reduction in the physiologic lordosis of the spinal column and induces stretching of the cauda equina, and this stretching may jeopardize blood perfusion and increase the vulnerability of the nerve fibers. This stretching also could be due to the *tethered cord syndrome* described by Pang and Wilberger[33] and Yamada.[34]

Finally, preexisting systemic disease such as diabetes may make some patients more vulnerable to ischemic damage. Kalichman and Calcutt[35] injected 2% and 4% lidocaine around the sciatic nerves of streptozotocin-diabetic rats and control rats. Injury was produced in all groups but was significantly greater in the diabetic group. They concluded that the risk of local anesthetic–induced nerve injury is increased in this diabetic animal model.

Infection

Fortunately, bacterial meningitis and epidural abscess now are rare complications of spinal and epidural anesthesia. Modern sterile "kits," close attention to aseptic technique, and perhaps the bacteriostatic effect of many local anesthetics deserve much of the credit. Of course, infection of the skin or subcutaneous tissues at the site of injection is an absolute contraindication to regional anesthesia. Bacteremia or viremia is more controversial since many septic patients undergo lumbar puncture without serious sequelae. Many anesthesiologists, however, fear that pathogens may be introduced into the subarachnoid space, thus breaching the blood-brain barrier. Most prefer to defer spinal anesthesia in the septic patient or at least wait until adequate antibiotic treatment has been administered.

Subarachnoid infection usually is not complicated by long-term neurologic deficit. However, adhesive arachnoiditis can follow infection. It is more commonly associated with trauma or chemical irritants are well as being idiopathic. This inflammatory response can obliterate the subarachnoid space with adhesion to the spinal cord and dense attachment of the arachnoid to the dura.

Local Anesthetic

Animal Data

Ample animal data show that all local anesthetics have the potential for neurologic injury. Gentili et al.[36] found that carbonate lidocaine and the two ester drugs, procaine and tetracaine, caused more neural damage than the amide drugs, bupivacaine, lidocaine, and mepivacaine. However, Kalichman et al.[37] later found that all local anesthetics, when injected around the rat sciatic nerve, produced reversible, concentration-dependent damage to the blood-nerve barrier with endoneurial edema that peaked at about 48 hours and then declined. More recently Kalichman et al.[34] examined the amide local anesthetics (lidocaine and etidocaine), as well as the ester-linked procaine and 2-chloroprocaine in the rat sciatic model. The authors concluded that these local anesthetics are similarly neurotoxic and that their toxicity parallels their anesthetic potency. They noted no difference between the amide and ester-linked drugs. Kroin and co-workers[39] conducted an interesting modification of the rat sciatic model using 1%, 2%, or 4% lidocaine with two different catheter injection systems. The injections were made three times a day for 3 days into a loose cuff around the sciatic nerve and into a doubly slit catheter positioned 3 mm from the nerve. Axonal degeneration was produced in a concentration-dependent fashion with the cuff system whereas little damage was produced with the slit catheter. The authors postulated that the severe damage produced with the cuff injection system probably reflected a longer exposure to the local anesthetic whereas the slit catheter allowed rapid dilution with the interstitial fluid. Ready et al.[40] injected a variety of local anesthetics with concentration limited only by their solubility (up to 32% lidocaine). Pathologic changes were noticed in the cord and in the cauda equina after treatment with lidocaine concentrations of 4% and higher. Lambert et al.[41] conducted an in vitro, electrophysiologic study of desheathed frog sciatic nerves with solutions of hyperbaric 5% and 1.5% lidocaine, 1.5% plain lidocaine, and 7.5% dextrose. The nerves were exposed for 15 minutes and then washed with Ringer's solution. Nerve conduction recovery after the wash was then measured, with only a 7% recovery of the action potential after 5% hyperbaric lidocaine, compared with 53% and 69% in the 1.5% hyperbaric and 1.5% plain lidocaine groups, respectively. It was concluded that high concentrations of lidocaine were potentially neurotoxic when directly exposed to nerve tissue.

Human Data

In the early 1980s, case reports surfaced linking the use of 2-chloroprocaine with persistent neurologic deficit and adhesive arachnoiditis after inadvertent subarachnoid administration of doses intended for the epidural space.[42,43] Gissen and associates[44] used an in vitro model to demonstrate that the toxicity seen was probably because of a combination of low pH of the anesthetic solution and the addition of sodium bisulfite.

More recently the reports of cauda equina syndrome after continuous spinal anesthesia have heightened awareness of the potential for neurotoxicity with regional anesthesia. Continuous spinal anesthesia has been used clinically since it was first described by Dean in 1907.[45] However, the technique often was complicated by the occurrence of postdural puncture headache secondary to the relatively large dural hole produced by the spinal needle. In 1987, Hurley and Lambert[46] described the first of a new generation of microbore catheters that could be inserted with small-gauge needles, thus hopefully minimizing the incidence of postdural puncture headache. The new catheters proved popular and one manufacturer packaged a kit with hyperbaric 5% lidocaine included. Then in 1991 Rigler et al.[47] and Schell and co-workers[48] published two series of case reports that documented cauda equina syndrome after continuous spinal anesthesia. Five of the six cases reported were with the new spinal microcatheters, whereas the last was with a standard epidural catheter. The cases were notable in that relatively high doses of local anesthetic were given. Five of the six cases were with hyperbaric 5% lidocaine and one with tetracaine. The authors speculated that "maldistribution" of the local anesthetic may have led to excessive local anesthetic administration, resulting in relatively poor mixing with the cerebrospinal fluid and toxic exposure to the nerves of the cauda equina. Fabricated mechanical models of the dural sac have shown that sacral pooling of the hyperbaric local anesthetic is likely, especially with a caudally directed catheter.[49,50] The authors urged the use of lower concentrations of local anesthetic and alternative baricities to alleviate the problem of sacral pooling. However, in 1992 the United States Food and Drug Administration (FDA) responded by withdrawing approval for the spinal microcatheters.

In 1992 Drasner et al.[51] reported a case of cauda equina syndrome after the accidental subarachnoid injection of 20 ml of 2% lidocaine intended for the epidural space. The use of shock wave lithotripsy in this case clouded the search for the cause of the neurologic damage.

Most recently, Schneider and associates[21] documented four cases of transient lumbosacral monoradiculopathy after exposure to "normal" clinical doses of subarachnoid hyperbaric 5% lidocaine. The authors speculated that the lithotomy position may have stretched fibers of the cauda equina and increased their vulnerability to this relatively concentrated local anesthetic.

Local Anesthetic Additives

Vasoconstrictors

Epinephrine and, to a lesser extent, phenylephrine are added to local anesthetic solutions to prolong the duration of the block. Epinephrine also is added to aid in the detection of intravascular injection. Both agents can reduce neural blood flow, and epinephrine has been linked to the anterior spinal artery syndrome, as discussed earlier in this chapter. Epinephrine is easily oxidized and is thermolabile, and therefore requires the addition of an antioxidant and the maintenance of an acid milieu. Many practitioners avoid the preservative by adding the epinephrine just before administering the block.

Dextrose

Dextrose is added to increase the baricity of the local anesthetic solution. Osmolarity is increased to 800 when 7.5% dextrose is added to 5% lidocaine. Wildsmith[52] speculated that the unsheathed nerves of the cauda equina may be vulnerable to the dehydrating effects of such a hyperosmolar solution, especially if mixing with the cerebrospinal fluid is poor.

Methylparaben

Methylparaben is added to local anesthetics as an antibacterial agent, and is found only in multidose vials that are susceptible to contamination. Although methylparaben has not been associated with neurotoxicity, it is metabolized to para-aminobenzoic acid, which is a known allergen.

Metabisulfite

Metabisulfite is one of a number of agents added to local anesthetic solutions to prevent the oxidation of epinephrine. As discussed above, Gissen et al.[44] found that metabisulfite was neurotoxic when combined with the acidic 2-chloroprocaine. Wang and co-workers[53] tested 2-chloroprocaine and metabisulfite in a rabbit model. High doses of the local anesthetic failed to produce neurologic damage, but metabisulfite caused hind limb paralysis in 50% of the animals.

Bicarbonate and Carbon Dioxide

Sodium bicarbonate has become a popular additive to local anesthetics. By alkalinizing the solution, a greater proportion of the local anesthetic will be in its nonionized form and the neural membrane will be penetrated by more molecules of anesthetic. This theoretically results in a block with faster onset, a more profound depth, and a wider spread. Whether this happens is a matter of considerable debate. In any event, bicarbonate has not been linked to any reports of neurotoxicity to date, although a theoretical risk exists from the increased osmolarity.

Carbonated local anesthetics are not available in the United States. Gentili and associates[37] found carbonated 2% lidocaine to be the most toxic of all the lidocaine preparations they studied.

Opioids

There has been an explosion of interest in neuraxial-applied opioids in the last decade, with thousands of publications touting their benefits and with few evaluating their potential for neurologic damage. Rawal and co-workers[54] administered large and small doses of butorphanol, sufentanil, and nalbuphine to sheep intrathecally every 6 hours for 3 days. They concluded that butorphanol in doses of 0.075 and 0.375 mg/kg and sufentanil in a dose of 7.5 mg/kg were neurotoxic. Nalbuphine produced histopathologic changes similar to those of controls.

Meperidine has local anesthetic properties and has been used alone for cesarean delivery and urologic procedures. Fentanyl has some local anesthetic properties, but not in clinically relevant doses.[55]

Only morphine in its preservative-free form (epidural and spinal) and recently sufentanil (epidural) have been approved by the FDA for perispinal use.

Summary

1. Local anesthetics can be neurotoxic by a variety of mechanisms, including toxicity of the drug itself. However, overwhelming clinical evidence shows that most of the approved formulations are safe, although it may be time for a reevaluation of 5% lidocaine in 7.5% dextrose. Certainly if 2% lidocaine is adequate in the epidural space, the 5% concentration is excessive for the subarachnoid space.
2. The recent attention paid to the unfortunate complications after continuous spinal anesthesia has focused a reevaluation of all the local anesthetics, their additives, and their routes and means of administration. It is curious that when a new local anesthetic agent was evaluated in the past, most attention was paid to its local anesthetic action and evaluation of its systemic side effects with scant attention paid to the therapeutic:toxic ratio of the target organ itself. Certainly, local anesthetic action may be seen as a limited, reversible toxicity.
3. The subarachnoid space will receive increased attention in the future. We have only begun to explore the usefulness of intrathecal antibiotics, chemotherapy agents, α-agonists, antinausea agents, narcotics, and endorphins. The need for a standardized animal model for the evaluation of drugs and their additives and a mechanism for delivery is evident.

References

1. Vandam LD: *Some aspects of the history of local anesthesia.* In: Strichartz GR, editor: *Local anesthetics,* New York, 1987, Springer-Verlag.
2. Wildsmith JAW. *The history and development of local anesthesia.* In: Wildsmith JAW, Armitage EN, editors: *Principles and practice of regional anesthesia,* New York, 1987, Churchill Livingstone.
3. Holmstedt B, Fredga A: Sundry episodes in the history of coca and cocaine, *J Ethnopharmacol* 1981; 3:113.
4. Freud S: Uber coca, *Zentralbl Ges Ther* 1884; 2:289.
5. Fink BR: *History of neural blockade.* In: Cousins MJ, Bridenbaugh PO, editors: *Neural blockade in clinical anesthesia and management of pain, ed 3,* Philadelphia, 1988, JB Lipincott Company.

6. Bull CS: The hydrochlorate of cocaine as a local anesthetic in ophthalmic surgery, *NY Med J* 1884; 40:609.
7. Hall RJ: Hydrochlorate of cocaine, *NY Med J* 1884; 40:643.
8. Corning JL: Spinal anaesthesia and local medication of the cord, *NY Med J* 1885; 42:483.
9. Quinke H: Die lunbal punction des hydrozephalus, *Berl Klin Wochenschr* 1891; 28:929.
10. Bier A: Versuche uver cocainisirung des ruckenmarkes, *Dtsch Z Chir* 1899; 61:361.
11. Mattison JB: Cocaine poisoning, *Med Surg Res* 1891; 17:645.
12. Eggleston C, Hatcher RA: A further contribution to the pharmacology of the local anesthetics, *J Pharmacol Exp Ther* 1919; 13:433.
13. Einhorn A: On the chemistry of local anesthetics, *MMWR* 1889; 46:1218.
14. Löfgren N: Studies on local anesthetics: Xylocaine a new synthetic drug, doctoral dissertation. Faculty of Mathematics and Natural Sciences, University of Stockholm, 1948, Ivar Haeggstroms, Stockholm, 13.
15. Dripps RD, Vandam LD: Long term follow-up of patients who received 10,098 spinal anesthetics, *JAMA* 1954; 156:1486.
16. Phillips OC, Ebner H, Nelson AT, Black MH: Neurologic complications following spinal anesthesia with lidocaine, *Anesthesiology* 1969; 30:284.
17. Kane RE: Neurologic deficits following epidural or spinal anesthesia, *Anesth Analg* 1981; 60(3):150.
18. Dawkins CJM: An analysis of the complications of extradural or spinal anaesthesia, *Anaesthesia* 1969; 24:554.
19. Usubiaga JE: Neurological complications following epidural anesthesia, *Int Anesthesiol Clin* 1975; 13:1.
20. Selander D: *Nerve toxicity of local anesthetics.* In: Löfström JB, Sjöstrom U, editors: *Local anesthesia and regional blockade.* Amsterdam, 1988, Elsevier Science Publishers BV (Biomedical Division).
21. Schneider M, Ettlin T, Kaufmann M, et al: Transient neurologic toxicity after hyperbaric subarachnoid anesthesia with 5% lidocaine, *Anesth Analg* 1993; 76:1154.
22. Ferguson FR, Watkins KH: Paralysis of the bladder and associated neurological sequelae of spinal anaesthesia (cauda equina syndrome), *Br J Surg* 1937; 25:735.
23. Nicholson MJ, Eversole UH: Neurological complications of spinal anesthesia, *JAMA* 1946; 132(12):679.
24. Bromage PR: Nerve injury and paralysis related to spinal and epidural anesthesia, *Reg Anesth* 1993; 18(suppl):65.
25. Oswalt K: Medical/legal issues in regional anesthesia, *ASRA Newsletter* 1989; November 4.
26. Cousins MJ, Bromage PR: *Epidural neural blockade.* In: Cousins MJ, Bridenbaugh PO, editors: *Neural blockade in clinical anesthesia and management of pain,* Philadelphia, 1988, JB Lippincott.
27. Kane RE: Neurologic deficits following epidural or spinal anesthesia, *Anesth Analg* 1981; 60:150.
28. Dohi S, Matsumiya N, Takeshima R, Naito H: The effects of subarachnoid lidocaine and phenylephrine on spinal cord and cerebral blood flow, *Anesth Analg* 1989; 68:312.
29. Mitchell P, Goad R, Erwin CW, et al: Effect of epidural lidocaine on spinal cord blood flow, *Anesth Analg* 1989; 68:312.
30. Davies A, Solomon B, Levene A: Paraplegia following epidural anaesthesia, *Br Med J* 1958; 2:654.
31. Urguhart-Hay D: Paraplegia following epidural analgesia: case report, *Anaesthesia* 1969; 24:461.
32. Ackerman WE, Juneja M, Knapp RK: Maternal paraparesis after epidural anesthesia and cesarean section, *South Med J* 1990; 83:695.
33. Pang D, Wilberger JE: Tethered cord syndrome in adults, *J Neurosurg* 1982; 57:32.
34. Yamada D, Zinke DE, Sanders D: Pathophysiology of "tethered cord syndrome," *J Neurosurg* 1981; 54:494.
35. Kalichman MW, Calcutt NA: Local anesthetic induced conduction block and nerve fiber injury in streptozotocin-diabetic rats, *Anesthesiology* 1992; 77:941.
36. Gentili F, Hudson AR, Hunter D, Kline DG: Nerve injection injury with local anesthetic agents: a light and electron microscopic, fluorescent microscopic horse-radish peroxidase study, *Neurosurgery* 1980; 6:263.
37. Kalichman MW, Powell HC, Myers RR: Quantitative histologic analysis of local anesthetic-induced injury to rat sciatic nerve, *J Pharmacol Exp Ther* 1989; 250:406.
38. Kalichman MW, Moorhouse DF, Powell HC, Myers RR: Relative neural toxicity of local anesthetics, *J Neuropathol Exp Neurol* 1993; 52:234.
39. Kroin JS, Penn RD, Levy FE, Kerns JM: Effect of repetitive lidocaine infusion on peripheral nerve, *Exp Neurol* 1986; 94:166.
40. Ready LB, Plumer MH, Hasche RH, et al: Neurotoxicity of intrathecal local anesthetics in rabbits, *Anesthesiology* 1985; 63:364.
41. Lambert LA, Lambert DH, Strichartz GR: Potential neuro-

toxicity of lidocaine and dextrose solutions used for spinal anesthesia, *Reg Anesth* 1992; 17(suppl):164.

42. Ravindran R, Bond VK, Tasch MD, et al: Prolonged neural blockade following regional analgesia with 2-chloroprocaine, *Anesth Analg* 1980; 59:447.
43. Reisner LS, Hochman BN, Plumer MH: Persistent neurologic deficit and adhesive arachnoiditis following intrathecal 2-chloroprocaine injection, *Anesth Analg* 1980; 59:452.
44. Gissen AJ, Datta SD, Lambert DH: The chloroprocaine controversy II: Is chloroprocaine neurotoxic? *Reg Anesth* 1984; 9:135.
45. Dean HP: Discussion on the relative value of inhalation and injection methods of inducing anesthesia, *Br Med J* 1907; 5:869.
46. Hurley RJ, Lambert DH: Continuous spinal anesthesia with a microcatheter technique, *Reg Anesth* 1987; 12:54.
47. Rigler ML, Drasner K, Krejcie TC, et al: Cauda equina syndrome after continuous spinal anesthesia, *Anesth Anals* 1991; 72.275.
48. Schell RM, Brauer FS, Cole DJ, Applegate RL: Persistent sacral root deficits after continuous spinal anesthesia, *Can J Anaesth* 1991; 38:908.
49. Lambert DH, Hurley RJ: Cauda equina syndrome and continuous spinal anesthesia, *Anesth Analg* 1991; 72:817.
50. Ross BK, Coda B, Heath CH: Local anesthetic distribution in a spinal model: a possible mechanism of neurologic injury after continuous spinal anesthesia, *Reg Anesth* 1992; 17:69.
51. Drasner K, Rigler ML, Sesler DI, Stoller ML: Cauda equina syndrome following intended epidural anesthesia, *Anesthesiology* 1992; 77:582.
52. Wildsmith JA: Catheter spinal anesthesia and cauda equina syndrome: an alternative view (letter to the editor), *Anesth Analg* 1991; 73:368.
53. Wang BC, Hillman DE, Spielholz NI, Turndorf H: Chronic neurologic deficits and Nesacaine-CE: an effect of the anesthetic, 2-chloroprocaine, or the antioxidant, sodium bisulfite? *Anesth Analg* 1984; 63:445.
54. Rawal N, Nuutinen L, Raj PP, et al: Behavioral and histopathologic effects following intrathecal administration of butorphanol, sufentanil, and nalbuphine in sheep, *Anesthesiology* 1991; 75:1025.
55. Power I, Brown DT, Wildsmith JAW: The effect of fentanyl, meperidine and diamorphine on nerve conduction in vitro. *Reg Anesth* 1991; 16:204.

13

Cardiac and Central Nervous System Toxicity of Local Anesthetics

A 28-year-old primigravida at term is admitted in active labor. She requests epidural analgesia for pain relief. After placement of the catheter into the epidural space, the anesthesiologist injects a dose of local anesthetic. About 30 seconds after this injection, the patient starts to convulse. The electrocardiogram shows ventricular dysrhythmias. Discuss the management.

Recommendations by Ram S. Ravindran, M.D.

The use of epidural analgesia to relieve the pain of labor and delivery has become a common practice. Likewise, epidural anesthesia frequently is used for cesarean sections. One of the serious complications associated with this technique is systemic toxicity. Although it is a rare complication, it is potentially life threatening. Therefore anyone providing anesthesia to a pregnant patient should be familiar with the causation, pathophysiologic characteristics, prevention, and treatment of this condition.

Incidence of Systemic Local Anesthetic Toxicity

In nonpregnant patients who receive epidural anesthesia, the incidence rate of systemic local anesthetic toxicity ranges from 0.2% to 0.35%, but in pregnant patients the incidence rate is about 1%.[1] Notice that systemic toxic reactions can occur during the administration of paracervical or pudendal block as well.

Higher Incidence in Pregnant Patients

In pregnant patients the epidural veins are markedly enlarged. During placement of the epidural needle, injury to the epidural veins occurs in 10% of the attempts. Recognized intraepidural placement or migration of the epidural catheter occurs in 4% to 8% of patients.[2] However, it occurs only in 2% to 4% of nonpregnant patients.

During labor and delivery, with the epidural catheter in place, the parturients tend to move around in bed. They also are transferred to the delivery room or surgery room with the catheter in place. Subjecting them to such movements might result in migration of the catheter into the intravascular space.[3] A decreased level of serum protein is noticed during pregnancy. Because of its presence, a higher fraction of the highly protein-bound local anesthetic is present in an unbound state. This could contribute to a greater toxic potential of local anesthetics in parturients than in nonpregnant patients.

Causation of Toxic Reactions

Systemic local anesthetic toxicity results from an excessive amount of local anesthetic in the blood or from brief exposure of the heart and brain to a high concentration of the local anesthetic. A high concentration of a local anesthetic in the blood primarily results from inadvertent intravascular injection. Rarely it results from injection of an excessive amount of the local anesthetic in a highly vascular space like the epidural space, intercostal space, or axillary sheath. The magnitude of absorption of the local anesthetic depends on (1) the total mass of the drug injected, (2) the vascularity of the space, and (3) whether vasoconstricting drugs are added to the local anesthetic.

In pregnant patients, in the event of inadvertent venous injection, because of the increased blood flow through lumbar veins (vertebral venous plexus), the heart and brain may be exposed to a high concentration of local anesthetic.[1] However, in this situation the concentration of the local anesthetic in the peripheral venous sample may not be as high. In the case of unintended venous injection, the patient manifests signs and symptoms of toxicity within a minute or two of injection, but with venous absorption several minutes might elapse.

Effect of Systemic Toxicity

Excessive levels of local anesthetic in the blood affect the functioning of the central nervous system (CNS), the heart, and the peripheral vasculature. The effect on these systems can indirectly affect the well-being of the fetus and newborn. High levels of the local anesthetic may get across the placenta and can directly affect the fetus and newborn. Local anesthetics block conduction of neural impulses by blocking the conduction of sodium. At toxic levels depression of inhibitory pathways of the CNS occurs first. This results in stimulation of excitatory pathways and development of seizures. With very high levels generalized depression of all organ systems occurs.

In the cardiovascular system, a toxic level of local anesthetic first causes depression of myocardium followed by dilatation of smooth muscles of the peripheral vasculature. Depression of the conductance system in the heart causes loss of automaticity, prolongation of the P-R interval, widening of the Q-R-S complex, and triggering of various ventricular dysrhythmias.

Systemic toxicity of the local anesthetic is further increased by an increase in carbon dioxide pressure (P_{CO_2}), a decrease in pH, concomitant administration of other depressant drugs, potency of the local anesthetic used, and physiologic status of the patient.[4] Preexistent sympathetic neural block could further add to the cardiovascular compromise. The rate of injection also can affect the toxicity. Rapid, inadvertent, intravenous injection of the local anesthetic can produce toxic reactions at a lower blood level.[5]

Central Nervous System Toxicity

The earliest manifestations of systemic local anesthetic toxicity are noticed in the CNS. Progressive increase in the blood level of local anesthetic results in the development of the following signs and symptoms: tinnitus, light-headedness, metallic taste, circumoral numbness, slurred speech, nystagmus, talkativeness, feeling "something funny," and tremors. While the local anesthetic level increases further, full-blown seizure with tonic-clonic convulsions ensues. Sometimes generalized CNS depression can induce cardiorespiratory arrest.

Massive overdose of the local anesthetic sometimes causes generalized depression unpreceded by excitatory CNS symptoms. This is manifested by coma, hypotension, bradycardia, and apnea. In general, CNS toxicity of a local anesthetic correlates well with its potency (Table 13-1). Thus the relative toxicity of bupivacaine, etidocaine, and lidocaine is about 4 : 2 : 1, which is similar to their potency in blocking peripheral nerves.[6] During subconvulsant stages, no significant changes are noticed in the electroencephalogram. However, in the preconvulsant and convulsant stages, an increase in the alpha and delta activity occurs, particularly in the amygdaloid area. From there, the seizure activity spreads to other areas.

Cardiovascular Toxicity

A high blood level of a local anesthetic can affect the functioning of the cardiovascular system by (1) inhibiting the conduction of neural impulses along the conducting system of the heart, (2) depressing myocardial contractility, and (3) dilating the smooth muscles of the peripheral vasculature. Preexistent sympathetic block could affect cardioaccelerator fibers and peripheral sympathetic nerves, and could potentially aggravate the cardiac compromise.

In general the CVS is more resistant to the toxic effects of local anesthetic than is the CNS. However, if CVS toxicity were to occur, it is potentially more lethal and is harder to treat than CNS toxicity. The CVS toxicity, like the CNS toxicity of a lo-

TABLE 13-1

Correlation Between Local Anesthetic Property and CVS and CNS Toxicities for Various Local Anesthetics

Agent	Relative Anesthetic Potency	Convulsive Threshold (Cats) (mg/kg)	CNS Relative Toxicity	Lethal Dose (Dogs) (mg/kg)	Relative Lethal Dose
Procaine	1	35	1.0	85	1.0
Chloroprocaine	1	—	—	30	2.8
Prilocaine	2	22	1.5	30	2.8
Mepivacaine	2	17	2.0	30	2.8
Lidocaine	2	15	2.3	30	2.8
Etidocaine	4		—	22	4.0
Bupivacaine	8	4	8.0	11	8.0
Tetracaine	8	—	—	13	6.5

CVS, cardiovascular system; CNS, central nervous system.

cal anesthetic, is proportional to its potency in blocking peripheral nerves. In addition to the potency of a local anesthetic, several other factors affect CVS toxicity: rate of injection, the site of inadvertent venous injection, the acid-base status of the patient, pregnancy, hyperkalemia, and importantly, concentration of the anesthetic used.

After inadvertent intraepidural venous injection, a pregnant patient is more likely to manifest significant cardiovascular compromise than is a nonpregnant patient. During pregnancy, the blood flow through the epidural-azygos venous channel is high. Sometimes streaming of the local anesthetic could occur in the epidural venous system. As a result, after an inadvertent epidural venous injection, during the first pass through, the heart and the brain may be exposed to a significant concentration of local anesthetic (Fig. 13-1). Highly protein-bound local anesthetics like bupivacaine are present in an unbound form to a greater extent in a pregnant patient than in a nonpregnant patient. Studies in sheep have shown that the ratio between cardiovascular collapse and convulsive threshold for a local anesthetic is lower in pregnant animals than in nonpregnant animals.[7] The CNS toxicity may be decreased by prior treatment with barbiturates or benzodiazepines.

Treatment of Central Nervous System Toxicity

In the majority of the cases involving unintended intravenous injection, if the amount of local anesthetic injected is small (<3 ml), no significant complications result. Accidental intravenous injection is recognized by the presence of preconvulsant signs and symptoms. Further injection of the local anesthetic is stopped and the patient is carefully observed for any manifestations of toxic reactions. The

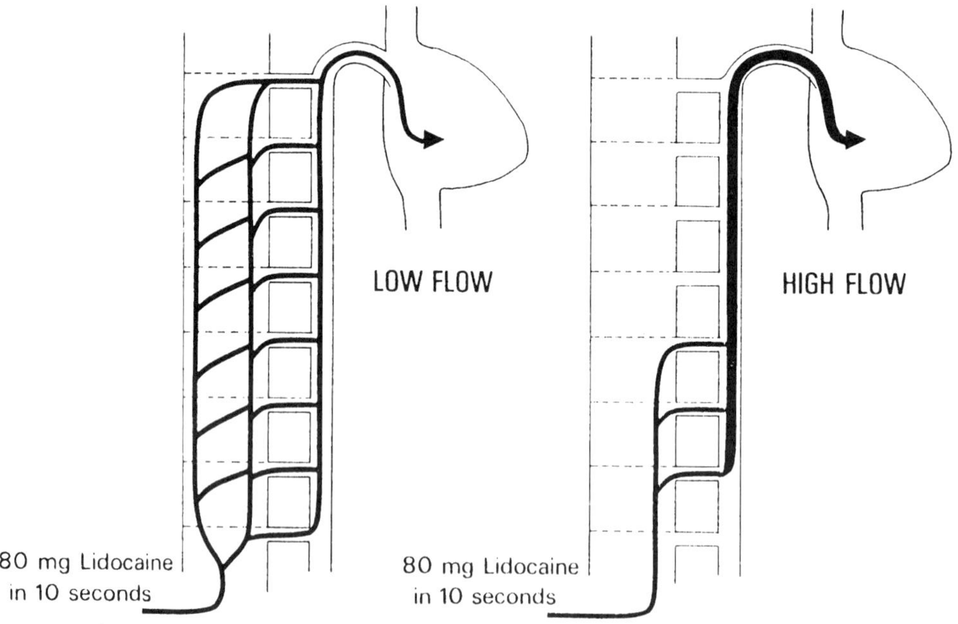

Fig. 13-1.

Vena caval compression associated with pregnancy can cause a "bolus" effect after inadvertent epidural venous injection. *(From Bromage PR:* Epidural analgesia, *Philadelphia, 1979, WB Saunders.)*

epidural catheter is removed and a new one is placed at a different location.

If accidental intravenous injection occurs during the top-up injection (<5 ml), the blood level may be high enough to trigger a seizure episode. Generally the seizure activity in this situation is short lived and self-terminating. During the second pass through the brain, the concentration is much lower on account of redistribution, and seizure activity ceases.

The CNS toxic reaction that follows a test dose injection generally is mild. The patient is informed and reassured. Supplemental oxygen is administered via mask. The airway is maintained and respiration is supported. Precautionary steps are taken to treat any serious toxic reactions. If the seizure persists, measures to control seizure activity like administration of succinylcholine, midazolam, or ultra-short acting barbiturates must be undertaken.

If inadvertent intravenous injection follows the second top-up dose or administration of a large volume of local anesthetic for perineal anesthesia or for cesarean section, one should be prepared to manage convulsions and cardiorespiratory arrest. The management of this situation is discussed in a subsequent section of this chapter.

Pathophysiology of Cardiovascular Toxicity

Local anesthetics depress transmission of impulses via the cardiac conduction system by blocking the sodium channels. This blockade generally occurs during systole and dissipates during diastole. However, different anesthetics dissipate during diastole at different rates. Bupivacaine becomes firmly attached to the sodium channels and does not dissipate during diastole. In subconvulsive levels local anesthetics generally do not significantly affect the functioning of the cardiovascular system. At these levels slight tachycardia and hypertension are noticed. Local anesthetics cause vasoconstriction or vasodilatation of the smooth muscles in the peripheral vasculature, depending on the concentration. At low concentration they cause vasoconstriction. It has also been noticed that local anesthetics, by their action on the central autonomic centers, can affect cardiac rhythm and peripheral vasomotor tone. The clinical effects of subconvulsive levels of local anesthetic include slight depression of myocardium and minimal increase in heart rate and blood pressure. Minimal changes are noticed in the electrocardiogram (ECG) tracing.

At convulsant and supraconvulsant levels of local anesthetic, significant changes in myocardial neural conduction, myocardial contractility, and peripheral vasomotor tone are noticed. A progressive rise in the local anesthetic level causes prolongation of the P-R interval, widening of the Q-R-S complex, bradycardia, and even asystole. Cardiac contractility and stroke volume are greatly diminished. Systemic vascular resistance is decreased. The addition of epinephrine to local anesthetic might minimize the cardiodepressant effect of a high concentration of local anesthetic. The cardiovascular toxicity is further increased by hypoxia and the lactic acidosis that follows generalized convulsions. Unintended injection of long-acting amide-type local anesthetics, in some cases, might cause irreversible cardiac arrest.

Cardiovascular Toxicity with Various Local Anesthetics

The ester type of local anesthetics like 2-chloroprocaine are likely to induce less toxic reactions than the amide type of local anesthetics. This is because they are more rapidly metabolized. Clinical experience suggests that highly protein bound and highly lipid-soluble local anesthetics, if accidentally intravenously injected, could produce cardiac depression that is not easily reversible, or even death. Reports of deaths associated with the use of 0.75% bupivacaine and the subsequent investigative results prompted the Food and Drug Administration to issue a recommendation that 0.75% bupivacaine should not be used in parturients.[8] Subsequent investigations in various animals have yielded the following results:

- In vitro atrial muscle studies have shown that bupivacaine is more cardiotoxic than equipotent levels of lidocaine.[9]
- Under conditions of hypoxia and lactic acid, bupivacaine is more cardiotoxic than any other local anesthetic.
- When a lethal dose of a local anesthetic is administered, a higher percentage of animals receiving bupivacaine develop ventricular dysrhythmias.[10]
- Even when convulsant doses of equipotent local anesthetics are administered, bupivacaine is more likely to produce ventricular dysrhythmias than is lidocaine.
- Intracerebroventricular injection of a subconvulsant concentration of bupivacaine produces ventricular dysrhythmia and cardiac depression.[11]

Thus several animal studies confirm the increased cardiotoxic potential of bupivacaine. This toxicity is further enhanced during pregnancy.

Treatment of Severe Cardiovascular Toxicity of Local Anesthetics

When epidural anesthesia is administered to a pregnant patient, the anesthesiologist should be prepared to handle a severe toxic reaction in the patient's room. Effective therapy should be initiated within 15 seconds of occurrence of a seizure or cardiorespiratory arrest. The recommended resuscitative steps include the following:

1. Summon help to manage cardiopulmonary resuscitation (CPR). Effective management of cardiorespiratory arrest requires the involvement of several people.
2. Administer oxygen by mask.
3. Maintain the patient's airway with the placement of oral or nasal airways.
4. Monitor ECG for development of ventricular dysrhythmias and asystole.
5. If the patient is apneic, ventilate the patient's lungs with bag and mask.
6. Control seizures with administration of a small amount of succinylcholine (80 mg), midazolam (0.1 mg/kg), or barbiturate (100 mg).
7. Place the patient in the supine position and insert a firm board under the patient.
8. Elevate the patient's lower extremities and shift the uterus to the left; these measures will improve the venous return.
9. Correct hypotension and bradycardia with administration of liberal amounts of ephedrine (10 to 25 mg), epinephrine (0.1 to 0.2 mg), calcium chloride (500 mg), atropine (0.5 to 1.0 mg), phenylephrine, and other cardioactive drugs.
10. Institute CPR if the blood pressure is low or in the presence of cardiorespiratory arrest.
11. Correct ventricular dysrhythmias with administration of bretylium (5 to 10 mg/kg) or by application of defibrillatory shock.
12. In a desperate situation, while CPR is being performed, expeditious delivery of the infant might improve fetal and maternal outcome.[12]

Prevention of Systemic Toxicity

Systemic local anesthetic toxicity generally follows inadvertent intravenous (IV) injection of a significant amount of local anesthetic. However, in most cases this is preventable. Various experts have recommended several different methods to identify the intravascular placement of the epidural catheter. It must be remembered that these techniques are not 100% sensitive or specific.

Aspirate Blood from the Catheter

Aspirate for blood from the epidural catheter, both before and after injection of any volume of local anesthetic. Aspiration must be done before bandages are applied. If the tip of the catheter is up against the wall of the vein, there might be a negative aspiration of blood. Using a multiple-hole catheter tip might avoid this problem. In about 10% of parturients placement of epidural needle could cause some bleeding from the traumatized veins. This might result in aspiration of blood-tinged fluid, even if the catheter is not in the vein. Clearing the catheter with administration of 2 ml of saline and then reaspirating fluid through the catheter will confirm or rule out intravascular placement of the catheter.

Test Dose

Inject a test dose consisting of 3 ml of a local anesthetic and 15 μg of epinephrine before any injection of local anesthetic. It has been observed that intravenous injection of 15 μg of epinephrine transiently raises the heart rate by at least 10 beats per minute.[13] Notice that this rise in the heart rate lasts for only 10 to 30 seconds. Therefore it is recommended that the anesthesiologist monitor the pulse with pulse oximetry or ECG while the test dose is injected. By causing vasoconstriction, epinephrine might minimize the vascular absorption of the local anesthetics. (Epinephrine, 15 μg as a test dose, is not used in laboring patients in the editor's institution because of the possibility of maternal tachycardia from uterine contraction.)

Use the Lowest Effective Concentration

Whenever possible, the lowest concentration of a local anesthetic, in the smallest effective volume, should be used in the epidural space. Significant toxic reactions are unlikely to occur if bupivacaine 0.125% or lidocaine 0.5% is used as a continuous IV infusion. Continuous-infusion technique offers greater safety over the intermittent bolus technique.

Use Less-Toxic Local Anesthetic

Since cardiorespiratory arrest is less likely to occur with chloroprocaine or lidocaine, it may be prudent to use 2% lidocaine or 2% lidocaine with epinephrine instead of 0.5% bupivacaine. Ropivacaine, which still is under investigation, seems to be a better alternative to bupivacaine.

Fractional Dosing

A large volume of anesthetic is used to institute perineal anesthesia or to raise the level of anesthesia for cesarean section. In these situations, it is recommended that the local anesthetic be administered in increments not exceeding 5 ml. By using this technique, inadvertent injection of a large volume of local anesthetic is avoided.

Close Monitoring of the Patient

Maintenance of verbal contact with the patient during injection of local anesthetic cannot be overemphasized. While injecting the local anesthetic, the patient should be urged to notify the operator if she experiences "racing of the heart" or other symptoms of mild toxic reactions. If possible, heart rate should be monitored with pulse oximetry or ECG. The patient's vital signs should be closely watched for 15 minutes after each injection.

Suspect Intravenous Injection

If the patient does not develop sensory anesthesia with administration of 10 to 12 ml of a local anesthetic, the possibility of intravenous injection should be considered. One should keep in mind that venous injections of increments of lidocaine or chloroprocaine sometimes may not produce subjective symptoms.

Be Prepared for Successful Resuscitation

Sometimes, in spite of observing all of the recommended precautions, toxic reactions do occur.[14] Therefore anyone administering epidural anesthesia should always be mentally prepared to handle such situations. An epidural cart should be fully equipped with all resuscitative equipment and drugs. An oxygen source and suction apparatus should be immediately available. The nurse who is monitoring the patient should be authorized to administer ephedrine IV and oxygen if the patient develops significant hypotension and if the anesthesiologist is unavailable immediately. It is desirable to conduct periodic drills involving the anesthesiologist, obstetrician, nurses, and personnel who are ancillary in the management of anesthetic emergencies.

Management of the Presented Case

In the case cited at the beginning of the chapter, the patient probably received more than 5 ml of bupivacaine anesthesia without the benefit of a test dose. Since she developed tachyarrhythmias, she should be treated like one who has a serious toxic reaction. The patient's airway should be maintained and protected. She should receive 100% oxygen. If the patient stops breathing, she should receive mask-ventilation by bag and mask first. If the seizure persists, it should be controlled with the IV administration of 1 mg/kg of succinylcholine and 5 mg of midazolam, and the patient should be intubated. Fetal heart rate and maternal ECG should be closely monitored.

Depending on the type of arrhythmia, she should receive bretylium or defibrillatory shock. One should anticipate that prolonged CPR would be needed to restore the patient to her normal state. If CPR is ineffective or if fetal distress is present, then expeditious vaginal or abdominal delivery should be considered.

Summary

The use of epidural anesthesia to relieve the pain of labor and delivery has become very popular. One of the serious complications associated with administration of epidural anesthesia is the occurrence of CNS and cardiac toxicity. In the majority of these cases the cause of toxic reaction is unintended intravascular injection. This complication potentially is life threatening. By taking proper preventive measures the incidence of this complication can be minimized. This will include the following:

1. Aspirating blood from the catheter
2. Using a test dose of anesthetic (in the laboring patient this is controversial)
3. Using the lowest effective concentration of anesthetic
4. Using a less toxic local anesthetic
5. Fractional dosing of the anesthetic
6. Close monitoring of the patient
7. Suspecting IV injection

However, in spite of incorporating all of the precautionary steps, toxic reactions can and do occur. A person involved in the administration of epidural anesthesia should be well prepared to handle such a complication.

References

1. Bromage PR: *Pharmacology: epidural analgesia,* Philadelphia, 1979, WB Saunders.
2. Leighton BL: *Anesthetic complications: intraoperative.* In Norris MC, editor: *Obstetric anesthesia,* Philadelphia, 1992, JB Lippincott.
3. Ravindran RS, Albrecht W, McKay M: Apparent intravascular migration of epidural catheter, *Anesth Analg* 1979; 58:252.
4. Thigpen JW, Kotelko DM, Shnider SM, et al: Bupivacaine cardiotoxicity in hypoxic-acidotic sheep, *Anesthesiology* 1983; 59:A204.

5. Moore DC, Bridenbaugh LD, Thomson GE, et al: Factors determining dosages of amide type local anesthetic drugs, *Anesthesiology* 1977; 47:263.
6. Liu P, Feldman HS, Covino BM, et al: Acute cardiovascular toxicity of intravenous amide local anesthetics in anesthetized ventilated dogs, *Anesth Analg* 1982; 61:317.
7. Crandell JT, Kotelko DM: Cardiotoxicity of local anesthetics during late pregnancy, *Anesth Analg* 1985; 64:204.
8. Albright GA: Cardiac arrest following regional anesthesia with etidocaine or bupivacaine, *Anesthesiology* 1979; 51:285.
9. Block A, Covino BG: Effect of local anesthetic agents on cardiac conduction and contractility, *Reg Anesth* 1981; 6:55.
10. Sage DJ, Feldman HS, Arthur GR, et al: The cardiovascular effects of convulsant doses of lidocaine and bupivacaine in the conscious dog, *Reg Anesth* 1985; 10:175.
11. Heavner JE: Cardiac dysrhythmias induced by infusion of local anesthetics into the lateral cerebral venticle of cats, *Anesth Analg* 1986; 65:133.
12. Marx GF: Cardiopulmonary resuscitation of late-pregnant women, *Anesthesiology* 1982; 56:156.
13. Colonna-Romano P, Lingaragu N, Godfrey SD, et al: Epidural test dose and intravascular injection in obstetrics: sensitivity, specificity, and lowest effective dose, *Anesth Analg* 1992; 75:372.
14. McLean BY, Rottman RL, Kotelko DM: Failure of multiple test doses and techniques to detect intravascular migration of an epidural catheter, *Anesth Analg* 1991; 74:454.

14

Drug Interactions in Obstetric Patients

A 21-year-old primigravida with a history of severe preeclampsia is admitted to the labor floor. Magnesium sulfate is administered intravenously (IV) as follows: 4 g loading dose IV and then 1 g/hr by continuous infusion. After 8 hours of poor labor, emergency cesarean section is performed for acute fetal distress, with the patient receiving general anesthesia. Succinylcholine, 100 mg given IV is used for tracheal intubation. Anesthesia lasts 1 hour 20 minutes, after which the patient makes no effort at spontaneous ventilation. The patient has previously received uneventful general anesthesia. Discuss the drug interactions.

Recommendations by Jaya Ramanathan, M.D.
John G. D'Alessio, M.D.

This case represents one of the classic examples of drug interactions in pregnancy, familiar to obstetric anesthesiologists practicing in busy perinatal centers.

Before the discussion of specific drug interactions in pregnancy, a brief description of the definitions of various types of drug interactions is necessary. These are addition, synergism, potentiation, and antagonism.[1] The term *addition* is defined as the combined effects of one half dose of a drug with one half dose of another equipotent drug is the same as the entire dose of either drug (i.e., $2 + 2 = 4$). *Synergism* is defined as the type of drug interaction in which the combined effects of the two drugs are far greater than when each drug is used alone (i.e., $2 + 2 > 4$). *Potentiation* occurs when the action of one drug is enhanced by another drug, which does not have an action on its own (i.e., $2 + 0 = 3$). *Antagonism* is perhaps the easiest term to understand: the drugs have opposing actions (i.e., $2 + 2 < 4$).

During pregnancy the average number of drugs ingested by the woman varies from 1.3 to 11.[1] In addition to iron and vitamin supplements, pregnant women use many nonprescription drugs such as antiemetics, antihistamines, antiallergy medications, and analgesics. While the number of drugs administered to any patient increases, so does the potential for adverse interactions.

When discussing the drug interactions in pregnancy, one cannot ignore the physiologic changes of pregnancy that profoundly affect the drug absorption, distribution, metabolism, and elimination. During pregnancy, the plasma volume increases by 45% and cardiac output by 40% with significant increases in renal, uterine, and pulmonary blood flow.[2] However, the hepatic blood flow remains unaltered. The total body water at term is increased by 8 liters, 60% of which is accounted for by the products of conception.[3] Therefore the apparent volume of distribution is increased significantly, resulting in lower plasma drug levels. The significant decreases in plasma protein concentrations—specifically, albumin levels—can lower the bound fraction of drugs. This results in increased free fractions of drugs and enhanced pharmacologic response. The increased pulmonary blood flow and alveolar ventilation can alter the pulmonary uptake of drugs and anesthetic agents administered by inhalation. Progesterone enhances the activity of hepatic microsomal enzymes and increases the biotransformation of certain drugs.[4] However, since hepatic blood flow remains unchanged, the hepatic extraction ratio is not altered in pregnancy.[5] Effective renal plasma flow is increased by 25% and glomerular filtration rate by 30% to 60% and therefore renal clearance is rapid.[6]

Specific Drug Interactions

Anesthetic Induction Agents

Barbiturates and benzodiazepines frequently are used for sedation, hypnosis, and induction of general anesthesia. Thiopental and midazolam act synergistically, with 50% to 70% reduction in induction doses. The combination should be used with caution in a patient with a full stomach.

Ketamine is another commonly used induction agent in obstetric anesthesia. Benefits include stable hemodynamics and minimal respiratory depression. Ketamine is a potent bronchodilator and frequently is used for anesthetic induction in asthmatic patients. In combination with methylxanthines, cardiovascular side effects such as dysrhythmias may be accentuated. The seizure threshold is lowered by high levels of both methylxanthines and ketamine.[7] Therefore the combination should be used with caution in patients with a history of seizure disorders. Lithium often is used in the treatment of manic depressive disorders, with sedation as a frequent side effect. Ketamine administered to the patient receiving lithium can prolong the actions of ketamine.[8] Barbiturate action also may be prolonged by ketamine.

Antiasthmatic Drugs

Asthma affects 0.5% to 1.5% of pregnancies and progresses to status asthmaticus in 0.2% of cases.[9] About one third of parturients will experience worsening, improvement, or no change from the nonpregnant state.[10,11] Exacerbation of symptoms often is noticed after the twenty-ninth week of pregnancy and into the postpartum period. Thus it is essential that appropriate therapy be continued throughout the pregnancy and in the immediate postpartum period. As has been noted in patients with epilepsy, risks to both the mother and the fetus increase in the presence of asthma.

Oral *theophylline* preparations are commonly

used for prophylaxis and treatment of asthma in spite of the narrow therapeutic window. Interactions with many drugs used in pregnancy are common with this drug. Frequent measurements of plasma concentrations are necessary due to increasing maternal weight and volume of distribution, and normal clearance.[12] A drug interaction of note includes decreased clearance of theophylline when combined with cimetidine or beta blockers. Plasma levels of theophylline rise unpredictably and do so within the first day of combined therapy. Ketamine and other sympathomimetic drugs may induce tachycardia in the susceptible patient. Ketamine and theophylline may interact to lower the seizure threshold whereas either drug alone will not do so.[7] If the parturient is using a theophylline preparation, it should be continued; however, acute administration adds little if any benefit to β-agonists.[13] *β-Adrenergic agonists* also are frequently prescribed for pregnant asthmatics. Parenteral administration is discussed in the section on tocolytics below. Inhaled preparations of β-agonists, because of the small dose and minimal systemic absorption, are less likely to interact with other medications.

Inhaled *corticosteroids* and *cromolyn sodium* are two other classes of drugs used in asthma treatment. Again, because of the very low administered dose and minimal systemic absorption, drug interactions of significance are minimal. Therefore, inhaled medications should be the first line of therapy in pregnant women with asthma.

Antiepileptics

Epileptic disorders are encountered in 0.5% of all pregnancies. Epilepsy increases the risk of preeclampsia, hemorrhage, and difficult delivery.[14,15] In addition, the risks of fetal malformations, preterm delivery, low birth weight, and fetal mortality were two to four times higher in these women.[14] About 50% of epileptic patients will experience an increase in seizure activity during pregnancy[16] and thus close control of plasma levels of antiseizure medications is essential.[17] Pregnancy-induced hepatic changes increase the metabolism of phenytoin but decreased protein binding raises free levels of drug. The two effects possibly counteract each other.

Phenytoin is the most frequently administered anticonvulsant and also the drug with which the largest number of significant drug interactions are observed. Chronic administration of phenytoin may cause peripheral neuropathies which should be evaluated and documented before initiation of regional anesthesia.[18] Benzodiazepines and barbiturates will increase free plasma levels of phenytoin and potentially cause overdose reactions. In addition, the combination will increase the risk of significant sedation. Cimetidine will inhibit metabolism of phenytoin and increase plasma levels.[19] When general anesthesia is administered, interactions with muscle relaxants are numerous. Defasciculating doses of d-tubocurarine (dTC) will be enhanced in effect and can result in significant neuromuscular blockade and loss of protective airway reflexes.[20] Chronic phenytoin use will decrease the duration of vecuronium and doxacurium by 50% whereas that of atracurium is not affected.[21,22] Acute administration will cause unpredictable prolongation of vecuronium block.[21] Succinylcholine metabolism is not affected.

Epileptic seizure activity suppression by valproic acid is another source of frequent drug interactions. Interference with hepatic metabolism is the mechanism of prolonged action of barbiturates, benzodiazepines, and opioids.[23] The time interval between doses should be increased. A second effect of chronic valproic acid use is thrombocytopenia and inhibition of platelet aggregation. Thrombocytopenia also is noticed with *carbamazepine*. Both adequate platelet counts and function should be verified before the administration of neuraxial anesthetic techniques. *Phenobarbital* is known to induce enhanced hepatic enzyme function and speed metabolism of many classes of drugs. Local anesthetic agents and regional anesthesia techniques generally are safe when applied using standard precautions.

Antihypertensives

Current therapy of preeclampsia includes use of several classes of antihypertensive agents. Chronic therapy utilizes alpha methyldopa and beta blockers in addition to bedrest. *α-Methyldopa* acts by interfering with the synthesis of dopamine and by behaving as a false neurotransmitter in place of norepinephrine.[24] The decrease in central nervous system (CNS) norepinephrine and dopamine concentrations cause a small but significant decrease in mean alveolar concentration (MAC) for the volatile anesthetic agents.[25] In combination with the decreased MAC observed in pregnancy, this may cause prolonged awakening from general anesthesia and exaggerated hypotensive effects.

β-adrenergic blockers such as labetalol frequently are used because of their mixed alpha and beta blocking effects (1:3 oral, 1:7 IV). Interactions of significance in the preeclamptic population include the risk of congestive heart failure in those receiving nifedipine because of the combined negative inotropic effects. Oral labetalol in combination with cimetidine results in increased bioavailability of labetalol. Nitroglycerin and β-blocker may result in profound hypotension. Interactions of *nifedipine* include those with magnesium with the possibility of significant hypotension due to the combined calcium channel blocking actions of both drugs. A similar mechanism may be responsible for hypotension seen with the use of volatile inhalation anesthetics.[26] Cimetidine administered to decrease gastric acidity will increase plasma levels of nifedipine and potentiate the hypotensive response. This may be due to inhibition of the hepatic P-450 microsomal enzyme system. Epidural anesthesia may interact with the vasodilating properties of nifedipine to produce more severe hypotension. Slow initiation of epidural block and adequate volume loading should prevent this interaction from becoming significant.[27] Nifedipine may act as a direct myometrial relaxant with resultant prolongation of labor or postpartum bleeding. Calcium channel blockade will directly antagonize the uterotonic effects of prostaglandin F2-α and may aggravate postpartum bleeding.[28]

Trimethaphan acts primarily as a ganglionic blocking agent with concomitant direct vasodilating properties. Trimethaphan in large doses will prolong the effects of succinylcholine and nondepolarizing neuromuscular blocking agents.[29] The mechanism of this effect is inhibition of pseudocholinesterase and decreased sensitivity of the postjunctional membrane to acetylcholine.[29] Potentiation of the customarily used hypotensive agents is frequent and may be severe.

Illicit Drugs

Cocaine use ranges from 7.5% to 45% in the obstetric population.[30,31] The half-life is the same as in the nonpregnant patient (20 to 60 minutes) due to the increased volume of distribution but decreased plasma cholinesterase activity.[32] Progesterone may increase the cardiac toxicity and myocardial depression of cocaine.[33,34] Cocaine predisposes the parturient to preterm labor, placental abruption, cerebrovascular accidents, and severe thrombocytopenia.[35] Drug interactions include the following: (1) increased incidence of hypotension secondary to epidural anesthesia; (2) possible decreased response to indirect acting sympathomimetic agents due to depletion of catecholamine stores; (3) amino-ester local-anesthetic cocaine may compete for metabolism by plasma cholinesterase with drugs such as trimethaphan thus increasing the likelihood of toxicity of both drugs; (4) epinephrine in local anesthetics used for test dose may act synergistically, resulting in severe hypertension and decreased uteroplacental blood flow; (5) halothane and ketamine may potentiate arrhythmogenic and myocardial toxicity potential of cocaine; and (6) succinylcholine degradation may be prolonged by interfering with plasma cholinesterase. Antagonism of cocaine-induced hypertension and myocardial ischemia is best achieved with the mixed α- and β-blocker labetalol. Hydralazine may lower maternal blood pressure at the expense of uteroplacental blood flow.[36]

Amphetamines are CNS stimulants that act by α- and β-adrenergic agonist effect, similar in effect to ephedrine. A resurgence in amphetamine abuse has been noted. Acute use may cause hypertension and increase anesthetic requirements. Chronic abuse depletes central catecholamine stores and may lower MAC, as well as precipitate hypotension in the situation of sympathetic blockade. Direct-acting vasopressors such as phenylephrine should be used to treat hypotension.

Neuromuscular Blockers

Succinylcholine is a part of the standard rapid-sequence induction as practiced in modern obstetric anesthesia. However, many potential problems occur with its use. Degradation of succinylcholine proceeds normally by plasma cholinesterase despite the decreased levels of this enzyme in pregnancy.[37] Preeclampsia reduces the level of this enzyme to a greater degree. In addition, several drugs commonly used to treat preeclampsia interact to prolong the normal action. Magnesium acts to decrease neuromuscular transmission by reducing acetylcholine release and diminishing responsiveness of the muscle cell membrane.[38] No direct effect exists of magnesium on plasma cholinesterase.[39] Metoclopramide acts to inhibit pseudocholinesterase, as do trimethaphan and neostigmine.[40] (See the following case discussion below for further interactions.)

Nondepolarizing neuromuscular blockers are used to prolong muscle relaxation, to allow ease of surgical exposure, and to achieve a quiet operative field. The intermediate-acting drugs, atracurium and vecuronium, frequently are administered for cesarean section. Magnesium augments the neuromuscular blockade of these drugs by its effects on the neuromuscular junction. Other interactions of note include potentiation by antibiotics such as gentamicin, tobramycin, and clindamycin, as well as drugs such as lithium and furosemide.

Tocolytics

The commonly used tocolytic agents are ritodrine and terbutaline, β-*2-agonists,* and magnesium. Other drugs with tocolytic properties are the prostaglandin synthesis inhibitors, calcium channel blockers, and oxytocin antagonists. Use of this second group is not widespread. The β-2-agonists act by increasing intracellular cyclic adenosine monophosphate concentrations, decreasing free calcium levels, and preventing the action of contractile proteins. Side effects include CNS stimulation, tachycardia, hypotension, hyperglycemia, hypokalemia, and pulmonary edema. Concurrent administration of magnesium also may result in pulmonary edema,[41] presumably due to salt and water retention initiated by the β-agonist combined with a negative inotropic effect of magnesium.[42] Other factors such as maternal infection may play an important role.[43] Concurrent use of other sympathomimetic and anticholinergic drugs may worsen the hyperglycemia and tachyarrhythmias, and should be avoided. Vasopressors must be used with caution to avoid further increases in vascular resistance and inotropic state resulting in cardiac decompensation. *Corticosteroids* frequently are used in preterm labor patients to enhance fetal lung maturation. Acute therapy may exacerbate the hyperglycemia initiated by β-agonists. Other side effects include hypokalemia and fluid retention, which are manifestations of mineralocorticoid effects.

Magnesium sulfate frequently is administered as

a tocolytic and is the drug of choice for cardiac patients and diabetics. Since it exists as a divalent cation, magnesium interferes with the actions of calcium and acts as an inhibitor of calcium mediated functions. The drug interactions with β-2-agonists already have been alluded to and their effects on the myoneural junction are discussed later in this chapter.

Uterotonics

Oxytocin is a potent stimulant of myometrial contractile activity. Uses include stimulation of labor and control of postpartum uterine bleeding. Oxytocin may cause either hypertension or hypotension based on its use. Hypertension has been noticed with oxytocin use in some individuals despite the lack of contamination by vasopressin, which is common to the naturally derived mixture. However, hypotension is far more common and is dose related.[44] Rapid administration of oxytocin in combination with sympathetic block of regional anesthesia may precipitate severe hypotension. Antidiuresis is a complication of prolonged or rapid oxytocin administration. In addition, hyponatremia and hyposmolar states can occur, with risk of cerebral edema and hyponatremic convulsions.[45] Avoidance of free water administration is recommended. Oxytocin in combination with the *ergot alkaloids* can cause severe hypertension, particularly in the preeclamptic patient.[46] Administration of any of the vasoactive agents such as phenylephrine, ephedrine, or methoxamine can result in precipitous hypertension, myocardial ischemia, and cardiac failure.[47] Therefore vasopressors should be administered with caution.

Prostaglandin F2-α is used for control of postpartum hemorrhage. This agent significantly increases uterine tone. Interactions with other drugs include bronchoconstriction when used in combination with β-blockers and precipitation of asthma in susceptible individuals.[48] Pulmonary artery vasoconstriction with arterial hypoxemia is another common side effect.[49] Hypertension may occur when this drug is used alone or more commonly when used in combination with ergot alkaloids.

Some of the important drug interactions are listed in Table 14-1.

Allergy

A chapter on drug interactions in pregnancy is not complete without discussion of anaphylactic reactions and their management. Anaphylaxis is characterized by respiratory (asthma, laryngeal edema), cardiovascular (hypotension, cardiovascular collapse), gastrointestinal (vomiting, diarrhea, abdominal pain), and dermatologic (urticaria, angioedema) symptoms occurring alone or all at once. These highly reproducible reactions are mediated by specific antibodies. IgE on the surface of mast cells and basophils binds a foreign immunogen which initiates release of histamine, chemotactic factors, bradykinin, and platelet aggregating factor. This massive release of stored mediators leads to secondary and prolonged production of equally dangerous prostaglandins (thromboxane A2, PGE2, PGF2, PGI2) and leukotrienes.

In a sensitized individual, the onset may be delayed up to 20 minutes; however, more than 90% of patients manifest the reaction in 10 minutes or less.[50] Anaphylaxis in patients under general anesthesia may include any or all of the signs in Table 14-2. Cardiovascular collapse and cardiac arrest are seen in 68% and 11%, respectively, whereas bronchospasm was noted in 23%.[51] Mean arterial pressure and SVR may decrease without a concomitant increase in heart rate. The incidence of anaphylaxis in pregnancy is as common as in the nonpregnant population receiving medications, and is initiated by the same triggering agents. Virtually any parenterally administered drug has the potential to cause an anaphylactic reaction. Of the cases reported in the intensive care and operating room areas, 50% are

TABLE 14-1
Drug Interactions in Pregnancy

Drug Name		Interaction	Therapy
Anesthetic Induction Agents			
Barbiturates	Benzodiazepines	Synergistic sedative effects	Reduce dose of each drug by 30%-50%
Ketamine	Lithium	Prolonged ketamine effects	Avoid combining
Ketamine	Methylxanthines	Release of endogenous catecholamines Tachycardia Lowered seizure threshold	
Antiasthmatics			
Theophylline/aminophylline	Ketamine	Release of endogenous catecholamines Tachycardia Ventricular dysrhythmias Lowered seizure threshold	
Theophylline/aminophylline	Sympathomimetic drugs	Endogenous catecholamines in combination with exogenously administered exceed the toxic limit Tachycardia Ventricular dysrhythmias	Reduce doses of sympathomimetics administered for hypotension
Theophylline/aminophylline	Cimetidine	Elevated plasma levels of theophylline, reduced elimination of theophylline	Follow plasma levels more frequently
Antiepileptics			
Phenytoin	Benzodiazepines Barbiturates	Increased free plasma levels of phenytoin with possible excessive sedation, neurologic and cardiac toxicity	Decrease dose of drugs given for sedation for induction of general anesthesia
Phenytoin	dTC	Augmentation of neuromuscular block	Do not administer dTC for defasciculation
Phenytoin	Regional anesthetic techniques	Peripheral neuropathies may lead to postblock questions about local anesthetic neurotoxicity	Document pre-block degree and extent of neuropathic injury
Phenytoin	Vecuronium Doxacurium	Acute administration of phenytoin prolongs action of these NMBs Chronic administration shortens duration of effect by up to 50%	Monitor neuromuscular function when used in combination

Continued.

TABLE 14-1—cont'd

DRUG INTERACTIONS IN PREGNANCY

Drug Name		Interaction	Therapy
Valproic acid	Regional anesthetic techniques	Thrombocytopenia and depressed platelet function induced by valproic acid may lead to bleeding	Verify platelet count and function before initiating block
Carbamazepine	Regional anesthetic techniques	Thrombocytopenia induced by carbamazepine may lead to bleeding	Verify platelet count before initiating block
Antihypertensive			
α-Methyldopa	Inhalation anesthetics	Decreased MAC Decreased CNS norepinephrine levels	Reduce volatile anesthetic doses
β-Blockers	Nifedipine	Elevated risk of heart failure due to combined negative inotropic effects	
Nifedipine	Epidural anesthesia	Hypotension due to sympathetic blockade and calcium channel blocking actions	Initiate epidural blockade slowly with adequate fluid preloading
Nifedipine	Magnesium	Hypotension due to combined calcium channel blocking actions	Administer ephedrine
Nifedipine	Inhalation anesthetics	Hypotension due to combined calcium channel blocking actions May decrease uterine tone and increase risk of bleeding	
Nifedipine	Cimetidine	Severe hypotension and tachycardia Elevated levels of nifedipine due to blocked degradation	Increase frequency and decrease dose of nifedipine
Nifedipine	PGF2-α	Inhibition of uterotonic effects of prostaglandin	Administer small intravenous boluses of calcium 100-250 mg
Trimethaphan	Succinylcholine Nondepolarizing neuromuscular blockers	Prolonged action of succinylcholine	Inhibition of pseudocholinesterase Decreased sensitivity of the postjunctional membrane to acetylcholine
Illicit Drugs			
Cocaine, acute	Epinephrine in local anesthetics for regional anesthesia or test dose	Cocaine blocks reuptake of norepinephrine, combined with epinephrine exaggerated pressor effect is manifest	Avoid epinephrine

TABLE 14-1—cont'd

DRUG INTERACTIONS IN PREGNANCY

Drug Name		Interaction	Therapy
Cocaine, chronic	Regional anesthesia	Higher incidence of hypotension due to central catecholamine depletion	Careful fluid preload Progress slowly with sympathetic blockade Consider phenylephrine for hypotension
Neuromuscular Blockers			
Nondepolarizing neuromuscular blockers	Magnesium	Decreased quantal release and effect of acetylcholine at motor endplate	Reduce dose of nondepolarizing agent, monitor and assure full return of neuromuscular function
Nondepolarizing neuromuscular blockers	Aminoglycoside antibiotics	Direct effect of aminoglycoside at the neuromuscular junction	Pronounced effect with vecuronium, none with atracurium, reduce dose of vecuronium
Succinylcholine	Metoclopramide Trimethaphan Neostigmine Phenelzine	Decreased plasma cholinesterase function, reduced destruction of succinylcholine	Administer usual intubating dose of succinylcholine, assure return of neuromuscular function before further dosing
Succinylcholine	Magnesium	Decreased quantal release and effect of acetylcholine at motor endplate	Administer usual intubating dose of succinylcholine, assure return of neuromuscular function before further dosing
Psychiatric Drugs			
Lithium	Succinylcholine	See neuromuscular blocking agents	
Monoamine oxidase inhibitors	Indirect-acting sympathomimetics	Exaggerated hypertensive response to common doses due to increased stores of norepinephrine	Avoid indirect-acting agents, epinephrine, cocaine Use decreased dose of phenylephrine for hypotension
Monoamine oxidase inhibitors	Meperidine and other opioids	Hypertension, hyperthermia, seizures, coma; unknown mechanism	Avoid meperidine Use morphine or fentanyl for analgesia
Monoamine oxidase inhibitors	Regional anesthesia	Anticipate potential for hypotension possibly due to false neurotransmitter octopamine	Raise anesthetic level slowly, fluid preload, treat hypotension with phenylephrine, avoid epinephrine
Phenelzine	Succinylcholine	Inhibition of plasma cholinesterase	Monitor neuromuscular blockade

Continued.

TABLE 14-1—cont'd

Drug Interactions in Pregnancy

Drug Name		Interaction	Therapy
Tocolytic Agents			
β-Mimetic	Corticosteroids	Hyperglycemia Hypokalemia Congestive heart failure	Inhibition of insulin action Potassium forced intracellularly Fluid retention from β stimulation May be due to maternal infection
β-Mimetic	Magnesium	Congestive heart failure	
Magnesium	Succinylcholine Nondepolarizing neuromuscular blocking agents	Increased effect of a given dose of NMB due to direct magnesium effect on neuromuscular junction	Carefully monitor neuromuscular function Use regular intubating dose of succinylcholine to ensure paralysis for intubation
Magnesium	Inhalation anesthetics	Hypotension, prolonged awakening	Decreased MAC
Magnesium	Regional anesthesia techniques	Hypotension with decreased uteroplacental perfusion	Establish epidural blockade slowly Adequate hydration Ephedrine is the vasopressor of choice
Uterotonic Agents			
Ergot alkaloids	Ephedrine or phenylephrine	Severe hypertension	Synergistic α-agonist properties
Oxytocin	Free water	Antidiuretic effects Hyponatremia Hyposmolar states	Antidiuretic effects may occur at greater than 20 μu/min Decrease infusion rate Do not infuse in salt-free solutions
Oxytocin	Ergot alkaloids	Severe hypertension, especially in preeclamptic patients	Avoid combined use
Prostaglandin E and F series	Ergot alkaloids Vasopressor agents	Transient hypertension, may be severe in preeclamptic patients	PGF2 will increase uterine tone and stop hemorrhage without the use of ergot alkaloids
Prostaglandin E and F series	β-blockers	Severe bronchoconstriction, hypoxemia	Avoid combined use
Prostaglandin E and F series		Pulmonary artery vasoconstriction, accentuates hypoxic pulmonary vasoconstriction	Supportive therapy

dTC, d-tubocurarine; NMBs, neuromotor blocks; MAC, minimum alveolar concentration; CNS, central nervous system.

TABLE 14-2

Signs and Symptoms of Anaphylaxis

Organ System	Signs	Symptoms
Cardiac/vascular	Hypotension Cardiovascular collapse Decreased systemic vascular resistance Dysrhythmias	Dizziness Decreased level of consciousness
Pulmonary	Tachypnea Stridor Wheezing Laryngeal edema Pulmonary edema Respiratory distress Increased peak airway pressure Decreased oxygen saturation Increased pulmonary artery pressure	Chest tightness Retrosternal pressure
CNS		Sense of impending doom
Integument	Cutaneus rash Hives Angioedema	Metallic oral taste Tongue tingling and swelling

CNS, Central nervous system.

caused by muscle relaxants, 42.3% by hypnotic agents, and less than 5% by benzodiazepines, opioids, and neuroleptic agents.[52]

Induction Agents

Thiobarbiturates incite anaphylaxis in about 1 of 23,000 administrations and thus rarely are a cause.[53] A test dose of 25 to 50 mg of thiopental before the induction dose has been advocated in the past to avoid anaphylaxis. However, because of the explosive self-perpetuating response of anaphylactic reactions, this approach is not warranted. The imidazole drug etomidate does not release histamine and has been recommended as the drug of choice in patients with history of allergy to barbiturates.[54] Propofol, a substituted phenol, is packaged in a soybean oil, glycerol, and purified egg phosphatide emulsion. Patients allergic to egg proteins may be at increased risk of systemic reactions. In phase IV trials more than 25,000 patients received propofol, and no anaphylactic reactions were described.[55] However, Laxenaire et al. described 14 patients with documented allergic reactions to propofol and recommend that it not be used in individuals allergic to muscle relaxants or with multiple documented drug allergies.[56] Regardless of these findings, propofol also is recommended for the barbiturate-allergic individual.

Opioids

Opioids are an integral part of obstetric anesthetic practice and are administered by multiple routes for pain relief. Morphine, codeine, and meperidine release histamine from cutaneous mast cells and may cause bronchospasm. Meperidine and fentanyl are known to initiate anaphylaxis.[57,58] The IgE antibodies to meperidine cross-react strongly with morphine but only minimally with the synthetic piperidine opioid fentanyl, and presumably sufentanil and alfentanil. Anaphylactic reactions to epidurally administered fentanyl have been reported.[58]

Neuromuscular Blockers

Muscle relaxants are the most frequently implicated anesthetic drugs for causing anaphylaxis.[52] This is because of the presence of biquaternary ammonium ions in all neuromuscular blockers.[59] If a patient is allergic to one muscle relaxant, then all must be suspect. Succinylcholine is most frequently implicated followed by alcuronium, gallamine, d-tubocurarine, pancuronium, and atracurium.[59] Women are eight times more likely than men to be allergic, probably because of chronic exposure to the ammonium ion epitopes in cosmetics.

Local Anesthetics

True allergy to local anesthetics fortunately is rare. Most reported reactions generally are because of overdosage, the epinephrine in the local anesthetics, and vasovagal reactions. When allergic reactions are documented, frequently they are due to the preservatives methyl or propylparaben, para-aminobenzoic acid (PABA), or sulfites (bisulfite, metabisulfite) in the local anesthetics.[60,61] In patients with a true history of allergic reaction to local anesthetics, the amino-ester type drugs are highly suspect because of their degradation to PABA.[62] Thus if local anesthesia is deemed necessary, incremental drug challenge using the proposed local anesthetic can be initiated by a specialist. No cross-reactivity occurs between ester and amide local anesthetics, and allergy to one class does not preclude the use of the other. Whether a pregnant patient should be subjected to the risk of such testing is questionable.

Antibiotics

Antibiotics are commonly used in the parturient for chorioamnionitis. Penicillin precipitates an allergic response in 0.7% to 8% of patients whereas anaphylactic reactions occur in 0.015% of exposures.[63] The true incidence of anaphylactic reactions to cephalosporins in penicillin-allergic and nonallergic patients is not known but may occur, although less frequently than penicillins.[64] In combination the penicillins and cephalosporins precipitate an anaphylactic reaction in 0.13% of medical inpatients.[52] Aminoglycosides rarely are implicated in allergic reactions.[65]

Management of Anaphylaxis

If anaphylaxis is suspected and other likely causes of symptoms are excluded, therapy begins by immediately terminating administration of the suspected drug. The primary goals of therapy are to maintain adequate oxygen delivery to mother and fetus and reversal of systemic histamine effects. Administration of 100% oxygen via a secure airway, rapid volume expansion ($>$ 50 ml/kg is not uncommon), and epinephrine are the mainstays of therapy. Total cardiovascular collapse requires large doses of epinephrine (0.5 to 1 mg) for appropriate response. An infusion of epinephrine may be necessary.[66] If the patient is receiving β-blockers for control of preeclampsia, epinephrine will be less effective. Glucagon 1 mg bolus given IV will override the blocked receptors and allow an appropriate catecholamine effect. Repeat dosing of glucagon often is necessary. Secondary treatments include 0.5 to 1 mg/kg of diphenhydramine and hydrocortisone, 250 mg to 1 g. Fetal monitoring should be maintained if delivery is not imminent. Epinephrine, in large doses, is a potent uterine artery constrictor and may compromise the already stressed fetus, even in spite of an adequate maternal blood pressure. Resuscitation of the pregnant patient in cardiovascular collapse is complicated by the gravid uterus, which severely reduces venous return. The uterus must be displaced from the inferior vena cava to improve venous return. Delivery of the fetus may be necessary to relieve aortocaval compression and to save the mother and baby.

Anesthetic Management

This leads us to the case described at the beginning of this chapter. The patient was a severe preeclamptic on magnesium sulfate infusion who underwent cesarean section for acute fetal distress. In this patient, rapid-sequence induction with thiopental and succinylcholine caused delayed respiratory muscular activity at the end of surgery with no spontaneous attempts at ventilation.

The differential diagnosis in this case includes prolonged neuromuscular blockade and/or increased sensitivity to volatile anesthetics, opioids, and benzodiazepines. Other catastrophic events such as intracranial bleeding due to poorly controlled hypertension before tracheal intubation, cerebral edema, and eclamptic seizures should be kept in mind. The agent analyzer and oxygen analyzer common to many anesthesia machines should indicate the end-tidal anesthetic concentrations. Adequate removal of all volatile anesthetic agents by ventilation with 100% oxygen is necessary.

Degree of neuromuscular blockade should be evaluated using a nerve stimulator. Train of four with estimation of T4:T1 ratio and response to tetanic stimulation are essential. Differential diagnosis of prolonged neuromuscular blockade includes drug interaction with magnesium sulfate; pseudocholinesterase deficiency; atypical pseudocholinesterase; and concomitant administration of other drugs that interfere with the degradation of succinylcholine such as metoclopramide, trimethaphan, neostigmine, phenelzine, and echothiophate.

Earlier reports indicated that magnesium potentiated and prolonged the actions of both depolarizing and nondepolarizing muscle relaxants in patients with preeclampsia.[67,68] More recent studies show conflicting results. Baraka and Yazigi studied the interactions of magnesium and succinylcholine-vecuronium sequence in eclamptic patients receiving general anesthesia for cesarean delivery.[69] These authors found that magnesium did not affect the actions of succinylcholine whereas the duration of vecuronium was significantly prolonged. James et al. found that in nonpregnant patients, magnesium had no effect on the duration of action of succinylcholine.[70]

Pregnancy lowers plasma cholinesterase levels, but in the normal parturient the duration of action of succinylcholine is not significantly prolonged.[37] In the preeclamptic patient pseudocholinesterase concentrations decrease further to less than 50% of control values.[71] Reduction of pseudocholinesterase function to even very low levels by itself does not prolong succinylcholine block more than about 20 minutes.[37] Magnesium by itself does not affect plasma cholinesterase function. Centrally, magnesium acts as a general depressant.[67,68] At the presynaptic membrane, the magnesium ion (Mg^{++}) competes with calcium ion (Ca^{++}) to decrease the influx of Ca ions and the quantal release of acetylcholine. At the postsynaptic membrane, Mg^{++} decreases the sensitivity of acetylcholine receptors. The presence of abnormal neuromuscular function in preeclamptic women receiving standard doses of magnesium sulfate is well documented.[38]

The effects of Mg^{++} on myoneural junction, in combination with the decreased levels of plasma cholinesterase, could have prolonged the actions of a single dose of succinylcholine in this patient with severe preeclampsia.

Other drugs administered to parturients in the perioperative period may interact to prolong neuromuscular blockade. Metoclopramide recently has been shown to inhibit plasma cholinesterase.[40] The net effect of this drug interaction is to prolong the action of succinylcholine by 100%.

Summary

The management of this patient should include the following steps;

1. Continue mechanical ventilation and support circulation.
2. Monitor the neuromuscular block; if phase II block is present, reversal with standard doses of anticholinesterases may be helpful. However, we believe that such drugs can compound the problem further and therefore do not recommend their use.
3. Intravenous calcium chloride or gluconate may partially antagonize the neuromuscular blocking effects of magnesium. Since calcium also may reverse the anticonvulsant effects of magnesium, its use is not recom-

mended. However, calcium is indicated in the management of lethal overdose of magnesium to prevent or treat myocardial depression and cardiovascular collapse.[72]

4. Severe hypertension and tachycardia can occur in the preeclamptic patient on the ventilator. Sedatives and analgesics should be administered to enable her to tolerate the endotracheal tube. Antihypertensive therapy also should be continued during mechanical ventilation. Before extubation, full return of muscular function must be assured because the parturient continues to be at risk of aspiration.

References

1. Smith T: *Dangers and opportunities.* In Smith T, Corbascio A, editors: *Drug interactions in anesthesia, ed 2,* Philadelphia, 1986, Lea & Febiger.
2. Cheek T, Gutsche B: *Maternal physiologic alterations during pregnancy.* In Shnider S, Levinson G, editors: *Anesthesia for obstetrics, ed 3,* Baltimore, 1987, Williams & Wilkins.
3. Cupit G, Rotmensch H: *Principles of drug therapy.* In Gleicher N, editor: *Principles and practice of medical therapy in pregnancy,* East Norwalk, 1992, Appleton and Lange.
4. Krauer B, Krauer F: *Drug kinetics in pregnancy, Clin Pharmacokinet* 1977; 2:267.
5. Dvorchik B: Drug disposition during pregnancy, Biol Res Preg 1982; 3:129.
6. Davison J, Hytten F: Glomerular filtration during and after pregnancy, *J Obstet Gynaecol Br Commonw* 1974; 81:588.
7. Hirshman C, Krieger W, Littlejohn G, et al: Ketamine-aminophylline induced decrease in seizure threshold, *Anesthesiology* 1982; 56:464.
8. Rubin E, Wooten G: Lithium-ketamine interaction: an animal study of potential clinical and theoretical interest, *J Clin Psychopharmacol* 1982; 2:211.
9. Mabie W, Barton J, Wasserstrum N, et al: Clinical observations on asthma in pregancy, *J Matern Fetal Med* 1992; 1:45.
10. Turner E, Greenberger P, Patterson R: Managment of the pregnant asthmatic, *Ann Intern Med* 1980; 6:905.
11. Schatz M, Harden K, Forsythe A, et al: The course of asthma during pregnancy, postpartum, and with successive pregnancies: a prospective analysis, *J Allergy Clin Immunol* 1988; 81:509.
12. Pollowitz J: Theophylline therapy during pregnancy, *JAMA* 1980; 243:651.
13. Chieb J, Beecher N, Rees P: Maximum achievable bronchodilation in asthma, *Respir Med* 1989; 83:497.
14. Nelson K, Ellenberg J: Maternal seizure disorder, outcome of pregnancy, and neurologic abnormalities in the children, *Neurology* 1982; 32:1247.
15. Bjerkedal T, Bahna S: The course and outcome of pregnancy in women with epilepsy, *Acta Obstet Gynecol Scand* 1973; 52:245.
16. Knight A, Rhind E: Epilepsy and pregnancy: a study of 153 pregnancies in 59 patients, *Epilepsia* 1975; 16:99.
17. Dalessio D: Seizure disorders and pregnancy, *N Engl J Med* 1985; 312:559.
18. Lovelace R, Horwitz S: Peripheral neuropathy in long-term diphenylhydantoin therapy, *Arch Neurol* 1968; 18:69.
19. Hetzel D, Bochner F, Hallpike J, et al: Cimetidine interaction with phenytoin, *Br Med J* 1981; 282:1512.
20. Harrah H, Way W, Katzung B: The interaction of d-tubocurarine with antiarrhythmic drugs, *Anesthesiology* 1970; 33:406.
21. Ornstein E, Matteo R, Schwarts A, et al: The effect of phenytoin on the magnitude and duration of neuromuscular block following atracurium or vecuronium, *Anesthesiology* 1987; 67:191.
22. Ornstein E, Matteo R, Weinstein J, et al: Accelerated recovery from doxacurium-induced neuromuscular blockade in patients receiving chronic anticonvulsant therapy, *J Clin Anesth* 1991; 3:108.
23. Mattson R: *Valproate: interactions with other drugs.* In Dixon M, Woodbury J, Keffin P, Pippenger C, editors: *Antiepileptic drugs, ed 2,* New York, 1982, Raven Press.
24. Frohlich E: Methyldopa: mechanisms and treatment 25 years later, *Arch Intern Med* 1980; 140:954.
25. Miller R, Way W, Eger E: The effects of alpha-methyldopa, reserpine, guanethidine and iproniazid on minimum alveolar anesthetic requirement (MAC), *Anesthesiology* 1969; 29:1153.
26. Tosone S, Reves J, Kissin I, et al: Hemodynamic responses to nifedipine in dogs anesthetized with halothane, *Anesth Analg* 1983; 62:903.
27. Waisman G, Mayorga L, Camera M, et al: Magnesium plus

nifedipine: potentiation of hypotensive effect in preeclampsia? *Am J Obstet Gynecol* 1988; 159:308.

28. Forman A, Andersson K, Ulmsten U: Inhibition of myometrial activity by calcium antagonists, *Semin Perinatol* 1981; 5:288.
29. Gergis S, Sokoll M, Rubbo J: Effect of sodium nitroprusside and trimethaphan on neuromuscular transmission in the frog, *Can J Anaesth* 1977; 24:220.
30. George S, Price J, Hauth J: Drug abuse screening of child bearing age women in Alabama Public Health Clinic, *Am J Obstet Gynecol* 1991; 165:924.
31. Volpe J: Effect of cocaine use on the fetus, *N Engl J Med* 1992; 327:399.
32. Shnider S: Serum cholinesterase activity during pregnancy, labor and the puerperium, *Anesthesiology* 1965; 26:335.
33. Plessinger M, Woods J: Progesterone increases cardiovascular toxicity to cocaine in non-pregnant ewes, *Am J Obstet Gynecol* 1990; 163:1659.
34. Morishima H, Pederson H, Finster M, et al: Bupivicaine toxicity in pregnant and nonpregnant ewes, *Anesthesiology* 1985; 63:134.
35. Burkett G, Yasin S, Palow D: Perinatal implications of cocaine exposure, *J Reprod Med* 1990; 35:35.
36. Vertommen J, Hughes S, Rosen M, et al: Hydralazine does not restore uterine blood flow during cocaine-induced hypertension in the pregnant ewe, *Anesthesiology* 1992; 76:580.
37. Viby-Mogensen J: Correlation of succinylcholine duration of action with plasma cholinesterase activity in subjects with the genotypically normal enzyme, *Anesthesiology* 1980; 53:517.
38. Ramanathan J, Sibai, Pillai R, et al: Neuromuscular transmission studies in preeclamptic women receiving magnesium sulfate, *Am J Obstet Gynecol* 1988; 158:40.
39. Kambam J, Perry S, Entman S, et al: Effect of magnesium on plasma cholinesterase activity, *Am J Obstet Gynecol* 1988; 159:309.
40. Kao Y, Turner D: Prolongation of succinylcholine block by metoclopramide, *Anesthesiology* 1989; 70:905.
41. Katz M, Robertson P, Creasy R: Cardiovascular complications associated with terbutaline treatment for preterm labor, *Am J Obstet Gynecol* 1981; 139:605.
42. Hankins G, Hauth J, Kuehl T, et al: Ritodrine hydrochloride infusion in pregnant baboons II: sodium and water compartment alterations, *Am J Obstet Gynecol* 1983; 147:254.
43. Benedetti T: Life-threatening complications of betamimetic therapy for preterm labor inhibition, *Clin Perinatol* 1986; 13:843.
44. Weis F, Markello R, Mo B, et al: Cardiovascular effects of oxytocin, *Obstet Gynaecol* 1975; 46:211.
45. Eggers T, Fliegner J: Water intoxication and syntocinon infusion, *Aust NZ J Obstet Gynaecol* 1979; 19:59.
46. Spielman F, Herbert W: Maternal cardiovascular effects of drugs that alter uterine activity, *Obstet Gynecol Surv* 1988; 43:516.
47. Buxton A, Goldberg S, Hirshfeld J, et al: Refractory ergonovine-induced coronary vasospasm: importance of intracoronary nitroglycerin, *Am J Cardiol* 1980; 46:329.
48. Smith A: The effects of intravenous infusion of graded doses of prostaglandins F2a and E2 on lung resistance in patients undergoing termination of pregnancy, *Clin Sci* 1973; 44:17.
49. Eklund B, Carlson L: Central and peripheral circulatory effects and metabolic effects of different prostaglandins given IV to man, *Prostaglandins* 1980; 20:333.
50. Delage C, Irey N: Anaphylactic deaths: a clinicopathologic study of 43 cases, *J Forensic Sci* 1972; 17:525.
51. Laxenaire M, Moneret-Vautrin D, Vervloet D: The French experience of anaphylactoid reactions, *Int Anesthesiol Clin* 1985; 23:145.
52. Jick H: Adverse drug reactions: the magnitude of the problem, *J Allergy Clin Immunol* 1984; 74:555.
53. Beamish D, Brown D: Adverse responses to I.V. anesthetics, *Br J Anaesth* 1981; 53:55.
54. Watkins J: Etomidate: an immunologically safe anesthetic agent, *Anaesthesia* 1983; 38:34.
55. McLeskey C, Walawander, Nahrwold M, et al: Adverse events in a multicenter phase IV study of propofol: evaluation by anesthesiologists and postanesthesia care unit nurses, *Anesth Analg* 1993, 77:S3.
56. Laxenaire M, Mata Bermejo E, Moneret-Vautrin D, et al. Life-threatening anaphylactoid reactions to propofol (Diprivan), *Anesthesiology* 1992; 77:275.
57. Bennet M, Anderson L, McMillan J, et al: Anaphylactic reaction during anesthesia associated with positive intradermal skin test to fentanyl, *Can J Anaesth* 1986, 33:75.
58. Zucker-Pinchoff B, Ramanathan S: Anaphylactic reaction to epidural fentanyl, *Anesthesiology* 1989; 71:599.
59. Didier A, Cador D, Bongrand P, et al: Role of the quaternary ammonium ion determinants in allergy to muscle relaxants, *J Allergy Clin Immunol* 1987; 79:578.

60. Schwartz H, Sher T: Bisulfite sensitivity manifesting as allergy to local dental anesthesia, *J Allergy Clin Immunol* 1985; 75:525.
61. Simon R, Green L, Stevenson D: The incidence of sulfite sensitivity in an asthmatic population, *J Allergy Clin Immunol* 1982; 69:118.
62. Nagle J, Fuscaldo J, Fireman D: Paraben allergy, *JAMA* 1977; 237:1594.
63. Idsoe O, Guthe T, Willcox R, et al: Nature and extent of penicillin side-reactions with particular reference to fatalities from anaphylactic shock, *Bull World Health Org* 1968; 38:159.
64. Ong R, Sullivan T: Detection and characterization of human IgE to cephalosporin determinants, *J Allergy Clin Immunol* 1988; 81:222.
65. Kraft D: *Other antibiotics.* In DeWeck A, Bundgaard H, editors: *Allergic reactions to drugs,* Berlin, 1983, Springer-Verlag.
66. Levy J: *Management of anaphylaxis, ed 2,* Boston, 1992, Butterworth-Heinemann.
67. Giesecke A, Morris R, Dalton M: On magnesium, muscle relaxants, toxemic parturients and cats, *Anesth Analg* 1968; 47:689.
68. Ghoneim N, Long J: Interaction between magnesium and other neuromuscular blocking agents, *Anesthesiology* 1970; 32:23.
69. Baraka A, Yazigi A: Neuromuscular interaction of magnesium with succinylcholine-vercuronium sequence in the eclamptic parturients, *Anesthesiology* 1987; 67:806.
70. James M, Cork R, Dennett J: Succinylcholine pretreatment with magnesium sulfate, *Anesth Analg* 1986; 65:373.
71. Kambam J, Mouton S, Entman S: Effect of preeclampsia on plasma cholinesterease Activity, *Can J Anaesth* 1987; 34:509.
72. Bohman VR, Cotton DB: Supralethal magnesemia with patient survival, *Obstet Gynecol* 1990; 76:984.

15

Anesthesia for Vaginal Delivery

A 28-year-old primigravida at term is admitted in early labor. The cervix is only 3 cm dilated and 90% effaced. The obstetrician wants to help decrease the pain of labor for the patient by administering narcotics. Discuss the management of the patient.

Recommendations by Mukesh C. Sarna, M.D., F.R.C.A., F.F.A.R.C.S.
Nancy E. Oriol, M.D.

Genesis 3,16: In sorrow thou shall bring forth children.

Lumbar epidural analgesia is a safe and highly efficacious means of providing pain relief to the laboring patient.[1] However, in certain situations it may be contraindicated or the necessary expertise and armamentarium may be unavailable. A number of alternative techniques have been employed toward this end and these are presented below. Before adoption of a particular method of labor analgesia, consideration must be directed to the safety of the method for the mother and fetus and its effects on labor.

Nonpharmacologic Methods

Psychoprophylaxis

Of the various methods of psychoprophylaxis developed, the Lamaze technique is the one most commonly employed.[2] The basis of psychoprophylaxis is the Pavlov conditioned reflex. It is thought that most parturients have been conditioned to believe that labor is painful, and thus they must first be deconditioned. Reconditioning involves an explanation in simple terms of the labor and delivery process and instruction in relaxation and breathing exercises. This process helps to allay anxiety and dispel some of the fear that may have been born out of ignorance. A well-informed patient approaches labor with realistic expectations knowing that it is not going to be an entirely pain-free process and that other forms of pain relief would be available should she require further analgesia. The breathing exercises during a contraction force the patient to concentrate on this activity and thus distract her attention away from the pain of contractions.

It has been shown that psychoprophylaxis helps to decrease the amount of analgesia requested by the mother, although most of the women who have had Lamaze training do require other means of pain relief.[3] Neonatal outcome was shown to be similar in women who had had Lamaze training compared with a group of unprepared mothers.

Trancutaneous Electrical Nerve Stimulation

Transcutaneous electrical nerve stimulation (TENS) is a simple noninvasive technique that has undergone evaluation in labor analgesia. The apparatus provides electrical stimulation to surface electrodes that may be applied on either side of the spine at the level of the nerve roots, transmitting painful stimuli. For the laboring parturient, one set of pads is applied on the back at the T10-L1 level for the first stage and at the S2-S4 level for the second stage of labor. The intensity and duration of electrical stimulation may be varied to optimize the analgesia.

The exact mechanism by which TENS provides analgesia is not clear. One theory involves the Melzack and Wall *gate theory of pain.*[4] It has been suggested that TENS stimulates the larger A-β nerve fibers, which modulate noxious stimuli transmitted by the smaller A-α and C fibers at the substantia gelatinosa in the spinal cord. Another theory suggests that TENS may work by release of endogenous opioids, although generally it is agreed that the analgesia is not reversible by naloxone.[5]

Use of TENS has achieved only a modest success rate in alleviating the pain of parturition.[6] It is more effective in relieving back pain in the first stage of labor and much less effective in the second stage.[7] A study by Harrison et al. suggested that women who have short labors were the most suitable for TENS analgesia.[8]

No adverse effects of TENS on the mother or on the fetus have been reported. Its main disadvantage is its low efficacy. It may cause electrical interference with the fetal heart recording.[9]

Hypnosis

Hypnosis as a method of pain relief in labor is suitable for a selected group of women, that is, those with a high susceptibility to hypnosis. It is a time-consuming process requiring multiple sessions with the mother in the antenatal period. During these sessions increasing levels of trance are induced in the subject. As a result the parturient may be able to induce self-hypnosis during labor.

In a nonrandomized study Davidson showed that hypnosis shortened the first stage of labor, provided better analgesia, and made labor a more pleasant experience.[10] A more recent randomized study did not show any analgesic effects of hypnosis.[11] Furthermore, mothers in the hypnosis group had longer labors. However, labor was believed to be more satisfying for women using hypnosis.

No adverse effects of hypnosis on neonatal outcome have been reported. A trial by Moya and James demonstrated better blood pH values of the neonatal cord born to women in the hypnosis group compared with those in the cyclopropane group.[12]

This modality of labor analgesia is not suitable for women who have a low susceptibility to hypnosis and is contraindicated in women who have a history of psychiatric illness.[13]

Acupuncture

Acupuncture (ACP) is an ancient system of Chinese medicine that only recently has been applied toward providing anesthesia and analgesia.[14] Its role in obstetric practice has been evaluated with disappointing results. In a pilot study, Wallis et al. examined the efficacy of ACP in 21 volunteer parturients.[15] Nineteen of these patients were judged to have inadequate analgesia. They concluded that any benefits from ACP in obstetrics in Western patients were likely, at best, to be modest. Abouleish and Depp studied the effects of ACP in 12 parturients and inferred that it could not be recommended as a routine method since the analgesia was inconsistent, unpredictable, and incomplete.[16] Neither study reported any adverse effects of ACP on the mother or neonate, or on the course of labor. The mechanism by which ACP provides analgesia is not clear, although the suggestion is that it may be via release of endogenous opioid-like peptides and serotonin.[17]

Pharmacologic Methods

Nitrous Oxide

Nitrous oxide (N_2O) is a weak anesthetic agent but a potent analgesic. Its low blood gas solubility is a desirable property since it ensures a fast onset of action and a rapid elimination. It may be administered to the laboring parturient either by an anesthetic machine or by a dedicated apparatus, several of which have been designed.[18] The apparatus most commonly used in the United Kingdom is the one developed by Tunstall called the Entonox apparatus. Entonox is an acronym for N_2O and oxygen. A mixture of 50% N_2O in oxygen is administered to the parturient from a premixed cylinder containing the two gases in equal proportions. The delivery system contains a demand valve which permits flow of gas only when a negative pressure is generated by the subject's inspiratory effort. This has been instituted as a safety feature so that should a woman be rendered unconscious she would be unable to initiate further flow of gas.

Method of Administration

It is important that expectant mothers receive instruction in the proper use of this technique in the prenatal period. Obtaining adequate analgesia is dependent on the parturient commencing inhalation of the gas approximately 45 seconds before the onset of a contraction and continuing to inhale through the contraction.[19] In the second stage, two to three deep inhalations of the gas before an expulsive effort help to decrease the pain associated with the stretching of the perineal tissues.

Efficacy of Nitrous Oxide Analgesia

About 50% of women given intermittent Entonox find the analgesia satisfactory.[20] This compares favorably with the analgesia provided by meperidine, which has been shown to be adequate in less than 25% of cases. Continuous administration of N_2O by nasal cannula was done to provide sustained concentrations of the gas in the maternal blood and thereby improve the quality of analgesia. In a field trial, however, only a marginal benefit could be demonstrated with this technique.[21]

Intermittent inhalation of N_2O does not lead to its accumulation in maternal or fetal tissues. Experimental evidence suggests that continuous inhalation for 5 minutes is not associated with depression of protective airway reflexes.[22] However, the combined effects of administration of opioids and sedatives may place the parturient at risk for aspiration of gastric contents. The effects of Entonox inhalation on the maternal circulation recently have been described.[23] The rise in cardiac output, heart rate, and blood pressure accompanying uterine contractions was blunted by the administration of Entonox. A close association existed between the analgesic effects and the cardiovascular effects.

Entonox analgesia has several disadvantages. It has a satisfaction rate of only about 50%. Several women object to the use of a face mask. An alternative to this is a disposable mouthpiece.[24] The Entonox cylinder requires storage precautions. Excessive cooling below −7° C can lead to separation of nitrous oxide and oxygen. The former, being heavier, would settle at the bottom of the tank. Were such a cylinder inadvertently used, pure oxygen initially would flow, followed by 100% nitrous oxide. Several precautions have been proposed to prevent such a calamity.[25] These include storage of the cylinder horizontally in an environment where the temperature is maintained between 10° C and 45° C. Should cooling occur accidentally or during transport, the cylinder should be kept for at least 2 hours in a room with a temperature above 10° C and then inverted three times before use.

Volatile Anesthetic Agents

Various inhalational anesthetic agents have been employed in subanesthetic concentrations to provide analgesia during labor. Although low concentrations are used, it should be appreciated that physiologic changes of pregnancy have been shown to lower the minimum alveolar concentration of these agents.[26] The parturient also is considered to be at greater risk of aspiration of stomach contents. Thus it is imperative that the mother be closely observed during administration of these agents when used alone or especially in combination with sedatives and narcotics. Methoxyflurane inhaled intermittently in concentrations of 0.35% was shown to be superior to trichloroethylene in the laboring parturient.[27] A study comparing methoxyflurane with systemic analgesics demonstrated a better analgesic profile with a shortened labor in the group of women receiving methoxyflurane.[28] Use of low concentrations of this agent has not been associated with neonatal depression. Concerns have been expressed regarding the potential for nephrotoxicity in both mother and fetus due to inorganic fluoride released by metabolism of methoxyflurane.[29,30] This has led to its decreased use in obstetric anesthesia. Recently enflurane and isoflurane have been evaluated as labor analgesics. Enflurane in concentrations of 0.25% to 1.25% was shown to provide satisfactory analgesia for labor.[31] This agent also has been compared with Entonox.[32] In this randomized study pain scores were significantly lower in mothers receiving 1% enflurane, although drowsiness was more frequent in this group.[32] None of the women considered the smell of enflurane to be unpleasant.

Similar results of analgesic efficacy and drowsiness were reported in a randomized study comparing 0.75% isoflurane and Entonox.[33] Wee et al. have compared the effects of Entonox alone versus the combination of Entonox and 0.2% isoflurane for analgesia in the first stage of labor.[34] The latter resulted in lower pain scores, and drowsiness was not found to be a problem. There was a higher acceptance rate for the mixture. No adverse effects of isoflurane were reported in the neonates.

Paracervical Block

Paracervical block (PCB) once was a popular method of analgesia in the first stage of labor, but it has fallen into disfavor because its use is associated with a high incidence of fetal bradycardia and acidosis. This technique involves injection of local anesthetic in the cervical fornices where the nerves supplying the uterus and the cervix may be blocked. It is a simple technique, familiar to many obstetricians who employ it for minor gynecologic surgery. It is not associated with maternal hypotension and has a relatively high success rate.[35]

As stated in the paragraph above, the chief disadvantage of PCB is its deleterious effects on the fetus. Bradycardia has been reported in up to 50% of cases.[36] The mechanism for this is not clear. High fetal levels of local anesthetics leading to direct myocardial depression were believed to be causative, but sensitive assays measuring fetal blood levels of local anesthetics show that this is not the case. Hypertonicity of the uterus has been demonstrated with PCB, and it has been suggested that this may compromise uteroplacental flow, which leads to fetal bradycardia and acidosis.[37] High doses of local anesthetics have been demonstrated to have a vasoconstrictor effect on isolated uterine artery preparations.[38] Since these vessels lie in close proximity to the uterine nerves, it is possible that a local vasoconstrictor effect may decrease blood flow to the placenta. Other complications of this method include accidental injection into a uterine vessel, injection into the fetus, vaginal laceration, and infection.

If PCB is employed for labor analgesia, fetal heart rate should be continuously monitored and facilities for acid-base evaluation should be available.[39] Furthermore, the dose of bupivacaine 0.25% should be restricted to 10 ml and the injection should not be made deeper than 3 mm in the cervical fornix.

Pudendal Nerve Block

The pudendal nerves are the main sensory nerves of the perineum, being derived from the anterior roots of the second, third, and fourth sacral nerves. In the second stage of labor, pudendal nerve block (PNB) alleviates the pain associated with stretching and frequent tearing of perineal tissues that accompanies descent and expulsion of the fetus. It will not, however, provide analgesia for the pain of uterine contractions. For instrumental delivery of the fetus, PNB also is useful.

The PNB technique has several disadvantages. Principal among these is the high failure rate, approaching 50%.[40] Maternal toxicity is an ever-present problem since high concentrations and volumes may be employed to achieve a satisfactory bilateral block. Maternal convulsive reactions have been reported when 40 ml of 1% lidocaine were used for PNB at a Scottish hospital.[41] Few data exist on the fetal effects of PNB, although it has been suggested that placental transfer of local anesthetics may be similar to that seen with conventional epidural analgesia.

Systemic Analgesia

Among the modalities of pain relief available in obstetrics, systemic medications (primarily opioids) are the most commonly employed.[42] Benzodiazepines, barbiturates, and phenothiazines also have been used as sedatives and anxiolytics.

Opioids

Many opioids have been used as analgesics in labor. Meperidine is the one that is most commonly used and one that has been most extensively reviewed. The dose range is 50 to 100 mg given intramuscularly, which provides analgesia for 3 to 4 hours. It has a low efficacy and poor patient satisfaction rates.[20] This is due to the fact that with these doses, complete analgesia is not obtained. Increasing doses do provide better analgesia but are associated with higher incidence of side effects in the mother and fetus. Maternal side effects include nausea, vomiting, delayed gastric emptying, respiratory depression, and disorientation. Neonatal effects of meperidine have been extensively studied. They are primarily related to the dosage and the timing of administration. In a study by Shnider and Moya it was pointed out that the percentage of neonates with depressed respiration born within 1 hour of administration of meperidine to the mother was no different when compared with a group of women who had not received any analgesics in labor.[43] However, when the drug to delivery interval (DDI) was 2 to 3 hours, a significant increase occurred in the number of newborns with depressed respiration. It is believed that the amount of drug transferred across the placenta increases with time. Measurement of urinary levels of meperidine metabolites in the neonate has shown that fetal exposure to meperidine is highest after a DDI of 2 to 3 hours.[44] Meperidine also has an active metabolite, normeperidine, and both the parent compound and the metabolite have longer half-lives in the neonate than the adult. Thus the fetus may have depressed respiration at birth because of the effects of meperidine, whereas low neurobehavioral scores may be the result of normeperidine. Studies evaluating subtle neonatal indices have demonstrated prolonged effects of meperidine. Administering meperidine to the mother in labor has been shown to adversely affect the infant's attempts at breast feeding and habituation to noise, and to cause periods of wakefulness in the infant.[45,46]

Morphine. In equianalgesic doses, morphine produces greater respiratory depression in the newborn than does meperidine. This has been attributed to the poorly developed blood-brain barrier in the neonate.[42] Morphine, being less lipid soluble than meperidine, crosses the adult blood-brain barrier less effectively. However, it more readily penetrates the immature blood-brain barrier of the fetus. Thus the dose of morphine that is considered adequate for maternal analgesia may be excessive for the fetus and neonate. For this reason, use of morphine is no longer popular in obstetrics.

Fentanyl. Fentanyl is a potent synthetic opioid that has undergone some evaluation in obstetrics. It has a rapid onset of action, with analgesia occurring within 5 minutes of intravenous administration and lasting for about 45 minutes. It is highly protein bound, which may limit its transfer across the placenta. In fact, in human and sheep studies, the maternal:fetal ratio of fentanyl has been shown to be about 3:1.[42] In a clinical trial using hourly or as-needed bolus doses of fentanyl of 50 to 100 μg in laboring women, effective analgesia was provided with no adverse effects occurring in the neonates.[47] A decrease in the beat-to-beat variability was noted in the fetal heart tracing, which lasted for about 30 minutes. A controlled randomized study has compared the effects of fentanyl and meperidine in labor analgesia.[48] Patients rated both the regimens as being equivalent in their efficacy. Maternal side effects including sedation, nausea, and vomiting were greater in the meperidine group. Acute depressant effects of the opioids on the neonate were greater in the meperidine group, whereas no difference occurred in the neurobehavioral scores in the two groups.

Sufentanil. Sufentanil is a potent synthetic opioid characterized by a high lipid solubility and a high affinity for the μ-receptor. It should, therefore, have a rapid onset of action and a low incidence of side effects. A study comparing the efficacy of intrathecal, epidural, and intravenous use of 10 μg of sufentanil in labor analgesia failed to demonstrate a benefit of the epidural and intravenous route.[49] To our knowledge this is the only study that has explored the use of sufentanil given IV in the laboring parturient.

Summary

1. From the discussion in this chapter it may be concluded that lumbar epidural analgesia is the most efficacious means of administering analgesia to a mother in labor.
2. When an anesthesiologist is presented with a parturient in whom regional analgesia is contraindicated, alternative methods, although less effective, may be considered. It is important that such mothers be referred to the anesthesiologist well ahead of time since an opportunity then exists for a formal consultation. During this consultation the various methods of analgesia should be presented to the parturient along with their risks and benefits. Then the mother, obstetrician, and anesthesiologist can agree upon the optimal analgesic regimen during labor.
3. However, when an anesthesiologist is intro-

duced to a parturient in labor in whom a regional procedure is contraindicated, the modality that would be most readily available would be systemic analgesia by opioids. Fentanyl has an attractive pharmacokinetic profile in both mother and fetus, and may be given by either intermittent boluses or by a patient-controlled analgesia system.[50] A transient loss in the beat-to-beat variability may be expected on the fetal heart rate tracing. Both mother and newborn should be monitored for signs of respiratory depression and naloxone should be available.

References

1. Reynolds F: Epidural analgesia in obstetrics, *BMJ* 1989; 299:751.
2. Lamaze F: *Painless childbirth: psychoprophylactic method*, London, 1958, Burke.
3. Scott JR, Rose NB: Effect of psychoprophylaxis (Lamaze preparation) on labor and delivery in primiparas, *N Engl J Med* 1976; 294:1205.
4. Melzack R, Wall PD: Pain mechanisms: a new theory, *Science* 1965; 150:1971.
5. Long DM: Fifteen years of transcutaneous electrical stimulation for pain control, *Stereotact Funct Neurosurg* 1991; 56:2.
6. Augustinsson LE, Bohlin P, Bundsen P, et al: Pain relief during delivery by transcutaneous electrical nerve stimulation, *Pain* 1977; 4:59.
7. Bundsen P, Peterson LE, Selstram U: Pain relief in labor by transcutaneous electrical nerve stimulation: a prospective matched study, *Acta Obstet Gynecol Scand* 1981; 60:459
8. Harrison RF, Shore M, Woods T, et al: A comparative study of transcutaneous electrical nerve stimulation (TENS). Entonox, pethidine + promazine and lumbar epidural for pain relief in labor, *Acta Obstet Gynecol Scand* 1987; 66:9.
9. Bundsen P, Ericson K: Pain relief in labor by transcutaneous electrical nerve stimulation: safety aspects, *Acta Obstet Gynecol Scand* 1982, 61.1.
10. Davidson JA: An assessment of the value of hypnosis in pregnancy and labor, *BMJ* 1962; 951.
11. Freeman RM, Macaulay AJ, Eve L, et al: Randomized trial of self hypnosis in for analgesia in labor, *BMJ (Clin Res Ed)* 1986; 292:657.
12. Moya F, James LS: Medical hypnosis for obstetrics, *JAMA* 1960; 174:2026.
13. Wahl CW: Contraindications and limitations of hypnosis in obstetric analgesia, *Am J Obstet Gynecol* 1962; 84:1869.
14. Bonica JJ: Acupuncture anesthesia in the People's Republic of China, *JAMA* 1974; 229:1317.
15. Wallis L, Shnider SM, Palahniuk RJ, Spivey HL: An evaluation of acupuncture analgesia in obstetrics, *Anesthesiology* 1974; 41:596.
16. Abouleish E, Depp R: Acupuncture in obstetrics, *Anesth Analg* 1975; 54:83.
17. How does acupuncture work? *BMJ (Clin Res Ed)* 1981; 283:746 (editorial).
18. Moir DD, Thorburn J: *Obstetric anesthesia and analgesia, ed 3,* London, 1986, Bailliere Tindall.
19. Waud BE, Waud DR: Calculated kinetics of distribution of nitrous oxide and methoxyflurane during intermittent administration in obstetrics, *Anesthesiology* 1970; 32:306.
20. Holdcroft A, Morgan M: An assessment of the analgesic effect in labor of pethidine and 50 percent nitrous oxide in oxygen (Entonox), *J Obstet Gynaecol Br Commonw* 1974; 81:603.
21. Arthurs GJ, Rosen M: Acceptability of continuous nasal nitrous oxide during labor: a field trial in six maternity hospitals, *Anaesthesia* 1981; 36:384.
22. Cleaton-Jones P: The laryngeal closure reflex and nitrous oxide-oxygen analgesia, *Anesthesiology* 1976; 45:569.
23. Westling F, Milsom I, Zetterstrom H, Ekstrom-Jodal B: Effects of nitrous oxide/oxygen inhalation on the maternal circulation during vaginal delivery, *Acta Anesthesiol Scand* 1992; 36:175.
24. Dolan PF, Rosen M: Inhalational analgesia in labor: face mask or mouth piece? *Lancet* 1975; ii:1030.
25. Cole PV, Crawford JS, Doughty AG, et al: Specifications and recommendations for nitrous oxide/oxygen apparatus to be used in obstetric analgesia, *Anaesthesia* 1970; 25:317.
26. Palahniuk RJ, Shnider SM, Eger EI: Pregnancy decreases the requirement for inhaled anesthetic agents, *Anesthesiology* 1974; 41:82.
27. Rosen M, Mushin WW, Jones PL, Jones EV: Field trial of methoxyflurane, nitrous oxide and trichloroethylene as obstetric analgesics, *BMJ* 1969; 3:263.

28. Barber IJ, Barnett HA, Williams CH: Comparison of methoxyflurane and parenteral agents for obstetric analgesia, *Anesth Analg* 1969; 48:209.
29. Creasser CW, Stoelting RK, Krisna G, Peterson C: Methoxyflurane metabolism and renal function after methoxyflurane analgesia during labor and delivery, *Anesthesiology* 1974; 41:62.
30. Clark RB, Beard AG, Thompson DS, Barclay DL: Maternal and neonatal plasma inorganic fluoride levels after methoxyflurane analgesia for labor and delivery, *Anesthesiology* 1976; 45:88.
31. Abboud TK, Shnider SM, Wright RG, et al: Enflurane analgesia in obstetrics, *Anesthesiology* 1981; 60:133.
32. McGuinness C, Rosen M: Enflurane as an analgesic in labor, *Anaesthesia* 1984; 39:24.
33. McLeod DD, Ramayya GP, Tunstall ME: Self-administered isoflurane in labor: a comparative study with Entonox, *Anaesthesia* 1985; 40:424.
34. Wee MYK, Hasan MA, Thomas TA: Isoflurane in labor, *Anaesthesia* 1993; 48:369.
35. Moir DD, Thorburn J: *Obstetric anesthesia and analgesia, ed 3,* London, 1986, Bailliere Tindall.
36. Liston WA, Adjepon-Yamoah KK, Scott DB: Foetal and maternal lignocaine levels after paracervical block, *Br J Anaesth* 1973; 45:750.
37. Vasicka A, Robertazzi R, Raji M, et al: Fetal bradycardia after paracervical block, *Obstet Gynecol* 1971; 38:500.
38. Greiss FC, Still JC, Anderson SG: Effects of local anesthetic agent on the uterine vasculature and myometrium, *Am J Obstet Gynecol* 1976; 124:889.
39. Jagerhorn M: Paracervical block in obstetrics: an improved injection method, *Acta Obstet Gynecol Scand* 1975; 54:9.
40. Scudamore JH, Yates MJ: Pudendal block: a misnomer? *Lancet* 1966; i:23.
41. Moir DD, Thorburn J: *Obstetric anesthesia and analgesia, ed 3,* London, 1986, Bailliere Tindall.
42. Coalson DW, Glosten B: Alternatives to epidural analgesia, *Semin Perinatol* 1991; 5:375.
43. Shnider SM, Moya F: Effects of meperidine on the newborn infant, *Am J Obstet Gynecol* 1964; 89:1009.
44. Kuhnert BR, Kuhnert PM, Tu AL, Lin DCK: Meperidine and normeperidine levels following meperidine administration during labor II: fetus and neonate, *Am J Obstet Gynecol* 1979; 133:909.
45. Brackbill Y, Kane J, Manniello RL, Abramson D: Obstetric meperidine usage and assessment of neonatal status, *Anesthesiology* 1974; 40:116.
46. Hodgkinson R, Bhatt M, Wang CN: Double blind comparison of the neurobehavior of neonates following the administration of different doses of meperidine to the mother, *Can Anaesth Soc J* 1978; 25:405.
47. Rayburn W, Rathke A, Leuschen MP, et al: Fentanyl citrate analgesia during labor, *Am J Obstet Gynecol* 1989; 161:202.
48. Rayburn WF, Smith CV, Parriott JE, et al: Randomized comparison of meperidine and fentanyl during labor, *Obstet Gynecol* 1989; 74:604.
49. Camann WR, Denney RA, Holby ED, Datta S: A comparison of intrathecal, epidural and intravenous sufentanil for labor analgesia, *Anesthesiology* 1992; 77:884.
50. Gavelin RJ, Janzen JA: IV fentanyl PCA during labor, *Can J Anaesth* 1992; 39:1116.

16

Epidural Anesthesia for Vaginal Delivery

A 30-year-old primigravida at term is in active labor. The cervix is 100% effaced and 5 cm dilated. Epidural analgesia is requested by the patient and her obstetrician.

Recommendations by J. Stephen Naulty, M.D.

Relief of Labor Pain

Analgesia for labor, since its inception, has been a controversial subject. In 1849, 1 year after the introduction of inhalation anesthesia, Channing clearly stated the dilemma that still confounds obstetric anesthesiologists today. He wondered whether it is ". . . reasonable to provide analgesia for a process which is not always painful and which can come to a successful conclusion (delivery) in the absence of analgesia."[1] Lumbar epidural analgesia and anesthesia have become commonly employed methods of labor pain relief. The frequent and widespread use of this technique has increased the controversy surrounding its use during labor.

On first inspection, lumbar epidural block offers many advantages for labor analgesia. The patient remains awake throughout labor. The insertion of a catheter into the epidural space allows the careful titration of analgesic effect to provide the minimum amount of analgesia needed to produce comfort during labor. As is discussed later in this chapter, changing the local anesthetic and dosing regimen can alter the onset and intensity of blockade. Depending on the clinical situation, epidural analgesia can provide rapid and profound, or gradual, muted pain relief. The presence of a catheter allows analgesia to be maintained for as long as needed and to the exact extent required by the obstetric situation. This flexibility is ideal for a dynamic situation like labor where analgesic requirements can change drastically within a few fetal heartbeats. Unfortunately, clinicians have not always used this potential to its fullest extent.

However, the advantages of epidural block are offset by some potential disadvantages. Epidural analgesia can adversely affect both mother and fetus. Concerns include effects on labor itself and changes in maternal hemodynamics. The absorption of local anesthetics by the fetus may produce observable and occasionally deleterious changes in the newborn. The existence and significance of the disadvantages of epidural analgesia have produced a sometimes acrimonious controversy. The most important consideration guiding the decision to institute epidural analgesia in this patient is the potential adverse effects of the technique on her hemodynamics and on labor itself.

Potential Adverse Effects of Epidural Analgesia

The benefits of epidural analgesia must be weighed against potential adverse effects during labor. The ways in which analgesia during labor can affect the mother and fetus are many, but they can be divided into *direct* and *indirect* effects. *Direct* effects are those produced by anesthetic drugs including the following:

- Drug effects on uterine muscle itself
- Changes in catecholamine release
- Impairment of the expulsive forces produced by voluntary and involuntary skeletal muscular activities in the second stage of labor

Indirect effects are those induced by the impact of anesthetic drugs and techniques on the physiology of the parturient that secondarily impair labor. Such actions include the following:

- Decreased uteroplacental perfusion, produced by maternal hypotension secondary to sympathetic blockade during epidural analgesia
- Alterations in oxytocin metabolism
- Impaired reflex activity (bearing down)

Direct Effects

Uterine Muscle and Catecholamines

Local anesthetic agents commonly employed in obstetrics produce constriction of uterine muscle. With the blood concentrations of local anesthetic normally achieved during lumbar epidural analgesia, this effect is not noticeable. However, a direct intravenous injection will elevate uterine baseline tone and the force of contractions. This rise may be of a magnitude and duration that could produce fetal distress.

The direct effects of neural blockade and decreased catecholamine release on uterine smooth muscle, however, are noticeable. Uterine innervation, both sympathetic and parasympathetic, does not initiate contractions. It merely serves to regulate the intensity and duration of contraction. Sympathetic stimulation decreases, whereas parasympathetic stimulation increases, the force and duration of uterine contraction. Therefore the effects of neural blockade depend on the balance of sympathetic to parasympathetic blockade produced. During the epidural analgesia currently used for labor, more sympathetic blockade is produced than parasympathetic (the converse is true for caudal blockade). Therefore the overall *direct* effect of modern segmental epidural blockade is to *increase* the force and duration of uterine contractions.

Skeletal Muscle

The most controversial area of interaction between obstetric analgesia and labor involves the potential effects of reductions in skeletal muscle strength. Local anesthetics can produce significant motor blockade. The potential effects of motor impairment include the following:

- Decrease in expulsive forces generated by maternal Valsalva maneuvers
- Inability of the mother to alter her position with intense motor blockade
- Reduced pelvic floor muscle tone

The reported incidence rate of operative delivery in patients receiving epidural analgesia varies from less than 10% to more than 93%. Depending on the bias of the investigators, these results have been credited to or blamed on labor epidural analgesia. Variations in practice patterns in obstetrics greatly increase the difficulty in controlling the many factors that determine whether an obstetrician will choose forceps or cesarean delivery. Additionally, patients who are more likely to require operative delivery also may be more likely to request epidural block for relief of labor pain. In contrast, patients with adequate pelvic dimensions who experience short, painless labors are the least likely to receive epidural analgesia.

Some recent studies have attempted to control these and other confounding variables (i.e., the indications for forceps delivery; the experience, skill, and philosophy of the obstetrician; and the acceptable duration of the second stage of labor). In general these studies reveal that infusions of dilute concentrations of local anesthetics are associated with minimal if any significant motor blockade in the second stage of labor.

Indirect Effects

Decreased Uteroplacental Perfusion

The most commonly observed effect of obstetric analgesia or anesthesia on labor and delivery is a transient decrease in uterine contractility secondary to decreased uterine perfusion. This change may occur without hypotension and is thought to be because of a decrease in cardiac output, which in turn is because of decreased preload and contractility.[2] It may, if placental perfusion is significantly impaired, be sufficient to produce transient fetal distress. Small doses of ephedrine (5 to 10 mg given intravenously) will easily reverse the decreases in both preload and contractility. If fetal distress is evident, this treatment may quickly restore the fetal condition.

Labor Pain

To provide pain relief to our patient, one must understand the pain process and the role of epidural injections of analgesic drugs in modulating this process. Stimulation of nerve receptors by tissue trauma produces a characteristic pattern of impulses. Nervous impulses arising from these receptors travel as "packets" of neural firings, which are conducted primarily in small myelinated and unmyelinated nerves. These packets have a frequency and duration specific for the type of pain experienced, like the digital "words" that form the basis of computer architecture.

Afferent somatic and visceral sensory nerve fibers carry the "encoded" information that arises from noxious stimuli. The nerves enter the spinal cord primarily through the dorsal roots corresponding to the embryonic dermatomes from which the involved tissues developed: the tenth, eleventh, and twelfth thoracic nerves in the case of uterine pain, and sacral roots for perineal pain.

Central Nervous System

On entering the central nervous system, pain information–bearing nervous impulses undergo a complex modulatory process in the posterior horn of the spinal cord. Many neurotransmitters,[3] notably enkephalins, polypeptides (substance P), serotonin, γ-aminobutyric acid, dopamine, and epinephrine, participate in the processing of pain impulses. The interaction between these neurotransmitters determines if a painful stimulus will ultimately produce the sensation of pain. If sufficient inhibitory modulation takes place, the sensation will be perceived as something other than pain (i.e., pressure or pruritus).

Applying local anesthetics, inhibitory neurotransmitters or their analogues (i.e., opioids), or antagonists of excitatory neurotransmitters (clonidine) to the spinal cord by epidural injection can diminish the transmission of pain to consciousness. This action forms the physiologic and pharmacologic basis for the use of opioids and other drugs in the central nervous system to produce analgesia.

Technique

If after a careful consideration of the risks and benefits of epidural analgesia outlined above, it is decided that this technique will be performed, several issues must be addressed:identification and cannulation of the epidural space, the drug(s) to be employed, and the management of analgesia throughout labor.

Epidural Cannulation

Many methods have been described to identify and cannulate the epidural space. Any technique with which one is facile is probably satisfactory, but the technique should recognize the alterations in maternal anatomy and physiology induced by the pregnancy. Ligaments may be less well defined and obesity and edema may make identification of bony landmarks difficult. The epidural vasculature is engorged in pregnancy, and intravascular cannulation is more likely. Finally, the dose of local anesthetic drugs needed to produce analgesia in pregnancy is reduced,[4] probably secondary to membrane effects of progesterone or its metabolites.

Intrapartum Management

The successful insertion of an epidural catheter and the injection or infusion of analgesic drugs frequently is the easiest part of the technique. Often the successful management of epidural analgesia for labor and its complications requires considerably more effort. The truly skilled anesthesiologist can manage these problems and make the technique work even in the most difficult situations. The most common of these problems are atypical blocks: any epidural that does not yield the expected results (analgesia of an appropriate degree and location). These atypical blocks can be inadequate or too extensive.

Inadequate Analgesia

The primary cause of inadequate analgesia after insertion of a lumbar epidural catheter and the injection of an appropriate amount of drug is improper placement of the epidural catheter. If adequate doses of drug have been injected through the catheter but the expected degree of comfort has not developed, one should promptly remove and replace the catheter. This is the only reliable and uniformly successful remedy for the situation where the *epidural was working for a while, but now she's not comfortable.* Injection of larger-than-necessary doses of analgesic drugs in high concentrations to *make the catheter work* is doomed to failure and is fraught with hazard.

The usual reason for failure of an epidural catheter to provide adequate pain relief is unrecognized intravascular catheter placement.[5] A misguided attempt to produce analgesia with inappropriately high doses of local anesthetic can lead to significant systemic toxicity, including seizures and cardiac arrest. If one suspects intravascular placement, one can inject 1 to 2 ml of air through the catheter while listening to maternal heart sounds with a Doppler device.[6] If one hears a distinct change in maternal heart sounds after injecting the air, the catheter is in a blood vessel. If the catheter is intravascular, one should remove and replace it. If the Doppler test is normal and the catheter is thought to be in the epidural space, one spould carefully inject small doses of drug (0.125 to 0.25% bupivacaine 5 to 10 ml) to intensify the block.

Patients whose fetus presents in the occiput posterior location or who progress rapidly to the second stage of labor frequently require extra local anesthetic to obtain adequate pain relief. However, if reasonable doses of local anesthetic fail to relieve the pain, replacement of the catheter will be necessary. At best, it will be an unreliable anesthetic for further possible emergency surgical manipulations.

Dural Puncture

The incidence of placement of an epidural needle into the subarachnoid space (the *wet tap*) varies with the facility, technique, and experience of the person performing the anesthetic. When this complication arises there are several options. A catheter can be reinserted in the epidural space at another interspace and used successfully. However, local anesthetic may pass from the epidural space through the dural puncture into the subarachnoid space, producing greater than expected blockade. I prefer to place a subarachnoid catheter deliberately. The location of the catheter is certain. I then use reduced doses of local anesthetic and opiates to provide labor analgesia.

Drugs

However, if in our patient the epidural space is successfully cannulated without the difficulties discussed earlier, one must next decide what type of drugs are to be injected to produce analgesia. This is far from a routine, one must consider the patient's and obstetrician's expectations, the force and frequency of her contractions, and the expected course of labor. Local anesthetics remain as the mainstays of epidural analgesia, but adjuvants such as catecholamines and opiates play an important role.

Local Anesthetics

Epidural injection of local anesthetics is widely used for the relief of labor pain. The exact mechanism by which epidural injections of local anesthetics produce analgesia is poorly understood. They decrease both the number and frequency of afferent nerve firings in the vicinity of the spinal cord. These drugs most effectively reduce or eliminate somatic pain. A consequence of their action is a decrease in efferent nerve activity, leading to motor blockade. The ideal local anesthetic for labor then would reliably produce analgesia and sensory blockade while preserving motor function. In addition, minimal uptake into the maternal and fetal circulation is highly desirable. Successful epidural analgesia for labor requires sensory blockade to at least the tenth thoracic dermatome.

Inducing this type of block with local anesthetics alone requires the administration of 10 to 15 ml of potent local anesthetics.[7] These large doses can lead to both maternal and fetal local anesthetic toxicity. For any given patient, the obstetric anesthesiologist strives to choose the least toxic drug that will yield effective analgesia with minimal maternal and fetal side effects.

Bupivacaine

Bupivacaine is an extremely useful local anesthetic in labor, but several concerns exist regarding its safety. Intravenous injection of bupivacaine may incite seizures, ventricular arrhythmias, and death. In one parturient, cardiac arrest followed intravenous injection of 25 mg of bupivacaine.[8] To ensure maternal safety, one should not give more than 20 mg of bupivacaine as a single bolus and one should inject all local anesthetics as fractionated doses. Injection of an initial large bolus does not speed onset or improve the quality of pain relief. A slow, controlled induction of epidural analgesia can greatly reduce the risk of local anesthetic toxicity and is an essential element of safe practice. Despite these safety concerns, bupivacaine is an excellent local anesthetic for labor analgesia. It produces relatively greater sensory block than motor block. This difference becomes more evident with more dilute concentrations of bupivacaine.[9]

Ropivacaine

Ropivacaine is a local anesthetic with structure and properties similar to bupivacaine. However, in animals ropivacaine appears to be less toxic than bupivacaine while retaining many of the latter drug's desirable characteristics. Limited experience is available with ropivacaine in pregnancy.[10] It appears to be a promising drug that may supplant bupivacaine.[11,12]

Lidocaine

Lidocaine provides a more rapid onset of analgesia (about 12 minutes) than bupivacaine. It has been extensively employed for labor analgesia. When given by bolus administration, significant motor block develops quickly. Continuous infusions of lidocaine also produce motor block, although at a slower rate.[13] I use lidocaine for the following:

- To provide profound motor and sensory block (i.e., emergency forceps deliveries)
- To induce analgesia rapidly (i.e., the multipara with tumultuous labor)
- To supply blockade of short duration (i.e., patients with persistent occiput posterior presentation, to facilitate rotation of the fetal head)

2-Chloroprocaine

2-Chloroprocaine is an ester local anesthetic that rapidly produces intense motor and sensory blockade. This drug also undergoes rapid hydrolysis in plasma, with a fetal half-life of about 40 seconds.[14] These properties make 2-chloroprocaine unique because even with large, rapidly administered boluses of the drug, placental transfer is small and maternal systemic toxicity is unlikely. However, 2-chloroprocaine has several undesirable characteristics that preclude its routine use. Motor block develops rapidly, even with dilute infusions. Several authors have reported a high incidence of severe back spasm after the epidural injection of 2-chloroprocaine.[15,16] Tissue toxicity, including nerve and muscle tissue lysis, may be a problem, especially when large doses are given over a prolonged period. Finally, 2-chloroprocaine antagonizes the action of epidural opiates.[17] 2-Chloroprocaine is useful in situations similar to those in which lidocaine is employed. If fetal acidosis or distress appears to be likely, the lack of apparent fetal effects of 2-chloroprocaine may be an advantage.

Catecholamines

The catecholamine epinephrine often is added to local anesthetics to potentiate and prolong their effects. Recently, catecholamines also have been shown to potentiate epidural opioid analgesia.[18] The action of catecholamines long has been attributed to their ability to decrease uptake of local anesthetics into the systemic circulation. However, at least some of their action comes from analgesia produced by spinal cord α-receptor activation. Other α-agonists, most notably clonidine, are powerful neuraxial analgesics themselves.[19] The role of these drugs as labor analgesics is unclear. Their hemodynamic and uterine muscular effects may limit their usefulness in this setting.[20]

Opiates

Epidural opioids (even rapidly acting ones like fentanyl and meperidine) as sole analgesic drugs are inferior to dilute concentrations of local anesthetics.[21] Adding epinephrine to the opioid appears to increase the incidence of satisfactory analgesia slightly but not sufficiently to make this technique reliable. Epidural opioids reduce but do not eliminate visceral pain (first stage of labor). They have little effect on somatic pain (second and third stages of labor). In contrast, local anesthetics produce better somatic than visceral analgesia. The combination of these two effects provides better analgesia than either separately.

Opiate–Local Anesthetic Combinations

This combination of dilute epidural local anesthetics and opioids can produce profound analgesia. Epidural injection of a local anesthetic combined with an opioid generates a more rapid onset of more profound analgesia with little motor blockade. Pain relief then lasts longer than after either drug alone.[22] A combination of dilute concentrations of bupivacaine and opioids significantly lowers the risk of systemic local anesthetic toxicity. Using this method, one can induce analgesia with less than 20 mg of bupivacaine. Maintaining pain relief with a continuous infusion limits the bupivacaine dose to 10 to 15 mg/hr. This approach seems considerably safer than bolus injections of the larger doses of local anesthetic required in the absence of opioids. The disadvantages of this technique include the possibility of adverse maternal and fetal effects of epidural opioids. The most serious risk is the chance of maternal and fetal respiratory depression.

Further study and evaluation of large numbers of mothers and neonates can prove if the advantages of this technique outweigh the potential risks. Currently several apparently safe epidural local anesthetic–opiate regimens have been described and used in thousands of women.

Specific Drug Combinations

Fentanyl-Bupivacaine

Fentanyl was the first opioid widely employed as an adjunct to local anesthetics for labor analgesia.[23] Recently the use of increasingly dilute local anesthetic–opiate solutions has become popular.[24] The addition of fentanyl roughly doubles the analgesic efficacy of continuously infused bupivacaine (i.e., 0.0625% bupivacaine with fentanyl is as potent as 0.125% bupivacaine). An initial dose of fentanyl 50 μg combined with 0.25% or 0.125% bupivacaine can produce good initial analgesia in most laboring parturients. A continuous infusion of 0.125% bupivacaine with 1 to 2 μg/ml fentanyl at 10 to 15 ml/hr will maintain good pain relief throughout parturition. Further lowering the fentanyl dose or concentration of local anesthetic may not produce completely reliable analgesia. No adverse effects on either the mother or on the neonate have been attributed to this technique.

Sufentanil-Bupivacaine

Patients who receive sufentanil 5 μg with 10 ml of either 0.125%, 0.0625%, or 0.0312% bupivacaine have a significantly faster onset and longer duration of complete analgesia (a pain score of 0) than patients receiving either 0.25% or 0.125% bupivacaine alone, with a greatly reduced incidence of hypotension.[25] Patients who receive 0.0312% bupivacaine with 0.5 μg/ml sufentanil exhibit no observable motor block and can ambulate without assistance. Epidural injection of sufentanil 5 μg plus bupivacaine provides safe, excellent analgesia with extremely low concentrations of bupivacaine. I think epidural sufentanil 0.3 to 0.5 μg/ml provides more profound potentiation of bupivacaine than that observed with epidural fentanyl 30 to 100 μg. Extraordinarily low concentrations of bupivacaine (0.0625 to 0.0312%) will produce superb analgesia in more than 95% of parturients with sufentanil, but not with fentanyl. This should be the drug combination of choice in the described patient. An initial bolus of 10 ml of 0.125% bupivacaine with 5 μg sufentanil should be injected. If the epidural was established earlier in labor than in this patient (1 to 2 cm dilation), the initial dose of bupivacaine should be halved.

Methods of Administration

In addition to deciding what drug or combination of drugs to employ in this patient, one must also decide how the drugs are to be administered over the course of what may be a prolonged period of time. Until recently, intermittent bolus injection of local anesthetics was the most common way of providing labor analgesia. An increasing realization of the hazards of this method of administration, plus the development of reliable and inexpensive infusion pumps, has produced widespread interest in continuous epidural infusion techniques for the relief of labor pain. The use of continuous infusions of local anesthetics can produce reliable pain relief with similar or lower blood concentrations of local anesthetics than intermittent bolus injections of these drugs.[26] Infusion techniques also allow the intensity and extent of sensory block to be adjusted promptly. Most importantly, continuous infusion reduces the possibility of sudden disastrous complications (total spinal anesthesia, massive intravascular injection with cardiovascular collapse) that can follow injections of large doses of local anesthetics outside of the epidural space. If an epidural catheter enters a vein during a continuous infusion the analgesia merely ceases, without producing central, nervous, or cardiovascular toxicity.[27] If the catheter enters the subarachnoid space, the level of sensory and motor blockade slowly rises without the sudden onset of complete subarachnoid blockade, as may occur when using bolus techniques.[28] This technique is safe and simple, but continuous monitoring of the patient for improper catheter placement or pump malfunctions is essential. I highly recommend using a different type or model of pump than that used for magnesium or oxytocin infusions in the parturient. This precaution will minimize the dangers of someone adjusting the wrong pump.

In this patient, a continuous infusion of 0.05% bupivacaine with 0.5 μg/ml sufentanil at about 6 to 10 ml/hr should be initiated, with adjustment to the rate of infusion according to the patient's response.

Summary

1. The goal of the anesthesiologist during labor is to produce pain relief with minimal effects on the mother, fetus, and labor.
2. A thorough understanding of the nature of obstetric pain is necessary to achieve this goal.
3. Inserting an epidural catheter in the pregnant patient may be more difficult and hazardous than in the nonpregnant patient.
4. Selection of an analgesic drug regimen is determined by the patient's and obstetrician's expectations, the nature and severity of the pain experienced, and the course and expected outcome of labor. The initial drug and dosage should be tailored to the analgesic requirements of the patient at the time of initiation of analgesia.
5. Continuous infusion of opiates and dilute local anesthetics is the preferable method for managing normal painful labor. However, considerable attention must be paid to the patient during these infusions to optimize safety and analgesia.

References

1. Channing W: *A treatise on etherization in childbirth,* Boston, 1849, William D. Ticknor and Company.
2. Ramos-Santos E, Devoe LD, Wakefield ML, et al: The effects of epidural anesthesia on the Doppler velocimetry of umbilical and uterine arteries in normal and hypertensive patients during active term labor, *Obstet Gynecol* 1991; 77:20.
3. Otsuka M, Yanagisawa M: Pain and neurotransmitters, *Cell Mol Neurobiol* 1990; 10:293.
4. Flanagan HL, Datta S, Lambert DH, et al: Effect of pregnancy on bupivacaine induced conduction blockade in the isolated rabbit vagus nerve, *Anesth Analg* 1987; 66:123.
5. Ravindran R, Albrecht W, McKay M: Apparent intravascular migration of epidural catheter, *Anesth Analg* 1979; 58:252.
6. Leighton BL, Gross JG: Air: an effective indicator of intravenously located epidural catheters, *Anesthesiology* 1989; 71:848.
7. Shnider SM, Levinson G: *Anesthesia for obstetrics.* In Miller RD,

editor: *Anesthesia, ed 3,* New York, 1990, Churchill Livingstone.

8. Albright GA: Cardiac arrest following regional anesthesia with etidocaine or bupivacaine, *Anesthesiology* 1979; 51:285.
9. Naulty JS: Continuous infusions of local anesthetics and narcotics for epidural analgesia in the management of labor, *Int Anesthesiol Clin* 1990; 28:17.
10. Santos AC, Pederson H, Sallusto JA, et al: Pharmacokinetics of ropivacaine in nonpregnant and pregnant ewes, *Anesth Analg* 1990; 70:262.
11. Concepcion M, Arthur GR, Steele SM, et al: A new local anesthetic, ropivacaine: its epidural effects in humans, *Anesth Analg* 1990; 70:80.
12. Fleck JW, Moorhty SS, Daniel J, Dierdorf SF: Sensory, motor, and sympathetic block during epidural analgesia with 0.5% and 0.75% ropivacaine with and without epinephrine, *Reg Anesth* 1994; 19:18.
13. Abboud TK, Afrasiabi A, Sarhs F, et al: Continuous infusion epidural analgesia in parturients receiving bupivacaine, chloroprocaine or lidocaine: maternal, fetal and neonatal effects, *Anesth Analg* 1984; 63:421.
14. Phillipson EH, Kuhnert BR, Syracuse CD: Fetal acidosis, 2-chloroprocaine, and epidural anesthesia for cesarean section, *Am J Obstet Gynecol* 1985; 151:322.
15. MacArthur C, Lewis M, Knox EG, et al: Epidural anaesthesia and long-term backache after childbirth, *BMJ* 1990; 301:9.
16. Hynson JM, Sessler DI, Glosten B: Back pain in volunteers after epidural anesthesia with chloroprocaine, *Anesth Analg* 1991; 72:253.
17. Malinow AM, Mokriski BLK, Wakefield ML, et al: Anesthetic choice affects postcesarean epidural fentanyl analgesia, *Anesth Analg* 1988; 67:138.
18. Madsen KE, Stowe DF, McDonald DJ, et al: A comparison of epidural narcotics, with and without a test dose, to epidural lidocaine for extracorporeal shock wave lithotripsy, *Reg Anesth* 1990; 15:288.
19. Huntoon M, Eisenach JC, Boese P: Epidural clonidine after cesarean section: appropriate dose and effect of prior local anesthetic, *Anesthesiology* 1992; 76:187.
20. Nishikawa T, Haruhuni I, Asakura N, Hamaya Y: Effects of epidural clonidine added to lidocaine solution upon the requirements of sedatives during epidural anesthesia. *Masui* 1991; 40:717.
21. Caldwell LE, Rosen MA, Shnider SM: Subarachnoid morphine and fentanyl for labor analgesia: efficacy and adverse effects, *Reg Anesth* 1994; 19:2.
22. Naulty JS: Obstetrical analgesia. *Probl Anesth* 1988; 12:408.
23. Justins DM, Francis D, Houlton PG, et al: A controlled trial of extradural fentanyl in labour, *Br J Anaesth* 1982; 54:409.
24. Robinson DE, Leicht CH: Epidural analgesia with low dose bupivacaine and fentanyl for labor and delivery in a parturient with severe pulmonary hypertension, *Anesthesiology* 1988; 687:285.
25. Naulty JS, Griffith W, Barnes D, et al: Epidural PCA vs. continuous infusion of sufentanil bupivacaine for analgesia during labor and delivery, *Anesthesiology* 1990; 73:963.
26. Chestnut DH, Owen CL, Bates JN, et al: Continuous infusion epidural analgesia during labor: a randomized, double-blind comparison of 0.0625% bupivacaine/0.0002% fentanyl versus 0.125% bupivacaine, *Anesthesiology* 1988; 68:754.
27. D'Athis F, Macheboeuf M, Thomas H, et al: A comparative study of continuous and intermittent epidural analgesia for labour and delivery, *Can J Anesth* 1988; 35:234.
28. Daley MD, Rolbin MB, Hew E, Morningstar B: Continuous epidural anaesthesia for obstetrics after major spinal surgery, *Can J Anaesth* 1990; 37:S112.

17

Vaginal Delivery After a Previous Cesarean Section

A 31-year-old multigravida at term has had a previous cesarean delivery for breech presentation. She has requested a trial of labor *for vaginal delivery (also known as vaginal birth after cesarean delivery). When the cervix is 5 cm dilated with 100% effacement, the parturient requests an epidural anesthetic for pain relief. Discuss the pros and cons of epidural analgesia for this patient.*

Recommendations by Raymond Glassenberg, M.D.
Naomi Vaisrub, Ph.D.
Kenneth L. Rodino, M.D.
Samuel Glassenberg

Due to escalating pressure from public and professional sectors to reduce the rate of cesarean deliveries performed, increased emphasis has been placed on conducting vaginal trials of labor (VTOL) after previous cesarean sections. This presents a unique problem to the anesthesiologist, who must determine whether administering an epidural block is safe and efficacious, and if so, under precisely what circumstances. The two most important questions facing the anesthesiologist are (1) *Does an epidural block increase the risks from undetected uterine rupture?* and (2) *Does it ultimately increase the probability of failure for the vaginal trial?*

When presented with a parturient in labor who has previously undergone a cesarean section for breech presentation, the anesthesiologist must be aware of any special risks associated with administering an epidural block. Whereas the patient's

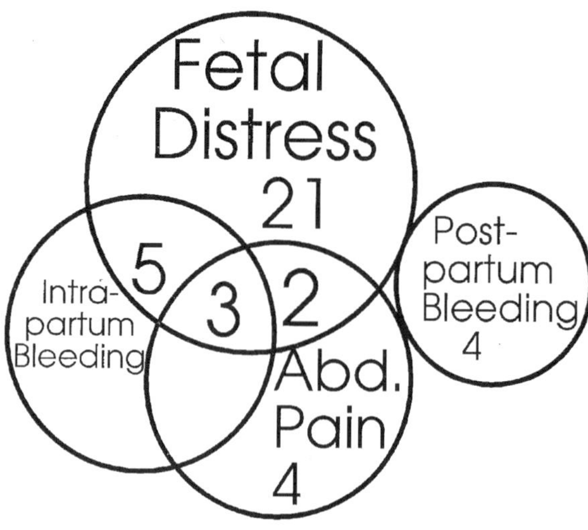

Fig. 17-1.
The Venn diagram shows the overlap of signs with symptoms in 39 cases of uterine rupture. Fetal distress occurred 31 times (21 + 5 + 3 + 2) followed by abdominal pain with 9 occurrences (4 + 3 + 2).

most immediate concern in this situation is likely to be pain relief, the anesthesiologist's major fear is that an epidural block will mask the pain of uterine rupture and thereby allow a potentially dangerous situation to proceed to catastrophic consequences. If hemorrhage should occur, delay in the diagnosis of uterine rupture in the presence of an epidural induced sympathetic block could result in uncontrolled hypotension, leading to both maternal and neonatal death. To elucidate any hazards connected with administering epidural blocks during vaginal trials of labor, the clinician must carefully separate unfounded fears from proven facts. For this review and the recommendations that follow, a number of topics have been examined that are germane to the central problem. These include the signs and symptoms of uterine rupture; the reported mortality from VTOL and elective repeat cesarean deliveries; the importance of the type of previous uterine scar and the original obstetric indication for the cesarean section; the pros and cons of using oxytocin augmentation during vaginal trials; the comparative success rates of VTOL conducted with and without concurrent epidural blocks; the relative risks of uterine rupture for the intact versus the scarred uterus; and finally, the management of uterine rupture.

What Are the Signs and Symptoms of Uterine Rupture?

Reported symptoms of uterine rupture include vaginal bleeding, abdominal pain unrelated to uterine contractions, and uterine tenderness. However, abdominal pain is not always a reliable symptom. After reviewing 20 cases of repeat cesarean sections performed because of severe lower abdominal pain, Case et al. found only one instance of uterine rupture.[1] Crawford observed that abdominal pain is not a common symptom of uterine rupture, and if peritoneal irritation occurs it will be obvious, even in the presence of a successful epidural block.[2] Signs of possible rupture are maternal tachycardia, maternal hypotension, and fetal bradycardia. In a review of 39 uterine ruptures, Johnson and Oriol found fetal distress to occur 79% (31/39) of the time (Fig. 17-1).[3]

How Does the Maternal and Neonatal Mortality from VTOL Compare with the Mortality from an Elective Repeat Cesarean Section?

Table 17-1 compares maternal and neonatal mortality in VTOL versus elective repeat cesarean section. Plauche' et al.[4] and Shy et al.[5] reviewed the incidence of rupture of previous cesarean section scars before labor and found between 7 and 19 uterine ruptures per 10,000 uterine scars (6/8573 to 5/2627). Lavin and co-workers[6] and Shy et al.[5] examined the incidence of uterine rupture in women permitted to labor after cesarean section and reported between 65 and 73 uterine ruptures per 10,000 VTOL (21/3214 to 35/4784). Thus, despite a threefold to twelvefold rise in uterine rupture during vaginal delivery after cesarean section, Lavin et al. did not observe any maternal deaths related to uterine rupture between the years 1930 and 1980.[6] In contrast, Shrinsky and Benson reviewed 658 cases of scarred uteri rupturing that produced a maternal mortality of 6.1% (40/658) and a neonatal mor-

TABLE 17-1

Maternal and Neonatal Mortality

Morbidity and Mortality	Incidence* Before 1980	Incidence† After 1980
Symptomatic rupture of the scarred uterus before labor	7 to 19 per 10,000 uterine scars	Unchanged
Symptomatic rupture of the scarred uterus allowed to labor	70 per 10,000 VTOL	47 per 10,000 VTOL
Maternal death from VTOL	3.8 per 10,000 VTOL	2.8
Maternal death from elective repeat cesarean sections	4.6 per 10,000 planned repeat cesarean sections	2.4
Maternal death from rupture of low-transverse scarred uterus	0-196 per 10,000 uterine scar ruptures	95
Maternal death from rupture of unscarred uterus	1296 per 10,000 unscarred uterine ruptures	Unchanged
Perinatal death from VTOL	119 per 10,000 VTOL	30
Perinatal death from elective repeat cesarean sections	158 per 10,000 planned repeat cesarean sections	40
Perinatal death from rupture of low-transverse scarred uterus	1200 to 3200 per 10,000 uterine scar ruptures	860
Perinatal death from rupture of unscarred uterus	7600 per 10,000 unscarred uterine ruptures	Unchanged

VTOL, Vaginal trials of labor.
*Data from Shy LL, Logerfo JP, Karp LE. Evaluation of elective repeat cesarean section as a standard of care: an application of decision analysis, *Am J Obstet Gynecol* 1981; 139:123.
†Rosen MG, Dickenson JC, Westhoff CL: Vaginal birth after cesarean: a meta-analysis of morbidity and mortality, *Obstet Gynecol* 1991; 77:465.

tality rate of 79% (388/493).[7] Subsequent to this 1978 report, Plauche' et al.[4] retrospectively studied 78 incidents of scarred uteri rupturing among 406,306 deliveries (Table 17-2); whereas maternal mortality had fallen to 0%, neonatal mortality was 24% (19/78). Despite the higher incidence of uterine rupture with VTOL and the greater than 9% probability of fetal death, if uterine rupture occurs, Shy and associates[5] predicted that for 10,000 planned trials of labor there would be 0.7 fewer maternal deaths and 39 (158−119) fewer perinatal deaths than if all 10,000 patients had an elective cesarean section. This is because uterine rupture accounts for 9.2% (11/119) of the perinatal mortality from VTOL, whereas prematurity accounts for 23% (37/158) of perinatal mortality from elective repeat cesarean section. Shy et al. used data from studies before 1980.[5] Rosen et al., using reports published after 1982, found almost no difference in perinatal mortality rates when comparing VTOL (30/10,000) to elective repeat cesarean sections (40/10,000).[8] Corrections were made to allow for prematurity and congenital anomalies, which still account for 26% and 31% of perinatal mortality (Fig. 17-2).[9] This review of 22,230 VTOL found an incidence of uterine rupture of 0.47% (105/22,230) and a fetal mortality rate of 8.6%(9/105) when uterine rupture occurs (Table 17-2). Thus fetal mortality from uterine rupture does not appear to have changed in the last 20 years. Rosen et al. did not find any difference in maternal mortality rates when comparing VTOL (2.8/10,000) to elective repeat cesarean sections (2.4/10,000). Maternal mortality statistics from 1970 to 1980 show that uterine rupture accounts for only 6% of overall maternal mortality (Fig. 17-3).[10] Maternal mortality from uterine rupture has fallen by half from 1.96% (1.8/92) to 0.95% (1/105) in the last decade.

TABLE 17-2

Reference	Incidence of Rupture	Mortality Rate: Maternal	Mortality Rate: Neonatal
Schrinsky and Benson[7]	$\frac{658}{3,107,637} = 0.021\%$*	$\frac{40}{658} = 6.1\%$	$\frac{388}{493} = 79\%$
Plauche' et al.[4]	$\frac{78}{406,306} = 0.019\%$*	0	$\frac{19}{78} = 24\%$
Lavin et al.[6]	$\frac{21}{3,214} = 0.65\%$†	0	$\frac{3}{21} = 14\%$
Rosen et al.[8]	$\frac{22}{5,436} = 0.4\%$†	0	$\frac{3}{22} = 14\%$
This review	$\frac{105}{22,230} = 0.47\%$†	$\frac{1}{105} = 0.95\%$	$\frac{9}{105} = 8.6\%$

*$\frac{\text{Uterine scar ruptures}}{\text{total deliveries}}$

†$\frac{\text{Uterine scar ruptures}}{\text{vaginal trials of labor}}$

‡Denominator based on 493 uterine ruptures for which neonatal mortality was expressed.

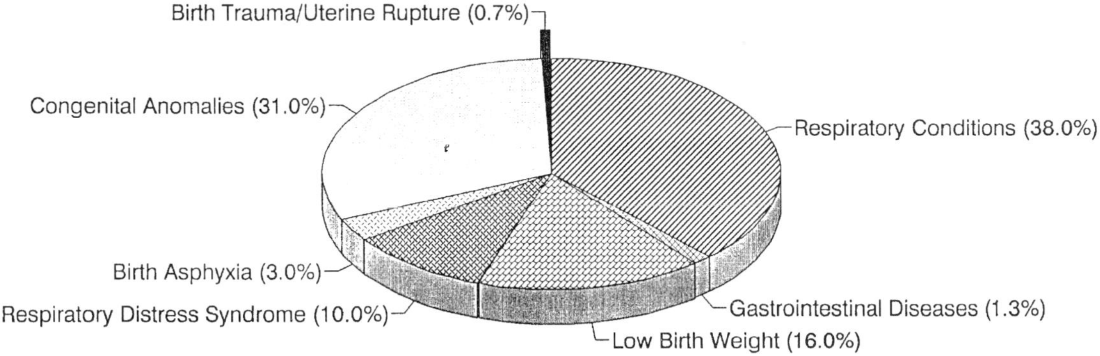

Fig. 17-2.
National health statistics reveal 23,450 perinatal deaths for the year 1992. The majority are due to congenital anomalies and complications associated with prematurity (low birth weight and respiratory distress syndrome).

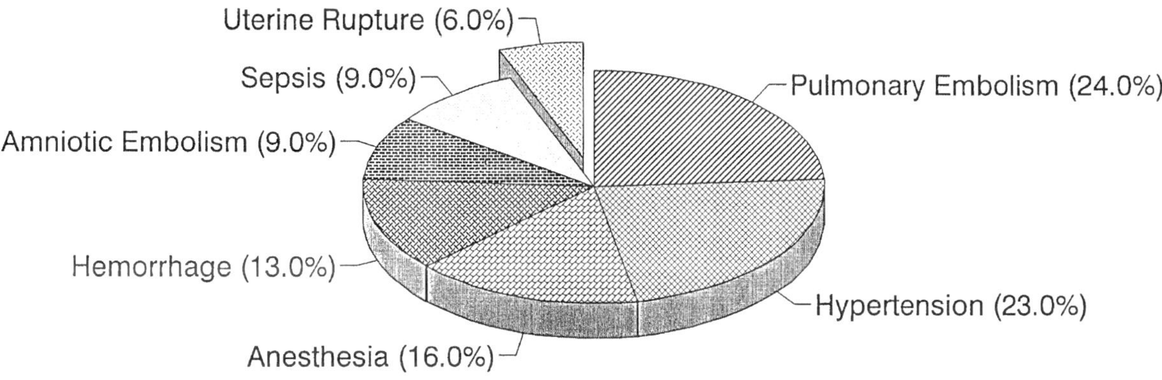

Fig. 17-3.
In the Confidential Enquiry series from the United Kingdom for the years 1970 to 1987, 48 of 843 deaths were due to uterine rupture.[10]

Should the Type of Previous Uterine Scar Influence the Decision to Allow VTOL?

When considering the influence on outcome of the type of uterine scar, Lawrence concluded that the classic scar had a 10 times' greater probability of rupture than that of the lower transverse scar.[11] Pedowitz and Schwartz found that for transverse, low vertical, and classic scars, the incidence rates of uterine rupture were 8.3% (22/266), 13.3% (20/150), and 18.2% (6/33), respectively, based on 48 cases of uterine scar rupture among 449 scarred uteri.[12] Plauche' and co-workers found that among 14 cases of uterine scar rupture, there was an incidence of 0.07% for rupture of the low vertical, 0.05% for the low transverse, and 0.02% for the classic when 8573 cesarean sections were performed.[4] He concluded, "No type of scar is exempt from the possibility of major rupture."[4]

Does the Obstetric Indication for the Primary Cesarean Section Affect the Outcome of VTOL?

Table 17-3 shows the outcome of VTOL grouped by previous obstetric indications. If the first cesarean section was performed for a recurring cause, such as cephalopelvic disproportion, there is a 33% to 67% chance that the vaginal trial will be successful.[6,13,14] With nonrecurrent causes (breech presentation, placenta previa, abruptio placentae, and fetal distress), there is a reported 70% to 100% chance of success.

Should Oxytocin Augmentation Be Used in a Previously Scarred Uterus?

In their report on vaginal deliveries in patients who previously had a cesarean section, Lavin et al. concluded that oxytocin stimulation of labor is contraindicated, and referenced the series of Meehan and associates[15] of 75 patients who received caudal anesthesia with 20 ml of 0.5% bupivacaine. Lavin et al. stated, "The only two cases of uterine rupture occurred among the patients who received oxytocin."[6] However, the study by Meehan et al. actually reported, "While two patients had scar dehiscence, neither patient had received Syntocinon."[15]

Flamm et al. have suggested that oxytocin improves the chances for vaginal delivery in VTOL if the primary section was for cephalopelvic disproportion.[14] A 72% success rate for VTOL occurred with pitocin augmentation, compared with only a 25% success rate without pitocin. Flamm et al. thus concluded, "There is no reason to believe that a given pressure achieved by augmentation is any more dangerous to a uterine scar than the same pressure achieved without augmentation."[14] This review of 3547 VTOL with oxytocin reveals a success rate of 70% (2473/3547) compared with a rate of 81% (5857/7261) in the 7261 VTOL in which patients did not receive oxytocin. The incidence of scar rupture was 0.42% (15/3547) in VTOL with oxytocin versus 0.15% (11/7261) without oxytocin (Table 17 4).

Does an Epidural Block Actually Increase the Risk of Uterine Rupture?

Lavin stated, "The available evidence suggests the relative safety of regional anesthesia."[6] However, the data for making this statement again were derived from the study of Meehan et al.,[15] and only 2% (75/3214) of the patients reviewed by Lavin et al. received a regional anesthetic.[6] Golan and coworkers[16] and Plauche' et al.[4] reported 7 of 116 cases of uterine rupture related to acute anteflexion of the maternal torso. These occurred while an

TABLE 17-3

Outcome of VTOL Grouped by Previous Obstetric Indications

Reference	CPD	Breech	Placenta Previa	Fetal Distress
Lavin et al.[6]	33.3% (543)*	—	85.7% (21)	68.4% (95)
Horowitz et al.[13]	40.0% (145)	—	84.0% (59)	76.0% (96)
Flamm et al.[14]	67.0% (107)	93% (61)	100% (12)	71.0% (24)

VTOL, Vaginal trials of labor; CPD, cephalopelvic disproportion.
*No. in parentheses indicates no. of cases.

TABLE 17-4

INFLUENCE OF EPIDURAL BLOCK AND OXYTOCIN ON OUTCOME OF VTOL

Reference	No. of VTOL	Epid†	UR	No Epid	UR	Oxy*	UR	No Oxy	UR
Carlsson et al.[17]	119	68/77	2	37/42		64/76	2	41/43	
Demianczuk et al.[18]	92	30/41		20/51	2	10/23	1	40/69	1
Meier and Porreco[19]	207	19/22		156/185		34/42		141/165	
Benedetti et al[20]	89					12/16		59/73	
Martin et al.[21]	162	27/44		74/118		17/25		84/137	
Uppington[22]	222	55/71	1	121/151	3				
Rudick et al.[23]	115	102/115	1						
Flamm et al.[14]	230	49/73		132/157		61/94		120/136	
Horenstein et al.[24]	292					31/58		186/234	
Finley and Gibbs[25]	1156								
Jarrell et al.[26]	216	6/13		137/203					
Stovall et al.[27]	272	114/153	1	102/119		98/133	1	118/139	
Molloy et al.[28]	1781								
Phelan et al.[29]	1796	183/244		1277/1552	5	547/793	2	913/1003	3
Flamm et al.[30]	1776	134/181	1	1180/1595	2	309/485	2	1005/1291	1
Ollendorf[31]	229	36/64		134/165		61/97		109/132	
Meehan and Magani[32]	1350	279/345	2	814/1005	4	349/431	3	744/919	3
Yetman and Nolan[33]	224								
Farmer et al.[34]	7598								
Johnson et al.[35]	110	37/51		37/59	2				
Sakala et al.[36]	237	76/87		124/150		49/73		151/164	
Flamm et al.[37]	3957					831/1201	4	2146/2756	3
TOTALS	22,230	1215/1581		4315/5552		2473/3547		5857/7261	
% Vaginal deliveries		77%		78%		70%		81%	

UR, Uterine rupture; Epid, epidural; VTOL, vaginal trials of labor; Oxy, oxytocin.

* $\frac{\text{Vaginal deliveries with oxytocin}}{\text{VTOL with oxytocin}}$

† $\frac{\text{Vaginal deliveries with epidural}}{\text{VTOL with epidural}}$

epidural anesthetic was administered with the patients in the sitting position. A summary of recent studies (Table 17-4) based on a total of 1581 patients undergoing VTOL with epidural anesthetics reveals a slightly higher incidence of uterine rupture with an epidural block 0.5% (8/1581) compared with parturients who did not receive epidural anesthesia 0.3% (18/5552).

Does an Epidural Block Increase the Chance of Failure of Labor Resulting in a Repeat Cesarean Section?

In our review of 15 studies involving a total of 7133 patients having VTOL showed a 77% (1215/1581) chance of vaginal delivery for those receiving an epidural block. The same outcome was observed for subjects not receiving an epidural anesthetic (4345/5552) (Table 17-4).

Should Oxytocin and Epidural Anesthetics Be Used in Combination in a Previously Scarred Uterus?

Table 17-5 reviews 5780 VTOL and shows an 86% (541/628) chance of vaginal delivery with the combination of oxytocin and epidural anesthetics compared with 69% (936/1357) using oxytocin alone. Epidural analgesia provides pain relief whereas oxytocin stimulation achieves adequate contractions for successful outcome. Table 17-6 presents a series of 105 uterine ruptures in which 24% (25/105) occurred with the combination, and 41% (43/105) occurred with oxytocin alone.

What Is the Incidence of Emergency Hysterectomy to Control Hemorrhage After Uterine Rupture?

In our series, 19% (20/105) of ruptures required an emergency hysterectomy. Uterine rupture accounts for 11.4% of all emergency hysterectomies[38] (Fig. 17-4).

In Contrast to Rupture of the Scarred Uterus, What Happens When the Intact Uterus Ruptures?

Schrinsky and Benson reviewed maternal and neonatal mortality after rupture of the intact uterus.[7] They found that before 1978 maternal mortality was 21% (258/1241), a figure which is 3.5 times the maternal mortality for rupture of the

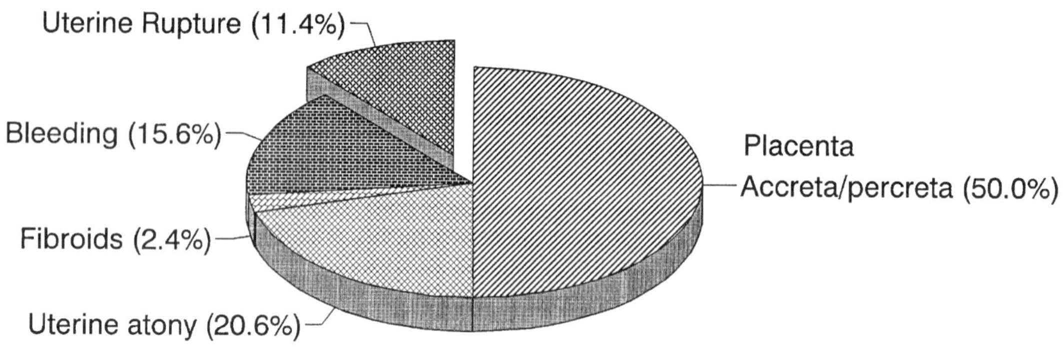

Fig. 17-4.

There were 123 emergency peripartum hysterectomies at LA County Hospital during the years 1985 to 1990. Uterine rupture ranked fourth in order of frequency.[38]

TABLE 17-5

Influence of Epidural Block, Oxytocin, and their Combination on the Outcome of VTOL

Reference	No. of VTOL	Epid	Oxytocin and Epid	Oxytocin	No Oxytocin and No Epid
Carlsson et al.[17]	119	17/18	51/59	13/17	24/25
Flamm et al.[14]	230	13/18	36/55	25/39	107/118
Stovall et al.[27]	272	43/50	71/103	27/30	75/89
Phelan et al.[29]	1796	60/66	123/78	424/615	853/937
Flamm et al.[30]	1776	47/64	87/117	222/368	958/1227
Meehan and Magani[32]	1350	139/170	140/175	209/256	605/749
Sakala et al.[36]	237	43/46	33/41	16/32	108/118
TOTALS	5780	362/432	541/628	936/1357	2730/3263
% Vaginal deliveries		84%	86%	69%	84%

VTOL, Vaginal trials of labor; Epid, epidural block.

TABLE 17-6

Incidence of Uterine Scar Rupture in VTOL with Epidural Blocks and Oxytocin

Reference	No. of VTOL	Epid	Oxy and Epid	Oxy	No Oxy and No Epid	Maternal Deaths Due to Scar Rupture	Fetal Deaths Due to Scar Rupture
Carlsson et al.[17]	119		2				
Demianczuk et al.[18]	92			1	1		
Demianczak et al.[19]	207						
Meier et al.[22]	222	1			3		1
Rudick et al.[23]	115	1					
Finley and Gibbs[25]	1156				1		1
Stovall et al.[27]	272		1				
Molloy et al.[28]	1781		4	2	2		1
Phelan et al.[29]	1796			2	3		1
Flamm et al.[30]	1776		1	1	1		
Meehan and Magani[32]	1350		2	1	3		3
Yetman and Nolan[33]	224				2		
Farmer et al.[34]	7598	2	15	30	14	1	1
Johnson et al.[35]	110			2			
Flamm et al.[37]	3957	—	—	4	3	—	1
TOTALS	20,775	4	25	43	33	1	9

VTOL, Vaginal trials of labor; Epid, epidural block; Oxy, oxytocin.

scarred uterus (21% versus 6.1%); and that neonatal mortality was 64.6% (620/960).[7] Plauche' et al. evaluated data from 1978 and determined that with a ruptured unscarred uterus, maternal mortality was 13% (21/162), whereas fetal mortality remained high at 76% (118/155).[4] Spontaneous uterine rupture was found to be associated with a threefold higher neonatal mortality than rupture of the scarred uterus (76% versus 24%) (Table 17-1). Plauche' et al. calculated the amount of blood loss that occurred with the rupture of an unscarred uterus, and found that it was between 1.2 and 1.9 times that which occurred if a scarred uterus ruptured. Clearly, rupture through a scar affords a less vascular plane than a spontaneous rupture. Because spontaneous rupture of an intact uterus has been observed in an older age group with a mean parity of 4.1, the clinician should replace the too general admonition to *beware of an epidural anesthesia for a vaginal trial of labor* with the specific caveat *beware of an epidural block in the multiparous parturient who has had four normal vaginal deliveries.*

What Parameters Should Be Followed to Guide Fluid and Blood Replacement if an Emergency Hysterectomy Is Performed to Control Hemorrhage?

During pregnancy, red blood cell mass increases from 1400 to 1800 ml and plasma volume increases from 2600 to 3700 ml. Therefore intravascular volume rises from 4000 to 5500 ml and hemoglobin concentration falls from 13 to 12 g/100 ml. During acute hemorrhage, even in the absence of intravenous infusion of fluid, these changes in blood volume help the parturient to maintain the hemoglobin concentration as well as the intravascular volume at a level 10% to 20% higher than the nonpregnant patient (Fig. 17-5). If the vascular volume

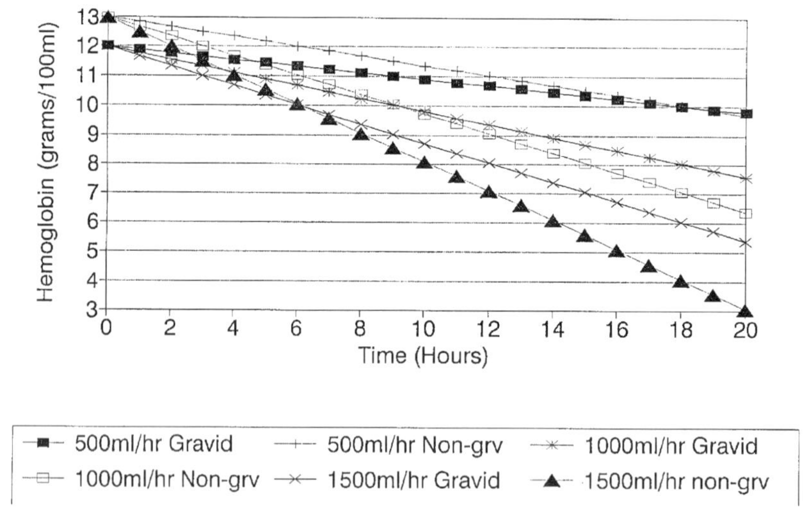

Fig. 17-5.

Hemoglobin concentration is calculated by solving the differential equation

$$d\,Hb/dt = (-Hb \cdot \text{blood loss})/(\text{intravascular volume} - \text{blood loss} \cdot t)$$

Blood loss is in milliliters per hour.

is expanded with crystalloid or colloid, the parturient with a hemoglobin concentration of 12 g/100 ml and a vascular volume of 5500 ml may not require a transfusion after a blood loss of 2000 ml/hr. The parturient starts with 12 g/100 ml × 5500 ml, or 660 g of hemoglobin. At the end of 2 hours, if the intravascular volume is expanded to 9400 ml, the parturient would loose 12 g of hemoglobin, leaving a hemoglobin concentration of 648/94, or 6.9 g/100 ml (Fig. 17-6). Blood is being lost at a falling hemoglobin concentration. If the calculation is made using a fixed hemoglobin concentration of 12 g/100 ml, the parturient would lose 12 g/100 ml × 4000 ml, or 480 g of hemoglobin. This leaves 660 − 480, or 180 g of hemoglobin in the circulation. If the vascular volume is maintained at 5500 ml, the final hemoglobin concentration would be 180/55, or 3.3 g/100 ml.

Therefore (1) it is difficult to predict the parturient's hemoglobin concentration at the end of 2 hours by estimating the blood loss; (2) the hemoglobin concentration of the parturient must be measured; (3) large volume expansions with crystalloid can lead to fluid overload; and (4) central venous pressure should be monitored.

How Low Should the Hemoglobin Level Be Allowed to Fall Before Replacement?

At a hemoglobin concentration of 12.5 g/100 ml with 100% arterial and 75% venous oxygen saturation, a cardiac output of 6 L/min, coupled with an extraction ratio of 25% (arterial content − venous content/arterial content) can supply 1000 ml of oxygen/min to meet metabolic requirements of 250 ml/min (Fig. 17-7, **A**). Depending on supply and demand, tissues can extract more oxygen, thereby lowering the venous oxygen content and increasing the extraction ratio from 25% at rest to 90% during acute stress.[39] When the he-

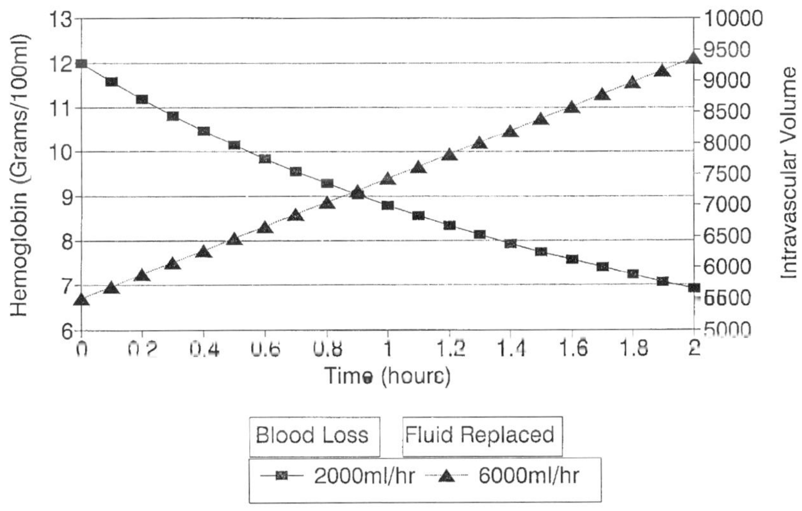

Fig. 17-6.
Hemoglobin concentration is calculated by solving the differential equation

d Hb/dt = (−Hb · blood loss)/(intravascular volume + (crystalloid − blood loss) · t) Crystalloid and blood loss are in milliliters per hour.

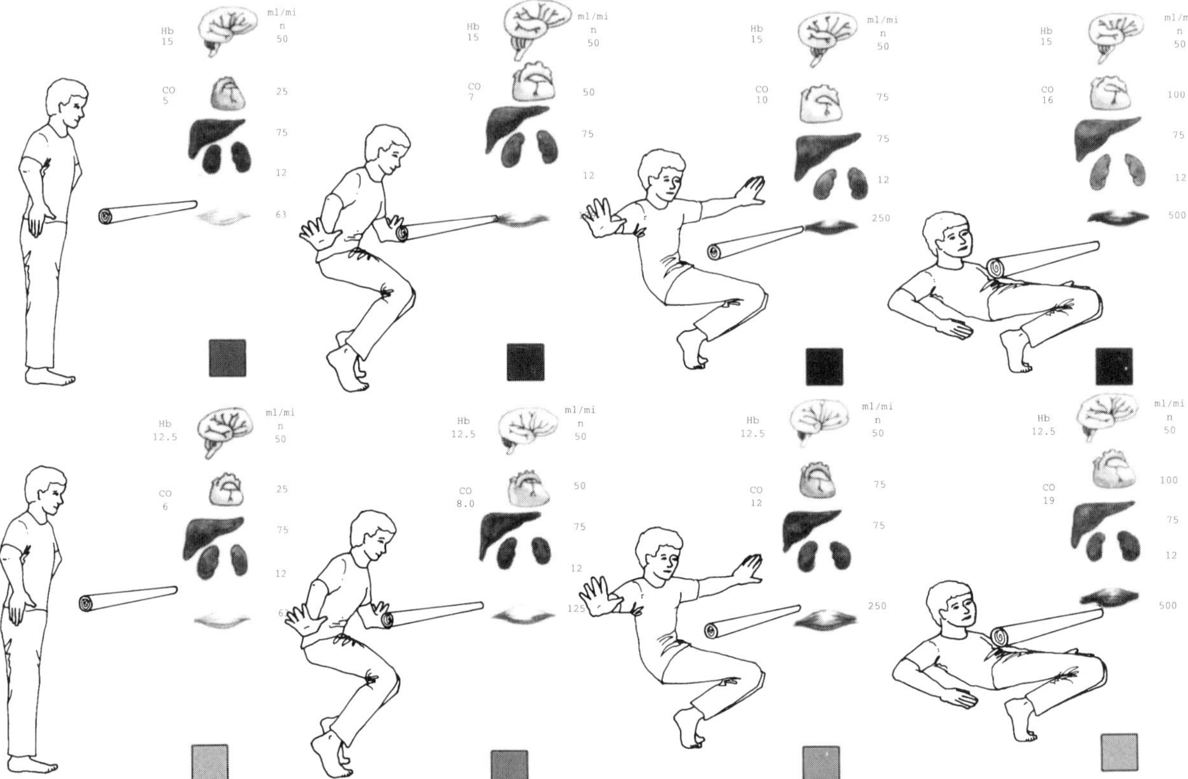

Fig. 17-7.

The hemoglobin concentration is represented by the shaded box in the lower right corner of each frame. **A** and **B,** The oxygen consumption is inversely proportional to the height of the limbo bar. Increases in exercise are reflected by greater blood flow to the coronary circulation, skeletal muscle, and skin. This dancer cannot change his extraction ratio from 25% and therefore must increase his cardiac output to match oxygen demand. A, Arterial oxygen content; v, venous oxygen content; CO, cardiac output in liters per minutes. Organ oxygen consumption in milliliters per minute.

moglobin concentration falls to 5 g/100 ml, a cardiac output of 15 L/min will deliver (6.7 ml/100 ml) × 15,000 ml/min, or 1000 ml of oxygen/min. If the extraction ratio remains at 25%, only 250 ml of oxygen/min can be used (Fig. 17-7, **B**). When the extraction ratio increases to 45%, the cardiac output can decrease to 8.3 L/min to meet a demand of 250 ml/min: (6.7 ml/100 ml) × (8300 ml/min) × (0.45) (compare Fig. 17-7, **B** with Fig. 17-8, **B**). If the hemoglobin concentration falls to 2.5 g/100 ml, a cardiac output of 15 L/min will deliver (3.35 ml/100 ml) × 15,000 ml/min), or 500 ml of oxygen/min. With an extraction ratio of 25%, only 125 ml of oxygen/min can be utilized—enough to supply the brain and heart, but not the liver, kidney, or skeletal muscle (Fig. 17-7, **B**). When the extraction ratio increases to 50%, 250 ml/min of oxygen will be available at a cardiac output of 15 L/min (Fig. 17-8, **B**). A higher extraction ratio enables a lower hemoglobin

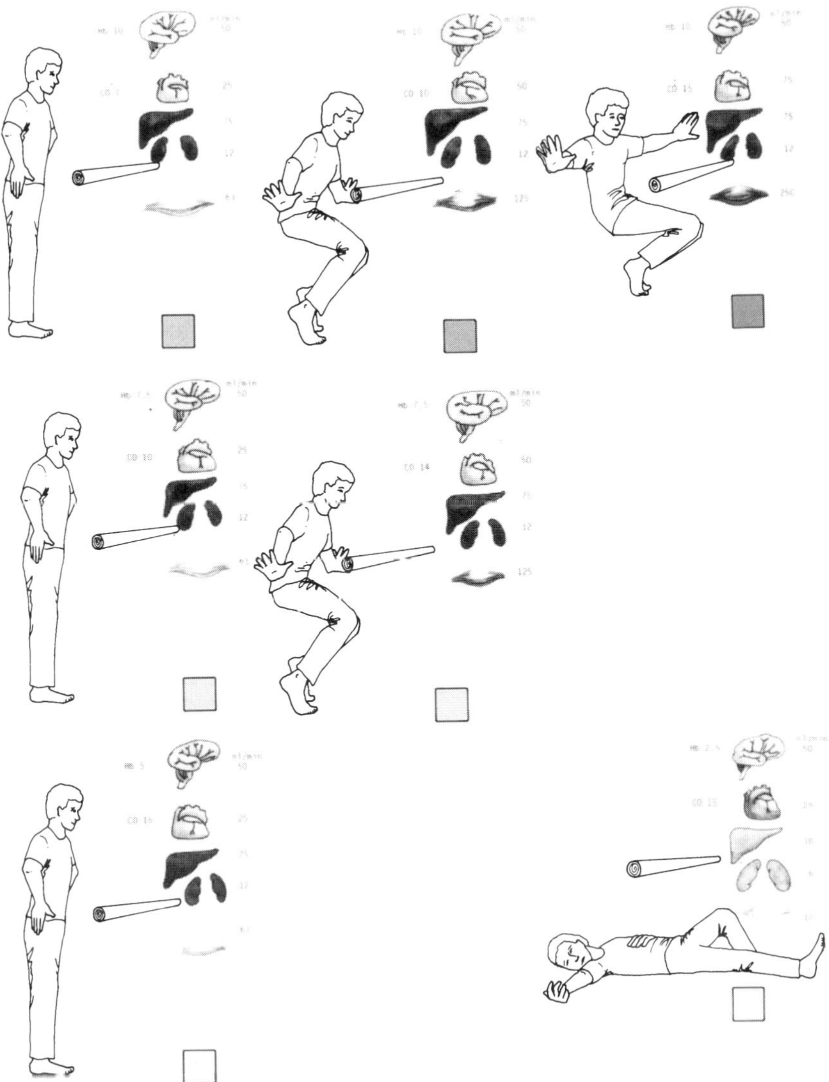

Fig. 17-7, cont'd.
For legend see opposite page.

concentration or cardiac output to meet metabolic requirements (Fig. 17-9). Therefore all of the oxygen supply data from Fig. 17-8 are plotted to the left of the oxygen delivery data from Fig. 17-7. A higher extraction ratio results in a lower mixed venous oxygen saturation (Fig. 17-10).

Hemoglobin concentration gives an indication of blood loss and fluid replacement. Arterial pH, mixed venous oxygen content, and cardiac output assess the adequacy of tissue perfusion. Blood should be replaced so oxygen supply is three to four times the demand, rather than to a specific hemoglobin concentration.

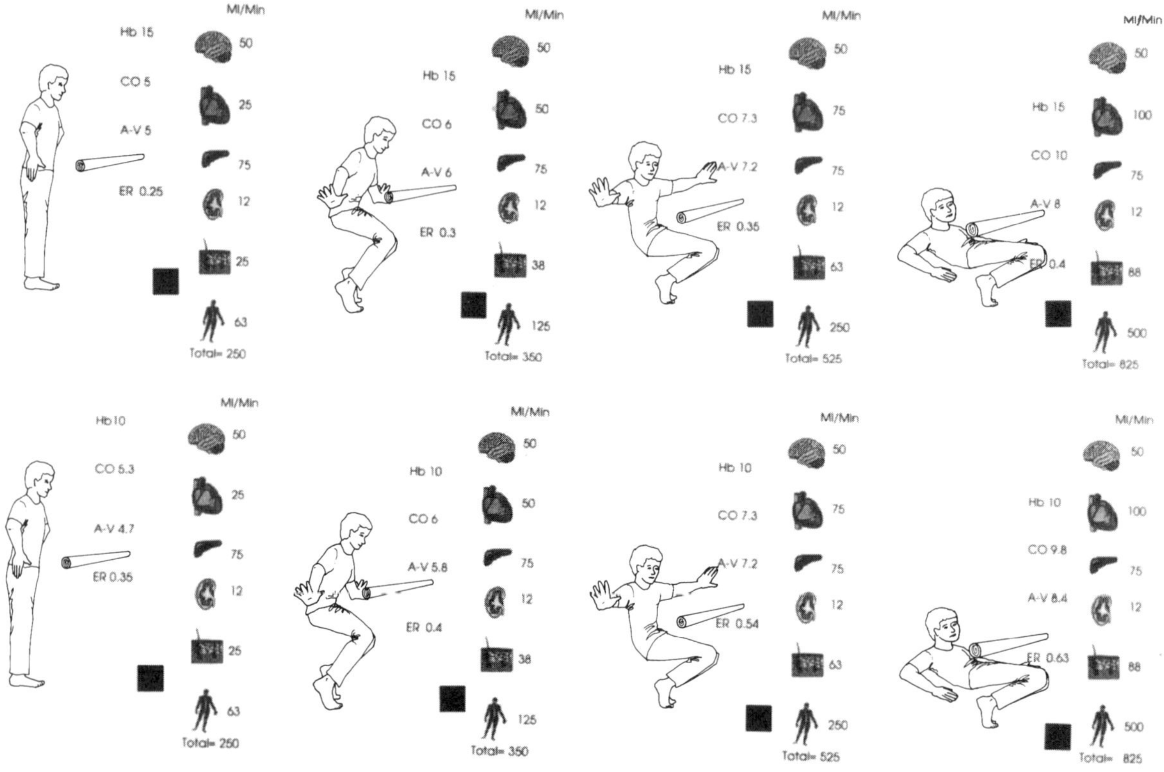

Fig. 17-8.
A and **B,** The limbo dancer can vary his extraction ratio as oxygen consumption increases, thereby performing the same tasks as the limbo dancer in Fig. 17-7, but at a lower cardiac output.

Summary

Should This Patient Receive an Epidural Block During Her Trial of Labor?

The patient under consideration had a previous cesarean section for breech presentation, a nonrecurring reason. According to Flamm et al., she should have a 93% chance of a successful vaginal trial.[14] Shy and associates believe that if the probability of a vaginal delivery is less than 0.45, a vaginal trial should not be attempted.[5] This patient has twice that chance of success, therefore a vaginal trial is not unreasonable; she should be allowed to have adequate analgesia during her course of labor, provided the following recommendations are met:

1. The previous type of cesarean section scar must be documented as a low cervical transverse. Although the works of Pedowitz and Schwartz[12] and Plauche' et al.[4] show that all types of uterine scars may rupture, the reported vaginal trials with epidural blocks have been performed primarily in women with low cervical transverse scars.[4,12]
2. An operating room must be in close proximity to the labor and delivery area.
3. The obstetrician and anesthesiologist must be present during the course of labor and deliv-

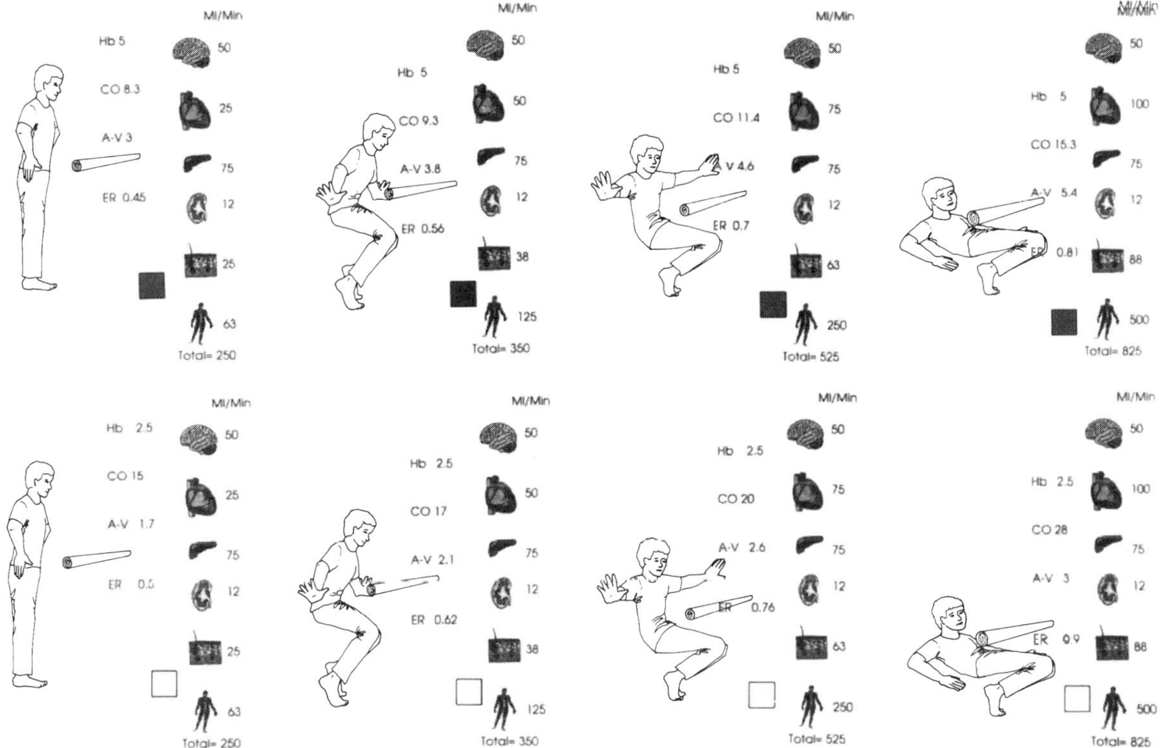

Fig. 17-8, cont'd.
For legend see opposite page.

ery and be prepared to perform an emergency cesarean section if the signs of uterine rupture occur, specifically fetal bradycardia, as shown by Johnson and Oriol.[3]

4. Two units of crossmatched blood should be available. Plauche' et al. estimated the mean blood loss at 2000 ml for 13 cases reviewed, with a mean of 4 U transfused.[4] Two units available within 45 minutes will buy time for the blood bank to crossmatch additional units as needed.
5. A 16-gauge intravenous catheter is the minimum size used in this class of patients.
6. Continuous fetal heart rate and intrauterine pressure monitoring must be performed.
7. Informed consent for an epidural anesthetic must be obtained by the anesthesiologist. There are only 1581 patients in the current world literature who have undergone vaginal trials with epidural blocks. The studies mentioned in this review (Tables 17-4 to 17-6) indicate that epidural blocks per se do not increase the risk of uterine rupture or failure of VTOL.
8. The epidural block should be performed with the patient in the lateral position, not in the sitting position. Golan et al.[16] and Plauche' et al.[4] reported seven cases of uterine rupture that occurred due to anteflexion of the maternal torso for epidural anesthesia.

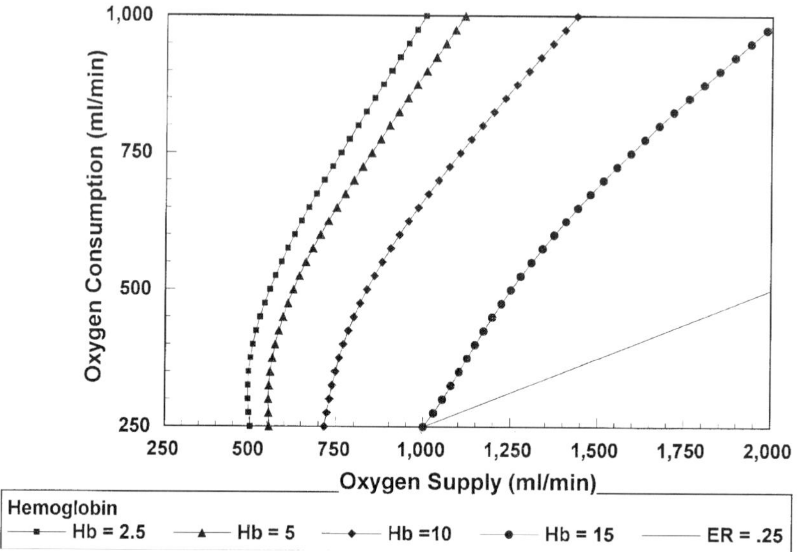

Fig. 17-9.

The oxygen supply-demand relationships illustrated in Figs. 17-7 and 17-8 are plotted. The slopes are equal to the extraction ratios and vary from 0.25 to 1.0. The data from Fig. 17-8 require multiple curves, each corresponding to a different hemoglobin concentration. The data from Fig. 17-7 are plotted as a single line with a slope equal to 0.25.

9. Low concentrations of local anesthetic should be used. Studies of Carlsson et al.[17] and Rudick et al.[23] employed concentrations of bupivacaine less than 0.4%.
10. During oxytocin stimulation, an intrauterine pressure catheter is essential. Flamm et al. concluded that oxytocin significantly improves the chances of success for the vaginal trial.[14]
11. A sensory level to at least the tenth thoracic dermatome should be provided for labor and vaginal delivery. This will also provide adequate pain relief after delivery, when uterine exploration is performed to rule out disruption of the prior uterine scar. Profound maternal hemorrhage after successful vaginal delivery must arouse suspicion of uterine rupture.
12. If fetal distress occurs during the course of labor, the epidural catheter should not be automatically redosed in preparation for cesarean section. At the time of fetal bradycardia, occult maternal blood loss may exceed 1000 ml. It may be more prudent to induce general anesthesia with ketamine than extend the level of the block. Of course, the choice of anesthesia will depend upon the cardiovascular status.
13. Hemorrhage accounts for 13% of all maternal mortality.[10] The management of an emergency hysterectomy requires large-bore intravenous lines to replace blood loss. An arterial line should be placed before the patient becomes hemodynamically unstable. This will enable the anesthesiologist to measure serial hemoglobin concentrations, clotting factors, and arterial pH. Placement of a pulmonary artery catheter allows for measurement of both mixed venous oxygen content and cardiac output.

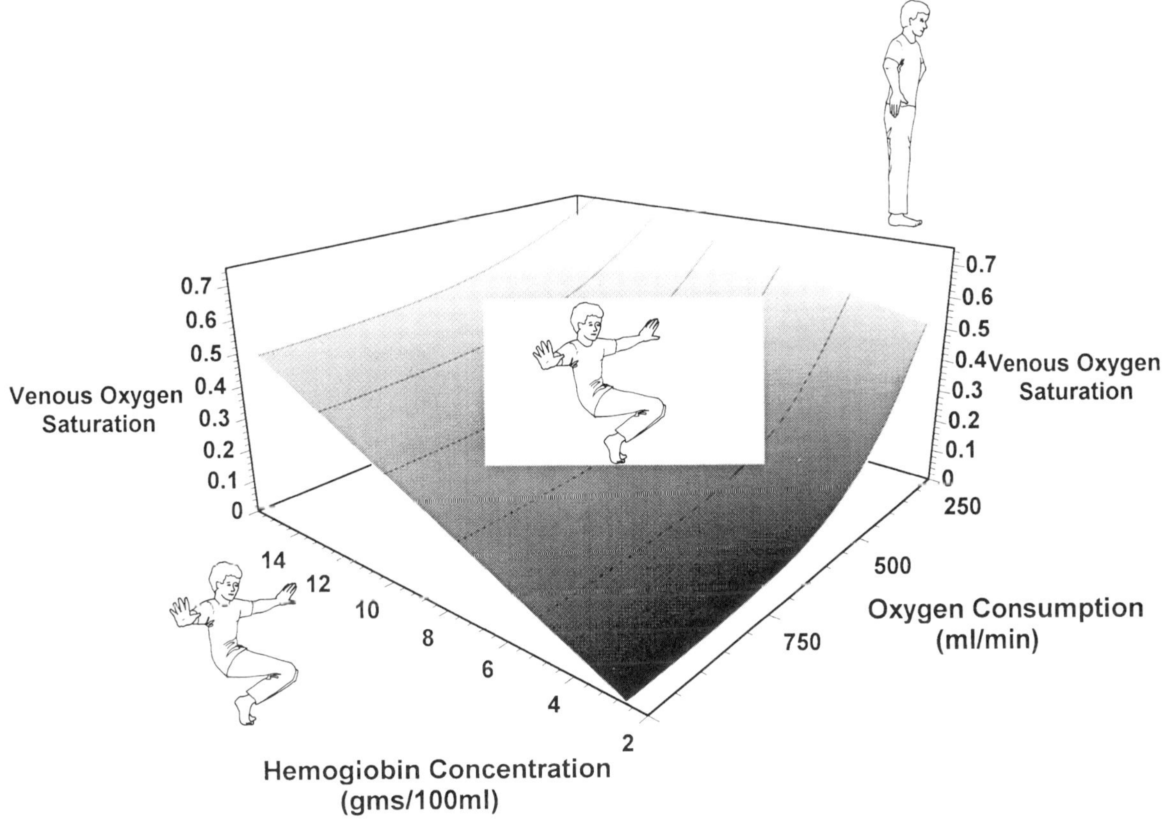

Fig. 17-10.
The mixed venous oxygen saturation is plotted as a function of oxygen consumption. The limbo dancer in Fig. 17-8 lowers his mixed venous oxygen saturation as oxygen consumption inceases. This is plotted as a curved surface influenced by the hemoglobin concentration.

References

1. Case B, Corcoran R, Jeffcoate N: Cesarean section and its place in modern obstetric practice, *Br J Obstet Gynaecol* 1971; 78:203.
2. Crawford JS: The epidural sieve and MBC (minimal blocking concentration): a hypothesis, *Anaesthesia* 1976; 30:1278.
3. Johnson C, Oriol N: The role of epidural anesthesia in trial of labor, *Reg Anesth* 1990; 15:304.
4. Plauche' WC, Von Almen W, Muller R: Catastrophic uterine rupture, *Obstet Gynecol* 1984; 64:792.
5. Shy LL, Logerfo JP, Karp LE: Evaluation of elective repeat cesarean section as a standard of care: an application of decision analysis, *Am J Obstet Gynecol* 1981; 139:123.
6. Lavin JP, Stephens RJ, Miodovnik M, et al: Vaginal delivery in patients with a prior cesarean section, *Obstet Gynecol* 1982; 59:135.
7. Schrinsky DC, Benson RC: Rupture of the pregnant uterus: a review, *Obstet Gynecol Surv* 1978; 33:217.
8. Rosen MG, Dickinson JC, Westhoff CL: Vaginal birth after cesarean: a meta-analysis of morbidity and mortality, *Obstet Gynecol* 1991, 77:465.
9. Wegman ME: Special article: annual summary of vital statistics—1992, *Pediatrics* 1993; 92:743.
10. Tindall VR, Beard RW, Sykes MK, et al: *Report on confidential enquiries into maternal deaths in the United Kingdom, 1985-1987,* London, 1991, Her Majesty's Stationery Office.

11. Lawrence RF: Rupture of the transverse uterine scar after lower segment cesarean section, *Br J Obstet Gynaecol* 1949; 56:1024.
12. Pedowitz P, Schwartz R: The true incidence of silent rupture of cesarean section scars: a prospective analysis of 403 cases, *Am J Obstet Gynecol* 1957; 74:1071.
13. Horowitz BJ, Edelstein SW, Lippman L: Once a cesarean always a cesarean, *Obstet Gynecol Surv* 1981; 36:592.
14. Flamm B, Dannett C, Fischermann E, et al: Vaginal delivery following cesarean section: use of oxytocin augmentation and epidural anesthesia with internal tocodynamic and internal fetal monitoring, *Am J Obstet Gynecol* 1984; 148:759.
15. Meehan F, Moolgoakera A, Stullworthy J: Vaginal delivery under caudal analgesia after caesarean section and other major uterine surgery, *Br Med J* 1972; 2:740.
16. Golan A, Sandbank O, Rubin A: Rupture of pregnant uterus, *Obstet Gynecol* 1980; 56:549.
17. Carlsson C, Nybell-Lindahl G, Ingemarson I: Extradural block in patients who have previously undergone cesarean section, *Br J Anaesth* 1980; 52:827.
18. Demianczuk NN, Hunter DJS, Taylor DW: Trial of labor after previous cesarean section: prognostic indicators of outcome, *Am J Obstet Gynecol* 1992; 142:640.
19. Meier PR, Porreco RP: Trial of labor following cesarean section: a two-year experience, *Am J Obstet Gynecol* 1982; 144:671.
20. Benedetti TJ, Platt L, Druzin M: Vaginal delivery after previous cesarean section for a nonrecurrent cause, *Am J Obstet Gynecol* 1982; 142:358.
21. Martin JN, Harris BA, Huddleston JF, et al: Vaginal delivery following previous cesarean birth, *Am J Obstet Gynecol* 1983; 146:255.
22. Uppington J: Epidural analgesia and previous caesarean section, *Anaesthesia* 1983; 38:336.
23. Rudick V, Niv D, Hetman-Peri M, et al: Epidural analgesia for planned vaginal delivery following previous cesarean section, *Obstet Gynecol* 1984; 64:621.
24. Horenstein JM, Eglinton GS, Tahilramaney, et al: Oxytocin use during a trial of labor in patients with previous cesarean section, *J Reprod Med* 1984; 29:26.
25. Finley BE, Gibbs CE: Emergent cesarean delivery in patients undergoing a trial of labor with a transverse lower-segment scar, *Am J Obstet Gynecol* 1986; 155:936.
26. Jarrell MA, Ashmead GG, Mann LI: Vaginal delivery after cesarean section: a five-year study, *Obstet Gynecol* 1985; 65:628.
27. Stovall TG, Shaver DC, Solomon SK, et al: Trial of labor in previous cesarean section patients, excluding classical cesarean sections, *Obstet Gynecol* 1987; 70:713.
28. Molloy BG, Sheil O, Duignan NM: Delivery after caesarean section: review of 2,176 consecutive cases, *Br Med J* 1987; 294:1645.
29. Phelan JP, Clark SL, Diaz F, et al: Vaginal birth after cesarean, *Am J Obstet Gynecol* 1987; 157:1510.
30. Flamm BL, Lim OW, Jones C, et al: Vaginal birth after cesarean section: results of a multicenter study, *Am J Obstet Gynecol* 1988; 158:1079.
31. Ollendorf DA, Goldberg JM, Minogue JP, et al: Vaginal birth after cesarean section for arrest of labor: is success determined by maximum cervical dilatation during the prior labor? *Am J Obstet Gynecol* 1988; 159:636.
32. Meehan FP, Magani IM: True rupture of the caesarean section scar (a 15 year review, 1972-1987), *E J Obstet Gynecol* 1989; 30:129.
33. Yetman TJ, Nolan TE: Vaginal birth after cesarean section: a reappraisal of risk, *Am J Obstet Gynecol* 1989; 161:1119.
34. Farmer RM, Kirschbaum T, Potter D, et al: Uterine rupture during trial of labor after previous cesarean section, *Am J Obstet Gynecol* 1991; 165:996.
35. Johnson C, Oriol N, Flood K: Trial of labor: a study of 110 patients, *J Clin Anesth* 1991; 3:216.
36. Sakala EP, Kay S, Murray RD, et al: Epidural analgesia: effect on the likelihood of a successful trial of labor after cesarean section, *J Reprod Med* 1990; 35:887.
37. Flamm BL, Newman LA, Thomas SJ, et al: Vaginal birth after cesarean delivery: results of a 5-year multicenter collaborative study, *Obstet Gynecol* 1990; 76:750.
38. Stanco LM, Schrimmer DB, Paul RH, et al: Emergency peripartum hysterectomy and associated risk factors, *Am J Obstet Gynecol* 1993; 168:879.
39. Dantzker DR, Foresman B, Gutierrez G: Oxygen supply and utilization relationships, *Am Rev Respir Dis* 1991; 142:675.

18

Trial of Forceps: Regional or General Anesthesia

A 25-year-old primigravida at term has remained fully dilated for more than 2 hours, even with effective pushing. The obstetrician has decided on a trial of forceps. *How does the clinician select the anesthetic and perform the technique? What are the contraindications to spinal anesthesia? Discuss the techniques of general anesthesia in such a case if spinal anesthesia is contraindicated.*

Recommendations by Joseph S. Mallon, M.D.
Stephen H. Rolbin, M.D.

Obstetric Considerations

Major causes of prolonged second-stage labor include the following: fetopelvic disproportion, which may be absolute or relative; malpresentations such as breech or brow; malpositions such as persistent occiput posterior; maternal exhaustion; and blockade of voluntary expulsive efforts of the mother by regional anesthesia. The major concern is rupture of the lower uterine segment. Whether operative delivery is vaginal or abdominal depends largely on the cause of the failure to progress.

Fortunately, with good antenatal and obstetric care the majority of major fetopelvic disproportions and malpresentations precluding vaginal delivery either are previously identified or are recognized, and rectified if possible, early in labor. The majority of *trials of forceps* under the circumstances presented will be for perceived minor degrees of fetopelvic disproportion, for malposition or soft tissue dystocia, and for maternal exhaustion. Unnecessary cesarean delivery can be avoided in most of these patients by a trial of forceps providing that (1) the cervix is indeed fully dilated; (2) the vertex is presenting; (3) the head is engaged; and (4) the position of the fetal head is known.

Unlike low forceps, the midforceps delivery is associated with significant maternal morbidity and fetal morbidity and mortality.[1-4] Maternal complications include hemorrhage from lacerations of the perineum, vagina, and uterus, and from uterine atony. Injury to bowel or uterus may require intra-abdominal repair. The neonatal risks of midpelvis instrumentation remain controversial. Fetal complications include the following: cephalohematoma, skull fracture, intracranial hemorrhage, facial or brachial nerve paralysis, cord compression, neonatal depression, asphyxia, and death. Major complications, although uncommon, are likely to occur simultaneously in both parturient and fetus. When difficult forceps delivery is anticipated, or if fetal distress is evident, the presence of a second anesthesiologist or other individual skilled in neonatal resuscitation is advisable.

Most trials of forceps will involve a midforceps application, possibly a rotational maneuver, followed by firm traction. Failure of one or two successful applications to result in descent of the fetus constitutes a *failure of forceps* and mandates immediate cesarean delivery. It is for this reason that a trial forceps should be carried out in an operating room with an anesthesiologist present in case an emergency cesarean section is required.

In a sense, every midforceps delivery constitutes a trial of forceps and it is important that the anesthesiologist maintains good communication with the obstetrician, is aware of the presumed cause of the prolonged labor, and knows whether the obstetrician anticipates any difficulty with the forceps delivery. No differences in adverse outcomes are seen whenever an operative delivery is performed successfully by midforceps when compared with those delivered by cesarean section after "failed forceps" or failure to progress in the second stage.[1-4]

In the past, second-stage labor without progression after 2 hours generally was terminated in the primigravida because the incidence of fetal and maternal complications increased if labor was permitted to continue beyond this point. As a result of changing obstetric practice, the arbitrary limitations of the duration of the second stage of labor have been extended when fetal monitoring confirms fetal well-being.[5] The American College of Obstetricians and Gynecologists has defined a prolonged second stage as longer than 3 hours in nulliparous women and longer than 2 hours in parous women with epidural anesthesia.[5]

Epidural anesthesia during labor is associated with an increased risk of instrumental vaginal delivery. There remains, however, controversy as to whether a causal relationship exists between epidural anesthesia and the incidence of instrumental deliveries.[6]

The Patient

The clinician can appreciate that after 2 to 3 hours of unproductive pushing this patient is likely to be physically and emotionally exhausted, in considerable pain and distress, probably disappointed or upset at failing to achieve a *natural* delivery, and now in fear of a perceived painful operative delivery. Considerable empathy, psychological support, and reassurances by the anesthesiologist are required.

If this is the first contact with the patient, the anesthesiologist may be under considerable pressure from both patient and obstetrician to administer the anesthetic without proper history or review of the course of labor, and indeed without informed consent. Such pressure must be firmly resisted. It only takes 2 or 3 minutes to ascertain pertinent medical and obstetric history from the chart, nurses, patient, and obstetrician. Particular notice should be taken of contraindications to any anesthetic contemplated. The administration and timing of any systemic narcotics and sedatives should be noted. Finally, evidence of fetal distress should be ruled out since its presence may greatly influence the choice of anesthetic technique.

In most trials of forceps, the operator is faced with inserting a space-occupying instrument into an already restricted pelvic area. Profound perineal and vaginal tract analgesia, plus pelvic floor muscular relaxation are required. Furthermore, it is necessary to block maternal expulsive efforts, which may interfere with the obstetrician's maneuvres or result in fetal or maternal trauma.

These anesthetic requirements can be met only by some form of regional anesthesia or by general anesthesia with full paralysis. No form of local anesthesia, including pudendal nerve block, will provide adequate relaxation, nor will it block the bearing-down reflex.

Regional Anesthesia Is the Method of Choice

Regional anesthesia is preferred over general anesthesia because it minimizes chances of maternal aspiration, enables the mother to be awake and the husband to be present for the delivery, and avoids neonatal drug-induced depression. We prefer to employ continuous lumbar epidural anesthesia for this patient. We believe it enables a more controllable level of anesthesia, with less precipitous drops in blood pressure, than does spinal anesthesia. Chances of a postspinal headache also may be less. Should the trial of forceps fail, the level of anesthesia usually can be extended for a subsequent cesarean delivery.

Nonetheless, spinal anesthesia is an acceptable alternative.[7] Compared with the initiation of epidural anesthesia, subarachnoid block is somewhat easier and quicker technically, with a more rapid onset of anesthesia. Neither the fetus nor the mother is exposed to significant systemic levels of local anesthetic. Notice that the "saddle block" technique, which is often employed for the second stage of labor (delivery), is inadequate for a midforceps rotation in which blockade to a sensory dermatome level of about at least T-10 is necessary. However, it is preferred to have a T-4 level, as this will be adequate for cesarean section should the trial of forceps fail.

Absolute contraindications to spinal and epidural anesthesia include the following: (1) patient refusal; (2) lack of full resuscitation equipment, drugs, or experience in the technique or treatment of its complications; (3) hypovolemic shock; (4) infection near the site of injection; and (5) coagulopathy.

Relative contraindications to regional techniques include (1) lack of cooperation of the patient due to pain, hysteria, or communication problems; (2) certain cardiovascular conditions in which a drop in blood pressure may be poorly tolerated, such as aortic stenosis or Eisenmenger's syndrome; and (3) preexisting neurologic or musculoskeletal disease. Each of these conditions must be evaluated individually and a regional technique must be acceptable to both patient and anesthesiologist.

A strong contraindication to regional techniques is acute fetal distress necessitating immediate delivery. When seconds count, we believe that the induction of general anesthesia most rapidly provides acceptable conditions for operative delivery, be it vaginal or abdominal. However, regional anesthesia should not be ruled out. Spinal anesthesia has been recommended when emergency delivery is required.[7,8] In addition, when overriding considerations are present such as a full stomach, a difficult intubation, or prolonged fetal distress that might have already resulted in the infant's condition being severely compromised, the clinician might choose a regional technique. In such circumstances, a spinal may be advantageous over an epidural technique, unless an epidural catheter is already in place.[8,9]

Before administration of regional anesthesia, the patient is taken to the delivery room. Anesthetic equipment and drugs are checked; we routinely keep on hand prepared endotracheal tubes, and all drugs necessary for emergency general anesthesia are kept drawn up and immediately available. It is especially important that ephedrine be prepared. A 16- or 18-gauge intravenous catheter must be in place, and ideally 1000 ml of a nondextrose-containing balanced salt solution is rapidly infused.

However, a recent reevaluation of the role of crystalloid preload in the prevention of hypotension associated with spinal anesthesia for elective cesarean section showed that hypotension cannot be eliminated by 20 ml/kg preload in the supine wedge condition.[10] Only a relatively small reduction occurs in the incidence of hypotension. The authors suggest that although volume and reload are recommended in elective cesarean sections, the requirement for a mandatory administration of a fixed volume could be abandoned for urgent cases.[10] However, this patient may require more fluids due to dehydration from prolonged labor, and if there is no urgent need to proceed, they should be given even though their merit is debatable. A baseline blood pressure should be obtained and oxygen administered at 10 L/min through a clear face mask.

The patient assumes the lateral decubitus position; the sitting position may be preferred for the markedly obese or in the presence of a marked lumbar lordosis. The lumbar area is prepped and the widest interspace below L-2 is chosen.

For epidural anesthesia, we administer 15 to 20 ml of either carbonated lidocaine (not available in the United States) or 25 ml of lidocaine hydrochloride alone or with epinephrine 1 : 200,000 in fractionated doses. The local anesthetic agent is administered slowly through the catheter. Excellent analgesia is provided by these doses.

If spinal anesthesia is selected, a 25- or 27-gauge whitacre spinal needle is used to minimize the incidence of headache. When cerebrospinal fluid (CSF) is recovered, the local anesthetic is injected without barbotage. It is important to inject between contractions to avoid a high spread. The local anesthetic is made hyperbaric with 5% to 7.5% dextrose. Epinephrine is not usually added, as a trial of forceps is a brief procedure. Tetracaine 7 to 10 mg will achieve the desired T-4 level. Lidocaine 50 to 75 mg or bupivacaine 11.25 to 15 mg also may be used, depending on the duration of the procedure.[11] Continuous spinal anesthesia is mentioned only for the sake of completeness. The authors believe that its use is contraindicated in clinical practice until there is more evidence of its safety.[12,13]

The patients are positioned with a wedge under the right hip and the legs are placed in the stirrups after attainment of T-10 level in the case of epidural technique, but immediately after subarachnoid block. Blood pressure is measured every minute for 10 minutes, then every 5 minutes. A decrease in blood pressure of greater than 20% or less than 100 mm Hg systolic is immediately treated with rapid infusion of fluids and 5- to 10-mg increments of intravenous ephedrine. Hypotension after application of the forceps must not automatically be assumed due to sympathetic blockade; evidence of hemorrhage and hypovolemia must be ruled out, both intrapartum and postpartum.

With successful delivery, the infant may require resuscitation because of the greater potential for trauma, depression, and neurologic injury.

General Anesthesia

General anesthesia is not the preferred technique for routine vaginal delivery. Its use should be reserved for situations in which anesthesia is necessary and regional anesthesia is contraindicated or inadequate.[14] Advantages of a general technique are a faster induction; less risk of maternal hypotension; and a rapid control of maternal airway, ventilation, and oxygenation. In the event of a failure of forceps, then a cesarean delivery can be performed without delay. The major risks are maternal aspiration, failure to control maternal airway, and drug-induced fetal depression.

During assessment of the patient's condition, careful attention must be paid to the airway, bearing in mind that mucosal edema of the upper airway may render the intubation more difficult. For the same reason, smaller endotracheal tubes are prepared, 5.0- through 7.0-mm tubes, rather than the more frequently used 7.5- or 8.0-mm tubes.

Premedication for this patient would be limited to a nonparticulate oral antacid (such as 30 ml of 0.3 M sodium citrate) to raise gastric pH. Other premedicants potentially useful in aspiration prophylaxis such as the H2 antagonists and metoclopramide have too long an onset of action to be of any benefit in this clinical setting. All anticholinergic drugs are contraindicated both as premedication and intravenously at induction because all cause rapid and marked relaxation of the lower esophageal sphincter, thus promoting reflux and aspiration.[15] All other hypnotics, sedatives, and opiates are contraindicated because of potential adverse effects on the fetus and lower esophageal tone.[15]

With the patient in the lithotomy position with left uterine displacement, oxygen is administered while the intravenous catheter is established, if it has not been established already, and the monitors are applied. Routine monitors for obstetric anesthesia include electrocardiogram, blood pressure cuff, peripheral nerve stimulator, pulse oximeter, capnograph, and temperature probe. In this situation the fetal heart rate also will be continuously monitored by an external transducer or internal electrode. The obstetrician will be completely prepared for operative delivery, and will have prepped and draped the perineum before induction to minimize the induction to delivery interval.

The necessity for precurarization in obstetrics has been seriously challenged, primarily on the evidence that succinylcholine-induced fasciculations raise lower esophageal sphincter pressure to a greater degree than intragastric pressure, thus providing a net protective effect against reflux.[16,17] If precurarization is used, the presence of fasciculations as an end point for intubation is lost, and the intubating dosage of succinylcholine must be increased. Finally, precurarization requires 3 minutes to be effective; such delay clearly is inappropriate if severe fetal distress occurs.

With respect to preinduction oxygenation, recently it has been shown that in healthy parturients, four maximally deep inspirations of 100% oxygen over 30 seconds are as efficacious in raising maternal arterial oxygen pressure (Pa_{O_2}) as the standard 3 minutes of oxygenation.[18] However, in one study using nonpregnant patients, oxygen desaturation decreased more quickly in patients preoxygenated with four breaths compared with those preoxygenated for 3 minutes.[19] Pregnant patients are expected to desaturate more quickly because of their decreased functional residual capacity and increased oxygen consumption. Without minimizing the importance of acute oxygenation, recognize that in the presence of severe fetal distress a 3-minute delay may be unjustified.

The mainstay in the prevention of maternal aspiration remains the rapid-sequence induction. Oral suction must be turned on and readily at hand. The endotracheal tube is prepared with a lubricated introducer inserted and preloaded syringe attached for rapid cuff inflation. Cricoid pressure is explained to the patient and applied by a trained assistant as pentothal 4 mg/kg of pregnant body weight (PBW) and succinylcholine 1.0 to 1.5 mg/kg PBW is injected rapidly into a freely flowing intravenous infusion. No attempt to ventilate the patient is made before intubation, nor should an oral airway be inserted. Laryngoscopy is delayed until fasciculations or the nerve stimulator indicate adequate paralysis; nothing is more conducive to active vomiting than instrumenting the airway of a lightly anesthetized and partially paralyzed patient.

Cricoid pressure is maintained until the endotracheal tube is in the trachea, the cuff is inflated, and auscultation has confirmed proper placement. At this point the obstetrician is permitted to proceed.

Propofol is a suitable alternative to pentothal as an induction agent for anaesthesia.[20-24] It assists in providing the smooth and rapid loss of consciousness required before intubation. Recovery times are shorter after propofol injections.[24] The rapid recovery time and lack of hangover may be a great advantage in the pregnant patient. There is no significant neonatal depression as assessed by Apgar scores and blood gas analysis.[23-25] One study has found a superior 1-minute Apgar score.[25] Another authority has shown that propofol is cleared rapidly from the neonatal circulation, and exposure through breast milk and colostrum is negligible compared with the placental transfer of the drug. There are no major adverse effects on the neonate.[26]

Anesthesia is maintained by ventilation with oxygen and nitrous oxide, with a minimum of 50% oxygen. Up to 0.5% halothane, 0.75% enflurane, or 1.0% isoflurane may be added without fear of suppressing uterine contractility. Intravenous agents are avoided until the fetus is delivered and the cord is clamped. Excessive maternal hyperventilation may adversely affect uteroplacental blood flow and should be avoided, bearing in mind that the normal arterial carbon dioxide pressure ($Paco_2$) in a parturient at term is about 30 to 33 mm Hg.

Propofol infusion anesthesia also has been used for cesarean section anesthesia. Initially concern was expressed about placental transfer of propofol, especially when induction to delivery times are long.[20,21] Several evaluations of this technique have been done and propofol appears to be a suitable induction and maintenance agent for elective cesarean section.[22,25,27]

Since the trial of forceps usually is a brief procedure, muscle paralysis is best maintained with succinylcholine. After delivery, the clinician can use any technique for repair of the episiotomy, using up to 70% nitrous oxide. Volatile agents in low concentrations may be continued if hemorrhage is not a problem. Isoflurane confers no special benefit and has been shown to accelerate the onset of phase-2 blockade when used with succinylcholine infusions.

The patient still is at risk for aspiration at extubation. This is minimized by delaying extubation until the patient is fully awake, follows commands, and meets all of the other regular criteria for extubation.

Postoperatively the patient requires the same duration and degree of recovery room care afforded to any surgical patient after general anesthesia.

Summary

The clinician has been asked to anesthetize a primigravida for a *trial of forceps*.

1. Regional anesthesia definitely is preferred over general anesthesia for the reasons outlined in this chapter. We prefer epidural anesthesia with insertion of an epidural catheter since it provides a more controllable level of anesthesia and allows easy extension of the blockade if cesarean delivery becomes necessary.
2. General anesthesia may be necessary in the case of inadequate block after regional anesthesia or in a situation of fetal distress.
3. Neonatal resuscitation may be necessary in such a situation.

References

1. Dierker LJ, Rosen MG, Thompson K, et al: The midforceps: maternal and neonatal outcomes, *Am J Obstet Gynecol* 1985; 152:176.
2. Dierker LJ, Rosen MG, Thompson K, et al: Midforceps deliveries: long term outcome of infants, *Am J Obstet Gynecol* 1986; 154:764.
3. Boyd ME, Usher RH, McLean FH, et al: Failed forceps. *Obstet Gynecol* 1986; 68:779.

4. Lowe B: Fear of failure: a place for the trial of instrumental delivery, *Br J Obstet Gynaecol* 1987; 94:60.
5. The American College of Obstetricians and Gynecologists Committee on Obstetrics: *Maternal and fetal medicine: obstetric forceps,* no. 71, 1989.
6. Chestnut DH: Epidural anesthesia and instrumental vaginal delivery, *Anesthesiology* 1991; 74:805.
7. Brownridge P: Spinal anaesthesia revisited: an evaluation of subarachnoid block in obstetrics, *Anaesth Intensive Care* 1984; 12:334.
8. Marx GF, Luykx WM, Cohen S: Fetal-neonatal status following caesarean section for fetal distress, *Br J Anaesth* 1984; 56:1009.
9. Ramanathan J, Ricca D, Sibai B, et al: Epidural versus general anesthesia in fetal distress with various abnormal fetal heart rate patterns, *Anesth Analg* 1988; 67:S180 (abstract)
10. Rout CC, Rocke DA, Levin J, et al: A re-evaluation of the role of crystalloid preload in the prevention of hypotension associated with spinal anesthesia for elective cesarean section, *Anesthesiology* 1993; 79:262.
11. Shnider SM, Levinson G, Ralstan DH: *Regional anesthesia for labour and delivery.* In Shnider SM, Levinson G, editors: *Anesthesia for obstetrics, ed 3,* 1993, Baltimore, Williams & Wilkins.
12. Rigler ML, Drasner K, Krejcie T, et al: Cauda equina syndrome after continuous spinal anesthesia, *Anesth Analg* 1981; 72:275.
13. Rigler ML, Draser K: Distribution of catheter-injected local anesthetic in a model of the subarachnoid space, *Anesthesiology* 1991; 75:684.
14. Cohen SE: *Inhalation analgesia and anaesthesia for vaginal delivery.* In Shnider SM, Levinson G, editors: *Anesthesia for obstetrics, ed 3,* Baltimore, 1993, Williams & Wilkins.
15. Cotton BR, Smith G: The lower oesophageal sphincter and anaesthesia, *Br J Anaesth* 1984; 56:37.
16. Conklin KA: Should precurarization be used in obstetrics? *Anesthesiology* 1984; 60:384.
17. Sellers WFS, Goddard RH: More about d-tubocurarine and succinylcholine in obstetrics, *Anesthesiology* 1984; 60:506.
18. Norris MC, Dewan DM: Preoxygenation for cesarean section: a comparison of two techniques, *Anesthesiology* 1985; 62:827.
19. Gambee AM, Hertkba RE, Fisher DM: Preoxygenated techniques: comparison of three minutes and four deep breaths, *Anesth Analg* 1987; 66:468.
20. Gin T, Gregory MA, Chan K, et al: Maternal and fetal levels of propofol at caesarean section, *Anaesth Intensive Care* 1990; 18:180.
21. Gin T, Gregory MA, Oh TE: The hemodynamic effects of propofol and thiopentone for induction of caesarean section, *Anaesth Intensive Care* 1990; 18:175.
22. Gregory MA, Gin T, Yau G, et al: Propofol infusion anesthesia for caesarean section, *Can J Anaesth* 1990; 37:514.
23. Moore J, Bill KM, Flynn RJ, et al: A comparison between propofol and thiopentone as induction agents in obstetric anesthesia, *Anaesthesia* 1989; 44:753.
24. Valtonen M, Kanto J, Rosenberg P: Comparison of propofol and thiopentone for induction of anaesthesia for elective caesarean section, *Anaesthesia* 1989; 44:758.
25. Richardson M, Abboud TK, Zhu MD, et al: Propofol as an induction and maintenance agent for caesarean section: maternal and neonatal effects. *Anesthesiology* 1991; 75:A1077 (abstract).
26. Dailland P, Cochshott ID, Lirzin JD, et al: Intravenous propofol during cesarean section: placental transfer, concentrations in breast milk and neonatal effects. *Anesthesiology* 1989; 71:827.
27. Finster M, Pedersen H, Strobel AF, et al: Propofol: induction and maintenance of anesthesia for cesarean section. *Anesthesiology* 1992; 77:A997 (abstract).

19

Anesthesia for Postpartum Hemorrhage

A 29-year-old multigravida has a normal, spontaneous vaginal delivery without any anesthesia in a birthing room. Profuse vaginal bleeding begins 30 minutes later and is discovered by the nurse during a routine check. The diagnosis of retained placenta is made by the attending obstetrician. The anesthesiologist is called to evaluate the patient's condition for an emergency examination under anesthesia and possible extraction of placenta. What would be the anesthetic management?

Recommendations by Katsuo Terui, M.D.

Obstetric hemorrhage still remains one of the leading causes of maternal mortality, although its incidence has declined due to the better prenatal care and improved availability of intensive care and blood products during the peripartum period.[1,2] Mortality from hemorrhage is 1.3 per 100,000 live births.[1] Postpartum hemorrhage is the major cause of blood loss in obstetrics. The most frequent causes of postpartum hemorrhage are cervical or vaginal lacerations and uterine atony.[3,4] The next most frequent cause is retained placenta or placental fragments: its incidence is 1% of all vaginal deliveries.[3] Predisposing factors and causes of immediate postpartum hemorrhage are presented in Table 19-1. In the case described above the diagnosis is retained placenta. A thorough description of the management plan of this case is discussed first, followed by a brief description of the management of other causes of postpartum hemorrhage.

Retained Placenta

During the normal process of delivery, uterine contraction is necessary for the cessation of hemorrhage once the placenta is detached from the en-

TABLE 19-1

PREDISPOSING FACTORS AND CAUSES OF IMMEDIATE POSTPARTUM HEMORRHAGE

- Trauma to the genital tract
  - Large episiotomy including extensions
  - Lacerations of perineum, vagina, or cervix
  - Ruptured uterus
- Bleeding from placental implantation site
  - Hypotonic myometrium: uterine atony
    - Some general anesthetics: volatile anesthetics
    - Poorly perfused myometrium: hypotension, hemorrhage
    - Overdistended uterus: large fetus, twins, hydramnios
    - After prolonged labor
    - After very rapid labor
    - After oxytocin-induced or -augmented labor
    - High parity
    - Uterine atony in previous pregnancy
    - Chorioamnionitis
  - Retained placental tissue
    - Avulsed cotyledon, succenturiate lobe
    - Abnormally adherent: accreta, increta, percreta
- Coagulation defects intensify all of the above

Modified from Cunningham FG, MacDonald PC, Grant NF, et al: *Abnormalities of the third stage of labor.* In: *Williams obstetrics,* ed 19, East Norwalk, CT, 1993, Appleton & Lange.

dometrium, because endometrial arteries and veins are left open until the uterus contracts. When the placenta or its fragment is left inside the uterus, this contraction mechanism does not work effectively, resulting in persistent bleeding. This type of hemorrhage due to retained placenta or uterine atony from retained products of the placenta can be massive because it is an arterial bleeding.

Evaluation of the Patient and Fluid Replacement

Removal of the retained placenta should be performed as soon as possible to control bleeding. The anesthesia team should be notified immediately and should discuss the situation with the obstetrician or midwife. While obtaining pertinent obstetric and medical history from the patient and medical staff, the anesthesia team has to assess the urgency of the situation by estimating the blood loss from drapes and sponges, and by observing the vital signs. Because of the increased blood volume during pregnancy (45% above prepregnant level at term), vital signs may remain relatively normal despite significant blood loss. Sometimes the patient may have normal blood pressure with tachycardia to compensate for the blood loss. Thus decreased blood pressure may imply significant or acute blood loss. When the patient needs prompt fluid replacement as in this case, large-bore peripheral intravenous (IV) lines should be established immediately and fluid replacement should be started using crystalloid and colloid solution (albumin, hetastarch) while the patient is evaluated. Clear, nonparticulate antacid (0.3 mol/L sodium citrate 30 ml) given orally, as well as metoclopramide 10 mg given intravenously, is administered to prepare for the anesthetic management for manual exploration of the uterus. Blood transfusion may be necessary depending on the situation, and at least two units of packed red blood cells (PRBC) should be ordered from the blood bank. In the case described at the beginning of this chapter, the blood bank should be informed of the potential need for the additional units of PRBC.

Management of Urgent Massive Transfusion

If transfusion of blood is urgently necessary without sufficient time to perform complete three-phase cross-match, type-specific, partially cross-matched blood can be given first. This takes 1 to 5 minutes and eliminates serious hemolytic reactions from errors in ABO typing. ABO-Rh typing alone results in a 99.8% chance of compatible transfusion, whereas complete cross-matching raises this to 99.95%.[5] When the situation is more urgent, type-specific, uncross-matched blood may have to be transfused. Rarely, O-negative blood is used in emergency transfusion when typing or cross-matching is not available. O-negative PRBC is preferred to O-negative whole blood because PRBC have smaller amount of plasma, which contains anti-A and anti-B antibodies. If more than two units of O-negative, uncross-matched whole blood are required during emergency transfusion, then O-negative blood will be necessary throughout the resuscitation of the patient to prevent major intravascular hemolysis of subsequent donor cells of the patient's own blood type.[5] Type-specific blood can be transfused to the patient only after transfused anti-A and anti-B has fallen to low enough levels.

If bleeding tendency is observed without clot formation during transfusion of multiple units of PRBC, dilutional thrombocytopenia, low coagulation factors such as V and VIII, disseminated intravascular coagulation (DIC), or hemolytic transfusion reaction should be suspected. For patients having a massive transfusion of close to 10 to 15 units of PRBC, or for those with a tendency toward clinical bleeding, prothrombin time, partial thromboplastin time, platelet counts, and fibrinogen levels need to be checked to determine the need for transfusion of fresh frozen plasma, platelet, or cryoprecipitate. Commonly used blood products and their effect on blood counts and laboratory results are summarized in Table 19-2.

Massive transfusion can also cause citrate intoxication. Citrate used for blood preservation chelates calcium ions and may result in hypocalcemia. Signs and symptoms of hypocalcemia include central nervous system (CNS) or muscle irritability, hypotension, narrow pulse pressure, and prolonged Q-T interval. Citrate intoxication rarely is observed in healthy adult patients in whom citrate is quickly metabolized by the liver, but may be observed when the patient has preexisting liver disease or hypothermia, or when citrate-containing blood is quickly transfused (faster than about 1 U blood/5 min). Calcium administration may become necessary on these occasions. Other complications of massive transfusion include metabolic acidosis followed by metabolic aklalosis from citrate load, hypothermia from infusion of inadequately warmed blood products, and hyperkalemia. These complications of massive transfusion have to be anticipated to prevent them or to treat them promptly.

Removal of Retained Placenta

Manual extraction of the retained placenta may be tried in the birthing room. If manual extraction is unsuccessful because of the patient's inability to tolerate painful intrauterine manipulation, adequate pain relief may be enough to extract the retained placenta successfully. Pain relief with intravenous fentanyl with sedation using IV midazolam sometimes is all that is necessary to aid in extraction. While administering these medications one has to keep in mind that pregnant patients are sensitive to CNS depressants. Further intervention, if necessary, should be carried out in an operating room. Adequate pain relief for manual extraction of retained placenta, however, is best achieved by spinal or epidural anesthesia unless contraindicated. Regional anesthesia allows an obstetrician to explore and manipulate the uterus freely while avoiding the risk of maternal aspiration. If the patient is still hypovolemic, even with ongoing volume replacement or blood transfusion, general endotracheal anesthesia is indicated to avoid exacerbating hypotension and circulatory collapse. General anesthesia may also be indicated in the situation when manual extraction is unsuccessful due to inadequate uterine relaxation despite adequate pain relief.

TABLE 19-2

Blood Products Used for Postpartum Hemorrhage

Blood Component	Content in Each Unit	Effect
PRBC	Hct 70% to 80% in 300 ml volume Plasma 70 ml Total K load 5.5 mEq at expiration	Increased Hb level by 1 g/dl Increased Hct by about 3%
Whole blood	450-ml donor blood 65-ml anticoagulant Hct 40%, plasma 250 ml Total K load 15 mEq Decreased coagulation factors Lost platelets	Increased Hct Volume expansion
Platelet concentrates	Plasma 50 ml/each unit Usual adult dose, 6 U	Increased platelet count by 7000-10,000
FFP	Volume 200-280 ml More than 70% of procoagulant activity preserved Fibrinogen level, 1-2 mg/ml	2 U raise procoagulant by about 20% and fibrinogen level by about 52 mg/dl
Cryoprecipitate	Factor VIII 80-100 U Fibrinogen 100-250 mg vWF 40-70% of original plasma	2-4 U/10 kg will maintain fibrinogen level above 100 mg/dl

PRBC, Packed red blood cells; Hct, hematocrit; Hb, hemoglobin; K, potassium; vWF, von Willebrand factor; FFP, fresh frozen plasma.

Regional Anesthesia for Removal of Retained Placenta

Before providing regional anesthesia for this situation, the anesthesiologist has to make sure that adequate volume replacement has been provided and that vital signs are in a reasonable range. Anesthetic considerations for immediate postpartum patients are almost the same for those undergoing cesarean section except that there is no fetus to consider. The risk of aspiration is still present at immediate postpartum. Thus clear antacid should be given orally before providing anesthesia. Preoperatively, I also prefer to give metoclopramide 10 mg intravenously. Patients will still be sensitive to both local anesthetics and general anesthetics compared with nonpregnant patients. After the effect from an enlarged uterus is removed, the spread of intrathecal or epidural local anesthetic is more than pregnant patients. The exact mechanism for this is not clear, but the increased neuronal sensitivity may be the possible mechanism. If the patient has an epidural catheter in place for labor analgesia, adequate pain relief and relaxation of perineum are achieved by administering 2% lidocaine or 3% 2-chloroprocaine 10 to 15 ml via the epidural catheter, with the patient in a semisitting position to obtain sensory level of T-10 and good perineal anesthesia. Onset of epidural blockade can be hastened by adding bicarbonate to adjust pH; this technique is useful even in an emergency situation. We add 4 ml of sodium bicarbonate (0.48 mEq/ml) to 16 ml of 3% 2-chloro-procaine and achieve clinical onset within 5 to 10 minutes.

Spinal anesthesia may be given to patients who do not have a preexisting epidural catheter if no contraindication exists. For spinal anesthesia, hyperbaric 5% lidocaine 40 to 60 mg may be given since this is a relatively brief procedure. Regional anesthesia does not have any clinically significant effect on uterine smooth muscle. If the regional anesthesia technique is inadequate to extract retained placenta successfully, uterine smooth muscle relaxation becomes necessary. This can be achieved by volatile anesthetic agents with endotracheal intubation, or preferably by intravenous nitroglycerin. Potent volatile anesthetic agents have been used for uterine muscle relaxation. However, one has to be very careful: these patients may not tolerate deep general anesthesia with a high concentration of a volatile agent because of the associated hypovolemia. Also, it takes longer to achieve a deep anesthetic level with these agents for uterine relaxation compared with intravenous nitroglycerin.

Uterine Relaxation by Intravenous Nitroglycerin

The use of nitroglycerin (NTG) for uterine relaxation was first reported by Peng and others in 1989.[6] Because smooth muscle is present in the uterine cervix and corpus, NTG was administered to relax the cervix and uterus to extract retained placenta. The authors injected a bolus of NTG 500 μg intravenously in 15 patients with successful extraction in all cases. They were normovolemic patients and the observed decrease in blood pressure was clinically insignificant. Subsequently DeSimone and others refined the dosage and technique. They found that, in all 22 patients, NTG 50 to 100 μg IV bolus was effective in relaxing uterine musculature for successful manual extraction of retained placenta without significant side effects.[7] Most of the patients had epidural anesthesia and one received IV fentanyl for analgesia. Onset of uterine relaxation was 30 to 40 seconds after IV bolus and duration of action was about 1 minute. Since then IV NTG has been gaining widespread use for a variety of conditions that require prompt uterine relaxation, such as inverted uterus[8] and fetal head entrapment during vaginal or cesarean delivery.[9] This therapy has the advantages of quick onset and short duration of action. Systemic hypotension may be a possible side effect, especially for these hypovolemic patients. Careful monitoring of blood pressure and vital signs is mandatory for this therapy. It is our clinical experience that if adequate volume replacement has been provided with a large-bore IV line in place, the degree of hypotension is not clinically significant and its duration is very brief.

General Anesthesia for Removal of Retained Placenta

General anesthesia can be provided for manual extraction of retained placenta to relax uterine smooth muscle by volatile anesthetic agents and to provide pain relief. Now that intravenous NTG is gaining popularity for uterine relaxation, the need for general anesthesia is limited to the patients for whom regional anesthesia is contraindicated. The contraindications to regional anesthesia include significant hypovolemia, coagulation abnormality, infection, patient refusal, some neurologic disorders, and technical difficulties.

As stated earlier in this chapter, the patient who has just delivered is still at risk for aspiration pneumonitis, and appropriate prophylaxis with antacid, metoclopramide, or H_2 blocker is mandatory. Endotracheal intubation with rapid-sequence induction using cricoid pressure is necessary if examination of the patient's airway indicates that intubation will be easy. If her airway is recognized as being difficult for intubation, then the clinician should choose intubation with the patient awake using either direct laryngoscopy with topical oropharyngeal anesthesia, or fiberoptic intubation. Evaluation of the airway is the same as with other surgical patients, but special attention should be paid to the changes that take place during pregnancy. Edema of the airway mucosa is present during pregnancy and can be exaggerated in patients with preeclampsia or eclampsia. Engorged breasts may make laryngoscopy more difficult, especially with obesity and the normal weight gain during pregnancy. Proper positioning of the patient and the use of a short-handle laryngoscope are of great help.

Induction agents and their doses are adjusted according to the condition and volume status of the patient. Ketamine in small doses (1 mg/kg) often is used as an induction agent for hypovolemic patients because of its sympathomimetic effect. However, it is a direct myocardial depressant and this effect may be more prominent if peripheral vasoconstriction already is maximal in severely hypovolemic patients. Also, it can cause uterine hypertonus when more than 1.5 mg/kg is given intravenously, which can be unfavorable for the subsequent manual extraction of the retained placenta. Succinylcholine 1 to 1.5 mg/kg should be used to facilitate endotracheal intubation. Inhalation anesthetics such as enflurane or isoflurane (2 to 3 minimum alveolar concentration [MAC]) may have to be used for a brief period. This should be discontinued immediately after extraction of placenta to avoid further bleeding from uterine relaxation. Depending on the situation, oxytocin, methylergonovine, or prostaglandin $F_{2\alpha}$ will be necessary to contract the uterus after the procedure.

Some authors recommend the use of a small dose of ketamime (0.1 mg/kg) intravenously or inhalational agents for sedation and analgesia for this procedure. Constant communication with the patient is mandatory if this technique is used.

Other Causes of Postpartum Hemorrhage

Vaginal or Cervical Laceration

Bleeding from these lacerations or episiotomy sometimes can be severe enough to cause hemorrhagic shock and coagulopathy. This has to be suspected whenever bleeding is present despite the firmly contracted uterus. The problem related to this type of bleeding is that it is frequently undiagnosed or its severity is underestimated. A better environment (operating room) with good illumination and room may be necessary for adequate exposure and repair of these lacerations and for effective management of the patient's volume status and condition. Keeping good communication with the obstetrician is important under these circumstances to assess the amount of blood loss until the time of anesthesiologist's involvement, and to estimate the amount of ongoing bleeding. Anesthetic management of this problem essentially is the same as when the placenta is retained, except that no need exists for uterine relaxation. Adequate pain relief often is necessary for thorough examination and detection of the source of bleeding. This can be achieved either by regional anesthesia or general endotracheal anesthesia, depending on the patient's condition and situation as previously discussed. Intravenous sedation may not be enough for this procedure because it may take several hours for repair if the laceration is severe.

Uterine Inversion

Inversion of the uterus almost always is caused by the strong traction of an umbilical cord and vigorous fundal pressure after the delivery of the infant.[4] The incidence is low (1 in 6407 pregnancies in one report)[10] but this is an obstetric emergency that can cause exsanguination in a short period. The anesthesiologist should be notified immediately while the obstetrician is trying to replace the freshly inverted uterus by pushing it back to its normal position. Large-bore IV lines are essential and fluid resuscitation should be started immediately with crystalloid and colloid solutions, then with blood products as indicated.

If immediate manual replacement of the inverted uterus is unsuccessful because of the constricted cervix, uterine relaxation and repositioning can be achieved by tocolytics such as terbutaline, ritodrine, and magnesium sulfate. Recently IV NTG has been used for this purpose with success.[8] If these techniques fail, general endotracheal anesthesia may be necessary to relax the uterus with inhalation anesthetics. After the uterus is repositioned, uterine relaxant should be stopped immediately and oxytocin or other uterotonic agents should be started to contract the uterus and prevent further bleeding. Short-lasting NTG is beneficial from this point. The need for careful observation of blood pressure and vital signs is the same as when NTG is used for treating a retained placenta.

When the above-mentioned methods fail to reposition the inverted uterus, laparotomy for repositioning becomes necessary under general endotracheal anesthesia.

Uterine Atony

Uterine atony is one of the two most common causes of immediate hemorrhage, occurring in 2% to 5% of all deliveries.[34] It was the leading cause of maternal death in one report.[11] It can occur immediately or several hours after the delivery of the baby. An overdistended uterus or abnormal labor are the predisposing factors for uterine atony. For example, women with a large fetus, multiple fetuses, or polyhydramnios are prone to have hemorrhage due to uterine atony. Patients with vigorous uterine activity or with a weak labor pattern who require oxytocin augmentation also are likely to have uterine atony. Uterine atony also can be caused by retained placental tissues or amniotic fluid embolism. Patients on tocolytic drugs for preterm labor may have increased incidence of uterine atony. Severe postpartum hemorrhage due to uterine atony also has been described after the use of dantrolene.[12] A parturient can lose up to 2 L of blood in less than 5 minutes from uterine atony.[3] Thus immediate fluid resuscitation is mandatory. As stated above, uterine contraction is essential for ceasing hemorrhage. Uterine massage is performed through the abdominal wall. Oxytocin should be administered intravenously. For severe hemorrhage, ergot alkaloid (methylergonovine 0.2 mg) should be given intravenously or intramuscularly (IM). Prostaglandin $F_{2\alpha}$ 0.25 mg can also be given IM or directly into the myometrium. The possible and well-documented side effects of these agents must be understood because some of the can be life threatening. Oxytocin can cause vasodilatation and hypotension when it is administered rapidly, especially in hypovolemic patients. Intravenous ergonovine may cause vasoconstriction and severe hypertension, especially in a patient with preeclampsia or eclampsia. Thus methergine should usually be given IM. Prostaglandin $F_{2\alpha}$ may provoke bronchospasm, nausea and vomiting, or hypertension. Overdose of this agent caused cardiovascular collapse in one patient.[13] If such measures fail to stop bleeding, hypogastric artery ligation or emergency hysterectomy becomes necessary. This may be complicated by a large amount of bleeding, and appropriate anesthetic management is essential for maternal survival. This should include establishment of the airway with an endotracheal tube, use of multiple large-bore peripheral lines for rapid transfusion of blood products, insertion of a Foley catheter for measurement of urine output, central line for pressor administration and CVP measurement if necessary. Different measures should be used to preserve body temperature.

Uterine Rupture

Uterine rupture or dehiscence can occur not only postpartum but also anterpartum or intrapartum, and it is most commonly associated with a previous cesarean section scar, even with low transverse uterine incision. The incidence is rare (1 in 2,251 deliveries in one report)[4] but it may be increasing because of the trend for vaginal birth after cesarean section. Uterine rupture can also be associated with another myometrial scar, midforceps delivery, difficult delivery, prolonged labor with excessive oxytocin stimulation, grand multiparity, or trauma. The patient may complain of a sharp shooting pain in the abdomen and express the feeling that something was torn inside of her. Realize that some patients may not complain of a typical sharp pain or tenderness, but instead may complain of shortness of breath, which is from hemoperitoneum and diaphragmatic irritation.[4] Thus a high index of suspicion is critical for prompt diagnosis and treatment. Another important and specific finding of intrapartum uterine rupture is thought to be the loss of uterine contraction or intrauterine pressure if an intrauterine pressure catheter (IUPC) is used, but IUPC may not be as reliable as it was thought.[14] It is likely to be associated with fetal bradycardia and fetal distress due to uterine rupture of the placental implantation site or maternal hypotension from hemorrhage. Fetal heart tone can also be lost due to the rupture.

Immediate treatment includes prompt volume replacement and blood transfusion as needed, and operative delivery for distressed fetus and for repair of the ruptured uterus. Sometimes hysterectomy is necessary with or without hypogastric artery ligation to reduce bleeding. Anesthetic management is not different from other cases of obstetric hemorrhage such as retained placenta or uterine atony. If there is adequate volume replacement in the patient and if there is the luxury of several extra anesthesiologists, regional anesthesia can be provided with careful management of volume status and condition of the patient. Otherwise, general endotracheal anesthesia usually is indicated for this emergency procedure when fetal distress and maternal hemorrhage have occurred. It may be safer to have secured the airway with an endotracheal tube and mechanical ventilation when one is busy with volume resuscitation of the patient. This is applicable to other cases that may require cesarean hysterectomy. Management of postpartum uterine rupture is the same as antepartum or intrapartum uterine rupture except for the lack of fetal considerations. Again, one has to keep in mind that maternal physiologic changes during pregnancy take several weeks to return to the prepregnant state.

Summary

1. Maternal mortality from hemorrhage has decreased but still remains as one of the leading causes of maternal mortality. Retained placenta is the third most common cause of postpartum hemorrhage.
2. Prompt recognition and treatment are critical for the survival of the mother. Immediate treatment includes establishing large-bore IV lines and volume replacement with crystalloid and/or colloid solutions and blood products.
3. For analgesia for manual extraction of a retained placenta, the clinician can provide IV analgesics, regional anesthesia, or general anesthesia. Regional anesthesia can be used if the volume status of the patient is normal.
4. When uterine relaxation is required for extracting the placenta, IV NTG, 50 to 100 μg per bolus, is the drug of choice for normovolemic patients since NTG has a rapid onset and a short duration of action. Careful observation of blood pressure is mandatory.
5. General endotracheal anesthesia is used for hypovolemic patients. Parturients immediately af-

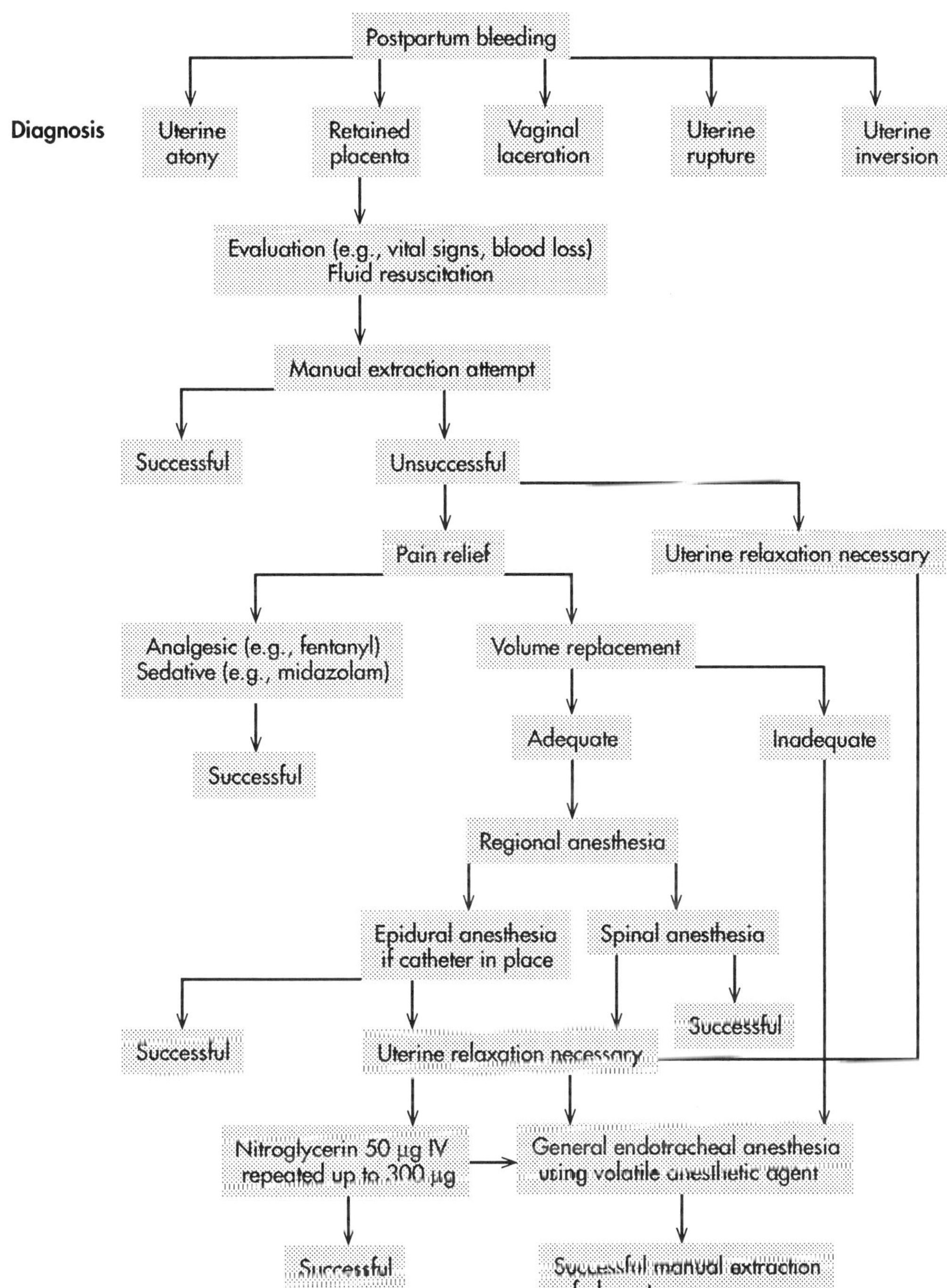

Fig. 19-1.

Management of the patient with a retained placenta.

ter delivery still are at increased risk for aspiration of gastric contents and thus need appropriate preparation and management.

A suggested management plan for a patient with a retained placenta is summarized in Fig. 19-1.

References

1. Rochat RW, Koonin LM, Atrash HK, et al: Maternal mortality in the United States: report from the maternal mortality collaborative, *Obstet Gynecol* 1988; 72:91.
2. Sachs BP, Brown DAJ, Driscoll SG, et al: Maternal mortality in Massachusetts: trends and prevention, *N Engl J Med* 1987; 316:667.
3. Biehl DR: *Antepartum and postpartum hemorrhage.* In Shnider SM, Levinson G, editors; *Anesthesia for obstetrics, ed 3,* Baltimore, 1992, Williams & Wilkins.
4. Cunningham FG, et al: *Abnormalities of the third stage of labor.* In Cunningham FG, McDonald PC, Gant NF, et al., editors: *Williams obstetrics, ed 19,* East Norwalk, CT, 1993, Appleton & Lange.
5. Miller RD: *Transfusion therapy.* In Miller RD, editor: *Anesthesia,* New York, 1990, Churchill Livingstone.
6. Peng ATC, Gorman RS, Shulman SM, et al: Intravenous nitroglycerin for uterine relaxation in the post partum patient with retained placenta, *Anesthesiology* 1989; 71:172.
7. DeSimone CA, Norris MC, Leighton BL: Intravenous nitroglycerin aids manual extraction of a retained placenta, *Anesthesiology* 1990; 73:787.
8. Altabef KM, Spencer JT, Zimberg S: Intravenous nitroglycerin for uterine relaxation of an inverted uterus, *Am J Obstet Gynecol* 1992; 166:1237.
9. Rolbin SH, Hew EM, Bernstein A: Uterine relaxation can be life-saving, *Can J Anaesth* 1991; 38:939.
10. Shah-Hosseini R, Evrard JR: Puerperal uterine inversion, *Obstet Gynecol* 1989; 73:567.
11. Gibbs CE, Locke WE: Maternal deaths in Texas, 1969-1973: A report of 501 consecutive deaths from the Texas Medical Association's Committee on Maternal Health, *Am J Obstet Gynecol* 1976; 126:687.
12. Weingarten AE, Korsh JI, Neuman GG, et al: Postpartum uterine atony after intravenous dantrolene, *Anesth Analg* 1987; 66:269.
13. Douglas MJ, Farquharson DR, Ross PL, et al: Cardiovascular collapse following an overdose of prostaglandin $f_{2\alpha}$: A case report, *Can J Anaesth* 1989; 36:466.
14. Rodriguez MH, Masaki DI, Phelan JP, et al: Uterine rupture: Are intrauterine pressure catheters useful in the diagnosis? *Am J Obstet Gynecol* 1989; 161:666.

20

Anesthesia for Cesarean Delivery

A 24-year-old primigravida is admitted to the hospital for primary elective cesarean delivery secondary to breech presentation. The patient is unsure as to what type of anesthesia is best for her and her baby.

Recommendations by Steven A. Lussos, M.D.

A healthy, nonobese, nonlaboring primigravida for elective cesarean delivery allows the broadest range of anesthetic choices. The decision will be based foremost on the maternal obstetric and medical history and physical examination findings. Institutional bias, maternal preferences, urgency of cesarean delivery, and the anesthesiologist's comfort level for a particular anesthetic technique all factor in to determine the appropriate anesthetic for cesarean delivery.

A detailed examination for each anesthetic technique is not practical here, therefore the reader is referred to recent review articles.[1-3] This chapter briefly overviews the wide range of anesthetic possibilities for cesarean delivery, in particular, spinal, epidural, combined spinal and epidural, and general anesthesia. Also discussed in this chapter are the particular needs of this patient and her optimal anesthetic.

Spinal Anesthesia

The advantages of using spinal anesthesia for cesarean delivery include the following:

1. Rapid onset of surgical anesthesia
2. Simplicity
3. Reliability (failure rate of about 2.8%)
4. Minimal fetal exposure to depressant medications
5. Denser and more reliable sacral nerve block than epidural anesthesia
6. Greater motor block than epidural anesthesia

7. Less shivering than epidural anesthesia
8. Parturient remains awake, hazards of aspiration are minimized
9. Allows for maternal participation in birth
10. Decreases stress response related to surgery

The disadvantages of using spinal anesthesia for cesarean delivery are as follows:

1. Greater risk of hypotension than epidural or general anesthesia
2. Intrapartum nausea and vomiting
3. Possibility of postdural puncture headache
4. Limited duration of action (unless continuous spinal or epidural techniques are used)

Contraindications to spinal anesthesia during cesarean delivery are listed below:

1. Patient refusal
2. Severe maternal hypertension or hypotension
3. Hypovolemia
4. Coagulation disorders
5. Active bacteremia or sepsis, localized infection over insertion site
6. Congenital cardiac disorders where hypotension may initiate or exacerbate right-to-left shunts and stenotic valvular heart disease
7. Some forms of neurologic disorders (e.g., multiple sclerosis)

Cardiovascular Effects

Maternal hypotension after induction of spinal anesthesia is avoidable, but the anesthesiologist must be actively involved in its prevention. Without preventative measures, maternal hypotension develops in up to 92% of parturients during spinal anesthesia for elective cesarean delivery.[4] Maternal hypotension may be defined as a decrease in systolic blood pressure to below 100 torr or by more than 30 torr from preanesthetic levels.[5] The higher the segmental sympathetic blockade and the rapidity with which it occurs (especially with levels greater than T-4), influence the incidence of hypotension[4] and associated emetic systems. More than a 46% decline from baseline arterial blood pressure, a 34% decline in cardiac output, and a 44% decline in stroke volume can be expected after spinal anesthesia when the sympathetic blockade coincides with the gravid uterus, impairing venous return in the supine position.[6] Acute volume expansion and left uterine displacement are helpful but usually are not sufficient to prevent maternal hypotension.[4] In nonlaboring patients under spinal anesthesia, most investigators observe maternal hypotension in 50% to 60% of parturients, despite these measures.[4,5]

Maternal hypotension (systolic blood pressure <80 mm Hg for 4 to 5 minutes) diminishes placental perfusion and intervillous blood flow (IVBF) to the point that fetal tissue hypoxia (asphysia) and bradycardia invariably result.[7,8] Fetal acidosis and tissue hypoxia may cause fetal brain injury and depressed motor performance. This is evidenced by lowered Apgar scores, prolongation of time to sustained respiration, fetal acidosis with hypercarbia, and increased neonatal base deficits at delivery.[9] Therefore sustained maternal hypotension diminishes fetal well-being by impairing placental exchange of oxygen, carbon dioxide, and fixed acids.

The healthy fetus may tolerate decreases in placental blood flow of 22% to 50% for relatively short periods of time.[1] Corke and associates[5] observed that short periods of maternal hypotension (less than 2 minutes) associated with spinal anesthesia for cesarean delivery, if promptly treated with ephedrine, were not harmful to the neonate, as assessed by Apgar scores and serial neurobehavioral examinations. Even this short period of hypotension resulted in mild fetal acidosis, although it was not statistically significant. Hollmen et al.[10] observed prolonged neurobehavioral changes (poor motor organization, depressed rooting and suckling reflexes) for 4 to 7 days in babies born to mothers who experienced prolonged periods of hypotension of 3 to 8 minutes during epidural anesthesia for cesarean delivery. Therefore the duration of hypotension, not necessarily the degree of hypotension, ultimately affects the condition of the newborn.[8]

Prehydration or acute volume expansion with 20 to 25 ml/kg (1.5 to 2.0 L) of lactated Ringer's solution over 15 to 20 minutes before spinal anesthesia is recommended. Crystalloid solutions should not contain dextrose for acute maternal volume expansion.[1] Maternal hypotension in an environment of maternal and fetal hyperglycemia leads to impaired uteroplacental perfusion, placental hypoxia, glycogenolysis, and anaerobic metabolism with lactate production, which may create a profound fetal and neonatal metabolic acidosis.[11] Furthermore, fetal hyperglycemia leads to a transient period of fetal hyperinsulinemia, which may result in neonatal hypoglycemia after delivery.

The laboring parturient is somewhat protected from developing hypotension, since the descent of the fetal head may lessen caval compression; but more importantly, each uterine contraction augments central blood volume with about 300 to 500 ml of blood.[4,6] Clark et al.[4] observed that after acute volume expansion, there was only a 14.7% incidence rate of hypotension in laboring parturients versus 52.8% in nonlaboring parturients after spinal anesthesia for cesarean delivery; they attributed this hemodynamic stability mainly to the maternal *autotransfusion* mechanism.

Vasopressors

Prophylactic intramuscular ephedrine is not a reliable means to avoid spinal or epidural anesthesia-related hypotension. Intravenous boluses or continuous infusions of ephedrine are effective ways to prevent or treat maternal hypotension after giving spinal anesthetics.[1] Intravenous ephedrine in 15-mg increments results in a 10- to 15-minute vasopressor effect, which improves IVBF.[12] In the nonlaboring parturient for elective cesarean delivery under spinal anesthesia, I begin giving 10 to 25 mg ephedrine in a bolus as the spinal anesthetic is being injected.[9,13] By the time the patient is repositioned into the left semilateral position with a right hip roll, the blood pressure cuff has cycled and maternal hypotension can effectively be prevented.[13] Further intravenous ephedrine, by bolus or infusion, should be given as soon as blood pressure begins to fall from baseline.[14] Ephedrine dosages up to 50 to 60 mg after the spinal anesthetic but before delivery do not cause adverse neonatal effects.[13] Prevention of maternal hypotension may be the most effective method in avoiding peripartum emetic symptoms,[1,14] although prophylactic metoclopramide also has been shown to be safe and effective.[13] Ephedrine remains the vasopressor of choice in the healthy parturient without ischemic heart disease, stenotic valvular heart disease, or severe maternal tachycardia (heart rate > 125 beats/min). Phenylephrine (in 40-μg bolus injections) is a reasonable alternative for management of post-spinal hypotension if there is no maternal history to suggest underlying uteroplacental insufficiency.[15]

Positioning

Successful spinal anesthesia for cesarean delivery usually requires a block of adequate intensity, duration, and a segmental level of T4. The best positioning technique for induction of spinal anesthesia is placing the parturient in the right lateral decubitus position, then immediately placing her in the left semilateral position with a wedge beneath the right hip. This avoids placing the parturient in the supine position while ensuring an adequate and symmetric local anesthetic distribution in the subarachnoid space.[16]

TABLE 20-1

SPINAL ANESTHETIC DOSAGES FOR CESAREAN DELIVERY

Drug	Dosage (mg)	Duration (min)
5% Lidocaine in 7.5% dextrose	60-80	45-75
1% Tetracaine in 10% dextrose	7-11	120-180
1% Tetracaine plus equal volume 10% procaine	6-10/60-100	120-180
0.75% Bupivacaine in 8.25% dextrose	12-15	90-129
0.5% Bupivacaine in 8.0% dextrose	12-15	90-120
	Dosage by Height Initial 152 cm	**Height Supplement**
Lidocaine	1.2 ml (60 mg)	
Tetracaine*	0.7 ml (7 mg)	0.1 ml/7.6 cm
TP mixture†	0.6 ml (6 mg)	
Bupivacaine	1.0 ml (7.5 mg)	0.1 ml/2.5 cm

TP, Tetracaine-procaine.
*Plus equal volume of 10% dextrose.
†Plus equal volume of 10% procaine.

Dosage Requirements and Regimens

Pregnancy is associated with an increased spread and potency of local anesthetics, so that 30% to 50% less drug is required for a given level of spinal or epidural anesthesia (Tables 20-1 and 20-2).[1] Hyperbaric local anesthetic solutions are advantagous since they tend to spread to the thoracic kyphosis at about the T-4 level, regardless of patient height. Norris[17] confirmed this finding using 1.6 ml of hyperbaric 0.75% bupivacaine in 8.25% dextrose for parturients between 146 and 178 cm (4 feet 11 inches and 5 feet 8 inches). Spread of sensory anesthesia ranged from T-7 to C-8 with a median level of T-3, with no correlation between sensory spread and height, weight, or body mass index. DeSimone et al.[18] compared 1.6 ml with 2.0 ml of 0.75% hyperbaric bupivacaine and found significantly more segmental spread with the latter: 22.6 versus 24.8 segments. The addition of 0.2 mg of epinephrine to hyperbaric bupivacaine speeds onset, and enhances the quality and duration of sensory analgesia and motor blockade.[19]

Tetracaine gives a profound motor blockade but often lacks adequate sensory anesthesia; therefore the majority of cases require supplemental intravenous opioids during cesarean delivery. A tetracaine-procaine (TP) mixture improves the quality of sensory anesthesia and increases spread to two to four segments, unless calculated dosage schemes are modified downward by 0.2 ml.[20] Hauch et al.[21] found that hyperbaric bupivacaine produces similar onset and quality of spinal anesthesia compared with a TP mixture. However, segmental spread was less than the TP mixture; this resulted in a less profound sympathetic blockade and hypotension. Furthermore, with hyperbaric bupivacaine, the motor block resolves coincidentally with the sensory blockade, whereas with the TP mixture, motor block often outlasts sensory blockade. Because of this, intrathecal bupivacaine may enhance patient satisfaction for cesarean delivery.

TABLE 20-2

SPINAL ANESTHESIA TECHNIQUE FOR CESAREAN DELIVERY

1. Sodium citrate 0.3 M, 30 ml within 30 min of procedure, metoclopramide 10 mg IV within 10 min of spinal administration
2. Acute volume expansion with a nondextrose-containing solution, 2000 ml
3. Monitoring ECG, blood pressure, pulse oximetry, face mask O_2 at 6-10 L/M until baby is delivered; obtain baseline vital signs
4. Place in right lateral decubitus position for induction of spinal anesthesia
5. Use of 22- to 25-gauge pencil-point needles, or 27-gauge quincke needle.
6. Hyperbaric bupivicaine, 0.75%, 1.6 ml (12 mg), in dextrose 8.25%, mixed with 0.2 ml fentanyl (10 μg), or 0.2 ml sufentanil (10 μg), or morphine 0.1 to 0.25 mg
7. In the healthy parturient, give 10-25 mg of ephedrine IV while spinal is being injected to prevent hypotension; cycle blood pressure every 1 min until baby is delivered
8. Immediately place the parturient supine with left uterine displacement during surgery until the baby is delivered
9. Subsequently administer 10-mg ephedrine increments and additional volume expansion if the maternal blood pressure drops from baseline until the baby is delivered; if administered dose of ephedrine begins to exceed 40-50 mg, recheck adequacy of left uterine displacement
10. *Goal is to prevent hypotension, rather than treat hypotension*

ECG, electrocardiogram; IV, intravenously; O_2, oxygen.

Intrathecal Opioids

Intrathecal or epidural opioids (Table 20-3), in combination with local anesthetics, improve the quality and prolong the duration of intraoperative analgesia. Opioids act selectively on nociceptors in the dorsal horn of the spinal cord, specifically in the substantia gelatinosa. Visceral nociceptive afferents may be blunted by an intrathecal μ agonist such as morphine and fentanyl.[2,22] Intrathecal preservative-free morphine sulfate 0.1 to 0.5 mg may provide postcesarean analgesia for 17 to 27 hours. Dosages greater than 0.5 mg increase the risk of life-threatening delayed respiratory depression. Intrathecal local anesthetic plus fentanyl 6.25 to 12.5 μg, or sufentanil 10 μg, can provide up to 2 to 4 hours of postoperative analgesia. However, intrathecal meperidine (25 mg/ml) as a sole agent, in doses of 1 mg/kg plus equal volume of 10% dextrose, can provide complete surgical anesthesia for cesarean delivery for up to 1 hour.[2]

Peripartum Emesis

Peripartum emetic symptoms can be markedly reduced after induction of anesthesia for cesarean delivery by avoiding maternal hypotension.[13,14] Presumably, hypotension results in relative brainstem hypoxia, which triggers vomiting. Supplemental oxygen by face mask will decrease emetic symptoms despite the presence of hypotension.[23] Conduction anesthesia to a level necessary for cesarean

TABLE 20-3

INTRATHECAL OPIOIDS FOR CESAREAN DELIVERY

Opioid	Dose	Onset (min)	Duration (hr)
Fentanyl	6.25-15 μg	5	2-4
Sufentanil	10-20 μg	5	3-5
Morphine	0.2-0.3 mg	30-40	12-27
Meperidine	1 mg/kg	3-4	1 (anesthesia), 6 (analgesia)

delivery results in vagal predominance in the upper gastrointestinal tract. Visceral pain from traction on the peritoneum or abdominal viscera (e.g., exteriorizing the uterus or stretching the lower uterine segment) may allow vagal afferents to trigger the vomiting center. This apparent autonomic imbalance, when coupled with an inadequate conduction block, may result in viscerally mediated emetic symptoms. An adequate local anesthetic dosage is essential to obtain a dense sensory afferent blockade. The addition of intrathecal and epidural opioids may enhance the quality of the sensory blockade and modulate nociceptive afferents mediating viseral pain.[22,24,25]

Peripartum emetic symptoms tend to be multifactorial in nature.[25] Cortical afferents may trigger the vomiting center. Olfactory, visual, gustatory, and psychological factors (e.g., anxiety) may predispose the parturient to emetic symptoms. Opioids may trigger the chemoreceptor trigger zone (CTZ) and sensitize the vestibular nucleus to the effects of motion. Metabolic disturbances also may trigger the CTZ. Therefore anesthetic-, hemodynamic-, surgical-, drug-, or patient-related factors may precipitate emesis, so prophylaxis is not always possible. Prophylactic antiemetics should be considered when intrathecal or epidural opioids are given, or if the parturient describes a history of postoperative emetic symptoms or motion sickness. The efficacy of droperidol, metoclopramide,[13] and scopolamine patches has been demonstrated in the parturient.[1,25]

Postdural Puncture Headaches

Postdural puncture headaches (PDPH) most often are related to needle size and cutting-type bevel tip or Quincke tip. The incidence of PDPH can be reduced by maintaining the bevel parallel to the longitudinally arranged dural fibers (to minimize dura tear) and using a paramedian approach to off-set dura and arachnoid entry sites to limit cerebrospinal fluid (CSF) leakage.[26] Probably of greater importance is using a pencil-point bevel-tipped spinal needle (Greene, Whitacre, and Sprotte needles), which tends to separate dural fibers instead of cutting them. Hurley et al.[27] at the Brigham and Women's Hospital, Boston, observed a 1.1% incidence rate of PDPHs with a 25-gauge Whitacre needle versus 4.8% with a 26-gauge Quincke, and 2.5% with a 27-gauge Quincke needle. PDPHs related to pencil-point needle tips tend to be milder and infrequently require epidural blood patches. Most PDPHs (85%) after spinal anesthesia are mild, self-limited, and resolve in 1 week. Conservative management schemes include bedrest, normal fluid intake, analgesics, and oral or intravenous caffeine. Epidural blood patch remains the specific treatment for PDPH that cannot be managed conservatively.

Epidural Anesthesia

Epidural anesthesia for cesarean delivery has several advantages, listed below:

1. Lower incidence and severity of maternal hypotension than spinal anesthesia[6,28]:
    a. Local anesthetics can be titrated slowly
    b. hemodynamic stability is useful for high-risk parturients with heart disease or preeclampsia
2. Avoids dural puncture
3. Catheter technique allows for indefinite maintenance of surgical anesthesia and is useful in repeat cesarean deliveries
4. Postopertive pain relief with epidural opioids, local anesthetics, or combination
5. Introperative blood loss of about half that associated with general anesthesia[29]
6. Allows for maternal participation in birth
7. Decreases the stress response related to surgery

The disadvantages of epidural anesthesia for cesarean delivery include the following:

1. Slower onset of surgical anesthesia compared to spinal anesthesia[30]
2. Greater likelihood of failure related to improper technique or inadequate dosing
3. Larger amount of local anesthetic and/or opioid required
   a. Potential for total spinal from inadvertent subarachnoid injection
   b. Potential for massive epidural or subdural injection
   c. Potential for intravascular injection (e.g., seizure, cardiovascular collapse)
   d. Greater neonatal drug exposure
4. Greater incidence of shivering compared with spinal anesthesia[30]

Contraindications to epidural anesthesia are listed below:

1. Patient refusal
2. Lack of operator skill in the performance of epidural anesthesia or the ability to treat potential complications (e.g., total spinal, seizure, cardiovascular collapse)
3. Localized cellulitis, dermatitis, or pustules overlying the intended puncture site, or acute generalized infections (e.g., septicemia, bacteremia)
4. Acute organic central nervous system disease, whether infectious or noninfectious
5. Hemodynamic instability of hypotension from severe blood loss and/or shock
6. Abnormalities in the clotting mechanism

Cardiovascular Effects

The gradual onset of epidural blockade with incremental dosing causes only minor alterations in maternal hemodynamics.[28] Compensatory sympathetic mechanisms remain intact longer and tend to allow hypotension to be more easily corrected. Reported incidences of hypotension, despite prehydration and left uterine displacement, range from 24% to 36%.[31] Healthy nonlaboring parturients are more susceptible to hypotension than their laboring counterparts,[31] as are those given pH-adjusted local anesthetics[32] or warmed lidocaine solutions. Prophylactic intramuscular ephedrine (25 to 50 mg) has been shown to be ineffective in preventing hypotension from epidural anesthesia.[31] Therefore intravenous ephedrine should be given while blood pressure begins to fall from baseline to avoid hypotension. Ramanathan et al.[33] included colloid prophylaxis during epidural anesthesia for cesarean section; they still observed a 25% to 30% incidence rate of maternal hypotension and similar intravenous ephedrine requirements as in their group given crystalloids. However, Lewis et al.[34] demonstrated that a 2-L crystalloid preload over 30 minutes reduces the incidence of postepidural hypotension to 6.7% in nonlaboring parturients for cesarean delivery.

Supplemental Oxygen

High inspired oxygen concentrations administered to the mother can improve fetal oxygen reserve and acid-base status during epidural anesthesia[35,36] and general anesthesia.[36,37] Ramanathan et al.[35] observed that umbilical vein and umbilical artery oxygen pressure (Po_2) values correlated closely with maternal arterial oxygen pressure (Pao_2) over a maternal Pao_2 range of 70 to 490 torr. Varying maternal fractional inspired oxygen concentration (Fio_2) from 21% to 100% resulted in a umbilical venous (UV) Po_2 range of 28 to 47 torr, and a umbilical artery (UA) Po_2 range of 15 to 25 torr. In this fetal Po_2 range the fetal oxyhemoglobin dissociation curve is nearly vertical; therefore small increases in fetal Po_2 can significantly increase fetal oxygen reserve by increasing fetal oxyhemoglobin saturation and total blood oxygen content. Improved neonatal oxygenation and acid-base status also may shorten the time to spontaneous respiration at delivery.[36] An oxygen face mask should be considered for all parturients during cesarean delivery, especially if fetal distress is present.

Choice of Local Anesthetics

Local anesthetics (LA) are weak bases (Tables 20-4 and 20-5). Commerically prepared solutions generally are acidic, which ionizes local anesthetics to maintain their solubility. *Alkalinization* or *pH adjustment* with sodium bicarbonate brings the solution pH toward the drug's pKa. This increases the uncharged, nonprotonated lipid-soluble concentration of local anesthetic, which tends to speed the onset of surgical anesthesia for cesarean delivery,[38] as well as increase the risk of hypotension.[32]

Choice of local anesthetic is important both for elective and emergency cesarean delivery. Three percent 2-chloroprocaine, an ester-linked local anesthetic, is preferred in the presence of fetal acidosis because of its rapid onset, short half-life, lack of significant toxicity, and fetal safety.[2] It is broken down by plasma cholinesterase to inactive metabolites. It provided excellent sensory and motor blockade for cesarean delivery, but its brief duration of action requires reinforcement dosages abo every 30 minutes. In the early 1980s cases o chronic adhesive arachnoiditis were reported in association with inadvertent dural puncture and administration of large volumes of 2-chloroprocaine intrathecally. It was shown that the combination of low solution pH (about 3.0) and the antioxidant sodium bisulfite could yield sulfurous acid and cause neurotoxicity.[39] Current solutions in use contain the antioxidant ethylene diamine tetraacetic acid (EDTA) with a solution pH between 2.7 and 4.0.

Lidocaine, mepivacaine, and bupivacaine are currently used amide-linked local anesthetics for cesarean delivery. Neonatal elimination half-lives for lidocaine and mepivacaine are about 3 and 9 hours, respectively. Previous concerns about the ability of lidocaine and mepivacaine to impair neonatal muscle tone have been overshadowed by recent studies that show either short-lived or no significant adverse neonatal neurobehavior effects when used over the short period required for cesarean delivery.[40] Mepivacaine tends to have a denser sensory block than either plain lidocaine or bupiva-

TABLE 20-4

Epidural Local Anesthetics for Cesarean Delivery

Agent	Ml/ Segment*	Vol (ml) for 18 Segments	Reinforcement Time (min)	Maximum Safe Dose† (mg/kg) Plain	+ Epi	Physicochemical Properties pKa	Protein Binding %	UV/MV Ratio
Lidocaine 2%	1-1.4	18-25	45-60	4	7	7.9	60-70	0.48-0.7
Mepivacaine 2%	1-1.4	18-25	45-60	4	7	7.6	70-80	0.57-0.69
Bupivacaine 0.5%	1.1-1.5	20-27	90	2.5	3.2	8.1	95	0.21-0.42
Etidocaine 1.5%	0.9-1.4	16-25	—	n/a‡	8	7.7	94	0.2-0.36
2-Chloroprocaine 3%	1-1.4	18-25	25-35	11	14	8.7	—	—

*Dosage guidelines for parturients 152-178 cm in height. Reinforcing doses should be one third to one half the initial dose.
†Manufacturers' recommendations.
‡n/a: etidocaine plain solution is not available.
Adapted from Lussos SA, Datta S: Anesthesia for cesarean delivery. Part II: epidural anesthesia, intrathecal and epidural opioids, venous air embolism, *Int J Obstet Anesth* 1992; 1:209.

caine; subjectively it seems comparable with lidocaine with epinephrine. Bupivacaine provides excellent motor and sensory anesthesia for cesarean delivery. Currently the 0.75% bupivacaine is not approved by the Food and Drug Administration for obstetric use because of previous maternal cardiotoxicity. The 0.5% bupivacaine solution has an excellent maternal and neonatal safety record, but usually requires the addition of epinephrine or supplementation with 50 μg of fentanyl to provide optimal conditions for cesarean delivery.[41]

Lidocaine with epinephrine (5 μg/ml = 1:200,000) is an extremely popular agent for cesarean delivery. Epinephrine tends to be slowly absorbed from the epidural space because of its local vasoconstrictor action.[42] Bonica et al.[42] observed that when LA solutions with epinephrine (80- to 120-μg amounts) are injected into and gradu-

TABLE 20-5

Epidural Anesthesia Technique for Cesarean Delivery

1. Sodium citrate 0.3 M, 30 ml within 30 min of procedure, metoclopramide 10 mg IV before epidural placement (optional)
2. Acute volume expansion with crystalloid, nondextrose-containing solution, 2000 ml
3. Monitoring NIBP and ECG for epidural block initiation
   Baseline vital signs
   Blood pressure and heart rate, pulse oximetry in the OR with vital sign measurement every 1-3 min until delivery, then every 5 min after delivery
4. Sitting or decubitus position for epidural placement; for topping up place parturient in semisitting position at 35° to 40° with 15° of left uterine displacement for 10-15 min to assure good sacral anesthesia, then lie supine with 15° left uterine displacement
5. LA:
   Administer 5-10 ml through needle after negative aspiration, wait 1-2 min
   Thread catheter 2-4 cm, assure negative aspiration, continue 3- to 5-ml increments of local anesthetic every 2-3 min until necessary volume injected
   Constant communication with the parturient with questioning relevant to detect an intravascular or subarachnoid injection of LA
   LA agents to obtain bilateral T-4 blockade (18 segments)

Agent	Volume
Lidocaine 2% (with epinephrine 1:200 K)	18-30 ml
Lidocaine 2% (plain)	18-25 ml
Bupivacaine 0.5%	18-25 ml
Mepivacaine 2%	18-25 ml
3% 2-Chloroprocaine	18-25 ml

   pH Adjustment
   1 mEq sodium bicarbonate per 10 ml lidocaine, mepivacaine, and 3% 2-chloroprocaine
   0.1 mEq sodium bicarbonate per 10 ml of bupivacaine
   Epidural opioids

Opioid	Dose
Fentanyl	50-100 μg
Sufentanil	20-30 μg
Morphine	3-5 mg
Meperidine	50 mg

6. If maternal blood pressure falls from baseline, treat with 10-mg increments of ephedrine and further volume expansion; phenylephrine in 0.5- to 1.0-μg/kg increments, when ephedrine contraindicated
7. *Goal is to prevent hypotension rather than treat hypotension*
8. Oxygen by face mask with 6- to 10-L flow rates.

IV, Intravenously; ECG, electrocardiogram; OR, operating room; NIBP, noninvasive; blood pressure; LA, local anesthetics.

ally absorbed from the epidural space, systemic β-adrenergic circulatory manifestations predominate. Epinephrine induces an increase in heart rate, stroke volume, and cardiac output, which are more than offset by marked decreases in total peripheral resistance, resulting in a decrease in mean arterial pressure (MAP).[42] For cesarean delivery, epidural administered dosages may contain between 100 and 125 μg of epinephrine. In parturients, 50 to 100 μg of epinephrine has had no significant effect on IVBF, provided that hypotension is avoided.[43,44]

Placental transfer of LAs is by passive diffusion; the rate and degree of passage vary according to the degree of plasma protein binding, ionization, and lipid solubility. These drugs are weak bases and therefore are more ionized in the fetus than in the maternal compartment, particularly when fetal acidosis is present. Amide local anesthetics are bound in plasma principally to α-1-acid glycoprotein, which is more concentrated in the mother than the fetus; hence the fetal:maternal (UV:MV) plasma concentration ratios of highly bound drugs are low (Table 20-4). Ion trapping in the fetus causes an increase in the UV:MV ratio. The distressed infant may be hypoxic and acidotic; compensatory physiologic mechanisms shunt blood from the fetal splanchnic, renal, and lung beds toward the fetal heart and brain, leading to further fetal myocardial and central nervous system depression, causing further acidosis and ion trapping as a vicious cycle develops. Therefore when cesarean delivery is imminent for the distressed fetus and epidural anesthesia is to be extended, amide LAs should be used with care. Optimally, pH-adjusted 3% 2-chloroprocaine could be used; this can rapidly achieve a surgical anesthetic level while minimizing the risk of ion trapping.

Transient hypotension does not appear to lead to ion trapping during epidural anesthesia, but significant hypotension associated with the supine semisitting position (35° to 40°) for sacral blockade under epidural anesthesia has resulted in higher neonatal bupivacaine levels, lower umbilical cord blood pH levels, and higher neonatal base deficits when compared with the lateral semisitting position.[45] Failure of epidural anesthesia results most frequently from inadequate blockade of the sacral roots S-2–4. Ensuring adequate anesthesia in this region will help alleviate visceral pain and emetic symptoms related to insertion of the bladder retractor and traction in the lower uterine segment or overlying peritoneum. Maternal positioning for epidural anesthesia affects both adequacy of anesthesia and fetal well-being.

Accidental Subarachnoid Injection

The ideal *test dose agent* is a controversial issue,[2] although agreement remains that it should be able to detect both intravascular and subarachnoid injection of local anesthetic without altering uteroplacental blood flow. The subarachnoid injection of even a portion of an intended epidural dose for cesarean delivery has the potential to produce *high* or *total spinal anesthesia*. Ascending numbness, dyspnea, and frequent shallow coughing may precede the loss of consciousness and protective airway reflexes. A total sympathectomy further predisposes the parturient to hypotension. Immediate airway management should include 100% oxygen by bag and mask, cricoid pressure, and probably tracheal intubation. Gentle laryngoscopy and tracheal intubation can be accomplished, usually without intravenous induction agents or muscle relaxants. Constant communication with and reassurance of the parturient are necessary since she may remain conscious; most often the parturient is amnestic of these events from brief cerebral hypoperfusion. Left uterine displacement, intravenous crystalloid hydration, and intravenous ephedrine bolus injections should be administered promptly to treat maternal hypotension. While respiratory and circulatory changes are being expediently controlled, continuous fetal heart rate monitoring may help determine whether an urgent cesarean delivery is necessary. If free flow of CSF occurs from the catheter, intermittent aspiration of CSF followed by lavaging with equal volumes of preservative-free normal saline in 10-ml increments has hastened the resolution of total spinal anesthesia. Saline exchange volumes up to 100 ml have been used without adverse maternal sequelae (my experience).

Accidental Intravenous Injection

An *accidental intravenous injection of LAs*, even in test dose amounts, may produce blood concentrations high enough to cause uterine artery vasoconstriction or uterine hypertonus leading to uteroplacental insufficiency.[2] Intravenous catheter insertion may complicate between 2.8% and 9.0% of epidural Placements Seizures resulting from toxic intravascular levels of LA may complicate between 1 in 9000 to 20,000 obstetric epidural anesthetics.[7] Life-threatening and even fatal maternal ventricular dysrhythmias and/or cardiac arrest have been reported after the inadvertent intravenous administration of bupivacaine and etidocaine. Intravascular catheter migration also may occur after satisfactory epidural analgesia, emphasizing the need for vigilance when topping up indwelling epidural catheters for cesarean delivery. Fractionated dosing in 3- to 5-ml increments of local anesthetics is essential to avoid serious complications; between dosages one should wait one to two circulation times (about 60 to 120 sec) while questioning the parturient about warning symptoms of tinnitus, altered sound perception, dizziness, perioral numbness, or metallic taste, which may suggest an intravascular injection of local anesthetic.

Shivering

Helbo-Hansen et al.[30] observed a ninefold increase in shivering with epidural compared with spinal anesthesia for cesarean delivery. Shivering can be unexpected and distressing to the parturient. Shivering is associated with increased oxygen consumption, carbon dioxide production, and cardiac work which may contribute to an elevated maternal base deficit. Postepidural shivering can be minimized by warming intravenous or LA solutions, or using LA mixed with opioids (e.g., fentanyl or sufentanil).[2]

Epidural Opioids

Despite an apparently adequate level of sensory anesthesia, up to one third of parturients under epidural anesthesia (Table 20-6) develop intraoperative

TABLE 20-6

Epidural Opioids for Cesarean Delivery

Opioid	Dose	Onset (min)	Duration (hr)
Morphine	3-5 mg	30-60	12-27
Diamorphone	2-5 mg	5-10	8
Hydromorphone	1.0 mg	10-20	6-12
Methadone	5.0 mg	15-20	6-8
Meperidine	25-50 mg	10-15	3-4
Fentanyl	50-100 μg	5-10	2-4
Sufentanil	20-30 μg	5-10	2-4
Butorphanol	1-4 mg	10-15	2-8

visceral discomfort.[46] Preston et al.[47] demonstrated a 7.5-fold reduction (7% versus 53%) in moderate-to-severe intraoperative pain when 1 μg/kg of fentanyl was added to 2% lidocaine with epinephrine epidurally. Paech et al.[48] also demonstrated improved intraoperative analgesia by adding 100 μg of fentanyl to 0.5% bupivacaine for cesarean delivery. Both studies noted good neonatal outcome with regard to Apgar scores, neonatal blood gases, time to sustained respiration, and/or neonatal neurobehavior evaluations. Capogna et al.[49] observed a fourfold reduction of visceral pain when epidural sufentanil was added to lidocaine with epinephrine for cesarean delivery. Epidural sufentanil is only two to three times more potent than epidural fentanyl. The optimal dosage of epidural sufentanil pre- or postcesarean delivery is in the 20- to 30-μg range to limit maternal complications and maintain fetal well-being.[2]

Epidural morphine 3.0 to 7.5 mg usually provides pain relief for 17 to 27 hours after cesarean delivery.[2] A 5.0-mg dose of preservative-free morphine in 10 ml of saline provides 23 hours (mean) of postcesarean analgesia, although 20% of women have pain relief for less than 12 hours.[50] Delayed respiratory depression (1:1100) always is a consideration when using epidural morphine, therefore hourly respiratory assessments by the nursing staff for 24 hours become necessary. Epidural hydromorphone (Dilaudid), 1.0 mg in 10 ml of physiologic saline, can provide postcesarean analgesia for 6 to 12 hours.[51] Interestingly, epidural 2-chloroprocaine or its metabolite 4-amino-2-chlorobenzoic acid tends to manifest a μ-receptor antagonism effect on fentanyl, but not butorphanol.[52] Therefore if epidural 2-chloroprocaine is used after cesarean delivery, analgesia should be begun with epidural butorphanol (2 to 3 mg).

My preference for postcesarean analgesia is an overnight continuous epidural fentanyl infusion at a rate of 1 μg · kg · hr with a patient control analgesia (PCA) mode that allows the parturient bolus capabilities equal to an additional 1 μg · kg · hr of fentanyl in divided doses.

Venous Air Embolism

During cesarean delivery, open uterine sinuses—especially during uterine incision, placental extraction, and uterine repair—give rise to the highest incidence of venous air embolism (VAE).[2] The reported incidence of VAE varies between 1.4% and 65% during cesarean delivery.[53,54] Even small VAE is potentially harmful since 25% of healthy individually have a patent foramen ovale and are at risk for paradoxical embolization. Massive VAE is potentially life-threatening by causing ventilation/perfusion mismatching, hemoglobin desaturation, and hypotension. A negative pressure gradient between the uterus and heart predisposes to VAE. Hypovolemia secondary to hemorrhage with placenta previa or abruptio placentae, regional anesthetic techniques, the horizontal or Trendelenburg positions, and uterine exteriorization may create such a gradient.[2] The triad of chest pain, dysrhythmias, and oxygen desaturation is suggestive of hemodynamically significant VAE. The incidence and potential for VAE may be reduced by the use of the 5° reverse Trendelenburg position[54] or by avoiding uterine exteriorization during hysterotomy repair.[2]

Combined Spinal-Epidural Anesthesia

About 10% to 25% of epidural blocks provide inadequate sacral analgesia for cesarean delivery.[55] Single-segment combined subarachnoid and epidural block (CSE) for cesarean delivery has been popularized in the United Kingdom and Sweden because it allows for the reliability and ideal operative conditions associated with spinal anesthesia (especially in the sacral roots), whereas a catheter in the epidural space allows for control of block height, flexibility in duration, and means for postoperative epidural opioid analgesia.

Rawal et al.[55] suggest performing the procedure with the parturient in the sitting position, entering the epidural space with an 16-gauge Tuohy needle (caudadly directed), then advancing a long, 26-gauge spinal needle into the CSF. To establish a spinal block from S-5 to T-8, a mean total dose of 8.0 to 8.5 mg of 0.5% hyperbaric bupivacaine was needed. The Tuohy needle is then rotated 180° cephalad and an 18-gauge catheter is advanced in the epidural space. On waiting 15 to 20 minutes to "fix" the spinal level, fractionated epidural doses of 1.5 to 2.0 ml per segment of 0.5% bupivacaine were administered to obtain a T-4–5 level for cesarean delivery. Mean induction delivery intervals (IDI) in the CSE group were 39 minutes. When they compared CSE with epidural bupivacaine block (without opioids) for cesarean delivery, they observed a threefold lower total bupivacaine requirement, with significantly lower maternal and fetal blood bupivacaine levels (although there were no adverse fetal effects in either groups as assessed by Apgar scores, neonatal blood gases, or serial neurobehavioral examinations). The CSE group also had a lower incidence of hypotension, with better overall surgical anesthesia and patient satisfaction.

Despite its advantages, CSE is a time-consuming technique and has a 4% failure rate[56] (which exceeds that of single-shot spinal anesthesia). In a recent case Myint et al.[57] reported on a cardiopulmonary arrest (responsive to naloxone) 40 minutes after 2.5 mg of diamorphine was administered epidurally in a parturient given CSE for elective cesarean delivery. The use of relatively hydrophobic epidural opioids postoperatively in CSE patients should be done with caution, since the previous dural puncture site may allow for direct CSF access.

General Anesthesia

The advantages of general anesthesia for cesarean delivery include the following:

1. Speed of induction (shorter induction delivery interval versus regional anesthesia)[9]
2. Reliability
3. Controllability
4. Reproducibility
5. Avoidance of hypotension associated with regional anesthesias[29]

Disadvantages of general anesthesia for cesarean delivery are listed below:

1. Risk of maternal aspiration on induction or emergence
2. Risk of failed tracheal intubation and hypoxemia
3. Potential for maternal awareness during light anesthesia
4. Neonatal depression secondary to maternally administered anesthetics during prolonged induction delivery interval

Indications for general anesthesia during cesarean delivery are as follows:

1. Active bleeding in a hemodynamically unstable parturient
2. Maternal coagulopathy
3. Severe fetal distress (e.g., prolapsed umbilical cord, persistent fetal bradycardia, shoulder dystocia)
4. Maternal sepsis
5. Certain neurological diseases or active central nervous system infections
6. Patient refusal of regional anesthetic techniques
7. Failed regional anesthetic techniques

The technique for general anesthesia for cesarean delivery is shown in Table 20-7.

TABLE 20-7

GENERAL ANESTHESIA TECHNIQUE FOR CESAREAN DELIVERY

Nonparticulate antacid: 30 ml 0.3 M sodium citrate (Bicitra) within 30-60 min of induction

Metoclopramide 10 mg IV

Left uterine displacement 15°—**journey tilt**

Prehydration (500-1000 ml lactated Ringer's)

Monitors: Fio_2 monitor; ECG; Spo_2; capnography with $ETco_2$ measurements; NIBP; peripheral nerve stimulator are essential, additional capabilities include esophageal temperature and stethoscope, and precordial Doppler ultrasound monitoring

Preoxygenation/Denitrogenation

3-5 min or 4 deep breaths of 100% O_2 (former preferred if time permits)

Attention to proper head positioning, airway equipment (various sizes) and suction ready

Begin oxygenation and apply monitors as patient is being prepped and draped

Induction

Begin IV induction only after surgeons are ready with scalpel in hand

Rapid sequence induction with cricoid pressure (Sellick's maneuver)

Thiopental 4 mg/kg (or ketamine 1.0-1.5 mg/kg, etomidate 0.3 mg/kg, or propofol 2.0 mg/kg)

Succinylcholine 1.0-1.5 mg/kg (avoid defasciculation, useful to see fasciculations)

Intubation with cuffed endotracheal tube, keep failed intubation protocol in mind

Maintenance

Before Delivery

50% O_2-N_2O plus 0.5 MAC isoflurane, enflurane, or halothane (keep total MAC about 1.0 with N_2O and volatile agent, analgesic, amnestic, but not complete anesthetic dosages desired to limit recall, permit relatively high Fio_2, minimizes intraoperative bleeding while maintaining myometrial responsiveness to oxytocin)

Succinylcholine 0.1-0.2% infusion (alternative vecuronium or atracurium)

Avoid hyperventilation or hypoventilation, maintain $ETco_2$ in 30-32 mm Hg range

Minute ventilation in 110-120 ml/kg/min range

Minimize IDI (optimally less than 8 min)

Minimize UDI (optimally less than 3 min)

After Delivery

Convert to pure O_2-N_2O-opioid technique plus benzodiazepines, discontinue or add additional volatile agent depending on the uterine response to oxytocin

Empty stomach with an oral gastric tube (if time did not permit preop Bicitra administration consider placement through gastric tube for some gastric protection on emergence)

Emergence

Awake extubation with intact airway reflexes

Administer reversal agents if nondepolarizing muscle relaxants used

Assess adequacy of reversal by clinical signs of neuromuscular recovery and peripheral nerve stimulator

IV, Intravenously; Fio_2, fractional inspired oxygen concentration; Spo_2, in pulse oximetry; $ETco_2$, end tidal carbon dioxide; NIBP, noninvasive blood pressure; O_2, oxygen; MAC, minimum alveolar concentration; N_2O, nitrous oxide; IDI, induction delivery intervals; UDI, uterine incision delivery intervals.

Cardiovascular Considerations

Tracheal intubation and extubation are associated with the greatest increases in cardiac output and arterial blood pressure; these changes are transient in nature and are deemed to be insignificant.[58] Such changes associated with induction of light general anesthesia tend to avoid the risk of hypotension associated with regional anesthetic techniques.[29,44] However, despite higher maternal blood pressure after induction of general anesthesia with thiopental, nitrous oxide, and succinylcholine, Jouppila et al.[44] observed a 35% decrease in placental blood flow. This reduction in IVBF seems to be well tolerated by the healthy fetus without a history of maternal uteroplacental insufficiency.[44] Before induction of general anesthesia, *Journey tilt,* or positioning the parturient with a 15° left uterine tilt in the 30 minutes before transportation to the operating room can help to minimize neonatal base deficits and metabolic acidosis from reduced uteroplacental perfusion related to aortocaval compression.[3]

Pulmonary Aspiration

Gastric stasis, increased gastric residual volume, decreased gastric pH, and lower esophageal sphincter (LES) tone predispose the parturient to esophageal reflux. Full-stomach considerations characterize the parturient from the eighteenth to the twentieth week of gestation, to at least 8 to 24 hours after delivery.[3] Mendelson's[59] classic article in 1946 reported 66 cases of maternal aspiration in 43,000 pregnancies (1:660 cases); 96% of these were related to gastric acid aspiration. Still today, pulmonary aspiration of gastric contents continues to be recognized as a leading cause of maternal morbidity and mortality for anesthesia.[60] A gastric pH of less than 2.5 and a gastric volume greater than or equal to 0.4 ml/kg (Roberts and Adamson unpublished data 1973, determined in rhesus monkeys), or almost 25 ml in adult females, poses a risk of acid aspiration pneumonitis.

Roberts and Shirley[61] observed in 100 parturients undergoing cesarean delivery that the presence of high gastric volume and low pH could not be excluded in any parturient, regardless of the time interval between last meal and onset of labor. Gibbs et al.[62] and Dewan et al.[63] reported that 30 ml of 0.3 mol/L sodium citrate given within 1 hour of induction of general anesthesia for cesarean delivery, increased gastric pH to more than 2.5 in all parturients. Gibbs et al.[62] also observed that about 80 minutes later, at the time of emergence and extubation, gastric pH remained above 2.5 in 96% of parturients. However, Dewan et al.[63] noted that 50% to 64% of parturients given sodium citrate over 1 hour before delivery had gastric aspirates that put them at risk for acid aspiration pneumonia. Furthermore, oral nonparticulate antacids do not significantly increase gastric volume.[61] Therefore *nonparticulate oral antacids should be mandatory; 30 ml of 0.3 mol/L of sodium citrate should be given within 30 minutes of induction of general anesthesia.*

Parturients have a reduced LES tone compared with nonpregnant women, whereas parturients with heartburn have a still weaker LES tone than those without. Hey and Ostick[64] observed that 80% of parturients with heartburn had moderate-to-severe esophageal reflux, compared with 30% of parturients without heartburn. Augmentation of gastric emptying and enhancing LES tone can be accomplished pharmacologically with *metoclopramide,* a dopamine antagonist. Metoclopramide accelerates gastric emptying by its direct effect on autonomic nuclei and sensitizes the gastric muscle to the effects of acetylcholine; it does not alter gastric pH. It increases LES tone in parturients with or without heartburn[64,65] and partially reverses the gastric stasis associated with labor or opioid usage.[3] Metoclopramid's central antiemetic effect results from its antidopaminergic action on the Chemotactic trigger zone.

Anticholinergic, (e.g., glycopyrrolate or atropine) frequently are administered before general anesthesia for cesarean delivery, since they may decrease gastric secretions and increase the pH of gastric contents. Unfortunately, they also decrease LES tone and increase the risk for gastroesphageal reflux. If anticholinergics are to be used, metoclopramide should be given before or in combination with them to reverse or neutralize their relaxant effect on the LES.[66] *Histamine (H_2) receptor antagonists,* such as cimetidine and ranitidine, inhibit basal gastric acid secretions to increase gastric pH and decrease gastric residual volume. Administering these drugs longer than 1 hour before induction seems to be necessary to derive any physiologic benefit.

Preoxygenation Techniques

Maternal Pao_2 below 100 mm Hg at the time of delivery is associated with prolonged time to sustained respiration and lower Apgar scores in neonates.[37] Increased oxygen demands and increased oxygen consumption in pregnancy, coupled with the parturient's decreased functional residual capacity, predispose the parturient to rapid hemoglobin desaturation during brief periods of apnea. Archer and Marx[67] showed that 1 minute of apnea produced a mean decrease in oxygen tension of 139 mm Hg in pregnant women versus 58 mm Hg in nonpregnant women. Norris and Dewan[68] compared preoxygenation techniques with 100% oxygen for 3 minutes versus four maximal deep breaths within 30 seconds of induction. The four-deep-breath group had a mean Pao_2 of 404 mm Hg versus 385 mm Hg in the 3-minute preoxygenation group. Either technique is acceptable to maximize maternal oxygen reserve when fetal distress is present and rapid induction of general anesthesia is necessary. Marx and Mateo[37] also observed that fetal oxygenation was highest and time to spontaneous respiration was lowest when maternal Pao_2 was greater than 300 mm Hg. This necessitated an inspired oxygen concentration of at least 65%. Moir[29] suggests that a maternal Fio_2 of 50% should be sufficient to bring the maternal Pao_2 close to the optimal 300-mm Hg value; this appears to give credence to the predelivery usage of 50% O_2/50% N_2O mixtures. The time required for a significant degree of maternal/fetal oxygen equilibrium ranges from 3 to 6 minutes[68]; high maternal Fio_2 exposure before delivery improves umbilical cord blood oxygenation and ultimately the neonate's condition at birth.[67]

Failed Tracheal Intubation

The *ACOG committee opinion*[60] specifically describes and alerts the obstetric care team of many anatomic and medical risk factors that may jeopardize the parturient if emergency cesarean delivery under general anesthesia is necessary. The obstetric care team has the responsibility to be aware of such risk factors, and once identified, they are advised to seek out consultants in anesthesia to devise an appropriate collaborative management plan to minimize the parturient's risk. When possible, early placement of intravenous lines and regional anesthetics are preferable to avoid general anesthesia in high-risk parturients.

Failed tracheal intubation in the obstetric population may complicate between 1 in 300[69] and 1 in 750[70] general anesthetics for cesarean delivery. Rocke et al.[70] evaluated parturients for difficult airway characteristics before elective or emergency cesarean delivery under general anesthesia. With the parturient seated upright, head in neutral position, oropharyngeal structures visible upon maximal mouth opening with tongue protruding (but without phonation) were assessed.

The following is the modified Mallampati airway classification[71]:

- *Class I*—soft palate, fauces, uvula, and tonsillar pillars are visible

- *Class II*—soft palate and fauces seen, tip of uvula is obscured
- *Class III*—soft palate and only base of uvula are seen
- *Class IV*—soft palate is not visible

The view at laryngoscopy as described by Cormack and Lehane[72] is as follows:

- *Grade A*—most of glottis is visible
- *Grade B*—only posterior extremity of the glottis is visible
- *Grade C*—no part of glottis is visible, only the epiglottis
- *Grade D*—not even the epiglottis is visible

Rocke et al.[70] found that there was a significant association between the modified Mallampati classification and the glottic view at larygoscopy and the difficulty at intubation. Compared with an uncomplicated Mallampati class I parturient, the relative risk of a difficult intubation was 3.2 times greater for class II parturients, 7.6 times greater for class III parturients, and 11.3 times greater for class IV parturients. Parturients with a short neck, receding mandible, or protruding maxillary incisors individually were also at increased risk for difficult intubations.

Interestingly, the two patients in this study who had true failed intubations were from the modified Mallampati class II and class III groups. Therefore a difficult airway or failed intubation algorithm is essential; a modified protocol set out by Malan and Johnson is useful when confronted with the unsuspected difficult or failed intubation[3] (Fig. 20-1). After three properly controlled attempts at intubation fail, further management is dictated by whether ventilation and oxygenation can be maintained by mask with cricoid pressure, together with the urgency of the cesarean delivery. In a *nonurgent setting,* the parturient should be allowed to awaken and proceed to awake intubation or regional anesthesia. If *fetal distress* is encountered and mask ventilation with cricoid pressure is possible while maintaining oxygenation, completion of the surgery is advisable. If failed intubation occurs while mask ventilation is impossible, the laryngeal mask airway (LMA) is an acceptable initial alternative to cricothyroidotomy. The LMA was developed to maintain airway patency.[73] Lifesaving oxygenation and ventilation (either spontaneous or positive-pressure ventilation), in the setting of failed tracheal intubation during cesarean delivery, has been reported.[74,75] Airway protection from regurgitation cannot be guaranteed in the parturient, and occasionally cricoid pressure must be released for reliable LMA insertion.[76] Nevertheless, the LMA may help facilitate passage of up to a 6.0-mm cuffed endotracheal tube once adequate oxygenation and ventilation has been restored for definitive airway protection. *Whereas endotracheal anesthesia is the safest for the parturient under general anesthesia, patients do not die from failure to intubate, they die either from failure to stop trying to intubate or from undiagnosed esophageal intubation.*[3] Therefore, capnography to detect carbon dioxide from expired gas is the most reliable means of confirming tracheal intubation, whereas pulse oximetry is invaluable to assess oxygen saturation.

Maternal Ventilation

Increased metabolic demands associated with pregnancy result in a 50% increase in maternal minute ventilation, a partially compensated respiratory alkalosis, and maternal arterial carbon dioxide pressure (Pa_{CO_2}) ranging between 28 and 32 mm Hg result at term. A direct correlation between maternal Pa_{CO_2} and fetal umbilical vein P_{O_2} has been observed.[3] Mechanisms explaining this phenomenon include the following:

1. Uterine artery and umbilical vessel vasoconstriction secondary to maternal hypocarbia and alkalosis
2. Increased intrathoracic pressure during hy-

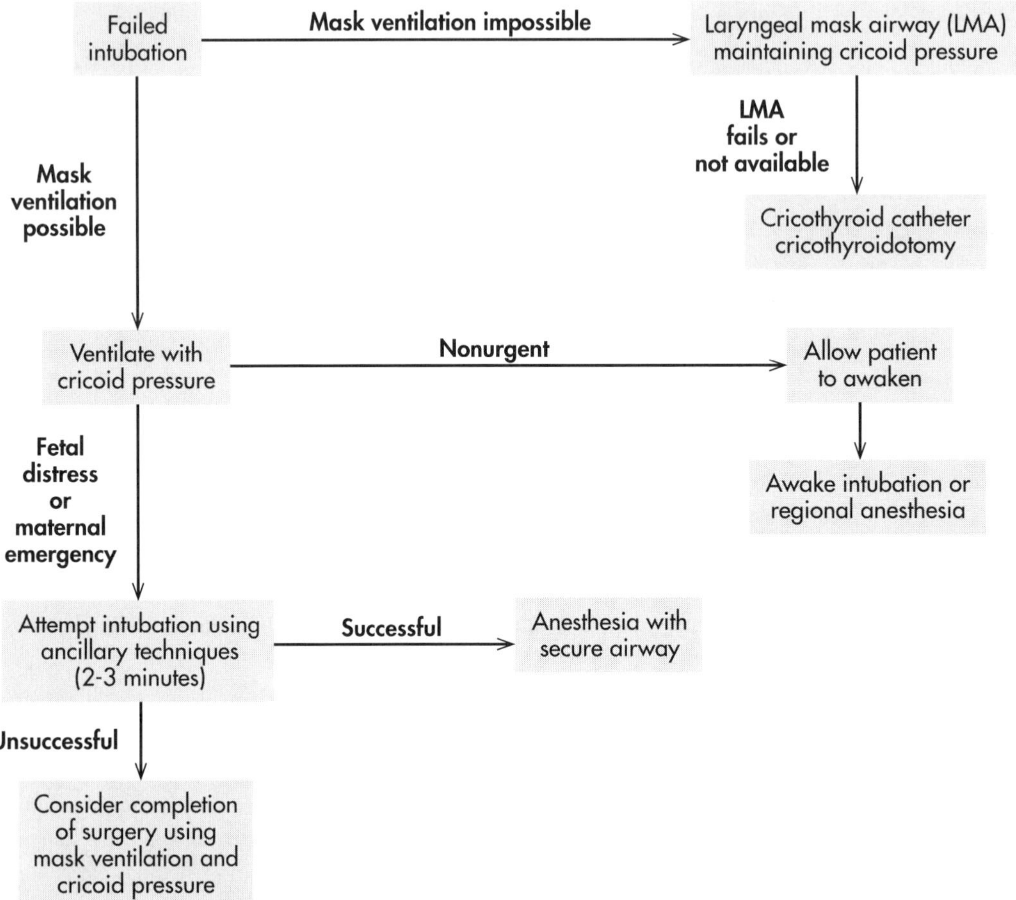

Fig. 20-1.

Failed intubation protocol. *(From Lussos SA, Datta S: Anesthesia for cesarean delivery. Part III: General anesthesia,* Int J Obstet Anes *1993; 2:112.)*

perventilation, which may reduce venous return, aortic pressure, and uterine blood flow up to 25%[77]

3. Alkalosis causing a shift to the left of the maternal oxyhemoglobin dissociation curve, which may impair oxygen release to the fetus

Maternal $Paco_2$ less than 23 to 25 mm Hg during general anesthesia impairs uteroplacental perfusion and is associated with a decrease in fetal Po_2, increased neonatal base deficits (acidosis), lower Apgar scores, and delays in the onset of spontaneous respirations.[3] Maternal $Paco_2$/end tidal ($ETco_2$) differences are small, between 0.03 and 0.6 mm Hg Pco_2.[78] Therefore $ETco_2$ monitoring is an excellent indicator of maternal $Paco_2$. There is also a direct correlation between maternal $ETco_2$ and fetal UV Po_2 values.[79] Monitoring $ETco_2$ is essential during general anesthesia and should be used to maintain a physiologic $ETco_2$ range from 30 to 32 mm Hg, using mechanical minute ventilation volumes in the 110- to 120-mg · kg · min range.[3]

Anesthetic Induction Agents

Intravenous induction agents used with certain dosage limitations can insure rapid maternal unconsciousness and limited fetal drug exposure if IDI can be minimized.

Thiobarbiturates (thiamylal and thiopental) rapidly cross the placenta with peak UV levels being detected by 90 seconds after injection, whereas peak UA levels are noted at 3.5 minutes.[80] The UV : MV ratio, a measure of placental drug transfer, remains less than 1 due to rapid maternal redistribution and tissue uptake of thiobarbiturates. The nonhomogenity of IVBF further decreases maternal arterial thiobarbiturate blood levels to lower diffusion gradients. With longer IDIs, the UV/MV ratio increases, as does the net transfer of thiobarbiturates to fetal tissue (increasing umbilical artery : umbilical vein ratios). But UA : UV ratios remain less than 1 due to extraction of thiobarbiturates from umbilical venous blood by the fetal liver, and by progressive dilution through circulatory admixture in the fetus. Repeated dosages of thiobarbiturates of as little as one third the initial dose rapidly increase fetal UV blood levels and risk fetal depression. Neonatal elimination half-life of thiopental is 11 to 43 hours. For laboring women, fetal thiobarbiturate exposure can be minimized by timing injection with the beginning of a uterine contraction. To avoid any significant degree of neonatal depression, it is best to limit maternal dosage of thiopental to 4 mg/kg.

Ketamine, a phencyclidine derivative, is useful when maternal hemorrhage or hypovolemia jeopardizes hemodynamic status, as well as for the parturient with asthma. Ketamine does not appreicably alter uterine blood flow. Optimal induction dosages are between 1.0 and 1.5 mg/kg for best neonatal outcome and limited maternal intraoperative awareness.

Propofol, or 2,6 diisopropylphenol, is solubilized in lecithin- containing formulation. Propofol has a short elimination half-life (81 minutes); this may allow the parturient to emerge less sedated from general anesthesia. Propofol also is associated with less emetic symptoms than thiopental. Its disadvantages include pain on injection and occasional involuntary muscle movements, and possibly a higher incidence of hypotension than with thiopental. Propofol rapidly crosses the placenta with UV : MV ratios of 0.6 to 0.72. Fetal tissue uptake and equilibrium occur rapidly with UA : UV ratios often exceeding 1.0 at delivery. It is also rapidly cleared by the neonate. Propofol is 1.6 times more potent than thiopental, therefore 2.5 mg/kg of propofol is equipotent to 4.0 mg/kg of thiopental. Propofol induction dosages of 2.0 to 2.5 mg/kg and limiting maximal infusion rates to 100 μg · kg · min have been associated with good neonatal outcomes.[81]

Etomidate is a carboxylated imidazole compound; its use is advantageous in the hemodynamically compromised or hypovolemic parturient, or the parturient with cardiovascular disease. It causes minimal myocardial depression and allows for stable hemodynamics. It has a short elimination half-life of 1 to 3 hours in the mother, but may be found in the neonatal urine up to 16 hours after delivery.[3] With etomidate there have been concerns of maternal as well as neonatal adrenocortical suppression, and the potential exists to impair neonatal extrauterine adaptation. Other concerns include higher incidence of postoperative emetic symptoms, pain on injection, and occasional myoclonic movements. The induction dose of etomidate is 0.3 mg/kg.

Midazolam is a poor induction agent for cesarean delivery, despite its superior amnestic quality and hemodynamic stability. Induction doses of 0.2 mg/kg tend to cause severe neonatal depression.

Neuromuscular Blocking Agents

Neuromuscular blocking agents are polar, quaternary ammonium compounds with low lipid solubility. Transplacental passage is minimal and neonatal effects are clinically insignificant when used in standard dosages.

Succinylcholine in doses of 1.0 to 1.5 mg/kg rapidly facilitates reliable intubating conditions during rapid-sequence inductions. Complete muscular relaxation occurs within 90 seconds and lasts an average of 6.2 minutes.[3] Plasma cholinesterase activity declines with pregnancy with a reduction of 15.6% in the peripartum period, 24.6% on the first postpartum day, and 32.3% on the third postpartum day. By the sixth week after delivery, enzyme activity returns to normal.[82] The parturient's expanded blood volume may account for these changes, therefore modification in induction dosages is not necessary. Parturients rarely have fasciculations or muscle pains after succinylcholine.[3] Succinylcholine produces inconsistent and unpredictable elevations in intragastric pressure. It also tends to increase LES pressure so barrier pressure is essentially unchanged, provided a preoperative anticholinergic has not been administered. Therefore the routine usage of a nondepolarizing muscle relaxant before the use of succinylcholine to prevent fasciculation and an associated rise in intragastric pressure is not warranted in the parturient. Prolonged neuromuscular blockade can be expected in the parturient who receives trimethaphan, magnesium sulfate, or who has an atypical pseudocholinesterase.

Nondepolarizing neuromuscular relaxants d-tubocurarine, gallamine, pancuronium, vecuronium, and atracurium produce minimal effects in the fetus when given to the mother. They cross the placenta slowly, with UV:MV ratios of 0.1 to 0.2, or 10% to 20%. There is one case report of neonate paralysis after the administration of 245 mg of d-tubocurarine over a 10-hour period to control status epilepticus in the mother.[3] All parturients given nondepolarizing muscle relaxants should be given a pharmacologic reversal agent before extubation.

Inhalation Agents

Pregnancy is associated with an increased sensitivity to volatile inhalation anesthetic agents. There is an inverse relationship between plasma progesterone levels and the minimum alveolar concentrations (MAC) of volatile anesthetics during pregnancy.[83] The MAC for volatile anesthetics are reduced between 25% and 40% with pregnancy.[84]

Nitrous oxide (N_2O) crosses the placenta rapidly; after 3 to 4 minutes of administration the mean UV:MV ratio is 0.83.[85] Fetal tissue uptake continues as IDIs increase, and by 15 to 19 minutes of maternal exposure, fetal tissue is 87% saturated.[85] Prolonged IDIs, along with inspired N_2O) concentrations of greater than 66%, may lead to neonatal depression. This may be manifested by reduced Apgar scores and prolonged time to sustained respiration, possibly reflecting fetal narcosis from diffusion hypoxia. Supplemental oxygen by a tight-sealing mask should be given to the neonate when prolonged maternal N_2O exposure occurs before birth. Limiting inspired N_2O concentrations to 50% before delivery minimizes this concern. Nitrous oxide does not cause uterine relaxation, therefore increasing inspired concentrations after delivery does not affect the uterus's response to oxytocin.

Modern *halogenated volatile anesthetics* when used in 0.5 MAC concentrations with 50% N_2O in oxygen provide light general anesthesia and adequate maternal amnesia before delivery.[29,86] Warren et al.[86] used a 50% mixture of N_2O/oxygen combined with either 0.5% halothane, 1.0% enflurane, or 0.75% isoflurane (combined 1 MAC equivalent), versus 50% N_2O alone during general anesthesia for cesarean delivery. No differences in neonatal outcome or maternal blood loss were observed in the four groups. Maternal recall occurred in 17% of the pure nitrous group and was absent in the combination groups. Equipotent concentrations of halogenated volatile anesthetics produce equivalent degrees of uterine relaxation; 0.5 MAC equivalent doses do not increase postpartum bleeding and allow the uterus to remain responsive to oxytocin. Usually MAC equivalent doses greater than 1 of volatile anesthetics are necessary to produce clinically significant uterine relaxation.

Maternal awareness during light general anesthesia consisting of unsupplemented oxygen/N_2O oxide ranges from 2% to 36%.[3] This can be minimized or prevented by using a volatile anesthetic in combination with N_2O in a total 1 MAC dose before delivery,[29,86] encouraging short IDIs, and using combinations of intravenous opioids and benzodiazepines immediately after delivery. The practice of turning off anesthetics at the time of uterine incision should also be discouraged.

Timing of Delivery

Prolonged IDIs allow for the time-dependent transfer of depressant inhalation and intravenous anesthetics to the neonate. If hypotension is avoided during regional anesthetic techniques, the length of the IDI is not a factor with regard to neonatal outcome.[87,88] However, significant maternal hypotension (> 2 minutes) during regional anesthetic techniques may impair neonatal blood gases despite short IDIs.[89] Crawford et al.[90] in 1976 demonstrated that during general anesthesia, IDIs of up to 30 minutes were not associated with detrimental effects on neonatal acid-base values, if one could maintain inspired oxygen concentrations of 65% to 70% while avoiding aortocaval compression and hypotension.

Possibly more important to the neonate, and beyond the control of the anesthesiologist, is the *uterine incision delivery interval* (UDI). Progressive fetal /asphyxia and clinically apparent neonatal depression are associated with prolonged UDIs, independent of the IDI.[91] Crawford and Davies[92] in 1975 postulated that during prolonged UDIs:

1. Uterine manipulation disrupts or impairs uteroplacental and umbilical cord blood flow
2. Exaggerated pressure on the uterus could enhance aortocaval compression
3. At this stressful time for the fetus, inhalation of amniotic fluid or meconium can occur as a result of gasping respirations in utero
4. Fetal head compression during difficult deliveries may further impair neonatal outcome

Datta et al.[87] 1981 observed that during general anesthesia, IDIs greater than 8 minutes, or UDIs greater than or equal to 180 seconds, resulted in lower 1-minute Apgar scores (less than 7) and neonatal UA acidosis. Bader et al.[88] also observed that prolonged UDIs during regional anesthesia results in elevated fetal UA norepinephrine levels and associated fetal acidosis.

Recovery and Emergence

Intubation does not always prevent pulmonary aspiration of gastric contents; aspiration may occur just before induction or during tracheal intubation, as well as immediately after extubation. Inadequate neuromuscular reversal or recurarization in the immediate postoperative period can be responsible for significant maternal morbidity. A peripheral nerve stimulator should be used along with clinical signs of adequate neuromuscular recovery before extubation. The parturient should be awake with intact pharyngeal reflexes before extubation and observed closely in the immediate postoperative period.

Case Scenerio Summary

1. There is a higher incidence of perinatal morbidity and mortality associated with breech as opposed to vertex presentations, even when corrected for prematurity and congenital abnormalities. Asphyxia from cord compression or intracranial hemorrhage from birth trauma exceed that of vertex deliveries. Most studies on breech deliveries focus on the neonate by comparing vaginal or cesarean birth outcomes, with little attention to the conduct of the particular anesthetic choosen.[93] In general, the breech fetus tends to deteriorate more rapidly than vertex fetus: this is believed to be related to a greater degree of in utero cord compression.[94] Even cesarean delivery of the breech infant can be difficult; a trapped head, despite a hysterotomy, can prolong the UDI. A taunt myometrium may require myometrial relaxation with a volatile agent or intravenous nitroglycerin. Therefore one must be prepared to induce general anesthesia, even in the presence of adequate regional anesthetic, or have intravenous nitroglycerin readily available.
2. The case provides little information except that the patient requires a primary elective cesarean delivery for breech presentation. It can be assumed that she is a healthy, nonobese woman with a normal-appearing airway (modified Mallampati class I or II). Since she is not in labor, she will be more prone to hypotension than a laboring parturient, therefore a full-volume loading and prompt intravenous ephedrine will be administered to avoid hypotension. Since the breech fetus is in general at greater risk of birth trauma and prolonged UDIs (both of which are beyond the obstetric anesthesiologist's control), efforts to minimize fetal exposure to depressant medications are desirable. Therefore avoiding general anesthesia for this elective breech cesarean delivery serves to minimize fetal drug exposure, whereas an awake parturient protects her own airway, thereby minimizing aspirations hazards. Either a spinal or an epidural anesthetic, as outlined in Tables 20-2 and 20-5, would be satisfactory for an elective breech cesarean delivery.

References

1. Lussos, SA, Datta S: Anesthesia for cesarean delivery. Part I: general considerations and spinal anesthesia, *Int J Obstet Anesth* 1992; 1:79.
2. Lussos SA, Datta S: Anesthesia for cesarean delivery. Part II: epidural anesthesia, intrathecal and epidural opioids, venous air embolism, *Int J Obstet Anesth* 1992; 1:208.
3. Lussos SA. Datta S: Anesthesia for cesarean delivery. Part III: General anesthesia, *Int J Obstet Anesth* 1993; 2:109.
4. Clark RB, Thompson DS, Thompson CH: Prevention of spinal hypotension with cesarean section, *Anesthesiology* 1976; 45:670.
5. Corke BC, Datta S, Ostheimer GW, et al: Spinal anesthesia for caesarean section: the influence of hypotension on neonatal outcome, *Anaesthesia* 1982; 37:658.
6. Ueland K, Gills RE, Hansen JM: Maternal cardiovascular dynamics I: cesarean section under subarachnoid block anesthesia, *Am J Obstet Gynecol* 1968; 100:4253.
7. Hon EH, Reid BL, Hehre FW: The electronic evaluation of the fetal heart rate II: changes with maternal hypotension, *Am J Obstet Gynecol* 1960; 79(2):209.
8. Ebner H, Barcohana J, Bartoshun AK: Influence of post spinal hypotension on the fetal electrocardiogram, *Am J Obstet Gynecol* 1960; 80:569.
9. Marx GF, Cosmi EV, Wollman SB: Biochemical status and clinical condition of mother and infant at cesarean section, *Anesth Analg* 1969; 48:986.
10. Hollmen AI, Jouppila R, Koivisto M, et al: Neurologic activity of infants following anesthesia for cesarean section, *Anesthesiology* 1978; 48:350.
11. Philipson EH, Kalhan SC, Riha MM, et al: Effects of mater-

nal glucose infusion on fetal acid-base status in human pregnancy, *Am J Obstet Gynecol* 1987; 157:866.

12. Hollmen AI, Jouppila R, Albright GA, et al: Intervillous blood flow during caesarean section with prophylactic ephedrine and epidural anesthesia, *Acta Anaesthesiol Scand* 1984; 28:396.
13. Lussos SA, Bader AM, Thornhill ML, Datta S: The antiemetic efficacy and safety of prophylactic metoclopramide for elective cesarean delivery during spinal anesthesia, *Reg Anesth* 1992; 17:126.
14. Datta S, Alper MH, Ostheimer GW, Weiss JB: Methods of ephedrine administration and nausea and hypotension during spinal anesthesia for cesarean section, *Anesthesiology* 1982; 56:68.
15. Moren DH, Perillo M, Laporta RF, et al: Phenylephrine in the prevention of hypotension following spinal anesthesia for cesarean delivery, *J Clin Anesth* 1991; 3:301.
16. Sprague DH: Effects of position and uterine displacement on spinal anesthesia for cesarean section, *Anesthesiology* 1976; 44:164.
17. Norris MC: Height, weight, and the spread of subarachnoid hyperbaric bupivacaine in the term parturient, *Anesth Analg* 1988; 67:555.
18. DeSimone CA, Norris MC, Leighton B, et al: Spinal anesthesia with hyperbaric bupivacaine for cesarean section: a comparison of two doses, *Anesthesilogy* 1988; 69:A670.
19. Abouleish EI: Epinephrine improves the quality of spinal hyperbaric bupivacaine for cesarean section, *Anesth Analg* 1987; 66:395.
20. Chantigian RC, Datta S, Burger GA, et al: Anesthesia for cesarean delivery utilizing tetracaine versus tetracaine and procaine, *Reg Anesth* 1984; 9(4):195.
21. Hauch MA, Hartwell BL, Hunt CO, et al: Comparative effects of subarachnoid hyperbaric bupivacaine and tetracaine-procaine for cesarean delivery, *Reg Anesth* 1990; 15:81.
22. Hunt CO, Naulty JS, Bader AM: Perioperative analgesia with subarachnoid fentanyl-bupivacaine for cesarean delivery, *Anesthesiology* 1989; 71:535.
23. Ratra CK, Badola RP, Bhargava KP: A study of factors concerned in emesis during spinal anaesthesia, *Br J Anaesth* 1972; 44:1208.
24. Ackerman WE, Juneja MM, Colclough GW, et al: Epidural fentanyl significantly decreases nausea and vomiting during uterine manipulation in awake patient undergoing cesarean section, *Anesthesiology* 1988; 69:A679.
25. Lussos SA, Johnson M: *Peripartum nausea and emesis.* In Ostheimer GW, editor: *Manual of obstetric anesthesia,* ed 2, New York: Churchill Livingstone.
26. MiHic DN: Postspinal headache and relationship of needle bevel to longitudinal dural fibers, *Reg Anesth* 1985; 10:76.
27. Hurley RJ, Hertwig LM, Lambert DH: Incidence of post dural puncture headache in the obstetric patient: 25 gauge Whitacre vs 26 and 27 gauge Quincke tip needles, *Reg Anesth* 1992; 17(3S):90.
28. Ueland K, Akamatsu TJ, Eng M, et al: Maternal cardiovascular dynamics. VI: cesarean section under epidural anesthesia without epinephrine, *Am J Obstet Gynecol* 1967; 114(6):775.
29. Moir DD: Anaesthesia for cesarean section: an evaluation of a method using low concentrations of halothane and 50% oxygen, *Br J Anaesth* 1970; 42:136.
30. Helbo-Hansen S, Bang U, Garcia RS, et al: Subarachnoid versus epidural bupivacaine 0.5% for cesarean section, *Acta Anaesthesiol Scand* 1988; 32:473.
31. Brizgys RV, Dailey PA, Shnider SM, et al: The incidence and neonatal effects of maternal hypotension during epidural anesthesia for cesarean section, *Anesthesiology* 1987; 67:782.
32. Parnass SM, Curran MJA, Becker GL: Incidence of hypotension associated with epidural anesthesia using alkalinized and nonalkalinized lidocaine for cesarean section, *Anesthesiology* 1987; 66:1148.
33. Ramanathan S, Masih A, Rock I, et al: Maternal and fetal effects of prophylactic hydration with crystalloids or colloids before epidural anesthesia, *Anesth Analg* 1983, 62:673.
34. Lewis M, Thomas P, Wilkes RG: Hypotension during epidural analgesia for cesarean section: arterial and central venous pressure changes after acute intravenous loading with two litres of Hartmann's solution, *Anaesthesia* 1983; 38:250.
35. Ramanathan S, Gandhi S, Arismendy J, et al: Oxygen transfer from mother to fetus during cesarean section under epidural anesthesia, *Anesth Analg* 1982; 61:576.
36. Fox GS, Houle GL: Acid-base studies in elective cesarean sections during epidural and general anesthesia, *Can Anesth Soc J* 1971; 18(1):60.
37. Marx GF, Mateo CV: Effects of different oxygen concentrations during general anesthesia for elective cesarean section; *Can Anaesth Soc J* 1971: 18:587.
38. DiFazio CA, Carron H, Grosslight KR, et al: Comparison of pH-adjusted lidocaine solutions for epidural anesthesia, *Anesth Analg* 1986: 65:760.

39. Gissen AJ, Datta S, Lambert D: The chloroprocaine controversy. II: is chloroprocaine neurotoxic? *Reg Anesth* 1984; 9:135.
40. Abboud TK, Moore MJ, Jacobs J, et al: Epidural mepivacaine for cesarean section, maternal and neonatal effects, *Reg Anesth* 1987; 12:76.
41. Gaffud MP, Bansal P, Lawton C, et al: Surgical anaglesia for cesarean delivery with epidural bupivacaine and fentanyl, *Anesthesiology* 1986; 65:331.
42. Bonica JJ, Akamatsu TJ, Berges MU: Circulatory effects of peridural block. II: effects of epinephrine, anesthesia, *Anesthesiology* 1971; 34:514.
43. Albright FA, Jouppila R, Hollmen AI, et al: Epinephrine does not alter human intervillous blood flow during epidural anesthesia, *Anesthesiology* 1981; 54:131.
44. Jouppila R, Jouppila P, Hollmen A, et al: Effects of the anesthetic method, epidural and general anesthesia, on intervillous blood flow in cesarean sections, *Reg Anesth* 1977; 2(4):2.
45. Datta S, Alper M, Ostheimer GW, et al: Effects of maternal position on epidural anesthesia for cesarean section, acid-base status, and bupivacaine concentrations at delivery, *Anesthesiology* 1979; 50:205.
46. Westmore MD: Epidural opioids in obstetrics: a review, *Anaesth Intensive Care* 1990; 18:292.
47. Preston PG, Rosen MA, Hughes SC, et al: Epidural anesthesia with fentanyl and lidocaine for cesarean section: maternal effects and neonatal outcome, *Anesthesiology* 1988; 68:938.
48. Paech MJ, Westmore MD, Speirs HM: A double-blind comparison of epidural bupivacaine and bupivacaine-fentanyl for caesarean section, *Anaesth Intensive Care* 1990; 18:22.
49. Capogna G, Celleno D, Tomassetti M: Maternal analgesia and neonatal effects of epidural sufentanil for cesarean section, *Reg Anesth* 1989; 14:282.
50. Leicht CH, Hughes SC, Dailey PA, et al: Epidural morphine for analgesia after cesarean section: a prospective report of 1000 patients, *Anesthesiology* 1986; 65:A366.
51. Chestnut DH, Choi WW, Isbell TJ: Epidural hypdromorphone for postcesarean analgesia, *Obstet Gynecol* 1986; 68:65.
52. Camann WR, Hartigan PM, Gilbertson LI, et al: Chloroprocaine antagonism of epidural opioid analgesia: a receptor-specific phenomenon? *Anesthesiology* 1990; 73:860.
53. Malinow AM, Naulty JS, Hunt CO, et al: Precordial ultrasonic monitoring during cesarean delivery, *Anesthesiology* 1989; 66:816.
54. Fong J, Gadalla F, Druzin M: Venous air embolism occurring during cesarean section: the effect of patient position, *Can J Anaesth* 1991; 38:191.
55. Rawal N, Schollin J, Wesstrom G: Epidural versus combined spinal epidural block for cesarean section, *Acta Anaesthesiol Scand* 1988; 32:61.
56. Randalls B, Broadway JW, Browne DA, et al: Comparison of four subarachnoid solutions in a needle-through-needle technique for elective cesarean section, *Br J Anaesth* 1991; 66:314.
57. Myint Y, Bailey PW, Milne BR: Cardiorespiratory arrest following combined spinal epidural anaesthesia for cesarean section, *Anaesthesia* 1993; 48:684.
58. Ueland K, Hansen J, Eng M, et al: Maternal cardiovascular hemodynamics. V: cesarean section under thiopental, nitrous oxide, and succinylcholine anesthesia, *Am J Obstet Gynecol* 1970; 108:615.
59. Mendelson CL: The aspiration of stomach contents into the lungs during obstetric anesthesia, *Am J Obstet Gynecol* 1946; 52:191.
60. ACOG Committee Opinion: Anesthesia for emergency deliveries. Committee on Obstetrics, Maternal and Fetal Medicine, No. 104, March 1992.
61. Roberts RB, Shirley MA: Reducing the risk of acid aspiration during cesarean section, *Anesth Analg* 1974; 53:859.
62. Gibbs CP, Spohr L, Schmidt D: The effectiveness of sodium citrate as an antacid, *Anesthesiology* 1982; 57:44.
63. Dewan DM, Floyd HM, Thistlewood JM, et al: Sodium citrate pretreatment in elective cesarean section patients, *Anesth Analg* 1985; 64:34.
64. Hey VMF, Ostick DG: Metoclopramide and the gastro-oesophageal sphincter: a study in pregnant women with heartburn, *Anaesthesia* 1978; 33:462.
65. Brock-Utne JG, Dow TGB, Welman S, et al: The effect of metoclopramide on the lower oesophageal sphincter in late pregnancy, *Anaesth Intensive Care* 1978; 6:26.
66. Brock-Utne JG, Rubin J, Downing JW, et al: The administration of metoclopramide with atropine: a drug interaction effect on the gastroesophageal sphincter in man, *Anaesthesia* 1976; 31:1186.
67. Archer GW, Marx GF: Arterial oxygen tension during apnoea in the parturient, *Br J Anaesth* 1974; 46:358.
68. Norris MC, Dewan DW: Preoxygenation for cesarean sec-

tion: a comparison of two techniques, *Anesthesiology* 1985; 62:827.

69. Lyon G: Failed intubation: six years' experience in a teaching maternity unit, *Anaesthesia* 1985; 40:759.
70. Rocke DA, Murray WB, Rout CC, et al: Relative risk analysis of factors associated with difficult intubation in obstetric anesthesia, *Anesthesiology* 1992; 77:67.
71. Samsoon GLT, Young JRB: Difficult tracheal intubation: a retrospective study, *Anaesthesia* 1987; 42:487.
72. Cormack RS, Lehane J: Difficult tracheal intubation in ostetrics, *Anaesthesia* 1987; 39:1105.
73. Brain AIJ: The laryngeal mask: a new concept in airway management, *Br J Anaesth* 1983; 55:801.
74. McClune S, Regan M, Moore J: Laryngeal mask airway for cesarean section, *Anaesthesia* 1990; 45:227.
75. Chadwick IS, Vohra A: Anaesthesia for emergency cesarean section using the brain laryngeal mask, *Anaesthesia* 1992; 44:261.
76. Ansermino JM, Blogg CE: Cricoid pressure may prevent insertion of the laryngeal mask airway, *Br J Anaesth* 1992; 69:465.
77. Levinson G, Shnider SM, de Lorimier AA, et al: Effects of maternal hyperventilation on uterine blood flow and fetal oxygenation and acid-base status, *Anesthesiology* 1974; 40:340.
78. Shankar KB, Mosely H, Kumar Y, et al: Arterial to endtital carbon dioxide tension difference during cesarean section anaesthesia, *Anaesthesia* 1986; 41:698.
79. Cook PT: The influence on foetal outcome of maternal carbon dioxide tension at cesarean section under general anesthesia, *Anaesth Intensive Care* 1984; 12:296.
80. Kosaka Y, Takahashi T, Mark LC: Intravenous thiobarbiturate anesthesia for cesarean section, *Anesthesiology* 1969; 31:489.
81. Gregory MA, Gin T Yau G, et al: Propofol infusion anaesthesia for cesarean section, *Can J Anaesth* 1990; 37:514.
82. Shnider SM: Serum cholinesterase activity during pregnancy, labor and puerperium, *Anesthesiology* 1965; 26:335.
83. Datta S, Migliozzi RP, Flanagan HL, et al: Chronically administered progesterone decreases halothane requirements in rabbits, *Anesth Analg* 1989; 68:46.
84. Palahniuk RJ, Shnider SM, Eger EI: Pregnancy decreases the requirement for inhaled anesthetic agents, *Anesthesiology* 1974; 41:82.
85. Marx GF, Joshi CW, Orkin LR: Placental transmission of nitrous oxide, *Anesthesiology* 1970; 32:429.
86. Warren TM, Datta S, Ostheimer GW, et al: Comparison of the maternal and neonatal effects of halothane, enflurane, and isoflurane for cesarean delivery, *Anesth Analg* 1983; 62:516.
87. Datta S, Ostheimer GW, Weiss JB, et al: Neonatal effects of prolonged anesthetic induction for cesarean section, *Obstet Gynecol* 1981; 58:331.
88. Bader AM, Datta S, Arthur GR, et al: Maternal and fetal catecholamines and uterine incision-to-delivery interval during elective cesarean, *Obstet Gynecol* 1990; 75:600.
89. Datta S, Brown WU: Acid-base status in diabetic mothers and their infants following general or spinal anesthesia for cesarean section, *Anesthesiology* 1977; 47:272.
90. Crawford JS, James FM, Crawley M: A further study of general anaesthesia for cesarean section, *Br J Anaesth* 1976; 48:661.
91. Crawford JS, Burton N, Davies P: Anaesthesia for cesarean section: further refinement of a technique, *Br J Anaesth* 1973; 45:726.
92. Crawford JS, Davies P: A return to trichloroethylene for obstetric anaesthesia, *Br J Anaesth* 1975; 47:482.
93. Thorpe-Beeston JG, Banfield PJ, Saunders NJ: Outcome of breech delivery at term, *Br Med J* 1992; 305:746.
94. Eilen B, Fleischer A, Schulman H, et al: Fetal acidosis and the abnormal fetal heart rate tracing: the term breech fetus, *Obstet Gynecol* 1984; 63(2):233.

21

Postoperative Pain Relief

A 35-year-old severely obese patient is scheduled for cesarean delivery. Discuss the different modes of postoperative pain relief that can be used for this patient.

Recommendations by Ferne B. Sevarino, M.D.

A commitment to postoperative analgesia has been mandated in the present health care environment. Whereas intrapartum analgesia has always been a large part of the practice of obstetric anesthesiology, analgesia is now managed throughout the peripartum period. The goal of peripartum analgesia is to provide safe and efficacious analgesia, allowing minimal effects that would influence the new mother's ability to bond with her newborn. The superimposition of surgical stress and the physiologic changes occurring with intraabdominal surgery provide additional challenges as they impact on the parturient's well being and postpartum outcome. The many physiologic perturbations associated with obesity exacerbate the normal physiologic changes of pregnancy, presenting the pain management specialist with a common high-risk scenario.

This chapter first reviews the pathophysiology association with obesity and discusses its impact on pregnancy. The stress of abdominal surgery in the obese parturient is reviewed and options for postoperative pain management are described. A discussion of the optimum management for the case presented above concludes this chapter.

Anesthesia in the Obese Patient

Physiology of the Obese Parturient

In the nonpregnant individual, obesity is defined as weighing 20% more than ideal body weight; and morbid obesity is weighing more than twice ideal body weight, or 100 lb more than ideal body weight (Metropolitan Life Insurance Tables). This definition, however, has not been extended to pregnancy, where physiologic weight gain is expected. Currently no weight standards exist for the obese parturient. As a result, it is difficult to compare most investigations examining outcome in the obese parturient.

Edwards et al. have reported an approximate 10% incidence of obesity in pregnancy.[1] Whereas most practitioners will identify a parturient as obese based on a subjective assessment of the patient's body habitus, greater than 220 lb (90 kg) at term is a generally accepted definition of obesity during pregnancy, and greater than 250 lb (114 kg) for massive obesity.

Respiratory

Obesity and pregnancy both alter pulmonary function. Obesity is associated with an increase in oxygen consumption and carbon dioxide production secondary to an increased body mass, thus increasing ventilatory requirements. Minute ventilation increases through an increase in the respiratory rate proportionally more than the tidal volume. This is because the work of breathing, already increased due to restricted abdominal movement and increased chest wall weight, is associated with frequent small tidal volumes rather than with larger tidal volumes. Pregnancy also presents an increase in oxygen consumption and carbon dioxide production. The increase in minute ventilation is required to meet these demands. This is achieved in the nonobese parturient by a proportionally greater increase in tidal volume than in respiratory rate.

Lung volumes and capacities also are affected by obesity. Functional residual capacity (FRC), total lung capacity, and inspiratory and expiratory reserve volumes all are decreased. Closing volumes increase, and in the supine position, may fall into the normal tidal range, leading to marked hypoxemia. Pregnancy also decreases FRC, IRV, and ERV. Whereas the magnitude of these changes in the obese gravida is not as great as in the nonobese gravida, the net degree of respiratory compromise is much greater in the obese than in the nonobese parturient. Obesity also increases thoracic kyphosis, and both pregnancy and obesity increase the lumbar lordosis, further resulting in respiratory compromise.

Arterial oxygenation in the nonobese parturient is normal or increased. In contrast, Eng and coworkers[2] have reported maternal arterial oxygen pressure ($Pa{O_2}$) averages of 85 mm Hg in the morbidly obese parturient. The $Pa{O_2}$ does not inversely correlate with weight, so this hypoxemia may not be clinically significant in the merely *obese* parturient. These patients would, however, be at greater risk for respiratory compromise with opioid use or after abdominal surgery, as would the morbidly obese.

Cardiovascular

Obesity and pregnancy both increase cardiac output and total blood volume. Cardiac output in pregnancy increases 35% to 45% by term, and in the immediate postpartum period may be increased yet another 80% over prelabor values. Blood volume increases by about 35% to 40%. In obesity, the increase in blood volume is directly related to the additional body mass of adipose tissue, which contains a large vascular bed. This increase in blood volume results in a concomitant increase in stroke volume and cardiac output. Blood volume and cardiac output in the morbidly obese individual are twice that predicted for ideal body weight. Obesity often is accompanied by hypertension; the obese parturient is at greater risk for hypertension, as well as the syndrome of pregnancy-induced hypertension (PIH), than her nonobese counterpart.

Pregnancy in the nonobese individual produces a significant cardiac stress, and obesity compounds this stress; when the increased incidence of hypertension and hypercholesterolemia associated with obesity is added to the equation, it is not difficult to understand why cardiac factors alone would place the obese patient into the category of *high-risk parturient.*

Gastrointestinal

Liver and gall bladder disease occur more commonly in the obese patient. Obese individuals are likely to have larger gastric volumes and a lower pH, as well as reduced rates of gastric emptying, than nonobese individuals. The change in the angle of the gastroesophageal junction associated with pregnancy and further decreased gastric emptying compound the risk for aspiration in obese parturients.

Effects of Obesity on the Obstetric and Anesthetic Course

As discussed in the introductory paragraphs, obesity in pregnancy is not clearly or consistently defined. As a result, the effects of this condition on pregnancy and anesthetic outcome have been difficult to determine. Reports have shown an increased incidence rate of hypertension (20% versus 2%), PIH (7% versus 4.5%), and gestational diabetes (10.5% versus 1.5%) in obese compared with nonobese patients, respectively.[3] Obesity increases the risk of death in pregnancy: the increased incidence of thromboembolism, specifically pulmonary embolism, is the major contributor to this increase. Finally, obesity is associated with a greater incidence of cesarean delivery, primarily due to the greater incidence of repeat cesarean delivery. Furthermore, obesity is a risk factor for surgical complications unrelated to pregnancy.[4]

Summary

Pregnancy is associated with pulmonary, cardiac, and gastrointestinal changes related to, or resulting from, anatomic and physiologic changes necessitated by the growing fetus. These changes are more pronounced in the obese parturient since these systems are further stressed to accommodate the increased body mass. The obese gravida is more likely than the nonobese gravida to develop complications of pregnancy, and is more likely to have an operative delivery. These patients are at increased risk for postoperative and postpartum complications. Furthermore, as is discussed later in this chapter, the obese patient warrants aggressive intraoperative and postoperative management of pain and surgical stress to minimize the risk of complications.

Postoperative Pain and Its Management

Effects of Surgical Injury and Pain

Physiologic responses to surgical injury result in metabolic derangement and changes to the pulmonary, gastrointestinal, and cardiovascular systems. Abdominal surgery is associated with decreases in tidal volume, vital capacity, and FRC. The obese individual, who preoperatively demonstrated increased closing volumes and a decreased FRC with mild hypoxemia when in the supine position, now is at great risk for pulmonary decompensation and significant hypoxemia.

Tachycardia, increased peripheral vascular resistance, increased cardiac work, and increased myocardial oxygen consumption all occur and are related to the increased sympathetic activity associated with pain. In the parturient at risk for myocardial disease, this could result in myocardial ischemia. Pain control with intravenous or neuraxial opioids can minimize or eliminate these changes.

Increased sympathetic activity results in decreased gastric motility and increased gastric secretion. This may further slow recovery in the obese individual. The hypermetabolic response to the surgical insult is compounded by the stress of pain itself. Increased cortisol and epinephrine secretion occur. Furthermore, increased secretion of antidiuretic hormone and aldosterone leads to salt and water retention. Parenteral opioid analgesia may decrease this sympathetic response, and epidural analgesia may eliminate it.[5,6]

Management of Postcesarean Pain

Studies have shown that providing improved analgesia, which minimizes perioperative stress, will enhance clinical outcome.[7] This also is true for parturients with different cardiac or respiratory problems, as well patients with severe PIH. As discussed in the introduction, the goal of postcesarean analgesia is to provide efficacious, safe analgesia in a manner which interferes minimally with maternal-infant interactions.

Intraoperative anesthetic management will directly impact postoperative analgesia. Most cesarean deliveries in the United States, especially the nonemergency surgeries, are performed under regional anesthesia. This provides the opportunity to maximize the benefits of the technique by extending its use into the postoperative period. This is achieved by using a continuous catheter technique or by administering a long-acting opioid. Regional techniques also allow for optimal preemptive analgesia.

The underlying principle of preemptive analgesia is that therapeutic intervention is made in advance of the pain stimulus rather than in reaction to it. Maximum efficacy of treatment requires some therapy until peripheral stimuli have decreased as the result of wound healing.[8] Studies have shown that preincisional administration of local anesthetic to the wound,[9] administration of opioid (neuraxially or parenterally[10,11]), or administration of nonsteroidal antiinflammatory drugs (NSAIDs)[12] will result in less postoperative pain. Practically, parenteral opioids are not routinely administered to the parturient before delivery, to eliminate the potential of respiratory compromise in the newborn. However, wound infiltration and preincisional use of neuraxial opioids should be considered in cesarean delivery. The intraoperative neuraxial use of a lipophilic agent, specifically fentanyl, has been shown to produce a reduction in visceral discomfort during abdominal manipulation associated with cesarean delivery.[13] Preincisional compared with postincisional use also reduced postoperative pain and analgesic use.[10]

As mentioned earlier, the choice of postoperative analgesia is influenced by the intraoperative technique chosen. Spinal anesthesia for intraoperative management would permit the use of a single dose of spinal opioid or opioid combination, which would be followed by oral or parenteral analgesics. Spinal morphine provides postoperative pain relief for 16 to 24 hours when given in doses of 0.2 to 0.5 mg.[14,15] The onset of analgesia requires 45 to 60 minutes, so it should be coadministered with a more lipophilic agent to achieve a preemptive effect. Early onset of respiratory depression does not occur since the vascular absorption from this dose is minimal. Late-onset respiratory depression may occur at 6 to 10 hours after administration. Experience with doses of less than 0.5 mg intrathecal morphine showed reduced respiratory effects, making respiratory monitoring—other than routine vital signs—unnecessary in the healthy patient.[16] Subarachnoid or epidural morphine administration is associated with other nonrespiratory side effects: pruritus in the obstetric population has been reported to occur with an incidence rate of 40% to 90%, and nausea and vomiting occurs in 20% to 60% of patients

TABLE 21-1

POSTOPERATIVE ANALGESIC THERAPY

Route	Drug	Dose	Duration
Epidural	Morphine	SD: 3-5 mg	16-24 hr
		CI: 70 μg/ml at 8-10 ml/hr	—
	Meperidine	SD: 50 mg	5-6 hr
		CI: 10 μg/ml at 8-10 ml/hr	—
	Fentanyl	SD: 50 μg	3 hr
	Hydromorphone	SD: 1 mg	17 hr
		CI: 10 μg/min at 8-10 ml/hr	—
Subarachnoid	Morphine	0.2-0.5 mg	16-24 hr
	Meperidine	10 mg	5-6 hr
	Fentanyl	12.5-20 μg	3 hr
	Sufentanil	5-7.5 μg	3 hr
IV-PCA	Morphine	Dose: 1-1.5 mg Interval: 6 min 4-hr maximum: 30 mg	—
	Meperidine	Dose: 10-15 mg Interval: 6 min 4-hr maximum: 300 mg	—
IV	Ketorolac	Loading dose: 30 mg Maintenance: 15 mg every 6 hr	—
Oral	Meperidine	100-150 mg every 3-4 hr	—
	Ibuprofen	400-800 mg every 3-4 hr	—

SD, single dose; CI, continuous infusion; IV, intravenous; IV-PCA, intravenous patient-controlled analgesia.

receiving spinal morphine.[16] Table 21-1 summarizes recommended treatment for side effects of therapy.

Subarachnoid administration of other opioids also is efficacious in parturients. Fentanyl, in doses of 12.5 to 20 μg, and sufentanil, in doses of 5 to 7.5 μg, provide a short duration of postoperative analgesia with minimal side effects. Meperidine 10 mg provides rapid onset of action with a duration of 5 to 6 hours.

After resolution of their analgesic effect, administration of all subarachnoid opioids in the postpartum patients requires the additional use of systemic analgesics. Intravenous patient-controlled analgesia (IV-PCA) with opioids has been used safely and efficaciously[17,18] in this population, as have parenteral NSAIDs.[19] The duration of analgesia with morphine, and at times with meperidine, may extend beyond the period that the patient is taking nothing by mouth, after which oral analgesics can be used.

Analgesic options in patients who have epidural anesthesia for their cesarean delivery include a single epidural dose of the opioids discussed above, with the dose adjusted for epidural use. Morphine administered in doses of 3 to 5 mg, meperidine 50 mg, or fentanyl 50 μg, will all provide analgesia of similar duration as that discussed with subarachnoid administration. The incidence of side effects also is discussed earlier in the chapter. The presence of an indwelling catheter allows the use of continuous epidural analgesia for postoperative analgesia. In the afebrile patient, the catheter may be left in place for up to 5 days. The uncomplicated cesarean delivery patient, with a 3- to 5-day postoperative hospital course, could be maintained on epidural analgesia until the day before discharge, at which time the patient's analgesic requirements can easily be met using oral NSAIDs.

The advantages of continuous postoperative epidural analgesia in the patient undergoing abdominal surgery include superior analgesia, early ambulation, earlier return of bowel function, and less pulmonary embarrassment than in patients receiving parenteral opioid analgesia.[7] In the low-risk, uncomplicated, cesarean delivery patient, the added complexity of providing this therapy usually precludes its use. Most of these patients are managed with a single dose of epidural opioid followed by intravenous or oral analgesics as are needed. The high-risk patient, including the obese parturient, is at increased risk for postsurgical complications, which may be minimized by using continuous epidural analgesia. These patients can also benefit from the use of patient-controlled epidural analgesia, which allows a lower continuous infusion with the use of *on-demand* dosing by the patient.[20,21]

Opioid infusions, including morphine 60 μg/ml or meperidine 10 μg/ml, provide excellent analgesias when administered at rates of 8 to 10 ml/hr. These drugs are associated with a high incidence of nausea, vomiting, and pruritus, which may impact negatively on patient satisfaction if not treated aggressively. Hydromorphone at concentrations of 10 μg/ml infused at a rate of 8 to 10 ml/hr provides excellent postoperative epidural analgesia with minimal side effects.[21,22]

In patients in whom regional anesthesia for cesarean delivery is not used, and for some patients who still are not taking anything orally when the effects of the administered neuraxial opioid resolve, IV-PCA opioid therapy may be effectively used for postoperative analgesia.[18] The recommended dosage for IV-PCA with meperidine is 10 mg with a lockout of 6 minutes and a 4-hour maximum of 300 mg; and for morphine, 1 mg every 6 minutes with a 4-hour maximum of 30 mg. Compared with morphine, meperidine for IV-PCA may have a depressant effect on the infant if the mother is nursing.[23] These effects are likely related to normeperidine levels and resolve without sequelae.

To summarize, all patients who have regional anesthesia for their surgical procedure should be administered a neuraxial opioid for optimum postoperative analgesia. The healthy parturient needs no special monitoring and may be discharged to a floor with routine postpartum patients, providing the epidural dose of morphine is less than 5 mg, the subarachnoid dose less than 0.5 mg, or an opioid other than morphine is used. If the manpower and equipment are available, continuous opioid infusions may be used. After resolution of the spinal opioid effect, analgesia is provided with parenteral or oral opioids, or NSAIDs. If regional anesthesia is not used, IV-PCA opioid therapy should be used. Table 21-2 summarizes the analgesic options that have been described.

The high-risk parturient, who is at greater risk for postoperative complications, will benefit from aggressive pain management. This may reduce surgical stress and the complications associated with abdominal surgery. For these patients, continuous epidural analgesia may be beneficial, even in light of the labor-intensive nature of the therapy.

TABLE 21-2
RECOMMENDATIONS FOR TREATMENT OF SIDE EFFECTS

Side Effects	Treatment
Nausea and vomiting	Metoclopramide 10 mg IV every 6 hr Droperidol 0.625 mg IV every 6 hr Ondansetron 4 mg IV every 6 hr
Pruritus	Naloxone 40 μg IV then 400 μg/L infused in maintenance intravenous fluid Diphenhydramine 25-50 mg IV
Respiratory depression	Naloxone 40-80 μg IV, repeat as needed, decrease or discontinue dose of ongoing therapy

IV, Intravenously.

Summary

For the reasons already discussed:

The morbidly obese patient presented at the beginning of the chapter is at increased risk—when compared with the nonobese parturient—for postoperative complications.

Aggressive postoperative analgesia may decrease these complications.

A regional technique is the choice for both intraoperative and postoperative management of this patient.

I would elect to use a catheter technique, that is, epidural anesthesia, for this patient's perioperative management. Epidural anesthesia allows the intraoperative advantage of greater control of both the level and duration of anesthesia (see Chapter 44 for a more in-depth discussion of intraoperative management), and postoperatively, one can utilize a continuous analgesic infusion.

Epidural opioid analgesia with hydromorphone would be the choice for this patient. One milligram should be given as a bolus in combination with the anesthetic agent before incision. An infusion would be started immediately postoperatively using a 10-μg/ml hydromorphone solution administered at 10 ml/hr via the lumbar epidural catheter. This therapy will allow the patient to be pain free, or to have minimal incisional pain, permitting early mobilization and decreased postoperative complications. This obese patient is at increased risk for respiratory compromise secondary to both surgery and the opioid therapy. Respiratory rates should thus be assessed every 2 hours for the first 12 hours postoperatively, then every 4 hours while the epidural infusion is maintained. Intermittent pulse oximetry, with Spo_2 recorded every 4 hours, will also be performed, and supplemental oxygen administered as needed. Side effects of therapy, if they occur, will be aggressively treated, as recommended in Table 21-2. Intravenous access will be maintained until the epidural infusion is discontinued.

In the case of an uneventful postoperative course, the epidural infusion will be maintained until the second postoperative day. At this time, the patient should be taking a full diet and will be provided with ibuprofen 400 to 800 mg orally on an as-needed basis for analgesia. If postsurgical complications occur, necessitating a delay in the return to a regular diet or a delay in hospital discharge, the infusion can be maintained until the fourth postoperative day. At this time IV-PCA opioid can be used if oral analgesia is not indicated or is inadequate.

To conclude, postoperative analgesia in the obese postoperative parturient is optimally provided with a continuous infusion of an epidural opioid analgesia. Other options for analgesia include single-dose neuraxial opioids or IV-PCA therapy.

References

1. Edwards LE, Dickes WF, Alton IR, et al: Pregnancy in the massively obese: course, outcome, and obesity prognosis of the infant, *Am J Obstet Gynecol* 1978; 131:479.

2. Eng M, Butler J, Bonica J: Respiratory function in pregnant obese women, *Am J Obstet Gynecol* 1975; 123:241.
3. Garbaciak JA Jr, Richter M, Miller S, et al: Maternal weight and pregnancy complications, *Am J Obstet Gynecol* 1985; 152:238.
4. Fisher A, Waterhouse TD, Adams AP: Obesity: its relation to anaesthesia, *Anaesthesia* 1975; 30:633.
5. Blunnie WP, McIlroy PDA, Merrett JD, et al: Cardiovascular and biochemical evidence of stress during major surgery associated with different techniques of anaesthesia, *Br J Anaesth* 1983; 55:611.
6. Breslow MJ, Jordan DA, Christopherson R, et al: Epidural morphine decreases postoperative hypertension by attentuating sympathetic nervous system hyperactivity, *JAMA* 1989; 261:3577.
7. Rawal N, Sjostrand U, Christoffersson E, et al: Comparison of intramuscular and epidural morphine for postoperative analgesia in the grossly obese: influence on postoperative ambulation and pulmonary function, *Anesth Analg* 1984; 63:583.
8. Woolf CJ, Chong M-S: Preemptive analgesia: treating postoperative pain by preventing the establishment of central sensititzation, *Anesth Analg* 1993; 77:362.
9. Trotter TN, Hayes-Gregson P, Robinson S, et al: Wound infiltration of local anaesthetic after lower segment caesarean section, *Anaesthesia* 1991; 46:404.
10. Katz J, Kavanagh BP, Sandler An, et al: Preemptive analgesia: clinical evidence of neuroplasticity contributing to postoperative pain, *Anesthesiology* 1992; 77:439.
11. Dahl JB, Hansen BL, Hjortso NC, et al: Influence of timing on the effect of continuous extradural analgesia with bupivacaine and morphine after major abdominal surgery, *Br J Anaesth* 1992; 69:4.
12. Engel C, Lund B, Kristensen SS, et al: Indomethacin as an analgesic after hysterectomy, *Acta Anaesthesiol Scand* 1989; 33:498.
13. Ackerman WE, Juneja M, Colclough GW, et al: Epidural fentanyl significantly decreases nausea and vomiting during uterine manipulation in awake patients undergoing cesarean section, *Anesthesiology* 1988; 69:A651 (abstract).
14. Abboud TK, Dror A, Mosaad P, et al: Minidose intrathecal morphine for the relief of postcesarean section pain: safety, efficacy, and ventilatory responses to carbon dioxide, *Anesth Analg* 1988; 67:137.
15. Abouleish E, Rawal N, Fallon K, et al: Combined intrathecal morphine and bupivacaine for cesarean section, *Proc Soc Obstet Anesth Perinatol* 1987; 19:16.
16. Chadwick HS, Ready LB: Intrathecal and epidural morphine sulfate for postcesarean analgesias: a clinical comparison, *Anesthesiology* 1988; 68:925.
17. Rayburn WF, Geranis BJ, Ramadei CA, et al: Patient-controlled analgesia for postcesarean section pain, *Obstet Gynecol* 1988; 72:136.
18. Harrison DM, Sinatra R, Morgese L, et al: Epidural narcotic and patient-controlled analgesia for post-cesarean section pain relief, *Anesthesiology* 1988; 68:454.
19. Bush DJ: Diclofenac for analgesia after cesarean section, *Anaesthesia* 1992; 47:1075.
20. Yarnell RW, Polis T, Reid GN, et al: Patient-controlled analgesia with epidural meperidine after elective cesarean section, *Reg Anesth* 1992; 17:329.
21. Parker RK, White PF: Epidural patient-controlled analgesia: an alternative to intravenous patient-controlled analgesia for pain relief after cesarean delivery, *Anesth Analg* 1992; 75:245.
22. Chestnut DH, Choi WW, Isbell TJ: Epidural hydromorphone for postcesarean analgesia, *Obstet Gynecol* 1986; 68:65.
23. Wittels B, Scott DT, Sinatra RS: Exogenous opioids in human breast milk and acute neonatal neurobehavior: a preliminary study, *Anesthesiology* 1990; 73:864.

22

Postdural Puncture Headache

A 25-year-old primigravida has an accidental dural tap while an epidural catheter is being placed for cesarean delivery. The catheter is relocated to another space and the rest of the procedure is uneventful. Twenty-four hours after delivery, the patient complains of a severe headache on arising from bed. It markedly improves as soon as she lies down. The obstetrician requests an anesthetic consultation.

Recommendations by Brian King, M.D., Ph.D.
William Camann, M.D.

The above case describes the typical symptoms seen in postdural puncture headache (PDPH), a frequent complication of accidental dural puncture and a less frequent complication of spinal anesthetics in obstetric populations. This chapter reviews PDPH and then considers the specific case.

History and Pathophysiology

August Bier first described PDPH in 1898 when he and an assistant, Dr. Hildebrandt, performed spinal anesthetics on each other.[1] Dr. Bier reportedly felt fine until the next afternoon when he began to develop the pounding headache and dizziness on arising, symptoms that are now known as hallmarks of PDPH. His symptoms forced him to remain bedridden for 9 days. Dr. Hildebrandt also experienced 3 to 4 days of headaches, malaise, nausea, and vomiting. Dr. Bier's hypothesis that the cause of their problems was a slow leak of cerebrospinal fluid (CSF) through a dural tear is virtually unchanged nearly 100 years later. Supporting studies have shown that CSF pressure is reduced in PDPH patients.[2,3] Furthermore, drainage of 20 ml of CSF from volunteers elicits a postural headache whereas its replacement with an equal volume of saline, or tilting to the horizontal position, relieves the headache.[4] Brownridge has hypothesized that loss of CSF volume through a dural tear causes traction on pain-sensitive intracranial structures with referral of pain to the frontal region via the trigeminal nerve and to the occipital region via the vagus and glossopharyngeal nerves.[5] Since intracranial volume must remain constant, loss of CSF volume and pressure also can lead to cerebral vasodilation, producing migraine-like pain.[6]

Clinical Presentation

Usually PDPH occurs after purposeful (spinal anesthetic or lumbar puncture) or accidental (during epidural catheter placement) puncture of the dura, although spontaneous dural tears have been reported. The defining feature of PDPH is a severe pounding headache that gets worse with standing and is relieved with recumbancy. As described in the landmark study of spinal anesthesia by Vandam and Dripps, the pain typically begins in the occipital area and spreads to the frontal area.[7] It also may spread to the neck and shoulders. Nausea and vomiting, blurred vision, diplopia, and auditory changes are less-common symptoms. Although PDPH can present soon after dural puncture, it most commonly presents 1 to 3 days later. Afflicted patients tend to stay in bed; the headache resolves spontaneously in 7 days in 70% of patients and in 6 weeks in 95% of patients. Data originally showed that PDPH is most common in young women, but this may be due to the fact that many young women who receive neuraxial anesthesia are laboring patients in whom the increased intraabdominal pressure might be expected to increase any CSF leak. Furthermore, postpartum patients become volume depleted due to blood loss and diuresis, which can reduce CSF production.

Postpartum Headache

Headache is a common occurrence in postpartum women, even when the dura is not touched. Grove followed 187 primigravida women who delivered without epidural or spinal analgesia for up to 6 days after delivery and found that 22% of spontaneous deliveries and 25% of forceps deliveries were followed by headache.[8] At the same hospital, in a different series in which 6% of PDPH followed accidental dural puncture, the incidence rate was 19% in patients who had epidural analgesia. The postural nature of PDPH usually can differentiate PDPH from other causes of headache (Table 22-1), but care must be taken to avoid misdiagnosis of other potentially disastrous causes.

Prevention

Recent years have seen dramatic decreases in the incidence of PDPH after spinal anesthesia due to appreciation of the effects of needle size and needle tip design. As is expected, a smaller needles makes a smaller dural hole and results in fewer patients with PDPH. This was clearly shown by Vandam and Dripps[7] and subsequently has been confirmed by many other investigators.[9,10] The effects of changing the needle tip design are less intuitive. Figure

TABLE 22-1
DIFFERENTIAL DIAGNOSIS OF POSTPARTUM HEADACHE

Infectious
Meningitis
Sinusitis
Circulatory
Cerebral hemorrhage (subdural, subarachnoid)
Cerebral infarction (cortical vein thrombosis)
Hypertensive (preeclampsia)
Migraine
Metabolic
Hormonal imbalance
Hypoglycemia
Electrolyte imbalance
Psychogenic (postpartum)
Other (e.g., tumor)

22-1 shows three commonly available tip designs for spinal needles. The Quincke needle is a cutting needle that is associated with a much higher rate of PDPH than either the Sprotte or Whitacre needles, which both have pencil-point designs. This is likely due to slow healing of the cut dural fibers after Quincke needle insertion. Pencil-point (blunt) tip needles can pass between dural fibers without cutting them, enabling the dural rent to seal more quickly after needle removal.[11] At our institution, the incidence rate of PDPH after spinal anesthesia using a 25-gauge Whitacre needle in pregnant patients is about 0.8%, a remarkably low figure.[12]

Other manipulations of spinal needles have been tried to minimize PDPH. These include entering the dura at an angle, such as with a paramedian approach, which results in a longer, more easily closed rent in the dura and overlapping holes in the dura and arachnoid membranes.[13,14] Some data show that inserting the bevel of a cutting needle, such as a Quincke needle, parallel to the longitudinal axis of the dura reduces the incidence of PDPH.[15,16] This is hypothesized to be due to a smaller, more easily closed hole in the dura since the dural fibers run longitudinally. Furthermore, using pencil-point spinal needles eliminates bevel direction as a concern.

Accidental puncture of the dura with a large-bore epidural needle is associated with about a 75% incidence rate of PDPH in obstetric patients.[17] A few steps can help avoid *wet taps.* Naturally, the needle should be advanced slowly while recognizing that the ligaments in parturients can present less resistance to the needle than in nonpregnant pa-

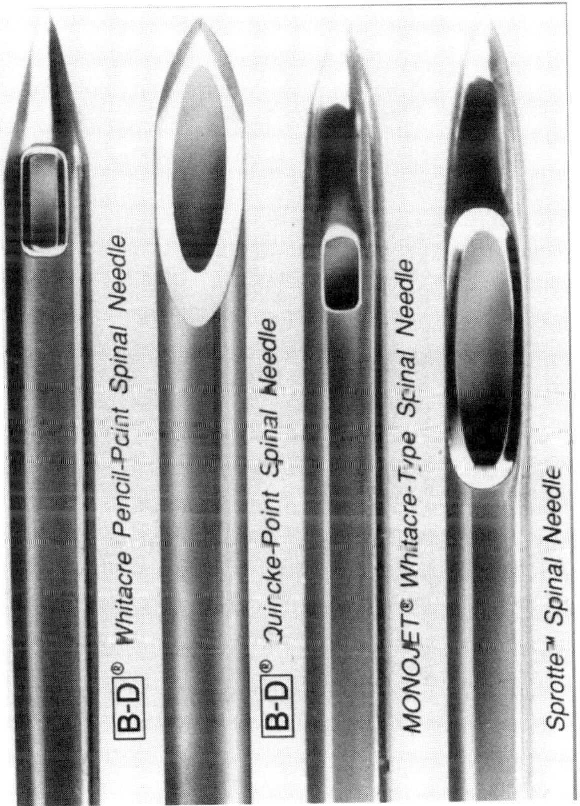

Fig. 22-1.
Spinal needle designs currently in use.

tients. If the needle has been advanced a considerable distance without a stylet and without finding a loss of resistance, the stylet should be inserted again before further advancement to dislodge any tissue that may be clogging the needle. Finally, avoid twisting the needle to change the bevel direction once a loss of resistance has been found. If a *wet tap* occurs, the epidural catheter should be placed at a different interspace with the catheter directed away from the dural puncture; this prevents the local anesthetic from entering the CSF, and thus produces the clinical features of spinal anesthesia rather than epidural anesthesia. Alternatively, a catheter could be purposefully placed into the subarachnoid space and the procedure continued using a continuous spinal anesthetic technique. Using a spinal catheter in this setting does not reduce the incidence of PDPH in parturients.[18] The value of prophylactic blood patches is discussed later.

Traditionally, patients were required to rest in bed for up to a day after dural puncture in the hope that PDPH could be avoided. However, recent studies have shown that avoidance of early ambulation is not preventative for PDPH and actually may increase the chance of undesired problems such as deconditioning and deep vein thrombosis.[19,20]

Treatment

Usually PDPH is self-limited and resolves spontaneously with only conservative treatment, in less than a week in most cases. Conservative therapy consists of bed rest, moderate hydration, and nonsteroidal antiinflammatory agents. The value of bed rest is to keep the headache under control until the dural rent, which is causing it, is repaired; hydration helps to increase CSF pressure and volume. Although a number of other treatments have been advocated for patients for whom conservative therapy of PDPH has failed, the most common alternative treatments are caffeine, epidural saline infusion, and epidural blood patch.

Caffeine

Caffeine has long been known to constrict cerebral blood vessels, and in fact it was once used as a treatment for migraine headaches.[21] A number of studies have shown that intravenous caffeine sodium benzoate can relieve PDPH, at least transiently. The mechanism is likely via constriction of cerebral blood vessels that have been dilated by decreased CSF pressure. Sechzer and Abel performed a double-blind, placebo-controlled study of caffeine sodium benzoate 500 mg (equivalent to 250 mg of caffeine base) and found that 15 of 20 of patients treated with caffeine had relief with a single dose, compared with 3 of 21 patients treated with placebo.[22] Camann et al. compared oral doses of 300 mg caffeine base with placebo in 40 postpartum PDPH patients; they found improvement in 18 of 20 caffeine-treated patients and in 12 of 20 placebo-treated patients.[23] However, 24 hours later no difference existed between groups, suggesting, as other studies have done, that the beneficial effect of caffeine is transient in many patients. To our knowledge, no study of repeated doses of caffeine over the course of several days has been done, but this may be limited by side effects from excessive caffeine intake. The caffeine content of some common products is shown in Table 22-2. A preliminary study indicates that a single dose of an oral theophylline preparation (Theodure, 200 mg) may offer longer lasting relief than caffeine therapy.[24]

Epidural Saline Infusion

Continuous or intermittent infusion of saline into the epidural space has been used as a treatment of PDPH with variable results. It is likely that epidural saline transiently decreases the transdural pressure gradient and thereby reduces CSF leak. However, other mechanisms may be involved since Usubiaga and co-workers found that the increase in epidural pressures after the injection of 10 to 20 ml of saline lasted only 3 to 10 minutes.[25] One

TABLE 22-2

Caffeine in Some Common Products

Product	Mg of Caffeine Base
Coffee (5 oz)	
Freeze-dried	66
Percolated	107
Drip grind	142
Tea (5 oz)	
Black	47
Green	32
Coca Cola (12 oz)	65
Pepsi Cola (12 oz)	43
Mountain Dew (12 oz)	55
No Doz tablets (each)	100
Vivarin tablets (each)	200

group has found that the prophylactic bolus of epidural saline can significantly reduce the incidence of PDPH in patients with accidental dural puncture,[26] but another group found no difference between treated and untreated patients.[27] In the two studies in which epidural saline bolus was compared with epidural blood patch, the blood patch was significantly more effective and was equally safe.[28,29] Therefore epidural saline boluses should not be used in the treatment of PDPH unless there is a reason to avoid an epidural blood patch, such as bacteremia or viremia.

Epidural Blood Patch

James Gormley, an anesthesiologist in Pennsylvania, noticed that bloody spinal taps were associated with a lower incidence of PDPH and hypothesized that the blood can patch the hole in the dura. He tested this in a patient with PDPH after spinal anesthesia for varicose vein stripping. Four days after the surgery, he performed a lumbar puncture at the same intervertebral space and found a pressure of about zero. The patient's headache was relieved after Dr. Gormley injected 15 ml of saline intrathecally. He then withdrew the needle into the epidural space and injected 2 ml of the patient's blood. The patient's headache did not return. Dr. Gormley then cured six of six *spinal headaches,* including one in himself, using this technique.[30]

The most common technique for performing epidural blood patches was introduced by DiGiovanni and Dunbar in 1970.[31] After prehydration with up to 1 L of Ringer's solution and the epidural injection of 10 ml of autologous blood, 41 of 45 PDPH patients had permanent relief of their headaches. Other than a mild, transient backache, there were no complications of the procedure and epidural blood patch was established as the treatment of choice for PDPH. The success rate has been shown in multiple studies to be greater than 90%.[32]

It seems likely that the immediate relief of headache pain experienced by patients having an epidural blood patch is related to the increase in CSF pressure caused by the increased epidural space volume. Thus the immediate mechanism is the same as in patients receiving an epidural saline bolus. Whereas the increase in pressure with saline is very transient, however, the increase with blood in the epidural space is more prolonged, with the subarachnoid pressure remaining at 70% of peak 20 minutes after injection of blood. The cellular and colloidal components of blood are much less likely than saline to escape the epidural space. Rosenberg and Heavner studied dog dura in vitro and found that injection of blood actually may force blood through the dural tear, forming a clot plug that can resist the increased pressure of CSF experienced by the lumbar dura when a patient sits or stands.[33]

Since it is known that at least 70% of patients with a *wet tap* by an epidural needle will develop PDPH, a number of trials of prophylactic blood

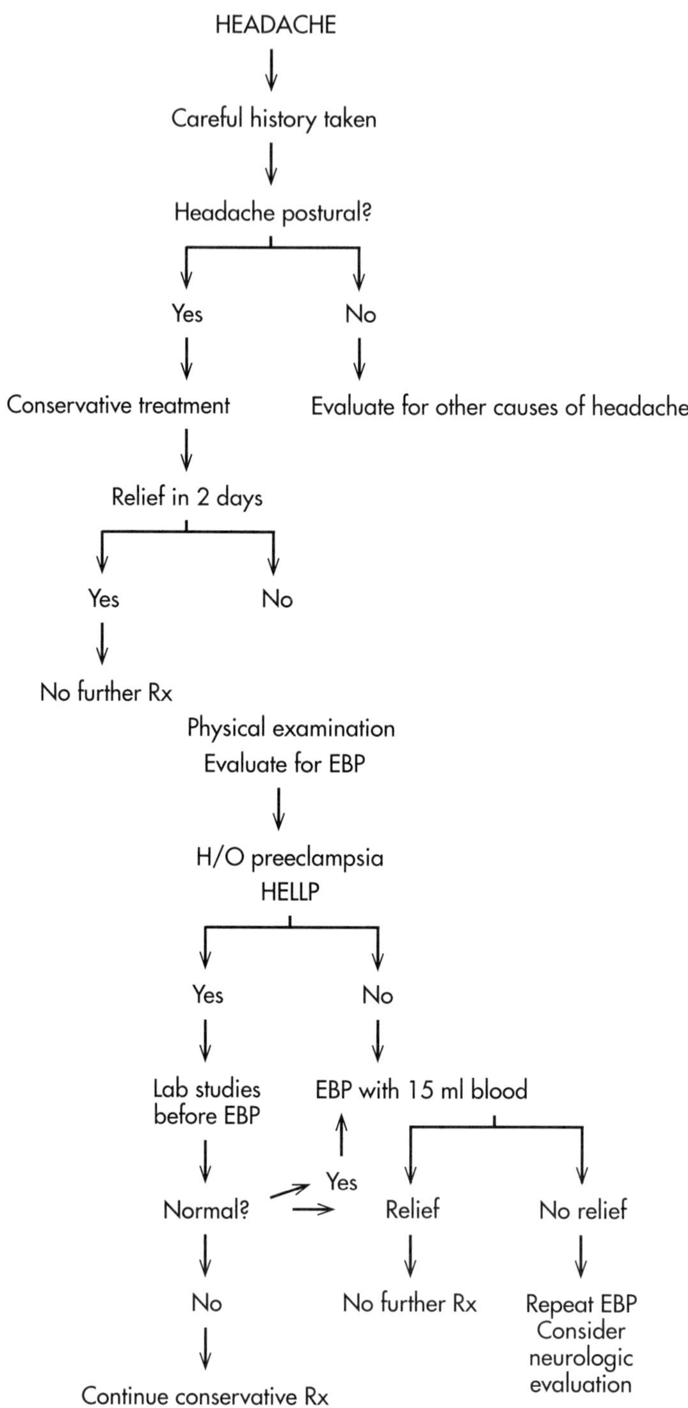

Fig. 22-2.

Care of headache in obstetric patients.

patches have been done. Unfortunately the results are widely variable. This may be partially related to the findings of Loeser and co-workers.[34] They found a 96% success rate of epidural blood patches when performed on PDPH patients more than 24 hours after the dural puncture, but only a 29% success rate when performed at less than 24 hours. Thus, immediately performing a blood patch after a dural puncture may not seal the dural rent. Colonna-Romano and Shapiro performed prophylactic blood patches in obstetric patients 2 to 14 hours after unintentional dural puncture and were able to decrease the incidence rate of PDPH from 80% to 21% by injecting 15 ml of blood.[35] In contrast, Palahniuk and Cumming failed to prevent PDPH with 5 to 10 ml of epidural blood.[36] It is likely that both time from dural puncture and volume of blood injected have effects on the efficacy of prophylactic epidural blood patches. If the obstetric patient has a successful epidural placement after an unintentional dural puncture, it may be useful to leave the catheter in place for a day and then inject blood just before removing the catheter. Some authors argue against this technique, because the chance of infection is high when blood is injected through a catheter that has been in position for a long time. The ideal blood volume for treatment of PDPH has been studied by Szeinfeld and co-workers, who used an imaging technique and 10 patients to conclude that 12 to 15 ml of blood is ideal.[37] Obviously, there is bound to be individual variability so that one should inject blood until the patient feels discomfort in the back or legs

The safety of epidural blood patches was once of great concern. When the technique first became popular, there was concern about side effects, ranging from permanent neurologic sequelae to closed epidural spaces, making later epidural catheter insertion impossible. It is now apparent that the technique is very safe in both the short and long term when not performed in patients with contraindications.[38,39] Contraindications are septicemia or bacteremia, local infection in the area of the back to be injected, bleeding tendencies due to platelets or clotting factors, and active neurologic disease. Back pain is the most common side effect, occurring in most patients. Radicular pain, transient temperature elevation, and neck pain occur with an incidence rate of 1% to 12%.

Summary

The 25-year-old primigravida with a headache, introduced at the beginning of this chapter, would be best treated with the following:

1. Conservative treatment should be given initially, once a thorough history-taking makes the problem likely to be PDPH.
2. With 2 days of bed rest and fluids, perhaps with caffeine-containing fluids such as coffee and cola, her symptoms may resolve.
3. If the headache persists, she should be reevaluated for an epidural blood patch. Fig. 22-2 shows a flow chart that can be useful in evaluating these patients.
4. An emergency autologous blood patch may be indicated in the presence of severe headache with nausea and vomiting, diplopia related to abducen nerve streching, or hearing loss due to streching of the auditory nerve.

References

1. Bier A: Versuche Ober Concaineisirung des ruckenmarkers, *Deutsche Z Chirugie* 1899; 51.361.
2. Dodd JE, Effid RC, Rauck Rl: Cerebral blood flow changes with caffeine therapy in postdural puncture headache, *Anesthesiology* 1989; 71:A679 (abstract).
3. Miyakawa Y, Meyer JS, Ishihara N, et al: Effect of cerebrospinal fluid removal on cerebral blood flow and metabolism in the baboon, *Stroke* 1977; 8P:346.
4. Kunkle EC, Ray BSd, Wolff HG: Experimental studies on

headache: analysis of the headache associated with changes in intracranial pressure, *Arch Neurol* 1943; 49:323.
5. Brownridge P: The management of headache following accidental dural puncture in obstetric patients, *Anaesth Intensive Care* 1983; 11:4.
6. Hattingh J, McCalden JA: Cerebrovascular effect of cerebrospinal fluid removal, *S Afr Med J* 1978; 54:780.
7. Vandam LD, Dripps RD: Long term followup of patients who received 10,098 spinal anesthetics, *JAMA* 1956; 61:586.
8. Grove LH: Backache, headache and bladder dysfunction after delivery, *Br J Anaesth* 1973; 45:1147.
9. Phillips OC, Ebner H, Nelson AT, Black MH: Neurologic complications following spinal anesthesia with lidocaine: prospective review of 10,440 cases, *Anesthesiology* 1969; 30:284.
10. White FH, Rodt SA, Vannes J, et al: Postdural puncture headache using 26 or 29 gauge needles in young patients, *Reg Anesth* 1988; 11:5.
11. Campbell DC, Douglas MJ, Pavy TJG, et al: Comparison of the 25 gauge Whitacre with the 24 gauge Sprotte spinal needle, *Can J Anaesth* 1993; 40:1131.
12. Hurley RJ, Hertwig LM, Lambert DH: Incidence of postdural puncture headache in the obstetric patient: 25 gauge Whitacre vs. 26 and 27 gauge Quincke tip needles, *Reg Anesth* 1992; 17:3S-90.
13. Hatfalve BI: The dynamics of post-spinal headache, *Headache* 1977; 17:64.
14. Ash WH: Lateral approach for spinal anesthesia, *Anesthesiology* 1955; 16:455.
15. Mihic D: Postpinal headache and relationship of needle bevel to longitudinal dural fibers, *Reg Anesth* 1985; 10:76.
16. Norris MC, Leighton BL, DeSimone CA: Needle bevel direction and headache after inadvertent dural puncture, *Anesthesiology* 1989; 70:729.
17. Hodgkinson R: Total spinal block after epidural injection into an interspace adjacent to an inadvertent dural puncture, *Anesthesiology* 1981; 55:593.
18. Norris MC, Leighton BL: Continuous spinal anesthesia after unintentional dural puncture in parturients, *Reg Anesth* 1990; 15:285.
19. Thormberry EA, Thomas TA: Posture and postdural puncture headache: a controlled trial in 80 obstetric patients, *Br J Anaesth* 1988; 60:195.
20. Vilming ST, SHarder H, Monstad I: Post lumbar puncture headache: the significance of body posture, *Cephalgia* 1988; 8:75.
21. Denker PG: The effects of caffeine on cerebrospinal fluid pressure, *Am J Med Sci* 1931; 181:675.
22. Sechzer PH, Abel L: Post spinal anesthesia headache treated with caffeine: evaluation with demand method (I), *Curr Ther Res* 1978; 24:307.
23. Camann WR, Murray RS, Mushlin PS, Lambert DH: Effects of oral caffeine on post dural puncture headache: a double blind, placebo controlled trial, *Anesth Analg* 1990; 70:181.
24. Swalbe SS, Schiffmiller MW, Marx GF: Theophylline for post dural puncture headache, *Anesthesiology* 1991; 75: A1082.
25. Usubiaga JE, Usubiaga LE, Brea LM, et al: Effect of saline injections on epidural and subarachnoid pressures and relation to post spinal anesthesia headache, *Anesth Analg* 1967; 46:293.
26. Crawford JS: The prevention of headache consequent upon dural puncture, *Br J Anaesth* 1972; 44:598.
27. Santos DJ, Barrett J, Lachia R, et al: Efficacy of epidural saline patch in preventing post dural headache, *Reg Anesth* 1986; 11:42 (abstract).
28. Bart AJ, Wheeler AS: Comparison of epidural saline placement and epidural blood patch in the treatment of post lumbar headache, *Anesthesiology* 1978; 48:221.
29. Trivedi NS, Eddi D, Shevde K: Prevention of headache following inadvertent dura puncture, *Reg Anesth* 1989; 14:51.
30. Gormely JB: Treatment of post spinal headache, *Anesthesiology* 1960; 21:565.
31. DiGiovanni AJ, Dunbar BS: Epidural injections of autologous blood for post lumbar puncture headache, *Anesth Analg* 1970; 49:268.
32. Crawford JS: Experience with epidural blood patch, *Anaesthesia* 1980; 35:513.
33. Rosenberg PH, Heavner JE: An In-vitro study of the effect of epidural blood patch on leakage through a dural puncture, *Anesth Analg* 1985; 64:501.
34. Loeser EA, Hill GE, Bennet GM: Time vs. success rate for epidural blood patch, *Anesthesiology* 1978; 49:147.
35. Colonna-Romano P, Shapiro BE: Unintentional dural puncture and prophylactic epidural blood patch in obstetrics, *Anesth Analg* 1989; 69:522.

36. Palahnuik RJ, Cumming M: Prophylactic blood patch does not prevent post lumbar puncture headache, *Can Anaesth Soc J* 1979; 26:132.
37. Szeinfeld M, Ihmeidan IH, Moser MM, et al: Epidural blood patch: evaluation of the volume and spread of blood injected into the epidural space, *Anesthesiology* 1986; 64:820.
38. Tarkkila PJ, Mirales JA, Palomaki EA: The subjective complications and efficacy of the epidural blood patch in the treatment of postdural puncture headache, *Reg Anesth* 1989; 14:247.
39. Carrie LES: Postdural puncture headache and extradural blood patch, *Anaesthesia* 1993; 71:179.

23

Neurologic Complications

A 32-year-old primigravida at term has an uneventful epidural analgesia for labor and delivery. At 24 hours after delivery, the patient complains of the inability to flex her left foot (foot drop) and hypoesthesia on the outer side of the left calf. Her obstetrician requests an anesthetic consultation. How would you evaluate the patient and make the differential diagnosis?

Recommendations by Kenneth W. Gerard, M.D., Ph.D.

Fortunately there was a time when babies were delivered without the use of a regional anesthetic, or one might think that all nerve damage was related to a regional anesthetic done during childbirth. Certainly, one might think that anesthesiologists would be at greater risk for malpractice claims for nerve damage in obstetrics with the increasing use of regional anesthesia. In fact, only 15% of all claims evaluated in the American Society of Anesthesiologists Closed Claims Study Database were for nerve damage.[1] In addition, only 8% of all claims that were made in obstetric anesthesia were related to nerve damage[2] (all of these cases were not related to regional anesthesia). Surprisingly, minor neurologic complications such as headache and backache represented 12% and 5% of the obstetric claims, respectively. Although the vast majority of neurologic complications in obstetric anesthesia are not related to anesthesia, it is important to be able to carefully evaluate and assist in an investigation into a neurologic complication. As an obstetrician previously stated, patients have a tendency to believe that their backaches or other discomforts are dated from and directly due to a previous spinal or block anesthesia. If a case of foot drop or paralysis occurs and the patient has received regional anesthesia, this will probably be accepted as the cause by the patient.[3]

Central Nervous System Complications

Neurologic complications that relate to regional anesthesia and obstetrics can be divided into two broad categories, central and peripheral. Central disorders tend to require more rapid treatment since the central nervous system has essentially no ability to regenerate after trauma. The peripheral nervous system can regenerate after injury at a rate of about 1 mm/day as long as the cell body is spared.[4,5] A partial list of various neurologic complications and their incidences is found in Table 23-1.

Headache

The most common complication after regional anesthesia is a postdural puncture headache, which generally does not require emergency treatment.[6] However, it should not be confused with rare but potential fatal causes for headache such as subdural hematoma, intracranial tumor, or subarachnoid bleeds.[7-9] In addition, cortical vein thrombosis (throbbing headache unrelated to position) and sinusitis are additional reasons for headache that need to be excluded.[10] (See Chapter 22 for a more complete discussion concerning postdural puncture headaches.)

Spinal Cord Compression and Ischemia

Spinal cord ischemia can be due to either a mass effect on the spinal cord or a loss of blood flow to the cord. Epidural abscesses and hematomas, lumbar disc protrusions, and tumors all can exhibit mass effects on the spine, but will vary in the rapidity of onset and severity of symptoms. In addition, presentation will depend on the region of the spinal cord that is compressed.

The spinal cord contains an H-shaped gray matter that is essentially comprised of cell bodies and synapses. The gray matter is surrounded by white matter, which contains ascending and descending fiber pathways. The sensory (ascending) pathways are both crossed and uncrossed in the spinal cord. Pain and temperature fibers enter the spinal cord and cross almost immediately to the other side of the cord to ascend to the brain. Proprioception and stereognosis remain on the same side of the spinal cord until they reach the brain stem and then cross over to the contralateral side. Fine touch is both crossed and uncrossed in the spinal cord, and results in its preservation in unilateral lesions of the spinal cord due to the maintenance of its pathways.

Motor fibers of the corticospinal pathway (descending) are simpler, crossing at the level of the brain stem and the spinal cord. The motor pathway is composed of two neurons that synapse in the anterior horn of the spinal cord. The upper motor neuron is from the brain cortex to the anterior horn. Lesions at this level result in spastic paralysis and hyperreflexia without fibrillations, fasciculations, or muscle atrophy. The lower motor neuron originates from the anterior horn and exits the spinal cord. Defects in the lower motor neurons result in flaccid paralysis, hyporeflexia, fasciculations, fibrillations, muscle atrophy, and the loss of the Babinski reflex.[11]

Back Pain

Back pain, or backache, is a symptom that is common to several serious complications that deserve prompt evaluation. More serious complications such as spinal epidural hematoma, abscess, tumor, and prolapsed discs can present with back pain. In addition, back pain can be unrelated to the spine and represent another medical emergency such as a dissecting aneurysm.[12]

Back pain is a common feature in pregnancy, with nearly 40% to 50% of all pregnant patients reporting some degree of back discomfort before delivery.[13] Sacroiliac joint dysfunction was the most common finding in patients with low back

TABLE 23-1

Incidence of Complications

Complication	Incidence	Percentage	Per/10,000	Reference
Central				
Cortical vein thrombosis	1-2/6000		3.3	Younker et al.[10]
Intradural tumors	0.3-1/10,000		0.3-1	Martin et al.[87]
Low back pain due to tumor		0.66	66	Martin et al.[87]
Epidural needle nerve trauma		0.07	7	Usubiaga[29]
Nerve trauma with spinal needle		0.04-0.89	40-89	Vandam and Dripps,[30] Phillips et al.[31]
Spinal/epidural abscess unrelated to anesthesia	1.96/10,000		1.96	Hlavin et al.[42]
Backache with epidural anesthesia	8/100		800	MacArthur et al.[18]
Lumbar disc herniation	1/10,000		1	Simon et al.[24]
Subarachnoid hemorrage (during pregnancy)	1-2/10,000		1-2	Donaldson[7]
Unrecognized dural puncture		0.2	20	Dawkins[88]
Epidural vein damage during epidural placement		3-9	300-900	Sage[35]
Spinal hemorrhage after lumbar puncture in anticoagulated patients		0.35	35	Owens et al.[36]
Peripheral				
Paresthesias and motor dysfunction	18.9/10,000		18.9	Ong et al.[89]
Femoral nerve palsies	2.8/100,000		0.28	Vargo et al.[80]
Lateral femoral cutaneous nerve	1.4/100,000		0.14	Vargo et al.[80]
Lumbosacral cord	1/2600		3.8	Hill[3]

pain, with the discomfort persisting up to 1 year after delivery.[14] Back pain always has been difficult to evaluate, and clinical studies reflect the same difficulty.

Patients who delivered without an anesthetic indicated the presence of backache, headache, and bladder dysfunction in 40%, 22%, and 14% of patients respectively, after delivery.[15] In addition, the number of patients with backache decreased to 25% and bladder dysfunction increased to 38% if forceps were used. All three complications commonly are associated with regional anesthesia, yet none of these patients had a regional anesthetic. Studies with small numbers of patients have not been able to demonstrate a relationship between backache and epidurals.[16] One prospective study of 855 women found back pain occurred during pregnancy in 49% of women, and the pain resolved within 6 months after delivery.[17] Also, patients with recurrent back pain from previous pregnancies continued to have pain up to 18 months after delivery.

Certainly the administration of regional anesthesia complicates the evaluation of postpartum back pain because there is the tendency for all back discomfort and headaches to be related to a previous regional anesthetic. A retrospective evaluation of 11,701 postpartum women indicated that there was new backache in 14%, which persisted for up to 1 year in 10% of women.[18] Postpartum backache occurred in 18.9% of the patients who received epidurals versus 10.5% of patients who delivered without an epidural. It was concluded that epidural anesthetics for labor that progressed to either delivery or cesarean section caused an increase in backache due to a stressed posture during labor. In comparison, patients who had epidural catheters placed for elective cesarean sections had significantly less backache. Perhaps this was related to the more concentrated local anesthetics used during this study. Additional muscle relaxation could have permitted postures that put additional strain on the back joints. A small retrospective study has challenged this conclusion by evaluating the risk of backache in women who had manual extraction of the placenta with either general or epidural anesthesia.[19] These circumstances resulted in 33% of women with backache in the epidural group and only 6% (one patient) with backache in the general anesthetic group. Since general anesthesia often is administered to promote uterine relaxation for placental extraction, this may simply reflect a more difficult placental extraction in the epidural group. Interestingly, in a follow-up article, the large retrospective study of 11,701 patients reported that the same epidural patients also have slightly more headaches, neckaches, migraines, and tingling in the hands and fingers.[20] This seems to support the suggestion that patients attribute unusual symptoms to epidural anesthesia.

Ultimately, additional prospective studies are needed to determine the relationship of backache with epidural anesthesia. However, it can be concluded that backache is common after delivery, and when an epidural is used for analgesia, patients may push harder, have their legs and back in unusual positions, and have more difficult procedures done that may not be possible in patients without this form of analgesia. Consequently, epidural anesthesia could indirectly contribute to back pain in the postpartum patient.

Chloroprocaine and Backache

Epidural chloroprocaine can be the cause of severe, deep burning and aching back pain after the administration of the current formulation, which contains disodium ethylenediaminetetraacetic acid (EDTA). EDTA replaced sodium bisulfite and methylparaben in 1987 because of the concerns that these preservatives were potential neurotoxins. The EDTA-containing solution has been demonstrated to cause backaches in volunteers and patients when used in large doses.[21,22] Back pain did not persist beyond 24 hours and was relieved with 100 to 150 μg of epidural fentanyl. Further study has demonstrated that volumes of greater than 25 ml of chloroprocaine containing EDTA resulted in significantly more backache than similar volumes of chloroprocaine with methylparaben.[23] Interestingly, alkalinization of chloroprocaine resulted in a 50% reduction of the number of patients who had back pain. Chloroprocaine for emergency cesarean sections still should be considered after alkalinization and in volumes of 25 ml or less. Personal experience with these restrictions has not produced any adverse effects.

Disc Herniation

The frequency of disc herniation during pregnancy is about 1 in 10,000.[24] Lumbar disc protrusions are the most common: 95% occur at the levels of L4-5 and L5-S1.[25] Most of the protrusions (60% to 85%) are posterolateral and result in symptoms of low backache and leg pain on the side of the disc herniation. Straining, coughing, or sneezing can aggravate the pain. Paresthesias and muscular weakness can occur with numbness over the affected dermatome (Table 23-2). Straight leg raising will stretch the nerve root over the herniated disc and reproduce the pain. Spasm of the erector spine muscle often is present and tender to palpation. In addition, spasm can cause loss of the lordotic curvature that is normally present. Disc protrusions have been reported to occur during pregnancy for the first time, and preexisting disc protrusions have been exacerbated during pregnancy.[26] Lastly, hormonal factors responsible for pelvic joint changes have been suggested to predispose pregnant women to disc bulging and herniation. Magnetic resonance imaging of 45 pregnant and 41 nonpregnant patients revealed disc bulging or herniation in 53% of pregnant and 54% of nonpregnant patients. This suggests that disc abnormalities are common in women of child-bearing years and probably not associated with hormonal changes associated with pregnancy.[27]

Nerve Trauma

Direct trauma to the spinal cord after spinal or epidural anesthesia is rare, especially if epidural or lumbar puncture is made below the conus medullaris. The spinal cord terminates in infants at the third lumbar vertebra, and rises during childhood to end between the first and second lumbar in 60% of adults or higher in 30% of adults. However, the spinal cord may remain extended to the third lumbar vertebra in as many as 10% of adults. Lastly, the spinal cord is largest at the levels of the brachial plexus (C5-T1) and the sacral plexus (L4-S3), narrowing the epidural space.[28] Consequently performing epidural punctures below the level of the second lumbar vertebra and spinal punctures below the third lumbar vertebra significantly increases the safety of the procedure. Certainly, epidural catheters are placed in the thoracic and cervical regions routinely in some institutions. This would not be a common practice if regular nerve trauma occurred. Nerve root trauma has been reported to occur in about 0.07% of patients after epidural anesthesia.[29]

TABLE 23-2
Neurologic Signs with Lumbar Disc Protrusions

Level	Reflex	Pain	Weakness	Sensory
L3-4	Knee jerk	Low back, upper sciatic, thigh, knee	Quadriceps(L2,3,4), Adductors(L2,3,4) (except adductor magnus)	L4
L4-5	Medial hamstring	Low back, sciatic distribution	Extensor hallucis longus (L5-S1)	L5
L5-S1	Ankle jerk	Low back, sciatic distribution	Soleus(S1-2) Gluteus maximus(L5,S1,2)	S1

Modified from Bakay L: *Neurosurgery.* In Nardi GL, Zuidema GD, editors: *Surgery: essentials of clinical practice,* Boston, 1982, Little, Brown and Company; and Felsenthal G: *Peripheral nervous system disorders and pregnancy.* In Goldstein PJ, Stern BJ, editors: *Neurological disorders of pregnancy,* Mount Kisco, 1992, Futura Publishing.

The incidence may be as low as 0.04% after traumatic lumbar puncture with a spinal needle.[30] In this series of 10,098 patients, four patients had pain with backache and spasm during lumbar puncture, with persistent postoperative complaints of up to 18 months' duration. In another series of 10,440 patients, an incidence rate of 0.89% was obtained when all paresthesias after a spinal anesthetic were documented as traumatic punctures.[31] Paresthesias with epidural catheter placement can be reduced by as much as 50% by simply placing the bevel of the epidural needle cephalad.[32]

When needle trauma occurs to the spinal cord or nerve roots, the result is severe lancinating pain, often in the distribution of the injured nerve root. The procedure should be discontinued immediately with the occurrence of pain and the removal of the offending needle or catheter. In addition, pain during injection also should signal a stop with an obligatory adjustment of the needle or catheter. A recent case report demonstrates the need to reevaluate the occurrence of pain during epidural catheter placement and catheter injection.[33] An obstetric patient experienced pain in the lower back, buttocks, and posterior thighs and calves during each of six injections (totaling 44 ml) through an epidural catheter that had been placed without incident for cesarean section. Postoperatively, the patient had complaints of severe back pain with radiation to the legs, urinary retention, left leg weakness, and hyperesthesia of both legs. An impressive syrinx involving the conus medullaris that extended from about T-11 to L-1 was found by magnetic resonance imaging. Although this fluid collection may have been present before epidural catheter placement, the postoperative neurologic deficits and history of three prior epidural trials are suggestive that the most recent procedure may have been responsible.

Hematoma

The formation of a hematoma in any of the three spaces (epidural, subdural, or subarachnoid) will result in spinal cord compression and eventual paralysis unless it is removed. Fortunately, the formation of a spinal hematoma seems to be extremely rare, despite the fact that blood vessel perforation occurred in nearly 3% to 9% of epidural procedures performed.[34,35] In addition, the majority of hematomas after spinal or lumbar puncture occurred in patients who had a coagulopathy, who received anticoagulation, or who had a difficult or traumatic catheter placement.[36] Interestingly, more than 100 spontaneous spinal epidural hematomas have been reported in the literature, resulting from as little as sneezing, lifting, or straining.[37]

Acute hemorrhage in the spinal canal usually presents with pain localized to the spinal cord segments adjacent to the hematoma. Pain may be radicular in nature and may mimic a herniated disc. The location of the hematoma will determine the progression to quadriplegia (cervical) or paraplegia (thoracic or lumbar). Sensory loss varies and the patient may have subjective complaints of numbness. Urinary retention, flaccid motor weakness, and the loss of deep tendon reflexes are common. Rapid surgical decompression can result in full recovery, depending on the degree of neurologic deficit and duration of the symptoms.

Preexisting coagulopathies should preclude the use of regional anesthesia until coagulation studies are determined. Thrombocytopenia is known to occur in obstetric patients with pregnancy-induced hypertension.[38] Bleeding times (although less than 10 minutes) were found to be significantly elevated in patients with severe pregnancy-induced hypertension compared with nonpregnant patients, despite platelet counts of greater than 200,000/mm[3,39]. Patients also may present as thrombocytopenic with no prior history of bleeding abnormalities; they represent undiscovered chronic cases of idiopathic thrombocytopenic purpura. However, these patients may be thrombocytopenic and have normal bleeding times due to larger and more competent platelets, which are seen with this disorder.[40] Low-dose aspirin is being used more frequently in patients to prevent pregnancy-induced hypertension[41]; however, bleeding time was found to be within normal limits after treatment with low-dose aspirin. Hence regional analgesia or anesthesia should not be contraindicated in this situation.

Spinal Epidural Abscess

Epidural abscesses in patients without regional anesthetics are relatively rare events, with an incidence of nearly 2 in 10,000.[42] Reports of abscess after epidural anesthesia are extremely rare, with only 1 of 505,000 patients with abscess in one large retrospective study. About 13% of patients who present with an abscess had a history of a previous spinal surgical procedure. The vast majority of patients (67%) had a compromised immune status due to diabetes, chronic renal failure, alcoholism, malignancy, or intravenous drug abuse. Consequently, pregnancy, which can be described as a state of immunosuppression necessary for fetal growth, would seem to put the mother at increased risk.[43] Extraspinal abscess sources are present in 60% of epidural abscess, suggesting that hematogenous dissemination of bacteria from other sites is responsible.[44] Gram-positive organisms have been isolated in nearly 80% of all abscesses. *Staphylococcus aureus* was the most common pathogen isolated in all studies. After epidural anesthesia, 100% of abscesses were from gram-positive organisms (82% *S. aureus,* and 18% *S. epidermidis*).[45] Spinal epidural abscesses were present in four stages, described as spinal ache, nerve root pain, weakness (including bowel and bladder dysfunction), and paralysis. The first three phases are highly variable and symptoms have appeared in as little as hours to weeks. Patients who had abscesses after epidural procedures presented with symptoms in as little as 3 days to as long as months after catheterization.[45] Consequently, patients with chronic abscesses had less fever, leukocytosis, and back pain than patients with acute abscesses, who had more severe back pain and an acute onset of paralysis.[46] Redness, tenderness, and swelling of the paravertebral muscles also may be present.[47] Magnetic resonance imaging and computed tomographic myelogram were equally sensitive, but neither was 100% accurate in the diagnosis of abscess tissue.[42] Early reports with MRI scans indicated that the margins of the abscess can have the appearance of cerebrospinal fluid.[48] The availability of MRI contrast may increase the sensitivity of this technique. Granulation tissue and pus generally are found with surgical decompressive laminectomy. Debriding and draining the area, and intravenous antibiotics remain the traditional management. Early intervention results in complete recovery in 50% to 70% of patients.[44-46]

Meningitis

Bacterial infection of the cerebrospinal fluid after epidural and spinal anesthesia remains rare, with only occasional case reports.[30,31,49] Traditionally, the placement of a regional anesthetic has been considered contraindicated in the presence of infection or sepsis, with the concern that the trauma caused by a spinal or epidural needle would allow bacterial seeding, resulting in meningitis or abscess. Since the vast majority of abscesses appear to be a result of hematogenous spread, this would seem to be a reasonable concern. Also, several recent cases of meningitis after epidural anesthesia report the presence of unusual organisms not commonly associated with meningitis.[50] *S. uberis* was found in vaginal cultures and considered the source in one case; and *S. sanguis,* a common mouth pathogen, was considered the source in the other.[51 52] *S. faecalis* also was responsible for meningitis after epidural catheter placement, and was thought to be due to an area of cellulitis at the site of catheter insertion.

Can a regional anesthetic catheter be placed with the presence of an infection? This is particularly important in patients who present with chorioamnionitis. Recently researchers attempted to answer this question by evaluating the risk of meningitis after dural punctures in rats during artificially created sepsis with *Escherichia coli*. Rats that were pretreated with gentamicin before dural puncture did not develop meningitis.[53] Thirty percent of rats that were bacteremic developed meningitis in the absence of pretreatment. One should note that *E. coli* is not a pathogen that commonly causes meningitis and the size of the dural tears made in the rats is significantly larger than that seen during regional anesthesia in patients. However, this suggests that if appropriate antibiotic coverage can be instituted before a regional anesthetic, then subsequent infection may be averted. Clinically, when epidurals were administered to 39 women with chorioamnionitis (40% had epidural procedures before antibiotics), no infectious complications were observed. In addition, 74 women in this study developed chorioamnionitis after epidural placement and received antibiotics at that time.[54] Consequently, the use of regional anesthesia during the time of chorioamnionitis probably can be instituted safely with some reasonable precautions.[55,56] Lastly, is a patient at greater risk for another complication, such as a failed general anesthetic induction, if the regional anesthetic is not performed? If antibiotic therapy can be initiated with the observation of a positive response to antibiotic therapy, then the safety of placing a regional anesthetic in the presence of an infection may be increased. Finally, one should consider the discontinuation of the regional technique if placement of the block is difficult or compromised by previous back surgery. Despite these precautions, the presence of abnormal flora that are not covered by the antibiotic therapy could result in an infection.

Anterior Spinal Artery Syndrome

Anterior spinal artery syndrome is the consequence of either a decrease in blood flow or thrombosis of the anterior spinal artery resulting in motor weakness or paralysis, and loss of pain and temperature perception. This devastating cause of paralysis is not as potentially reversible as the many other mass effects discussed. Ischemia is not seen with the posterior third of the spinal cord because it is supplied by two continuous posterior spinal arteries that make numerous anastomoses with the vertebral, cervical, intercostal, and lumbar arteries. The numerous anastomoses make ischemia to this section of the spinal cord rare. On the other hand, the anterior two thirds of the spinal cord is supplied by the single anterior spinal artery, which is divided into the cervical, thoracic, and lumbar segments.[57] The lumbar segments are supplied by the artery of Adamkiewicz (or the radicularis magna). In 85% of cases, the artery of Adamkiewicz originates between T-9 and L-2 and supplies the bulk of the conus medullaris, with a small ascending contribution by the internal iliac arteries. However, in 15% of cases, the origin is as high as T-5 and the internal iliac artery becomes the dominant blood supply to the conus medularis.[56] Under these circumstances, there is an increased risk of cord ischemia due to the fetal head compression of the branches from the internal iliac artery, which lie on the posterior wall of the pelvis and cross on the ala of the sacrum. One case report of anterior spinal artery syndrome postulated that an obstetric patient with diabetic scleredema, who already had a tenuous arterial blood flow to the spinal cord due to the scleredema, had a further reduction in blood flow as a result of the large volume of local anesthetic injected in the epidural space.[58]

Interestingly, the clinical consequences of the 15% minority for the origin of the artery of Adamkiewicz may be observed in the literature. In a prospective study of neurologic injuries in Nigerian women, Bromage noted that 15% did not recover and remained with spastic paralysis. None of the 34 patients who had neurologic deficits after delivery had received regional anesthetics.[56]

Cauda Equina Syndrome and Local Anesthetic Neurotoxicity

Cauda equina syndrome is a consequence of sacral nerve root injury, which is characterized by low back pain, a localized sensory loss in the perineal area, sphincter dysfunction with both fecal and urinary incontinence, and a varying degree of leg weakness.[59] Until recently, most reports of cauda equina syndrome with anesthesia occurred before 1940 and were associated with the anesthetic agent Stovaine (amylocaine). Additional reports with anesthetics piperocaine or tetracaine also were presented, but few additional cases of cauda equina syndrome have been reported until recently, with lidocaine.

Cauda equina syndrome with lidocaine was observed after continuous spinal anesthesia, initially with microcatheters but also after continuous spinals with 18- and 20-gauge epidural catheters. Microcatheters were removed from medical use with the hypothesis that they were responsible for nerve root damage due to the inadequate mixing of hyperbaric 5% lidocaine with the cerebrospinal fluid.[60] However, two other reports used preservative-free 2% lidocaine through epidural catheters; in one case it was used after neutralization with sodium bicarbonate.[61,62] More recently there has been a report of four cases of transient neurologic symptoms with hyperbaric 5% lidocaine after spinal anesthesia.[63] Patients were placed in the lithotomy position after a spinal anesthetic. The stretching of the cauda equina was thought to contribute to the transient neurologic deficits, which improved after several days. This last report precipitated an editorial suggesting caution when using hyperbaric lidocaine during procedures that may require stretching of the cauda equina, causing an increase in lidocaine's toxicity.[64] Although one should be aware of these potential complications that have surfaced with lidocaine, it seems premature to state that *hyperbaric lidocaine formulation carries us uncomfortably close to the brink of neurotoxicity* without further evaluations. Certainly there is a large worldwide experience with hyperbaric lidocaine that has not yielded a large number of patients with permanent neurologic deficits. Allergic reactions with thiopental, which could lead to anaphylaxis, are estimated to be about 1 in 30,000; yet this drug has been used as the primary induction agent for general anesthetics until recently.[65] It is the function of the anesthesia personnel to determine the risks associated with various anesthetics and to choose the best anesthetic for a patient based on those risks. Currently the risk of a neurologic deficit after lidocaine still seems to be significantly less than the risk of anaphylaxis with thiopental, and should still be considered when determining an anesthetic for an individual.

Adhesive Arachnoiditis

Adhesive arachnoiditis is an inflammatory condition that results in the obliteration of the subarachnoid space with adhesions to the spinal cord and dura. This condition can be idiopathic or can occur in response to either a chemical or an infectious irritant.[66] The occurrence of adhesive arachnoiditis after spinal anesthesia results in the proliferation of the meninges, causing progressive sensory and motor weakness over months and ultimately, paralysis.[67] Although rare, this syndrome is not forgotten. Subarachnoid cysts were found after magnetic resonance imaging in seven patients who had epidural catheters placed for childbirth in several South American countries.[68] Cyst formation was postulated to be a consequence of the local anesthetics that had contained preservatives.

Prolonged Block

Bupivacaine remains the most common local anesthetic used for the initiation and maintenance of epidural anesthesia during labor. Reports suggesting a prolonged anesthetic action with bupivacaine are in the literature.[69,70] The increased sensitivity of nerves to local anesthetics during pregnancy is well known. The increased progesterone levels during pregnancy have been demonstrated to preferentially increase the sensitivity of cardiac muscle to bupivacaine in comparison with lidocaine.[71] Therefore increased exposure of nerves to high concentrations of bupivacaine (0.5%), as suggested in these case reports, may result in prolonged blockade up to 48 hours. Certainly sensory loss that can be attributed to one or two nerve roots may represent isolated nerve damage to a single nerve.[72] One should be cautious about concluding that a neurologic deficit is a consequence of prolonged neurologic blockade. Certainly if the deficit is improving, then this may be a reasonable conclusion.

Peripheral Nervous System Complications

Nerve injury associated with anesthesia represented 15% of the claims in the American Society of Anesthesiologist Closed Claims Study data base. More than 90% of the claims represented damage to nerves outside of the spinal cord; the vast majority were from damage to the ulnar, brachial plexus, and lumbosacral nerve roots (34%, 23%, and 16%, respectively).[1] One conclusion that can be drawn from these data is that peripheral nerves are more exposed to trauma or compression, and anesthesia personnel need to be vigilant for the mechanisms of these injuries. Interestingly, only 36% of nerve injuries were claimed after regional anesthesia, and the standard of care was thought to be met in the majority of these injuries.

Lumbosacral plexus injuries were fairly common before the use of epidural anesthesia and fortunately were documented in the literature. Now the current popularity of epidural anesthesia would make isolating its contribution to any nerve injuries difficult. In addition, it is difficult to devise epidural studies that have balanced patient populations. There is an inherent selection of epidural anesthesia for patients having difficult or previously difficult deliveries due to its superior analgesia when compared with alternatives. There are a number of compressive peripheral nerve palsies to nerves of the lumbosacral plexus due to compression of these nerves by the fetal scalp or retractors as they pass through the pelvis. Also, the patient's position during labor can result in nerve compression, which is exacerbated during anesthesia. The most common of these compressions affect the femoral, sciatic, peroneal, and lateral femoral cutaneous nerves, although the obturator, superiorgluteal, genitofemoral, ilioinguinal, and iliohypogastric nerve compressions also have been described.[73,74]

Lumbosacral Neuropathy

Lumbosacral plexus lesions occur secondary to direct compression of the plexus by the fetal head or by obstetric forceps. An incidence as high as 1 in 2000 deliveries has been reported in the past. A recent review of 143,019 live births shows a decrease to 3.5 in 100,000. The relationship of the lumbosacral cord in the pelvis and its vulnerability to compression can be seen in the classic figure by Cole from his review titled *Maternal Obstetrical Paralysis* (Fig. 23-1).[75] In this 1946 review, the author notes that the earliest symptoms of pain referred to the sciatic nerve are easily overlooked due to the widespread use of sedative drugs and caudal anesthesia. Patients complain of numbness, dead feeling, an asleep foot, pins and needles, and thermal changes. In fact, all of these symptoms could be attributed to the initiation of an epidural catheter or a long-running continuous epidural catheter that may seem to be one sided. At the time the re-

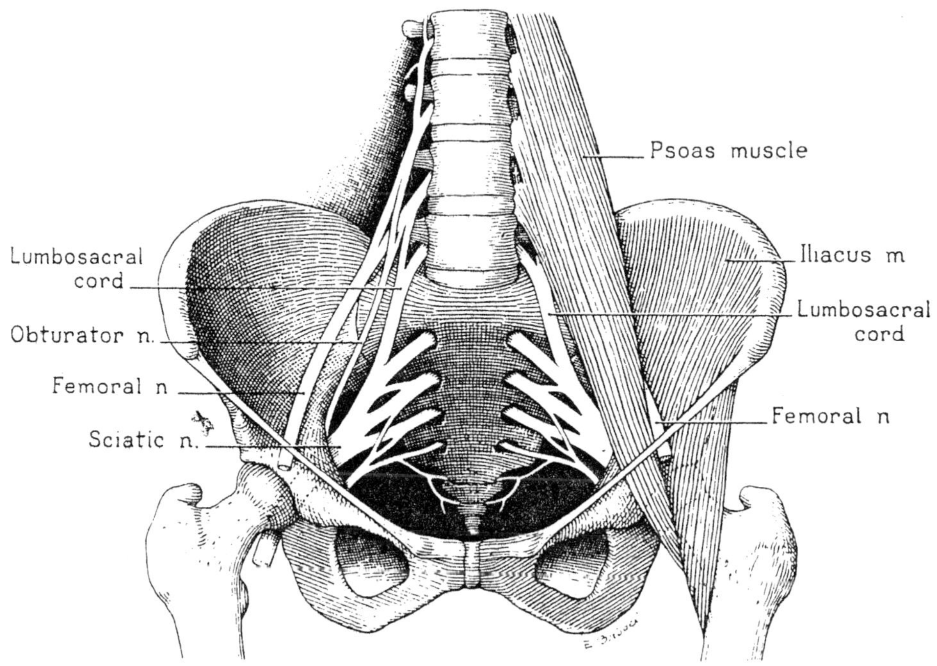

Fig. 23-1.

The relationship of the lumbosacral cord and femoral nerve to the pelvis and inguinal ligament. *(With permission from Cole JT: Maternal obstetric paralysis,* Am J Obstet Gynecol *1946; 52:372.)*

view was published, textbooks of obstetrics did not devote a great deal of attention to this complication, and this remains true today. Indeed, a recovery room nurse in our institution having her first child had the classic symptoms of sacral plexus compression with foot drop, and was told by the examining neurologist that it was related to a difficult epidural catheter placement.

Retrospective analysis of lumbosacral neuropathies show that two thirds of these complications are in nulliparous women with the baby in the vertex position (two of 73 cases were breech).[76] Anatomically, the patient may have a shallow anterior concavity of the sacrum so that the sacral promontory does not project into the birth canal. This results in the loss of the bony projections that act to protect against nerve injury.[3] Foot drop usually is unilateral and is manifest on the same side of the infant's brow during descent.[26] Postpartum complaints are of pain, numbness, or tingling with a heaviness or weakness in the affected leg. The patient may walk with a limp and have varying degrees of diminished touch and pain sensations with weakness and paralysis of the muscle groups that control the extensors of the toes and dorsiflexors of the ankle, causing foot drop.

Prognosis is determined by the level of the lesion. Consequently electrodiagnostic evaluation differentiates the level of the lesion by indicating if the foot drop is due to root, plexus, sciatic, or peroneal nerve injury. The more proximal the lesion, the worse the prognosis.[26] Treatment includes an orthosis to control foot drop and physical therapy to strengthen muscles and prevent contractures and disuse atrophy.

Peroneal Nerve Damage

The common peroneal nerve is composed of fibers from L-4,5,S-1,2 and splits off from the sciatic nerve in the middle of the posterior aspect of the thigh. The nerve travels lateral to the head of the fibula and is exposed to the risk of compression injury on the way to the anterior surface of the calf. During surgical procedures, care should be taken to prevent pressure on the peroneal nerve. In the lithotomy position, the common peroneal nerve can be at increased risk due to stretching, which can compromise its blood supply. One should be vigilant for additional mechanisms of peroneal nerve compression. One case report concluded that an epidural catheter placed for postoperative pain resulted in the patient acquiring peroneal nerve damage due to the patient's fibula resting against the bed rail postoperatively.[77] In addition, a case of bilateral peroneal nerve palsies were reported after natural childbirth due to prolonged pressure by the patient's palms against the upper lateral aspect of her legs.[78] Lastly, the sciatic nerve (L-4,5,S-1,2,3) exits the pelvis through the gluteal region and divides into the tibial and common peroneal nerves. Although elusive when attempting nerve blocks, direct intramuscular injections near or in the sciatic nerve are common and can result in foot drop from damage of the common peroneal nerve.[79]

Postpartum Femoral (Anterior Crural) Neuropathy

Femoral neuropathy was a frequent postpartum complication at the turn of the century, with an incidence as high as 4.7%, although now it is relatively rare.[80] In the review of Byrnes published in 1913, 84 of 136 cases of femoral neuropathies (62%) had their onset after delivery. Vaginal hysterectomies where the patient's legs were flexed, abducted, and rotated outward also were responsible for femoral neuropathies.[81] Femoral nerve injury remains a complication of vaginal hysterectomies, with three recent cases reported with bilateral components.[82] Femoral neuropathies are described primarily in primigravidas, often after a difficult delivery, with as many as 25% bilateral (most peripheral neuropathies are unilateral). The femoral nerve is the largest branch of the lumbar plexus and decends through the pelvis in the psoas major muscle. Motor and sensory changes are variable. Sensory changes in the femoral distribution can include anterior thigh pain and tenderness of the femoral nerve trunk. Motor changes can affect knee extension (quadriceps), hip flexion (iliopsoas), adduction (pectineus), and rotation (pectineus and sartorius). A woman with a postpartum femoral neuropathy is able to walk on flat surfaces but is unable to climb stairs or rise unassisted from a squatting position. The most reliable sign of a femoral neuropathy is the decrease or absence of the knee jerk. Compression of the femoral nerve can occur by several mechanisms. The femoral nerve is exposed as it passes over the pelvic brim (Fig. 23-1). Pressure can be placed on the nerve by self-retaining retractors, resulting in nerve injury.[83] In obstetrics, paralysis of the femoral nerve is thought to result from the flexion of the legs against the abdomen with abduction and outward hip rotation (lithotomy position).[84] This causes the femoral nerve and vessels to be compressed against the inguinal ligament at a near 90° angulation. Indeed, 26% of postpartum nerve damage in 34 Nigerian women were femoral neuropathies, probably due to the prevalence of a squatting position used for delivery.[85]

Meralgia Paresthetica

The lateral femoral cutaneous nerve, which contains only sensory fibers from L-2,3, can be compressed as it passes under the lateral border of the inguinal ligament. This can cause pain, numbness, or hyperesthesia that occurs along the anterolateral aspect of the thigh.[7] Meralgia paresthetica is seen most commonly in patients during the third trimester due to obesity and rapid weight gain during pregnancy. Symptoms usually resolve after delivery. This neuropathy can be seen after labor with an incidence of 1.4 in 100,000.[80]

Summary

1. As described in the beginning of the chapter, many neurologic deficits observed in the postpartum patient are related to the labor process or to a preexisting condition.
2. Postpartum neurologic complications, however, often are attributed to a regional anesthetic administered during the peripartum period. Consequently anesthesia personnel often are the first individuals to evaluated postpartum patients with such deficits. A working knowledge of the differential diagnoses can help prevent permanent neurologic sequelae.
3. Complications such as epidural hematoma and abscess need to be acted on quickly. The early involvement of a neurologist is important to coordinate the evaluation of a postpartum neurologic deficit and determine the age of neurologic deficits with electromyography.
4. Magnetic resonance imaging has become one of the best ways to evaluate the spinal cord for tumor, abscess, and hematoma.[86] The recent development of enhancers such as gadopentetare dimeglumine has improved the ability to delineate and characterize lesions that previously eluded detection with MRI.
5. Finally, the neurologist will be able to make regular assessments during the process of physical therapy, which will help assure the patient of improvement during rehabilitation.

References

1. Kroll DA, Caplan RA, Posner K, et al: Nerve injury associated with anesthesia, *Anesthesiology* 1990; 73:202.
2. Chadwick HS, Posner K, Caplan RA, et al: A comparison of obstetric and nonobstetric anesthesia malpractice claims, *Anesthesiology* 1991; 74:242.
3. Hill EC: Maternal obstetric paralysis, *Am J Obstet Gynecol* 1962; 83:1452.
4. Robbins SL, Cotran RS: *Pathologic basis of disease, ed 2,* Philadelphia, 1979, WB Saunders.
5. Dornette WHL: Compression neuropathies: medical aspects and legal implications, *Int Anesth Clin* 1986; 24:201.
6. Gerard KW, Fagreaus L: Postspinal headache, *Semin Anesth* 1990; 9:69.
7. Donaldson JO: *Neurologic complications.* In Burrow GN, Ferris TF, editors: *Medical complications during pregnancy,* Philadelphia, 1988, WB Saunders.
8. Edelman JD, Wingard DW: Subdural hematomas after lumbar dural puncture, *Anesthesiology* 1980; 52:166.
9. Beers RA, Cambareri JJ, Gerard SR: Acute deterioration of mental status following epidural blood patch, *Anesth Analg* 1993; 76:1147.
10. Younker S, Jones MM, Adenwala J, et al: Maternal cortical vein thrombosis and the obstetric anesthesiologist, *Anesth Analg* 1986; 65:1007.
11. Goldberg S: *Clinical neuroanatomy made ridiculously simple,* Miami, 1986, Medmaster.
12. Kao YJ, Zavisca FG, Tellez JM, et al: Backache after extradural anaesthesia in the postpartum period: dissection of a thoracic aneurysm, *Br J Anaesth* 1991; 67:335.
13. Diakow PR, Gadsby TA, Gadsby JB, et al: Back pain during pregnancy and labor, *J Manipul Physiol Ther* 1991; 14:116.
14. Berg G, Hammar M, Moller-Nielson J, et al: Low back pain during pregnancy, *Obstet Gynecol* 1988; 71:71.
15. Grove LH: Backache, headache, and bladder dysfunction after delivery, *Br J Anaesth* 1973; 45:1147.
16. Moir DD, Davidson S: Postpartum complications of forceps delivery performed under epidural and pudendal nerve block, *Br J Anaesth* 1972, 44.1197.
17. Ostgaard HC, Andersson GBJ, Wennergren M: The impact of low back and pelvic pain in pregnancy on the pregnancy outcome, *Acta Obstet Gynecol Scand* 1991; 70:21.
18. MacArthur C, Lewis M, Knox EG, et al: Epidural anaesthe-

sia and long term backache after childbirth, *Br Med J* 1990; 301:9.

19. Vickers RJ, May AE: Long-term backache after extradural or general anaesthesia for manual removal of placenta: preliminary report, *Br J Anaesth* 1993; 70:214.
20. MacArthur C, Lewis M, Knox EG: Investigation of long term problems after obstetric epidural anaesthesia, *Br Med J* 1992; 304:1279.
21. Stevens RA, Shester WL, Artuso AD, et al: Back pain after epidural anesthesia with chloroprocaine in volunteers: preliminary report, *Reg Anesth* 1991; 16:199.
22. Hynson JM, Sessler DI, Glosten B: Back pain in volunteers after epidural anesthesia with chloroprocaine, *Anesth Analg* 1991; 72:253.
23. Stevens RA, Urmey WF, Urquhart BL, et al: Back pain after epidural anesthesia with chloroprocaine, *Anesthesiology* 1993; 78:492.
24. Simon JN, Mokriski BK, Gillies BS, et al: Spinal cord compression following labor and delivery with epidural analgesia, *Reg Anesth* 1989; 14:256.
25. Bakay L: *Neurosurgery.* In Nardi GL, Zuidema GD, editors: *Surgery: essentials of clinical practice,* Boston, 1982, Little, Brown and Company.
26. Felsenthal G: *Peripheral nervous system disorders and pregnancy.* In Goldstein PJ, Stern BJ, editors: *Neurological disorders of pregnancy,* Mount Kisco, 1992, Futura Publishing.
27. Weinreb JC, Wolbarsht LB, Cohen JM, et al: Prevalence of lumbosacral intervertebral disk abnormalities on MR images in pregnant and asymptomatic nonpregnant women, *Radiology* 1989; 170:125.
28. Park WP: Factors influencing distribution of local anesthetics in the epidural space, *Reg Anesth* 1988; 13:49.
29. Usubiaga JE: Neurological complications following epidural anesthesia, *Int Anesth Clin* 1975; 13:1.
30. Vandam LD, Dripps RD: Long-term follow-up of patients who received 10,098 spinal anesthetics: failure to discover major neurological sequelae, *JAMA* 1954; 156:1486.
31. Phillips OC, Ebner H, Nelson AT, et al: Neurologic complications following spinal anesthesia with lidocaine: a prospective review of 10,440 cases, *Anesthesiology* 1969; 30:284.
32. Munoz HR, Dagnino JA, Allende M, et al: Direction of catheter insertion and incidence of paresthesias and failure rate in continuous epidural anesthesia: a comparison of cephalad and caudad catheter insertion, *Reg Anesth* 1993; 18:331.
33. Katz N, Hurley R: Epidural anesthesia complicated by fluid collection within the spinal cord, *Anesth Analg* 1993; 77:1064.
34. Vandam L: Neurological sequelae of spinal and epidural anesthesia, *Int Anesth Clin* 1986; 24:231.
35. Sage DJ: Epidurals, spinals and bleeding disorders in pregnancy: a review, *Anesth Intensive Care* 1990; 18:319.
36. Owens EL, Kasten GW, Hessel EA: Spinal subarachnoid hematoma after lumbar puncture and heparinization: a case report, review of the literature, and discussion of anesthetic implications, *Anesth Analg* 1986; 65:1201.
37. Scott BB, Quiling RG, Miller CA, et al: Spinal epidural hematoma, *JAMA* 1976; 235:513.
38. Schindler M, Gatt S, Isert P, et al: Thrombocytopenia and platelet functional defects in pre-eclampsia: implications for regional anesthesia, *Anaesth Intensive Care* 1990; 18:169.
39. Ramanathan J, Sibai BM, Vu T, et al: Correlation between bleeding times and platelet counts in women with preeclampsia undergoing cesarean section, *Anesthesiology* 1989; 71:188.
40. Writer WDR: *Hematologic disease.* In James RM, Wheeler AS, Dewan DM, editors: *Obstetric anesthesia: the complicated patient,* Philadelphia, 1988, FA Davis.
41. Walsh SW, Wang Y, Kay HH, et al: Low-dose aspirin inhibits lipid peroxides and thromboxane but not prostacyclin in pregnant women, *Am J Obstet Gynecol* 1992; 167:926.
42. Hlavin ML, Kaminski HJ, Ross JS, et al: Spinal epidural abscess: a ten-year perspective, *Neurosurgery* 1990; 27:177.
43. Levin ML, Horn J, Edred L, et al. *Infections of the nervous system during pregnancy.* In Goldstein PJ, Stern BJ, editors: *Neurological disorders of pregnancy,* Mount Kisco, 1992, Futura Publishing.
44. Curling OD, Gower DJ, McWhorter JM: Changing concepts in spinal epidural abscess: a report of 29 cases, *Neurosurgery* 1990; 27:185.
45. Ngan Kee WD, Jones MR, Thomas P, et al: Extradural abscess complicating extradural anaesthesia for caesarean section, *Br J Anaesth* 1992; 69:647.
46. Danner RL, Hartman BJ: Update of spinal epidural abscess: 35 cases and review of the literature, *Rev Infect Dis* 1987; 9:265.
47. Saady A: Epidural abscess complicating thoracic epidural analgesia, *Anesthesiology* 1976; 44:244.
48. Mamourian AC, Dickman CA, Drayer BP, et al: Spinal epidural abscess: three cases following spinal epidural injection

demonstrated with magnetic resonance imaging, *Anesthesiology* 1993; 78:204.

49. Scott DB, Hibbard BM: Serious non-fatal complications associated with extradural block in obstetric practice, *Br J Anaesth* 1990; 64:537.
50. Hoeprich PD: *Acute bacterial meningitis.* In Hoeprich PD, editor: *Infectious diseases,* Hagerstown, 1977, Harper & Row.
51. Ready LB, Helfer D: Bacterial meningitis in parturients after epidural anesthesia, *Anesthesiology* 1989; 71:988.
52. Berga S, Trierweiler MW: Bacterial meningitis following epidural anesthesia for vaginal delivery: a case report, *Obstet Gynecol* 1989; 74:437.
53. Carp H, Bailey S: The association between meningitis and dural puncture in bacteremic rats, *Anesthesiology* 1992; 76:739.
54. Vaddadi A, Ramanathan J, Angel JJ, et al: Epidural anesthesia in women with chorioamnionitis: a retrospective study, *Anesthesiology* 1989; 71:A863 (abstract).
55. Chestnut DH: Spinal anesthesia in the febrile patient, *Anesthesiology* 1992; 76:667 (editorial).
56. Bromage PR: *Neurologic complications of regional anesthesia for obstetrics.* In Shnider SM, Levinson G, editors: *Anesthesia for obstetrics,* Baltimore, 1993, Williams & Wilkins.
57. Adriani J, Naragi M: Paraplegia associated with epidural anesthesia, *South Med J* 1986; 79:1350.
58. Eastwood DW: Anterior spinal artery syndrome after epidural anesthesia in a pregnant diabetic patient with scleredema, *Anesth Analg* 1991; 73:90.
59. Jaradeh S: Cauda equina syndrome: a neurologist's perspective, *Reg Anesth* 1993; 18:473.
60. Rigler ML, Drasner K, Krejcie TC, et al: Cauda equina syndrome after continuous spinal anesthesia, *Anesth Analg* 1991; 72:275.
61. Ackerman WE, Andrews PJD, Juneja MM, et al: Cauda equina syndrome: a consequence of lumbar disc protrusion or continuous subarchnoid analgesia, *Anesth Analg* 1993; 76:898.
62. Drasner K, Rigler ML, Sessler DI, et al: Cauda equina syndrome following intended epidural anesthesia, *Anesthesiology* 1992; 77:582.
63. Schneider M, Ettlin T, Kaufmann M, et al: Transient neurologic toxicity after hyperbaric subarachnoid anesthesia with 5% lidocaine, *Anesth Analg* 1993; 76:1154.
64. de Jong RH: Last round for a "Heavyweight"? *Anesth Analg* 1994; 78:3.
65. Stoelting RK: Pharmacology and physiology in anesthetic practice, Philadelphia, 1987, JB Lippincott.
66. Vandam LD: *Complications of spinal and epidural anesthesia.* In Orkin RK Cooperman LH, editors: *Complications in anesthesiology,* Philadelphia, 1983, JB Lippincott.
67. Kane RE: Neurologic deficits following epidural or spinal anesthesia, *Anesth Analg* 1981; 60:150.
68. Sklar EL, Quencer FM, Green BA, et al: Complications of epidural anesthesia: MR appearance of abnormalities, *Radiology* 1991; 181:549.
69. Pathy GV, Rosen M: Prolonged block with recovery after extradural anagesia for labour, *Br J Anaesth* 1975; 47:520.
70. Cuerden C, Buley R, Downing JW: Delayed recovery after epidural block in labour: a report of four cases, *Anaesthesia* 1977; 32:773.
71. Moller RA, Datta S, Fox J, et al: Effects of progesterone on the cardiac electrophysiologic action of bupivacaine and lidocaine, *Anesthesiology* 1992; 76:604.
72. Bromage PR: An evaluation of bupivacaine in epidural analgesia for obstetrics, *Can Anaesth Soc J* 1969; 16:46.
73. King AB: Neurologic conditions occurring as complications of pregnancy, *Arch Neurol Psych* 1950; 63:611.
74. Massey WE, Cefalo RC: Neuropathies of pregnancy. *Obstet Gynecol Surv* 1979; 34:489.
75. Cole JT: Maternal obstetric paralysis, *Am J Obstet Gynecol* 1946; 52:372.
76. Murray RR: Maternal obstetrical paralysis, *Am J Obstet Gynecol* 1964; 88:399.
77. Cohen DE, Van Duker B, Siegel S, et al: Common peroneal nerve palsy associated with epidural analgesia, *Anesth Analg* 1993; 76:429.
78. Adornato BT, Carlini WG: "Pushing palsy": a case of self-induced bilateral peroneal palsy during natural childbirth, *Neurology* 1992, 12:936.
79. Ravindran MD, Viegas OJ: Transient lower extremity weakness in an obstetric patient unrelated to epidural anesthesia, *Anesth Analg* 1981; 60:527.
80. Vargo MM, Robinson LR, Nicholas JN, et al: Postpartum femoral neuropathy: relic of an earlier era? *Arch Phys Med Rehabil* 1990; 71:591.
81. Brynes CM: Anterior crural neuritis, *J Nerv Ment Dis* 1913; 40:758.
82. Hopper CL, Baker JB: Bilateral femoral neuropathy complicating vaginal hysterectomy, *Obstet Gynecol* 1968; 32:543.

83. Adelman JU, Goldberg GS, Puckett JD: Postpartum bilateral femoral neuropathy, *Obstet Gynecol* 1973; 42:845.
84. Donaldson JO, Wirz D, Mashman J: Bilateral postpartum femoral neuropathy, *Conn Med* 1985; 49:496.
85. Bademosi O, Osuntokun BO, Van de Werd HJ, et al: Obstetric neuropraxia in the Nigerian African, *Int J Gynaecol Obstet* 1980; 17:611.
86. Sze G: MR imaging of the spinal cord: current status and future advances, *Am J Roentgenol* 1992; 159:149.
87. Martin HB, Gibbons JJ, Bucholz RD: An unusual presentation of spinal cord tumor after epidural anesthesia, *Anesth Analg* 1992; 75:844.
88. Dawkins CJM: An analysis of the complications of extradural and caudal block, *Anaesthesia* 1969; 24:554.
89. Ong BY, Cohen MM, Esmail A, et al: Paresthesias and motor dysfunction after labor and delivery, *Anesth Analg* 1987; 66:18.

24

Sudden Fetal Distress

A 35-year-old primigravida at 42 weeks' gestation is admitted on the labor and delivery floor in active labor. Epidural anesthesia provides good relief of her labor pain. When she is 6-cm dilated, the fetal heart rate decreases at the end of a contraction, and the recording is interpreted as a late deceleration. The obstetrician performs a scalp capillary pH with findings of 7.08, 7.09, 7.08. The decision is made to perform an immediate cesarean section for fetal distress.

Recommendations by Andrew P. Harris, M.D.

The diagnosis of fetal distress during labor remains a leading cause of emergency cesarean sections, accounting for about one fourth of all cesarean sections.[1] The mortality secondary to anesthesia for emergency cesarean sections is greater than for all other obstetric anesthetics combined.[2] It is therefore important that all anesthesiologists who anesthetize patients for childbirth (1) become familiar with the underlying causes of fetal distress, (2) understand the various ways to diagnose fetal distress, and (3) have an algorithm to formulate a safe and reasonable anesthetic plan to be followed in such circumstances, taking into account both maternal and fetal outcome.

Etiology of Fetal Distress

Fetal distress can be defined as a pathophysiologic condition in which oxidative metabolic substrate (in acute circumstances, oxygen) becomes available to the fetus in quantities insufficient to sustain in utero life for a prolonged period of time. When this occurs, the fetus initiates various physiologic response mechanisms to maintain adequate oxygen delivery to vital organs, at the expense of oxygen delivery to nonvital organs. The result of decreased perfusion of nonvital organs initially, and all organs ultimately, is metabolic cellular and systemic acidosis. Since the transport of oxygen to the fetus is the critical determinant of whether acute fetal distress will occur, understanding that pathway is crucial to understanding the various etiologies of sudden fetal distress. Theoretically, the movement of oxygen from the environment to the fetal cellular level can be impeded anywhere along its course from the ambient environment to the fetal cellular level.

Delivery of Oxygen to the Intervillous Space

Oxygen from the ambient atmosphere is bulk-transported to the maternal alveoli, and crosses the maternal alveolar membrane into the pulmonary capillary blood. At this level, impairment of maternal ventilation and/or diffusing capacity will result in decreased maternal arterial oxygen pressure (PaO_2). Adequate pulmonary blood flow (i.e., cardiac output) and matching of ventilation and perfusion are necessary for normal maternal arterial oxygenation. Assuming that maternal arterial blood is oxygenated, this blood must be transported to the intervillous space. Bulk transport of oxygenated maternal blood to the intervillous space via the uterine vasculature is predominantly dependent upon two factors: the perfusion pressure gradient for the intervillous space (i.e., maternal uterine arterial pressure minus the greater of uterine venous pressure or intrauterine pressure), and the resistance of the uterine vasculature.

There are several ways impairment of the perfusion pressure gradient can occur. Systemic hypotension, reflected in lower uterine artery pressure, can result in decreased oxygen delivery to the intervillous space. Uterine venous pressure is increased significantly by inferior vena caval compression. Finally, intrauterine pressure can be increased during contractions and may interfere with normal perfusion if intrauterine pressures are excessive (i.e., frequent contractions, tetanic contractions, elevated uterine diastolic pressure).

Vasoconstriction of the uterine circulation, even in the presence of adequate blood pressure, will result in decreased intervillous blood flow. Changes in uterine vascular tone can occur as a response to many endogenous vasoconstrictors including epinephrine, norepinephrine, vasopressin, angiotensin II, and others. However, most intrapartum changes in uterine vascular tone occur secondary to sympathetically mediated vasoconstriction. Such vasoconstriction can be the result of any stimulus that increases sympathetic outflow, both through release of epinephrine from the adrenal medulla and the local release of norepinephrine in uterine vascular smooth muscles. Stimuli that result in increased sympathetic tone include (1) a reflex baroreceptor response to hypotension (even transient hypotension secondary to interior vena cava [IVC] compression), (2) a reflex chemoreceptor response to hypoxia or hypercarbia, and (3) a "stress" response to physical or emotional factors. It has been well demonstrated that such stress responses can significantly adversely affect intervillous blood flow[3] and fetal well-being.[4] Unlike measurable factors that affect the intervillous blood flow (i.e., blood pressure or intrauterine pressure), sympathetic tone cannot be measured directly at the present time.

The Placenta and Placental Vasculature

Oxygen in the intervillous blood diffuses across the placental membrane into the fetal villous circulation, which is the capillary network of the umbilical vessels. For the placenta to function adequately it must have a diffusion surface large enough to allow the amount of gas exchange required for fetal oxidative metabolism and growth, and the diffusion barrier itself must be relatively normal. There are circumstances in which the effective placental surface area is acutely decreased, such as placental abruption, when the intervillous space is not adequately filled with oxygenated maternal blood. In such cases, sudden intrapartum fetal distress can result. In disease processes such as postdates gestation, gestational diabetes, hepatoses of pregnancy, and toxemia of pregnancy, the placenta itself and/or the placental vasculature is abnormal to the point of chronically deficient oxygen transport. This chronic deficiency can be manifested as intrauterine growth retardation (IUGR). Fetuses with IUGR are at increased risk of superimposed acute fetal distress during labor.

Fetal Vasculature

The final pathway for oxygen that has traversed the maternal circulation and placenta is through the fetal umbilical vein and then to the fetal arterial circulation. Impairment of the fetal circulation of oxygen most commonly occurs secondary to extrinsic mechanical obstruction of the umbilical cord. When such obstruction occurs, fetal blood delivery to and from the placenta falls, with a resulting decrease in fetal oxygenation. Intrinsic vasoconstriction of the umbilical vasculature probably does not occur in utero to any appreciable extent,[5] since the extraabdominal umbilical vasculature is relatively devoid of α-adrenergic vasoconstrictive receptors. An additional mechanism active in the fetus to assure adequate oxygenation is that redistribution of fetal blood flow occurs during stress so that oxygenated blood preferentially flows to the heart, brain, adrenal glands, and placenta.[6]

Diagnosis of Fetal Distress

Current techniques are limited in their ability to optimally predict the presence of intrapartum fetal distress; although they are sensitive in general, they have a low positive predictive value. Thus, fearing a poor neonatal outcome (if fetal distress should indeed be present), the tendency is to "treat" patients who demonstrate any evidence of fetal distress, accepting that a certain proportion will not benefit from the treatment. There are two monitoring methods currently used to clinically diagnose intrapartum fetal distress: fetal heart rate analysis and fetal scalp pH testing.

Fetal Heart Rate Testing

Analysis of fetal heart rate frequently yields the first evidence of fetal distress. Heart rate patterns which either precede or are consistent with a diagnosis of fetal distress include the presence of late decelerations (especially nonreflex late decelerations), decreased fetal heart rate variability, and fetal tachycardia.[5] (See Chapter 9.) In the presence of a fetal heart rate tracing suggestive of fetal distress, a fetal scalp blood sample pH can be measured to confirm the diagnosis. Zalar and Quilligan[7] suggest that a fetal scalp blood sample pH greater than 7.25 is considered normal; pH between 7.20 and 7.25 should be repeated within 30 minutes; and a pH less than 7.20 indicates an immediate repeat of the measurement while beginning to implement medical or surgical delivery.

Epidural Anesthesia and Fetal Distress

No evidence supports that epidural analgesia or anesthesia in the absence of prolonged or profound hypotension contributes significantly to the incidence of fetal distress. In fact, by reducing or eliminating sympathetic innervation of the uterine circulation, one could argue that reflex baroreceptor-, chemoreceptor-, or stress-mediated vasoconstriction of the uterine arterial vasculature would occur to a lesser extent, tending to eliminate one potential cause of impeded oxygen flow to the fetus. In labor in preeclamptic patients, epidural anesthesia has indeed been shown to improve intervillous blood flow.[8]

Anesthetic Management

Anesthetic management for sudden fetal distress should be directed toward concurrently identifying and treating a reversible cause of fetal distress, while planning a safe anesthetic for the mother and fetus if the physiologic insult is not reversible.

Reversible Causes of Fetal Distress

Given the above outline of potential areas of maternal fetal oxygen flow impairment, a simple algorithm can be constructed for identifying reversible causes of fetal distress. Some examples of potential causes, their diagnosis, and their treatment are outlined in Table 24-1. Maternal blood pressure and oxygenation need to be checked and maternal position changed if umbilical cord compression is expected. If uterine hyperstimulation is present, tocolytic therapy (i.e., terbutaline 0.125 to 0.25 mg intravenously [IV]) may be useful. In the case presented in this chapter, the presence of late decelerations, without previous variable decelerations, makes the diagnosis of acute cord compression unlikely as a significant contributor to fetal distress. In this borderline postdates gestation, the most likely underlying cause of sudden fetal distress is uteroplacental insufficiency. Therefore left uterine displacement should be maintained, supplemental maternal oxygen administered if possible, and the patient reassured (to avoid undue psychologic stress) while being transported to the operating room for ceserean section. Tocolytic therapy may be useful in eliminating further contractions.

Choice of Anesthetic

The choice of anesthetic for emergency cesarean section should be based on (1) the urgency to treat the fetal distress, and (2) the presence of adequate epidural analgesia or anesthesia to begin a cesarean section. In general three categories of urgency can be defined.[9]

The first category (class I) are patients in whom the maternal and fetal physiologic makeup is stable and not life threatening to mother or fetus. Examples of these are given in Table 24-2. The anesthetic management for these patients would be similar to that chosen for patients undergoing elective cesarean section—that is, regional anesthesia is preferred over general anesthesia. Since conditions are stable, time is not of the essence in these cases.

TABLE 24-1

Causes, Diagnosis, and Treatment of Fetal Distress

Cause	Diagnosis	Treatment
Decreased maternal oxygenation	Measure S_AO_2	Supplemental O_2
Maternal hypotension	Measure blood pressure	Ephedrine, IV fluids
Uterine vasoconstriction	Suspect IVC occlusion	Left uterine displacement
	Suspect "stress" response	Reassure patient, relieve pain
Umbilical cord compression	Variable deceleration, sudden onset fetal bradycardia	Change maternal position Amniotic fluid infusion
Uterine hyperstimulation	Tocodynamometry	Tocolytic therapy

SAO_2, oxygen pressure; O_2, oxygen; IVC, intravenous catheter; IV, intravenous.

The second category (class II) of urgency would be patients in whom the underlying maternal and/or fetal physiologic makeup is not stable, but is not immediately life threatening to either mother or fetus. In these patients, anesthesia need not be administered immediately, but steps should be taken toward initiating adequate anesthesia for delivery (usually within the hour). Regional anesthesia would again be the preferred technique over general anesthesia. Spinal anesthesia, because of its speed of onset and excellence of block, might be preferable to initiating an epidural anesthetic.

Class III patients are those in whom the maternal and/or fetal physiologic makeup is unstable *and* immediately life threatening to one or the other. Examples of this situation are listed in Table 24-2. Fortunately this situation is the least common. Diagnoses include large maternal hemorrhage, uterine rupture, and severe fetal distress (characterized by an agonal fetal heart rate pattern). In these settings, a cesarean section would optimally start within several minutes. General anesthesia is preferred for speed, unless an epidural anesthetic level adequate to begin surgery is already in place. Surgery can be started in patients who have a good sensory block to the T-10 dermatone if supplemental intravenous analgesics (such as ketamine in repeated 10- to 20-mg doses IV) are given as necessary while the epidural is being topped up to bring the level up toward the more usual sensory level for cesarean section. If the epidural anesthetic is extended for cesarean

TABLE 24-2

Categories of Emergency Cesarean Section

Class	Examples	Preferred Anesthetic
I (Stable)	Chronic uteroplacental insufficiency Malpresentation with ruptured membranes (not in labor) Previous lower segment cesarean section (with or without labor) Preeclampsia	Epidural, spinal
II (Urgent)	Failure to progress during active labor Active herpes with ruptured membranes Nonbleeding placenta previa in labor Placental abruption without fetal distress Severe preeclampsia or HELLP syndrome Chorioamnionitis Previous classical cesarean section in active labor Cord prolapse without fetal distress	Epidural (extended from labor), spinal
III (Stat)	Agonal fetal distress Cord prolapse with fetal distress Placental abruption with fetal distress Massive hemorrhage Ruptured uterus	General, local, epidural (if working, with T-10 or higher level)

Stat, immediate; HELLP, hemolysis elevated live enzymes, low platelets.

section in the setting of probable fetal acidosis, the use of chloroprocaine should be considered, since it has a more rapid onset and is less subject to accumulation of significant fetal levels secondary to *ion-trapping* local anesthetics that occurs in an acidotic fetus. If an epidural anesthetic is not in place and working, general anesthesia should be induced after a careful airway examination and assessment of nothing-by-mouth status. When it is suspected that the airway will be difficult for intubation, a predetermined algorithm for handling this situation should be followed, such as that recommended by the ASA.[10] In addition, if the patient has eaten recently, awake intubation might be considered and attempted before a rapid-sequence induction. If the airway appears to be problematic and a general anesthesia cannot immediately be induced, the cesarean section can begin under local anesthesia if the surgical team is familiar with that technique and is willing to proceed. Although one study suggests that spinal anesthesia in emergency settings has a similar fetal outcome to general anesthesia[11] it is controversial.

The current case falls into class II. If the epidural anesthetic is indeed working, it should be extended for cesarean section. If there is any question of the epidural working, rapid spinal anesthesia should be considered. Prevention or treatment of hypotension with ephedrine (unless contraindicated) and volume expansion will be critical for better fetal outcome.

Neonatal Resuscitation

The incidence of neonatal depression will be higher in infants after cesarean section for sudden fetal distress. With that in mind, adequate resuscitative equipment and personnel should be called as soon as the diagnosis of sudden fetal distress is made and the cesarean section is planned.

Summary

1. Fetal distress is the result of inadequate oxygen delivery to the fetus.
2. Sudden fetal distress can arise from a variety of causes, some of which may be reversible.
3. The diagnosis of fetal distress is a result of tests which are relatively sensitive, but have poor positive predictive value. Surgery must proceed in all patients with the diagnosis of fetal distress to treat those in whom fetal distress is indeed present.
4. Reversible causes of fetal distress should be treated while preparing for emergency cesarean section.
5. The anesthetic plan should be based on urgency of the cesarean section, the presence or absence of a working epidural catheter, *and a careful history and airway examination of the mother.*
6. Neonatal resuscitation personnel and equipment must be immediately available.

References

1. Mor-Yosef S, Samueloff A, Modan B, et al: Ranking the risk factors for cesarean: logistic regression analysis of a nationwide study, *Obstet Gynecol* 1990;75:944.
2. Endler GC, Mariona FG, Sokol RJ: Anesthesia-related maternal mortality in Michigan, 1972 to 1984, *Am J Obstet Gynecol* 1988;159:187.
3. Shnider SM, Wright RG, Levinson G, et al: Uterine blood flow and plasma norepinephrine changes during maternal stress in the pregnant ewe, *Anesthesiology* 1979;50:524.
4. Myers RE: Maternal psychological stress and fetal asphyxia: a study in the monkey, *Am J Obstet Gynecol* 1975;122:47.
5. Parer JT: *Fetal heart rate.* In Creasy RK, Resnik R, editors: *Maternal-fetal medicine: principles and practice, ed 2,* Philadelphia, 1989, WB Saunders.
6. Harris AP: *Fetal physiology.* In Chestnut DH, editor: *Obstetric anesthesia: principles and practices,* St Louis, 1994, Mosby–Year Book.

7. Zalar RW, Quillivan EJ: *Techniques to evaluate fetal health.* In Pritchard JA, MacDonald PC, Gant NF, editors: *Williams obstetrics, ed 17,* Norwalk, Conn, 1985, Appleton-Century-Crofts.
8. Jouppila R, Jouppila P, Hollmen A, et al: Effects of segmental extradural analgesica on placental blood flow during normal labour, *Br J Anesth* 1978;50:563.
9. Harris AP: *Emergency cesarean section.* In Rogers MC, editor: *Current practice in anesthesiology,* ed 2, St. Louis, 1990 Mosby–Year Book.
10. Benumof JL: Management of the difficult adult airway, *Anesthesiology* 1991;75:187.
11. Marx GF, Luykx WM, Cohen S: Fetal-neonatal status following cesarean section for fetal distress, *Br J Anaesth* 1984; 56:1009.

25

Antepartum Hemorrhage

A 26-year-old primigravida at 39 weeks' gestation is admitted via the emergency room with active vaginal bleeding.

Recommendations by Markus C. Schneider, M.D.

Vaginal bleeding during pregnancy is among the familiar problems in obstetric units and can occur at any time throughout gestation. Because the clinical presentation of antepartum hemorrhage may be variable and assessment of blood loss may be difficult, expert obstetric and anesthetic management will contribute to improving the outcome for both mother and fetus. To effectively reduce maternal and fetal risks associated with antepartum bleeding, accurate diagnosis should be rapidly established. The approach to obstetric and anesthetic management is based on both maternal and fetal conditions; therefore good communication between practitioners of these two specialities is of paramount importance to improve patient care, safety, and outcome. Although delivery of a healthy baby will always represent the ultimate goal of such a joint management, therapeutic interventions have to focus primarily on the resuscitation of the parturient in the presence of life-threatening blood loss.

Mortality

Similar to the first half of the 20th century when hemorrhage represented one of the most important factors responsible for obstetric mortality,[1] antepartum and postpartum hemorrhages continue to contribute to maternal morbidity and mortality. The National Center for Health Statistics reported that 13.4% of all maternal deaths were caused by peripartum hemorrhage during the period of 1974 to 1978.[2] In a study analyzing different areas of the United States from 1980 to 1985, obstetric hemorrhage remained one of the leading factors of maternal mortality, contributing 10.8% of all direct maternal deaths[3]; this review pointed out that the mortality ratio associated with hemorrhage was almost fourfold higher in parturients older than 30 years of age than in younger pregnant women. Moreover, the maternal mortality ratio was somewhat higher for women of black and other nonwhite races. According to data published in the most recent *Report on Confidential Enquiries into Maternal Deaths in the United Kingdom 1985-87,* peripartum hemorrhage was the fourth major cause of maternal mortality from 1985 to 1987, reaching a mortality rate of 4.5 per million deliveries.[4] For this period, 10 maternal deaths from peripartum hemorrhage were documented: 4 of these cases were caused by placental abruption, and 6 by postpartum hemorrhage. Interestingly, contrary to previous years, there was no fatality attributable to hemorrhage from placenta previa.

Policies and Standards

Although uterine bleeding constitutes one of the most common obstetric complications, life-threatening hemorrhagic emergencies requiring immediate surgical intervention are rare (0.05% to 0.1%).[5] Still, the risk is real and ever present even if the frequency of disastrous complications can be reduced by careful prenatal counseling and expert peripartum management. Nevertheless, policies on how to care for patients presenting with massive bleeding should be defined in all labor and delivery rooms to allow prompt action. It is obvious that experienced obstetricians, anesthesiologists, and neonatologists should be on call; but easy access to a blood bank, laboratory facilites, and neonatal and obstetric intensive care units are equally important.

When dealing with a pregnant patient with active vaginal bleeding, both obstetric and anesthetic management should be based on a policy that includes the following key points:

1. Clinical assessment of the patient and the fetus
2. Defining severity and etiology of obstetric hemorrhage (Table 25-1)
3. Defining obstetric management options
4. Determining anesthetic management options.

These points are discussed separately in the context of the most pertinent causes of antepartum hemorrhage. Placental abruption and placenta previa are the most likely causes of vaginal bleeding after 20 weeks' gestation and account for one half to two thirds of all cases.[6] Both placental abruption and massive bleeding leading to hemorrhagic shock may be associated with disseminated intravascular coagulation (DIC). These important causes of obstetric bleeding are discussed in more detail, whereas this chapter refers to the rare event of uterine rupture only briefly. Other conditions predisposing to obstetric hemorrhage are only listed here since they are clinically less relevant: vasa previa, different forms of coagulation disorder, cervicitis,

TABLE 25-1

Differential Diagnosis of Antepartum Hemorrhage

	Placental Abruption	Placenta Previa	Uterine Rupture
Abdominal pain	Present	Absent	May be present
Blood	Old blood	Fresh blood	Fresh blood
Sudden fetal distress	Common	Uncommon	Common
DIC	Common	Rare	Rare

DIC, Disseminated intravascular coagulation.

polyps, and tumors. In many cases no apparent cause of bleeding is found.

Etiologies

Placental Abruption

Definition, Incidence, Risk Factors, Morbidity, and Mortality

Placental abruption is defined as premature separation of a normally implanted placenta from the uterus after 20 weeks' gestation and before delivery of the fetus. The overall frequency of placental abruption varies between 0.2% and 2.4%.[6] The recurrence risk in a subsequent pregnancy was estimated to be 9.1%.[7] In recent years the incidence of severe placental abruption associated with fetal demise has dropped from 1 in 500 to 1 in 850 deliveries.[8] About half of the cases result in preterm delivery of a premature neonate subjected to a perinatal mortality of 20% to 35%.[8] According to a follow-up study, 14% of surviving infants had significant neurologic deficits.[7]

The primary cause of placental abruption has not been identified, but a strong association exists with maternal hypertension, trauma,[9] sudden uterine decompression, short umbilical cord, aortocaval compression, uterine abnormalities, high parity and age, cocaine abuse, previous abruption, stressful physical work,[10] and, probably also, preterm premature rupture of membranes.[11] The impact of low-dose aspirin on the incidence of placental abruption is controversial, but recent data suggest that the risk may be increased among unselected healthy nulliparous women receiving 60 mg of aspirin per day.[12]

Clinical Course and Complications

The typical clinical manifestation of placental abruption is painful vaginal bleeding. In a prospective study external bleeding was observed in 78% of all patients.[13] In all other cases bleeding was concealed within the uterine cavity. Under such conditions, ongoing formation of a retroplacental hematoma may result in complete separation of the placenta from its attachment to the dicidua basalis and, ultimately, fetal death. Furthermore, maternal safety may be jeopardized by concomitant consumptive coagulopathy and hemorrhagic shock since the extent of intrauterine blood loss often is not recognized or is underestimated. As much as 4000 to 5000 ml of blood may be sequestered within the uterus.[6,14]

Fetal distress (60%), abnormal hypertonic uterine contractions (34%), and idiopathic preterm labor (22%) are pertinent signs of placental abruption.[13] These symptoms are very important as ultrasonographic evidence of a retroplacental hematoma may be missing in many cases. A study of patients with nonacute placental abruption showed that in only 25% of the cases the diagnosis was confirmed by ultrasound.[15] Currently the accuracy of sonography may have been improved due to high resolution scanners; nevertheless, a normal finding does not rule out a life-threatening abruption.[13] One should note that the primary goal of ultrasound examination in obstetric hemorrahge is to rule out the presence of placenta previa.[15]

Fetal death, maternal hypotension, and DIC are indices of severe placental abruption. In such a situation more than one half of the blood volume achieved in pregnancy may be lost invisibly within the uterine cavity; therefore hemorrhagic shock, if present, is seldom out of proportion.[14] Overt hypofibrinogenemia and elevated fibrin degradation products, along with laboratory evidence for consumption of various coagulation factors, occurred in about 30% of women in whom placental abruption was severe enough to kill the fetus.[14] These pathologic findings may be accompanied by thrombocytopenia—a common finding during and after massive transfusion therapy—and profuse bleeding from intravenous puncture sites, surgical incisions, and mucosal surfaces.

Severe placental abruption accompanied by hypovolemic shock and DIC may result in acute renal failure. Renal ischemia due to impaired blood perfusion, vasospasm, and to diffuse fibrin deposition are implicated in reversible tubular necorsis and, in some fatal cases, in cortical necrosis.[16]

The Couvelaire uterus is the result of widespread extravasation of blood into the myometrium and beneath its peritoneal serosa. Fortunately, uterine contraction after delivery rarely is hampered by myometrial hemorrhage to such an extent that hysterectomy is indicated to achieve control of blood loss because of uterine atony.[8]

Obstetric Management

Physical and gynecologic examination are completed by evaluation of the fetal heart rate and a diagnostic ultrasound examination (Fig. 25-1). Treatment is based on maternal and fetal assessments and the degree of placental separation which may be mild (I), moderate (II), or severe (III). Eighty five percent to 90% of abruptions are mild or moderate; severe abruptions only account for 10% to 15%.[17] If there are no life-threatening hazards for the mother or her baby as in mild placental abruption, a conservative approach is recommended. Such an attitude is favored for the fetus who is preterm because therapy with glucosteroids, which accelerates fetal lung maturation, can be initiated. Close observation of mother and fetus is mandatory, as are facilities for immediate surgical intervention and access to a specialized neonatal care unit. On the other hand, to improve the survival chances of the fetus, cesarean section may be indicated for patients presenting with massive bleeding and DIC. Fetal distress as a result of uteroplacental insufficiency after placental separation is another indication for emergent abdominal delivery. Prior therapy should focus on increasing uterine perfusion pressure by eliminating aortocaval compression by establishing a left lateral recumbent position. Other steps aimed at immediately improving residual placental function in a distressed fetus include correction of maternal hypovolemia, anemia, and hypoxemia. In the case of uterine hypertonicity or preterm labor, tocolytic therapy with β-receptor agonists is controversial. β-Receptor agonists are not recommended in parturients presenting with massive bleeding because they are likely to aggravate hypovolemia by peripheral vasodilation and to increase maternal tachycardia.[8] Parenteral magnesium sulfate in doses used for pre-

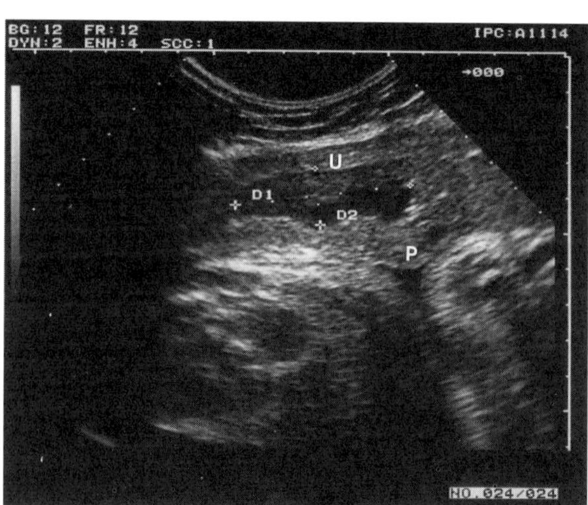

Fig. 25-1.

Placental abruption. Transabdominal ultrasound photograph showing an anterior placenta (P) separated from the uterine wall (U) by a retromembraneous bloodclot measuring 50.5 × 15.9 mm (✜ ··· ✜). *(Courtesy of Dr. Irène Hösli, University Women's Hospital of Basel, Basel, Switzerland.)*

eclampsia also has been administered without much tocolytic efficacy.[8] Vaginal delivery is the preferred method if the fetus is dead. Because DIC may develop within 8 hours after abruption complicated by fetal death[14] a timely delivery is critical. Unless the patient is in effective labor, the membranes should be ruptured and oxytocin augmentation should be instituted.[17] Cesarean section in a patient with severe coagulation defects carries a high risk of perioperative bleeding from the abdominal wall and uterine incisions, and even more so if obstetric hysterectomy should be necessary. Vaginal delivery restricts the problem of hemostasis to the placental implantation site where myometrial contraction and vascular retraction are the primary mechanisms of hemostasis,[8] to the perineal episiotomy site, and eventually to lacerations within the birth canal. Furthermore, pharmacologic stimulation to enhance myometrial contraction is well established and more easily achieved than control of diffuse bleeding because of DIC. Such a policy should help to reduce the risk of obstetric hysterectomy.

Placenta Previa

Definition, Incidence, Risk Factors, Morbidity, and Mortality

Placenta previa is a condition which occurs when the placental implantation site lies over or near the internal os of the uterus. Depending on the extent of encroaching, three types of placenta previa are differentiated as defined by Lavery[18]:

1. Total previa—the internal os is totally covered by the placenta
2. Partial previa—the internal os is partially covered by the placenta
3. Marginal previa—the placenta is proximate to the internal os and may lead to hemorrhage during cervical dilation caused by tearing of the placental attachment from the decidua.

The incidence of placenta previa at delivery varies from 0.4% to 0.6%.[19,20] The frequency increases with advanced maternal age, multiparity, and may be as high as 5% in the grand mulipara.[18] Other risk factors predisposing for faulty placentation include previous cesarean section, smoking during pregnancy, and prior spontaneous or induced abortion.[21] Placenta previa contributes significantly to maternal morbidity and perinatal mortality. Whereas maternal mortality secondary to this condition is expected to be minimal and was not documented at all in the *Report on Confidential Enquiries into Maternal Deaths in the United Kindom 1985-87*,[4] perinatal mortality still reaches almost 10% after third-trimester bleeding.[22] Prognosis for fetal outcome is even worse if bleeding occurs before the third trimester of pregnancy and may be as high as 67%.[22] The recurrence risk in a subsequent pregnancy is 4% to 8%.[18] Placental localization by transabdominal or vaginal ultrasound allows early identification of parturients at risk. Interestingly, in more than 90% of subjects with placenta previa in early gestation, placental migration resolves this condition by term.[23] Therefore an ultrasound diagnosis of placenta previa before 26 weeks' gestation is questionable.[17]

Clinical Course and Complications

The typical manifestation of placenta previa is painless third-trimester vaginal bleeding occurring in 90% of patients.[24] Commonly uterine activity is absent and diagnosis is supported by palpation of a large and soft uterus. With the presenting part of the fetus lying in the upper uterine segments, abnormal presentation may be encountered in 35% of all cases.[25] The risk of having a small-for-gestational age infant is increased in parturients presenting with a low-lying placenta: rates of 7.2% versus 0%[26] and 9.1% versus 2.7%[27] for low-lying versus normal placenta, respectively, have been reported. The probability of profuse hemorrhaging during the first episode is small and bleeding usually ceases spontaneously. Yet, any following hemorrhagic episode may result in significant blood loss and give rise to fetal compromise. Because blood lost from the placental implantation site does not enter maternal circulation and factors likely to trigger the coagulation cascade pass per vagina, DIC is rare and usually only occurs after a loss of large quantities of blood. Estimating blood losses is much easier with these patients rather than in patients with abruption, since all losses are visible in the case of placenta previa.

In parturients with placenta previa, abnormal implantation resulting in placenta accreta, increta, or percreta is more common. Placenta accreta is characterized by chorionic villi attached to the myometrial surface, placenta increta by villi invading the myometrium, and placenta percreta by villi penetrating the full thickness of the myometrium and sometimes even invading the uterine serosa.[28] The frequency of placenta accreta reportedly ranges from 1 in 2000 to 1 in 3750 deliveries.[28] This low incidence increases in parturients with placenta previa, and even more so in the presence of uterine scars; whereas placenta accreta was diagnosed in 7% of women with placenta previa presenting for primary cesarean section, the rate increased to 31% of subjects presenting with placenta previa who also have a history of one or more previous cesarean deliveries.[29,30] Recent data show that this condition predisposes to catastophic postpartum hemorrhage because abnormal adherence of the placenta to the uterine wall makes spontaneous separation impossible after delivery of the fetus.

Based on data collected at the Brigham and Women's Hospital, Boston, between 1983 and 1991, abnormal adherent placentation was the primary cause for emergency peripartum hysterectomy.[31] In this report the condition of abnormal placentation accounted for 64% of all gravid hysterectomies whereas uterine atony contributed only 21%. Although there was no maternal mortality, morbidity was very high, including the need for transfusion (87%), postoperative infection (50%), and intraoperative urologic injury (9%).[31]

Obstetric Management

Definite diagnosis of a placenta previa is commonly made by expert transabdominal ultrasonography (Fig. 25-2). The diagnostic accuracy is about

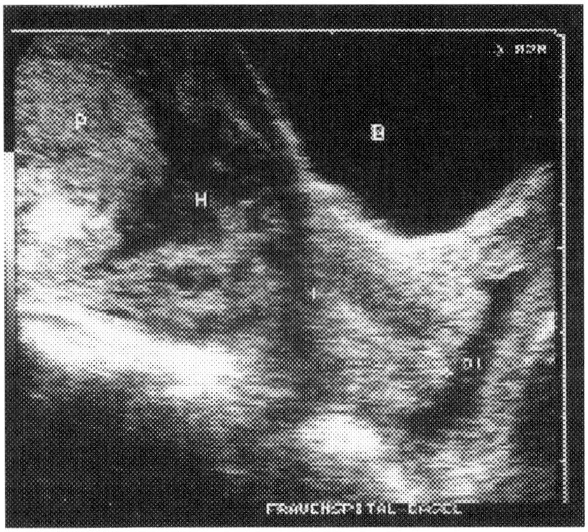

Fig. 25-2.

Placenta previa. Transabdominal ultrasound photograph showing a placenta previa (P) associated with a retroplacentar hematoma (H). The uterine cervix is directed sacrally and has a length of 35 mm (✤ ··· ✤). Urinary bladder (B). *(Courtesy of Dr. Irène Hösli, University Women's Hospital of Basel, Basel, Switzerland.)*

95% , with a false-negative rate of about 7%.[18] If done, vaginal examination should only be performed in the operating theater with the commitment to proceed to delivery after preparation for an immediate cesarean section in case of iatrogenic profuse bleeding. This so-called double setup is rarely required and carries all the risks of general anesthesia in an emergency situation. The time of the first bleed usually coincides with the period during which the lower uterine segment starts to elongate.[18] Because this usually takes place around 30 weeks' gestation, early delivery is better avoided with regard to fetal outcome, which is likely to be influenced by problems associated with prematurity.

All patients with significant bleeding should be hospitalized to enable close observation until 37 weeks' gestation. Expectant conservative therapy consists of bed rest, volume replacement, and blood transfusion in the case of severe anemia (hemoglobin level $<$ 8 g/100 ml) or shock. Continuous electronic monitoring of heart rate is important for fetal assessment and tocography allows for early detection of uterine contractions that may prompt further bleeding. In a laboring woman, when tocolytic therapy is warranted, magnesium sulfate or β-mimetic drugs, such as ritodrine or terbutaline, can be used. At the same time, glucosteroids are useful to accelerate fetal lung maturation.

Cesarean section is the preferred method of delivery in patients with placenta previa. In some cases of low-lying or marginal placenta previa, vaginal delivery may be successfully accomplished but should only be tried under optimal conditions for maternal and neonatal care.[18]

Uterine Rupture

Definition, Incidence, Risk Factors, Morbidity, and Mortality

Uterine rupture is defined as "complete separation of the wall of the pregnant uterus with or without expulsion of the fetus which endangers the life of the mother and/or fetus."[32] In contrast to complete disruption of the uterine cavity, incomplete rupture results in much lower morbidity and mortality. Incomplete rupture most commonly occurs in women with a history of previous cesarean section as a consequence of dehiscence of an uterine scar whereby the peritoneum remains intact.[33] The incidence of spontaneous uterine rupture is very low, ranging from 0.02% to 0.08%.[34] In the review of Plauché et al.[32] of 52,000 deliveries, the incidence of uterine rupture was 0.04%; the total number of 23 ruptures was composed of 14 cases of women (61%) in whom scar dehiscence was diagnosed whereas 9 cases (39%) resulted from rupture of an unscarred uterus. Although rupture of an intact uterus was characterized by increased blood loss and need for transfusion in comparison with incomplete rupture, in this report a similar fetal mortality of 35% was observed for both conditions, maternal mortality did not occur.[32] Clear evidence exists that the type of prior uterine incision influences the risk of future uterine rupture during vaginal birth after cesarean delivery; whereas the incidence of uterine rupture is about 4% for the classic vertical incision, it is less than 0.5% for the low transverse incision.[17] Therefore only parturients of the latter group should be encouraged to undergo a trial of labor and to have a vaginal delivery, provided that professional and institutional resources are available to immediately respond to acute intrapartum emergencies. According to guidelines issued by the American College of Obstetricians and Gynecologists, this means that authorized personnel should be present to perform a cesarean section within 30 minutes from the time the decision is made.[35]

Other clinical conditions apparently are associated with an increased frequency of uterine rupture. They encompass uterine distention due to macrosomia or hydramnios, grand multiparity, injudicious use of oxytocin, and direct trauma to the uterus by midforceps delivery or excessive fundal pressure.[33] Based on concerns about the theoretical possibility of masking pain associated with uterine scar dehiscence before rupture, epidural anesthesia once was implicated as a causative factor.[34] These reservations have largely subsided since a more recent study has shown that the sudden appearance of fetal distress is the most common sign in patients with uterine rupture, and that in 81% of patients, evidence of acute fetal distress precedes the onset of abdominal pain or vaginal bleeding.[36] Continuous electronic monitoring of the fetus therefore is recommended.

Clinical Course and Complications

The typical manifestation of uterine rupture is a sudden change of fetal heart rate pattern suggestive of fetal distress. This symptom often is accompanied by continuous tenderness over the lower uterine segment and abdominal pain that eventually "breaks through" a well-functioning epidural anesthetic. Commonly the pattern of uterine contractions changes and both a sudden increase in baseline uterine tone and a loss of intrauterine pressure may be indicative.[17] Passage of the fetus through the uterine wall may be reflected by alteration in the uterine contour and associated with symptoms typical of severe maternal hemorrhagic shock.[34]

Obstetric Management

Transabdominal ultrasound may be helpful in establishing the diagnosis of uterine rupture. In the presence of life-threatening hemorrhagic shock and severe fetal distress, immediate cesarean delivery should be performed. Repair of the ruptured uterus is a therapeutic option in patients with low parity and a desire for future childbearing; obstetric hysterectomy, though, is primarily recommended in patients with high parity and who do not desire future childbearing.[34] Persisting obstetric hemorrhage also can be controlled by ligation of the uterine arteries or the internal iliac arteries with the goal of avoiding unnecessary emergency hysterectomies.[37] Mechanical therapy (massage or compression of uterus) and/or manipulative treatment (insertion of a Foley balloon catheter into the lower uterine segment or packing of the uterine cavity with gauze) may obviate in some cases the need for immediate laparotomy and help to gain additional time before surgical intervention.[38]

Anesthetic Management

Assessment of Shock in Pregnancy

There is a consensus opinion that definitive management of profuse obstetric hemorrhage consists of emptying the uterus. Nevertheless, the urgency for achieving this goal is largely determined by the stability of the patients's cardiovascular system, the integrity of blood coagulation, and the postconceptional age and status of the fetus.[6] Before starting any therapy, estimation of the actual blood loss and the prehemorrhagic blood volume should be made as accurately as possible.[39] Because blood volume expands during pregnancy, hypotension and tachycardia are suggestive of severe hypovolemia. Profound hypovolemic shock—as characterized by a systolic blood pressure less than 80 mm Hg, marked tachycardia (120 to 160 beats/min), absent peripheral pulses, oliguria or anuria—corresponds to a loss that may exceed 40% of blood volume.[33] Since uteroplacental blood flow at term reaches about 600 to 700 ml/min per minute, unopposed uterine hemorrhage is striking. In case of severe hemorrhage, the primary goal of anesthetic management is to concentrate on maternal resuscitation by rapidly restoring maternal blood volume. This goal is achieved by immediate fluid resuscitation using two large-bore intravenous infusion lines (cannulae not less than 14 gauge or 16 gauge in diameter).

Monitoring of Volume Therapy

Volume therapy may be guided by control of central venous pressure. Central venous pressure is a relatively reliable tool to determine right ventricular preload and its response to rapid administration of fluids. Monitoring of arterial blood pressure using the Riva-Rocci technique may be inadequate in such a situation. Therefore insertion of a radial artery line for continuous measurement on a beat-to-beat basis seems justified; in addition, such a line is a prerequisite for repetitive control of arterial blood gas values and early detection of metabolic changes and acid-base abnormalities in shock. Insertion of a Foley catheter to measure urine output is of crucial importance because ongoing urine flow is one of the best tools to monitor effective plasma volume replacement.[40] Recording of pulmonary artery pressure and pulmonary artery wedge pressure as an approximation for left ventricular filling pressure is reserved for patients in whom straightforward volume therapy is complicated by left ventricular dysfunction or pathologic pulmonary problems. In such rare cases, determination of cardiac output by using a flow-directed pulmonary catheter may also be very informative. An important supplement to controlling aggressive fluid therapy is pulse oximetry, which not only provides information on arterial oxygenation, but also indicates pulmonary edema as a consequence of hypervolemia.

Diuresis and Diuretics

Loop or osmotic diuretics should not be used during the resuscitation period. Loop or osmotic diuresis would clearly negate the value of urine output as a guide for volume replacement therapy. In addition, induced diuresis increases the likelihood for the development of acute renal failure.[40] For the same reason, administration of balanced electrolyte solutions containing dextrose is discouraged since marked hyperglycemia with consequent osmotic diuresis may be induced.[40] Loop diuretics (furosemide 5 to 10 mg intravenously [IV]) are indicated only to initiate or accelerate the onset of fluid mobilization from the extravascular space, which starts about 24 hours after hemorrhage and operation.[40]

Guidelines for Volume Support

Despite the fact that "the amount of fluid given is often more important than the kind of fluid given,"[41] early use of properly crossmatched type-specific blood is important when hypovolemic shock is due to hemorrhage. Exceptionally, type-specific or Rh-negative type O blood *(universal donor)* may be transfused if blood of the proper type and crossmatch is not available.[42] However, initial maternal resuscitation is based largely on rapid infusion of lactated Ringer's solution. This allows time for accurate typing and crossmatching of blood. Furthermore, administration of balanced electrolyte solutions is essential for replacing the interstitial fluid deficit that accompanies severe hemorrhage. Current guidelines call for the infusion of 3 L of a balanced electrolyte solution for every 1 L of estimated blood loss, in addition to resuscitative transfusion therapy.[40] Extravascular fluid sequestration observed after resuscitation from hemorrhagic shock cannot be prevented by the administration of plasma. Albumin equilibrates at a rate approaching 500 ml/hr into the total extracellular fluid space, whereas intravascular albumin is degraded at a rapid rate.[42] Despite favorable changes of renal blood flow and plasma volume, albumin supplementation for hemorrhagic shock decreases glomerular filtration rate, sodium clearance, and urine output. Subsequently, an increased need for loop diuresis and an increased incidence of acute renal failure may be observed.[40] For these reasons, albumin should not be used in this setting. In contrast, administration of fresh frozen plasma is lifesaving in correcting severe coagulation defects induced by DIC. It is evident that in such a situation fresh frozen plasma always will have a favorable effect in terms of intravascular volume expansion. Finally, hydroxyethyl starch also can be used for acute intravascular volume expansion; it should be kept in mind, however, that neither the extravascular nor the intracellular fluid deficits will be corrected by a therapy using this colloid. Nevertheless, since plasma volume increases slightly in excess of the volume of hydroxyethyl starch administered, this supplementation may be helpful in "buying time" until blood is available. Dextran is no longer recommended.[4]

Pathophysiology and Therapy of DIC

Dealing with an increased bleeding tendency in a patient is always a challenge for the anesthesiologist. In obstetric patients presenting with antepartum hemorrhage, bleeding is most commonly the result of either placenta previa or placental abruption. In the case of placental abruption, maternal vessels supplying the placenta with blood are abruptly severed, causing part of the blood, which would have perfused the intervillous space, to escape into the uterine cavity, and forcing tissue thromboplastin and amniotic debris into the maternal circulation through open venous sinuses beneath the placental implantation site.[17] All of these events are considered to be contributory causes of coagulopathy, DIC, and abnormal platelet number and function. Clot formation as well as hemostasis depend on a variety of mechanisms, each of which may be independently impaired. In this setting the most pertinent feature is a generalized breakdown of coagulation and fibrinolysis accompanied by a progressive depletion of platelets. Pathologic range from small vessel occlusion due to microcirculatory thrombosis, resulting in distal organ ischemia and functional failure, to hemorrhage. Although identification and correction of the initiating stimulus are the ultimate goal of treatment, symptomatic therapeutic measures remain first priorities during the initial resuscitation phase. If hemorrhage is associated with laboratory evidence of DIC, at least two units of fresh frozen plasma should be a component of the initial therapy. Fresh frozen plasma contains factors V, VII, IX, XI, and XII that are synthesized by the liver, but also the regulatory proteins antithrombin III, protein C, and protein S, which may have therapeutic value in halting the coagulation cascade at two strategic points.[43] Cryoprecipitate, the best source of fibrinogen, may be administered when fibrinogen levels fall to less than 50 mg/dl.[43] If so, an average dose of up to 10 U may be required.[33] Platelet transfusion should be considered when platelet counts decrease to less than 80,000/μm^3 in association with bleeding or less than 30,000/μm^3 without bleeding.[33] Each platelet concentrate will increase the platelet count by about 10,000/μm^3 in the average 70-kg patient.[17] Because of the well-known hazards of blood transfusion therapy and because the risk of acquiring infectious diseases such as acquired immunodeficiency syndrome and hepatitis, one cannot entirely exclude a program fostering autologous blood donation of patients who are at increased risk of peripartum hemorrhage may be discussed to avoid the risks associated with donor blood.[33]

Cardiopulmonary Resuscitation

In the case of maternal cardiac arrest occurring before delivery of the fetus, cardiopulmonary resuscitation should be started immediately. Most of the standard procedures as defined by the American Heart Association should be applied without modification including airway management, defibrillation if ventricular fibrillation is present, pharmacologic therapy using standard drugs when clinically indicated, and last but not least, volume restoration.[44] Removing aortacaval compression by appropriate positioning of the pregnant patient is of paramount importance to increase the preload and to improve the efficiency of external cardiac massage. Open-chest heart massage and/or cesarean section may be required if standard measures are not successful. "Prompt performance of a perimortem cesarean section should be considered if initial attempts at cardiopulmonary resuscitation . . . have failed to restore effective circulation."[44]

Preanesthetic Checkup and Assessment

When called to see a patient who is actively bleeding, it is not possible to thoroughly determine the patient's past medical, surgical, and anesthetic history. Nevertheless, information about allergies to drugs, adverse anesthetic experiences, and time of the last food intake is needed. Preanesthetic assessment of the airway is of paramount importance and may subsequently influence anesthetic options. During the initial evaluation of the patient, oxygen can be administered via a face mask. Minimal monitoring includes blood pressure, heart rate, urine output, fetal heart rate, and if available, maternal arterial oxygen saturation. Laboratory tests should provide information about blood type, blood chemical values, hemoglobin level, hematocrit, white blood cell count, platelet count, and the actual coagulation profile (plasma fibrinogen concentration, factors V and VII, prothrombin time, partial thromboplastin time, fibrin degradation products, and bleeding time). While checking for the availability of blood (at least 2 U of packed red blood cells) and blood-derived products (at least 4 U of fresh frozen plasma), the hematologist as well as the blood transfusion service should be alerted.[4] Because parturients with antepartum hemorrhage are at risk to have to undergo a surgical procedure, oral administration of 30 ml 0.3 M sodium citrate (a nonparticulate antacid) is mandatory and may be accompanied by a prescription of metoclopramide (10 mg IV) and of a H_2-receptor blocking drug such as ranitidine (50 mg IV).

Regional versus General Anesthesia for Obstetric Emergencies

Anesthetic techniques used for operative vaginal or abdominal delivery depend largely on the urgency and the nature of the surgical procedure, maternal hemodynamics and volume status, and the results of actual coagulation studies. Epidural or spinal anesthesia is not recommended in patients presenting in shock or with established DIC. In these subjects, general anesthesia using a rapid-sequence induction (see the discussion later in this chapter) avoids the risk of epidural hematoma after accidental puncture of an epidural vessel; additionally, general anesthesia interferes to a lesser extent with blood pressure than does regional anesthesia and, for this reason, may be safer in a hemodynamically unstable patient. Furthermore, oxygenation of both mother and fetus may be optimized after endotracheal intubation unless problems related to difficult airway management are encountered. On the other hand, regional anesthesia is appropriate if results of clotting studies are normal, hypovolemia due to hemorrhage is being or has been corrected, and the fetal condition is acceptable for a spinal or epidural anesthetic.

Regional Anesthesia

Regional anesthetic procedures are not different from those performed in elective cases. The main advantages of spinal anesthesia include obtaining dense surgical anesthesia within a couple of minutes and a very low failure rate. Unfortunately, spinal anesthesia carries the disadvantage that a single injection may not work for another surgical procedure—for example, a subsequent obstetric hysterectomy. For such cases, established epidural anesthesia has been shown to be as safe as a general anesthetic in terms of maternal outcome and intraoperative blood loss.[45] To perform a continuous spinal anesthetic in such patients is almost impossible since small-bore catheters have been shown to be associated with cauda equina syndrome[46] and large-bore catheters produce an unacceptable rate of postdural puncture headache. When performing a spinal or epidural anesthetic, the potential for maternal hypotension should be anticipated and boluses of ephedrine (5 to 10 mg) should be given, or in presence of severe tachycardia, phenylephrine (50 to 100 μg) should be administered for treatment. Therefore prehydration is important: 10 to 20 ml/kg of lactated Ringer's solution should be administered in excess of the volume administered for blood replacement therapy. Correct positioning of the patient is an important prerequisite to reduce the incidence of hypotension due to aortocaval compression.

General Anesthesia

Before induction of general anesthesia, be sure of the following

- Anesthesia apparatus is working
- Endotracheal tube of appropriate size with cuff is prepared
- Two laryngoscopes are ready (one for the case of malfunction)
- Capnography is working
- Suction is available (in case of regurgitation)
- Monitors are attached to the patient (electrocardiogram, blood pressure cuff, pulse oximeter, nerve stimulator)
- Venous access is adequate for rapid fluid administration (two large-bore needles)
- All drugs are prepared for injection
- Urine catheter is in place (control of diuresis)
- Temperature probe is prepared.

After having preoxygenated the patient, anesthesia should be induced by an experienced anesthesiologist with the support of at least another staff person who applies cricoid pressure as soon as the patient falls asleep (Sellick's maneuver). As soon as a cuffed endotracheal tube is placed and its correct position confirmed by auscultation and capnography, cricoid pressure is released and the surgeon is told to start the intervention. A gastric tube then should be introduced for suctioning of the stomach.

What drugs can we use for *induction of anesthesia* for a shocked parturient?

- Thiopental at a reduced dosage (≤ 3 mg/kg IV)[33]
- Ketamine (0.5 to 1 mg/kg IV) for patients in shock (caveat: uterine tone may increase)[17]
- Etomidate (0.3 mg/kg IV) for patients with unstable hemodynamics
- Succinylcholine (1 to 1.5 mg/kg) for muscle relaxation

General anesthesia is maintained until the delivery of the baby by nitrous oxide in oxygen (up to 50%) and a potent volatile anesthetic (0.5 vol% halothane, 0.75 vol% isoflurane, 1 vol% enflurane).

After clamping of the cord, the potent volatile anesthetic should be discontinued to avoid uterine relaxation and replaced by drugs appropriate for *total intravenous anesthesia:*

- Midazolam (0.2 to 0.3 mg/kg IV) or
- Propofol (6 to 10 mg/kg/hr) and
- Fentanyl (0.2 to 0.3 mg IV) or other narcotics.

Muscle relaxation can be maintained by the following:

- Atracurium (0.2 to 0.3 mg/kg)
- Vecuronium (0.05 mg/kg) or
- Succinylcholine infusion.

The patient should only be extubated after full recovery from anesthesia and neuromuscular block. *Reversal of neuromuscular block* should be achieved by the administration of neostigmine (2.5 mg IV) with atropine or glycopyrrolate (1.25 mg or 0.5 mg IV, respectively).

Drugs used to enhance *uterine contraction* after delivery of the placenta include the following:

- Oxytocin, the standard first-line drug (2 to 5 U IV, 10 to 20 U in 1000 ml Ringer's lactate)
- Ergonovine or methylergometrine (0.2 mg IV or intramuscularly [IM])
- Prostaglandin PG $F_{2\alpha}$ (250 to 500 μg IM)

All of these drugs can also be injected intramyometrially by the obstetrician.

Summary

1. In this review several conditions resulting in life-threatening antepartum hemorrhage have been presented and obstetric and anesthetic management options have been discussed.
2. Although the ultimate goal of therapy consists of saving the lives of both mother and fetus, there can be no doubt that good maternal outcome should have priority. Immediate delivery of the fetus and placenta with simultaneous maternal resuscitation may be neccessary in patients with massive vaginal bleeding.
3. Consultation in the antepartum period and early notification from the obstetrician should make it possible to develop a joint plan of management, including the optimal location for delivery.[47]
4. Such institutions should have experienced obstetricians, anesthesiologists, and neonatologists on call, with easy access to a blood bank, laboratory facilities, and neonatal and obstetric intensive care units.
5. The authors of the *Report on Confidential Enquiries into Maternal Deaths in the United Kingdom 1985-87* recommend that "an agreed protocol for dealing with severe haemorrhage should be available in every maternity unit."[4] Such a preparation should contribute to further reducing maternal and fetal morbidity and mortality.

Acknowledgments

The author thanks Dr. Irène Hösli, obstetrician at the University Women's Hospital of Basel, for her invaluable help in preparing the ultrasound photographs, and Dr. Nenad Pavic, Acting Director of Obstetrics at the University Women's Hospital of Basel, for careful reading of the text and commenting on some pertinent issues of the manuscript.

References

1. Phillips OC, Hulka JF: Obstetric mortality, *Anesthesiology* 1965; 26:435.
2. Kaunitz AM, Hughes JM, Grimes DA, et al: Causes of maternal mortality in the United States, *Obstet Gynecol* 1985; 65:605.
3. Rochat RW, Koonin LM, Atrash HK, et al: Maternal mortality in the United States: report from the Maternal Mortality Collaborative, *Obstet Gynecol* 1988; 72:91.
4. Abrams ME, Metters JS, editors: *Report on confidential enquiries into maternal deaths in the United Kingdom 1985-87,* London, 1991; HMSO Publications Centre.
5. Chattopadhyay SK, Roy BD, Edrees YB: Surgical control of obstetric hemorrhage: hypogastric artery ligation or hysterectomy? *Int J Gynecol Obstet* 1990; 32:345.
6. Biehl DR: *Antepartum and postpartum hemorrhage.* In Shnider SM, Levinson JL, editors: *Anesthesia for obstetrics, ed 2,* Baltimore, 1987, Williams & Wilkins.
7. Abdella TN, Sibai BM, Hayes JM, et al: Relationship of hypertensive disease to abruptio placentae, *Obstet Gynecol* 1984; 63:365.
8. Lowe TW, Cunningham FG: Placental abruption, *Clin Obstet Gynecol* 1990; 33:406.
9. Kettel LM, Branch DW, Scott JR: Occult placental abruption after maternal trauma, *Obstet Gynecol* 1988; 71:449.
10. Schwartz RW: Pregnancy in physicians: characteristics and complications, *Obstet Gynecol* 1985; 66:672.
11. Vintzileos AM, Campbell WA, Nochimson DJ, et al: Preterm premature rupture of membranes: a risk factor for the development of abruptio placentae, *Am J Obstet Gynecol* 1987; 156:1235.

12. Sibai BM, Caritis SN, Thom E, et al: Prevention of preeclampsia with low-dose aspirin in healthy, nulliparous pregnant women, *N Engl J Med* 1993; 329:1213.
13. Hurd WW, Miodovnik M, Hertzberg V, et al: Selective management of abruptio placentae: a prospective study, *Obstet Gynecol* 1983; 61:467.
14. Pritchard JA, Brekken AL: Clinical and laboratory studies on severe abruption placentae, *Am J Obstet Gynecol* 1967; 97:681.
15. Sholl JS: Abruptio placentae: clinical management in nonacute cases, *Am J Obstet Gynecol* 1987; 156:40.
16. Silke B, Carmody M, O'Dwyer WF: *Acute renal failure in pregnancy.* In Bonnar J, MacGillivray I, Symonds EM, editors: *Pregnancy hypertension,* Baltimore, 1978, University Park Press.
17. Suresh MS, Kinch RA: *Antepartum hemorrhage.* In: Datta S, editor: *Anesthetic and obstetric management of high-risk pregnancy.* St. Louis, 1991, Mosby-Year Book.
18. Lavery JP: Placenta previa, *Clin Obstet Gynecol* 1990; 33:414.
19. Crenshaw C, Darnell Jones DE, Parker R: Placenta previa: a survey of twenty years experience with improved perinatal survival by expectant therapy and Cesarean delivery, *Obstet Gynecol Surv* 1973; 28:461.
20. Brenner WE, Edelman DA, Hendricks CH: Characteristics of patients with placenta previa and results of "expectant management," *Am J Obstet Gynecol* 1978; 132:180.
21. Taylor VM, Kramer MD, Vaughan TL, et al: Placenta previa in relation to induced and spontaneous abortion: a population-based study, *Obstet Gynecol* 1993; 82:88.
22. McShane PM, Heyl PS, Epstein MF: Maternal and perinatal morbidity resulting from placenta previa, *Obstet Gynecol* 1985; 65:176.
23. Rizos N, Doran T, Mikskin M, et al: Natural history of placenta previa ascertained by diagnostic ultrasound, *Am J Obstet Gynecol* 1979; 133:287.
24. Hibbard LT: Placenta previa, *Am J Obstet Gynecol* 1969; 104:172.
25. Silver R, Depp R, Sabbagha RE, et al: Placenta previa: aggressive expectant management, *Am J Obstet Gynecol* 1984; 150:15.
26. Newton ER, Barss V, Cetrulo CL: The epidemiology and clinical history of asymptomatic midtrimester placenta previa, *Am J Obstet Gynecol* 1984; 148:743.
27. Chapman MG, Furness ET, Jones WR, et al: Significance of the ultrasound location of placental site in early pregnancy, *Br J Obstet Gynaecol* 1979; 86:846.
28. Zahn CM, Yeomans ER: Postpartum hemorrhage: placenta accreta, uterine inversion, and puerperal hematomas, *Clin Obstet Gynecol* 1990; 33:422.
29. Clark SL. Koonings PP, Phelan JP: Placenta previa/accreta and prior cesarean section, *Obstet Gynecol* 1985; 66:89.
30. Arcario T, Greene M, Ostheimer GW, et al: Risks of placenta previa/accreta in patients with previous cesarean deliveries, *Anesthesiology* 1988; 69:A659.
31. Zelop CM, Harlow BL, Frigoletto FD, et al: Emergency peripartum hysterectomy, *Am J Obstet Gynecol* 1993; 168:1443.
32. Plauché WC, Von Almen W, Muller R: Catastophic uterine rupture, *Obstet Gynecol* 1984; 64:792.
33. Goldberg S, Norris MC: *Obstetric hemorrhage.* In Norris MC, editor: *Obstetric anesthesia,* Philadelphia, 1993, JB Lippincott.
34. Phelan JP: Uterine rupture, *Clin Obstet Gynecol* 1990; 33:432.
35. American College of Obstetricians and Gynecologists Committee on Obstetrics: *Maternal and fetal medicine: guidelines for vaginal delivery after a previous cesarean birth, publ no. 64,* Washington, DC, 1988.
36. Rodriguez MH, Masaki DI, Phelan JP, et al: Uterine rupture: are intrauterine pressure catheters useful in the diagnosis? *Am J Obstet Gynecol* 1989; 161:666.
37. Fehr H: Surgical management of life-threatening obstetric and gynecologic hemorrhage, *Acta Obstet Gynecol Scand* 1988; 67:125.
38. Floyd RC, Morrison JC: *Postpartum hemorrhage.* In Plauché WC, Morrison JC, O'Sullivan MJ, editors: *Surgical obstetrics,* Philadelphia, 1992, WB Saunders.
39. Lowe TW: Hypovolemia due to hemorrhage, *Clin Obstet Gynecol* 1990; 33:454.
40. Lucas CE, Ledgerwood AM: *Renal support.* In Fry DE, editor: *Multiple organ failure: pathogenesis and management,* St. Louis, 1992, Mosby-Year Book.
41. Hardaway RM: *Use of intravenous fluids in shock: introduction.* In Hardaway RM, editor: Shock: the reversible stage of dying, Littleton, 1988, PDG Publishing.
42. Shires GT, Shires III GT: *Use of intravenous fluids in shock.* In Hardaway RM, editor: *Shock: the reversible stage of dying,* Littleton, 1988, PDG Publishing.
43. Johnson PC: *Disseminated intravascular coagulation.* In Fry DE, editor: *Multiple system organ failure,* St. Louis, 1992, Mosby-Year Book.

44. Emergency Cardiac Care Committee and Subcommittees, American Heart Association: Guidelines for cardiopulmonary resuscitation and emergency cardiac care, part IV: special resuscitation situations, *JAMA* 1992; 268: 2242.
45. Chestnut DH, Dewan DM, Redick LF, et al: Anesthetic management for obstetric hysterectomy: a multi-institutional study, *Anesthesiology* 1989; 70:607.
46. Rigler ML, Drasner K, Krejcie TC, et al: Cauda equina syndrome after continuous spinal anesthesia, *Anesth Analg* 1991; 72:275.
47. ACOG commitee opinion: anesthesia for emergency deliveries. *American Society of Anesthesiologists Newsletter* 26, 1992.

26

Multiple Gestation

A 26-year-old primigravida is admitted to the high-risk unit with multiple gestation of about 36 weeks. On examination with ultrasound, she is found to be carrying triplets. The obstetrician requests an anesthesia consultation. Discuss the anesthetic management.

Recommendations by Catherine K. Lineberger, M.D.

The accepted incidence of spontaneous occurrence of multiple gestation is estimated at 1 in 90 pregnancies.[1] With increasing use of ovulation-stimulating drugs and in vitro fertilization techniques, the incidence of multiple gestation is increasing, with some studies showing rates as high as 22% in this group of patients.[2] Therefore obstetric anesthesiologists will be called upon to care for more and more women with multiple gestation.

Pathophysiologic Considerations in Multiple Gestation

Consideration of the physiologic changes occurring during pregnancy is important to optimal management of anesthetic for these women. Women with multiple gestations typically have larger, heavier uteri with more total intrauterine contents at any given point of gestation compared with singleton pregnancies.[3] Some of the physiologic changes of pregnancy may be more severe, and occur earlier in pregnancy in women with multiple gestations.

Women with multiple gestations are more likely to present with anemia at delivery and have increased blood loss with both vaginal and cesarean delivery.[4] Additionally, postpartum hemorrhage and uterine atony are more likely because of the overdistention of the uterus, which occurs with twin or higher-order gestations; therefore women with multiple gestation are more likely to require transfusion in the peripartum period than their singleton counterparts.

The presence of a *more than usually* enlarged uterus may result in decreased gastric emptying compared with singleton pregnancy. Additionally, the increase in symphysis-to-fundal height displaces the diaphragm even more cephalad, decreasing functional residual capacity further than in the usual singleton pregnancy and increasing maternal risk of hypoxemia during periods of apnea, such as during induction of general anesthesia.[4,5]

Another important mechanical effect of multiple gestation is that significant aortocaval compression may occur earlier in pregnancy and may be more severe than in a singleton pregnancy.[3,4] Aortocaval compression can even be present despite maintaining left uterine displacement if the uterus is particularly large. Awareness of this effect and attempts to avoid it are critical to preventing severe hypotension and decreased uterine perfusion during conduction anesthetics.

Multiple gestation pregnancies are also associated with an increased incidence of additional obstetric complications. These include a higher incidence of pregnancy-induced hypertension, preeclampsia, placenta previa, placental abruption, malpresentation, premature labor, and umbilical cord accidents compared with singleton pregnancies.[6] In addition, the incidence of fetal congenital anomalies is greater in multiple gestations compared with singleton gestations.

One of the most vexing problems in multiple gestations is that even with improved antepartum diagnosis, supervision, and care, the incidence of preterm delivery has not changed,[7] although perinatal survival has improved. The overwhelmingly predominant reasons for fetal loss continue to be intrauterine growth retardation and problems related to prematurity.[6]

Multifetal gestations (more than three fetuses) have worse outcomes than twins, although the numbers of these deliveries are too small for exact conclusions. Speculation exists that infant survival is at best that of triplets, and possibly less.[7] Although improvements in neonatal survival have been demonstrated in recent years, multifetal gestations must be considered high risk compared with their singleton counterparts.

In summary, obstetric anesthesiologists caring for women with multiple gestation often will be called upon to anesthetize high-risk women who have high-risk pregnancies. These women can be considered to have problems combining preterm delivery and possibly malpresentation in a patient whose physiologic reserve is minimal.

Twin Presentations and Modes of Delivery

Table 26-1 demonstrates the possible combinations of presentations of twin gestation, and the approximate incidence of the various types of presentation. For practical purposes regarding anesthetic management, all forms of twin presentation can be categorized as (1) vertex A/vertex B, (2) vertex A/nonvertex B, or (3) nonvertex presenting twin.

A detailed discussion of the preferred mode of delivery for various twin presentations is beyond the scope of this chapter. The preferred mode of delivery of twins, especially the delivery of a nonvertex twin B after a vertex twin A, is somewhat controversial,[8,9] and therefore obstetric anesthesiologists should be consulted early in the peripartum course of a woman presenting with multiple gestation. Most practitioners would agree upon the

TABLE 26-1

DISTRIBUTION OF TWIN PRESENTATIONS

Vertex-vertex	42.5%
Vertex-nonvertex	38.4%
Nonvertex	19.1%
Total	100%

Adapted from Adams DM, Chervenak FA: Intrapartum management of twin gestation, *Clin Obstet Gynecol* 1990; 33:52.

following indications for planned abdominal delivery: (1) conjoined twins, (2) nonvertex presentation of the first twin, and (3) more than twin gestation. Delivery of higher-order gestations (i.e., triplets or more) is almost always by cesarean section,[10] and therefore early obstetric anesthesia consultation should be obtained, preferably in the prepartum period. Although many obstetricians would accept vaginal delivery for vertex A-nonvertex B presentations, the obstetric anesthesiologist should be aware that the possibility of difficult twin delivery, particularly for the second twin, exists and there may be a need for emergent administration of anesthesia for cesarean section at any time during delivery of a multiple gestation.

The case presented is unusual in that spontaneous triplets are very rare, about 1 in 8000 pregnancies.[11] The survival of these babies to 36 weeks' gestation is also unusual, since the incidence of preterm labor is even higher in higher-order gestations than for twins. For example, the average delivery age for triplets is from 33 to 35 weeks,[7] and is unlikely to be older for higher-order gestations. Many women with multiple gestation require preterm delivery because of excessive uterine enlargement.[4]

Certainly in the case presented, with the potential for delivery of three viable infants, elective delivery, which optimizes the likelihood of adequate resuscitative care for each infant, would be desirable and should be undertaken at a center capable of such care. In all likelihood, the triplets in the case presented would be delivered by cesarean section.

Anesthetic Management

Analgesia for Labor and Delivery

Early consultation by anesthesia personnel is important in patients with multiple gestation because of the maternal and fetal high-risk situation they present. Labor and vaginal delivery are, for the most part, limited to women with twin gestations with the presenting twin in vertex position.

An anesthesiologist must consider several factors in making anesthetic choices for women in this circumstance. Knowledge of the anticipated delivery route and fetal age and maturity obviously is important. Assessing maternal comorbidities such as obesity, an anticipated difficult airway, or preeclampsia may affect anesthetic choices. Adequate personnel for delivery and resuscitation of more than one child must be available, and appropriate-level nursery care must be arranged. Monitoring fetal heart rate of both twins is necessary.

In preparation for providing analgesia for vaginal delivery for a parturient with twin gestation, several items must be prepared. Adequate intravenous access is important, and a blood specimen should be sent to the blood bank so that rapid cross-matching can be accomplished in the event of emergency cesarean section or postpartum hemorrhage. Administration of nonparticulate antacid and H_2-antagonists should be accomplished before any anesthetic administration.

In early or latent phase of labor, barring any other comorbidities, a small dose of narcotic can be employed for pain relief. Maternal desires are important, but epidural analgesia is the preferred method of pain relief for multiple gestation,[12] since it can provide the greatest flexibility for maternal analgesia and anesthesia, regardless of obstetric needs. Properly conducted epidural anesthesia provides the least exposure of the fetuses to anesthetic drugs, which may be a very important consideration in premature delivery.

Proper conduct of epidural analgesia for labor and delivery includes maintaining left uterine displacement during administration of local anesthetic and for the duration of the block. An appropriate bolus of isotonic fluid should be given intravenously before commencing the block, and slow, incremental dosing of the epidural blockade should be employed. This will minimize the likelihood of hypotension resulting from a sympathectomy in a patient with potentially inadequate venous return secondary to aortocaval compression, and minimizes the likelihood of toxic central nervous system effects if local anesthetic is accidentally injected intravascularly.

Appropriate choices of local anesthetic for initial administration of epidural analgesia include 0.25% bupivacaine or 1.5% lidocaine, 9 to 12 mL in 3- to 5-mL increments. An epinephrine-containing (15 μg) test dose can be used before administration of the bulk of the local anesthetic dose if the patient is not in labor, but it is not sensitive or specific if the patient is laboring. Incrementalization and gradual dosing of the local anesthetic administration provides safety in epidural dosing without the use of an epinephrine-containing test dose. Once the local anesthetic is administered, it is important to ensure that the block is bilateral and likely to function well for a cesarean delivery if necessary, so pinprick or other sensory testing should be carried out and checked intermittently during labor. Once the block is established, it can be maintained with a dilute solution of local anesthetic mixed with narcotic; a myriad of choices exist for this. It is important to maintain an adequate block at about the T-8 level for easy, rapid extension of the block for cesarean section, should this become necessary.

Ideally anesthesiologists should attend all twin deliveries. This allows for rapid administration of local anesthetic to provide adequate perineal analgesia for vaginal delivery or forceps delivery; this also allows for the administration of anesthesia for cesarean section should this become necessary. After the first twin is delivered, Twin B should be monitored for position and well-being. Occasionally, either external version of Twin B or breech delivery is attempted. This may require good uterine relaxation, which is not provided by regional anesthetics. Historically this has required induction of general anesthesia and administration of halogenated agents, but this is associated with the risks of general anesthesia in the parturient, such as aspiration and failed intubation.[13]

Intravenous nitroglycerin is being used with increasing frequency to provide uterine relaxation. In several cases it has been found to be efficacious with minimal hemodynamic effects, and of very brief duration, allowing normal uterine responses to oxytocin after delivery.[14] The usual doses reported have been 50-100 μg boluses, repeated as necessary. The use of intravenous nitroglycerin is supposedly contraindicated in patients who are volume depleted, but one must also consider the risks of inducing general anesthesia and administering volatile anesthetic agents to such a person. Additionally, at my institution early trials of sublingual nitroglycerin spray in 400 to 800 μg doses have been used with good efficacy.[15]

After delivery it is important to monitor the parturient for uterine tone and blood loss. Like all women with large, distended uteri, they are prone to develop uterine atony,[10] which should be promptly treated with infusion of oxytocin (20 U/L). Should this be ineffective, methergine or prostaglandin F2-α can be administered if there are no contraindications. Continued careful monitoring and ensuring adequate intravenous access for fluid resuscitation and blood transfusion are important, and obstetric anesthesiologists often are called upon to assist in this management.

Anesthesia for Cesarean Delivery

The anesthetic considerations for cesarean delivery include most of the recommendations discussed in the earlier section for labor analgesia.

The parturient with multiple gestation presenting for cesarean section is an ideal candidate for regional anesthesia for many reasons. Maternal benefits include the opportunity to be awake for the delivery, the ability to maintain a natural patent airway and avoid the risks of aspiration and hypoxemia, and with continuous techniques, hemodynamic stability is easier to achieve with regional than general anesthesia. Additional benefits include improved placental blood flow in circumstances of preeclampsia, which often is associated with multiple gestations. Benefits to the infants include less exposure to general anesthetic agents. This can be particularly important for premature infants, whose liver enzyme systems and blood-brain barriers are immature.

Preparation for administering anesthetics for cesarean section include several of the recommendations mentioned in the preceding section. These include adequate intravenous access (16-gauge catheter or larger), determination of preoperative hematocrit, and ensuring that crossmatched blood is available. Nonparticulate antacid and H_2-antagonists should be given, along with metoclopramide 10 mg intravenously, to reduce nausea and increase gastric motility once delivery is achieved.

A generous fluid bolus of at least 1000 to 1500 ml isotonic crystalloid should be administered before commencing the block. The parturient should be positioned in lateral decubitus position for the block if possible, to prevent aortocaval compression. Alternatively, the sitting position may be used, particularly if bony landmarks are difficult to palpate. Local anesthetic choices include 2.0% lidocaine (pH adjusted) with epinephrine 1 : 200,000 or 0.5% bupivacaine, the latter may be preferred if severe preeclampsia is present. I prefer to reserve 3% 2-chloroprocaine for situations requiring immediate reinforcement of an existing block, such as conversion of an epidural anesthetic from labor to cesarean section, because of its rapid onset and short duration. Fetal heart rate monitoring of all fetuses should be attempted and continued during the period when the patient is most vulnerable to the hemodynamic effects of sympathectomy. The patient should be closely monitored for early hemodynamic changes, and hypotension and/or bradycardia should be aggressively treated with increased left uterine displacement, administration of additional intravenous fluids, increments of ephedrine intravenously, and maternal administration of oxygen.

No large-scale studies exist to compare fetal or maternal outcomes regarding general versus regional anesthesia for cesarean section for multiple gestation, although there are many studies and reports[5,12,16-18] which document the safety of properly conducted regional anesthetics for these patients. Generally, epidural anesthesia is preferred over spinal anesthesia for these patients, although selected patients may tolerate a spinal without problem.[3] The use of epidural anesthesia allows for a more gradual onset of both the block, and most importantly, the associated sympathectomy. As mentioned earlier, a parturient with multiple gestation is likely to experience exaggerated aortocaval compression because of the markedly enlarged uterus. This is particularly true for higher-order multiple gestations. Spinal anesthetics may cause profound and rapid hypotension in these patients, which may be difficult to treat because of the severe aortocaval compression. One study found that spinal levels were higher in patients with multiple gestation compared with their singleton counterparts.[3] This was postulated to be due to the increased mass of the uterus and its contents compared with singleton pregnancy, causing engorgement of epidural veins and decreasing the size of the epidural and spinal spaces.

Most practitioners would recommend an epidural anesthetic for women with multiple gestation, particularly for those carrying higher-order pregnancies than twins. There may be certain instances when spinal anesthesia is necessary, such as if urgency for delivery precludes an epidural. If spinal anesthesia is chosen, meticulous attention to hydration, maintenance of left uterine displacement, and aggressive treatment of hypotension are required. General anesthesia, if desired by the patient or required by the circumstances, can be undertaken, although for the reasons listed earlier in this chapter, it is less desirable. If this is necessary, attention must be directed to avoiding aortocaval compression (by ensuring left uterine displacement), adequate prehydration, and minimizing induction-to-delivery time. All of the usual concerns regarding general anesthesia in the parturient are applicable to the parturient carrying multiple gestation, additionally remembering that functional residual capacity (FRC) is likely to be even smaller than in the parturient with a singleton pregnancy. Therefore adequate denitrogenation is essential before induction of anesthesia to prevent hypoxemia.

The recommendations regarding postpartum management after vaginal delivery of twins are similar to postpartum management after cesarean delivery of twins or higher-order gestation, with the added concern that blood loss after cesarean delivery is likely to be greater, and meticulous attention to volume replacement and treatment of uterine atony are important to maternal well-being.

These infants are likely to be small for gestational age, may require intubation or other airway management, and may have other associated anomalies. Additionally, certain conditions unique to multiple gestation may be present, such as discordant growth or twin-to-twin transfusion syndrome. It is important to ensure that adequate personnel and equipment are prepared for delivery of twins or higher-order gestations. The obstetric anesthesiologist will be busy caring for the mother and should not be the primary caretaker for the infants.

The parturient described in the case presentation almost certainly will be scheduled for elective cesarean section. The obstetric anesthesiologist should focus the preparation for this procedure on any coexisting medical or obstetric problems, a careful airway assessment, knowledge of prepartum hematocrit, and assurance that adequate intravenous access and blood products are available. An epidural anesthetic would be the preferred method of anesthetizing the patient. If possible, delivery should be elective, optimizing the likelihood that adequate nursing, obstetric, pediatric, and anesthetic personnel are available to treat all of the members of the rapidly increasing family.

Summary

1. Parturients carrying multiple gestation experience exaggerated physiologic changes of pregnancy compared with their counterparts carrying singleton pregnancies.
2. Properly conducted epidural anesthesia is the anesthetic of choice for cesarean section for multiple gestation, particularly for higher-order gestations.
3. Aortocaval compression is much more severe in these patients, and minimizing aortocaval compression is critical to optimal conduct of regional anesthesia in patients with multiple gestation.
4. Delivery of women carrying multiple gestations ideally should occur at institutions having adequate personnel and equipment to treat all the patients involved.
5. Chances of uterine atony are higher in this patient population and hence they should be followed closely in the postdelivery period.

References

1. Guttmacher AF: The incidence of multiple births in man and some of the other unipara, *Obstet Gynecol* 1953; 2:22.
2. Kurachi K, Aono T, Susuki M, et al: Results of HMG (Hurregon)-hCG therapy in 6,096 treatment cycles of 2166 Japanese women with anovulatory infertility, *Eur J Obstet Gynecol Reprod Biol* 1985; 19:43.
3. Jawan B, Lee JH, Chong ZK, et al: Spread of spinal anaesthesia for caesarean section in singleton and twin pregnan-

cies, Br J Anaesth 1993; 70:639.

4. McMorland GH, Effer SB: *Breech presentation, malpresentation, multiple gestation.* In Datta S, editor: *Anesthetic and obstetric management of high-risk pregnancy,* St. Louis, 1991, Mosby-Year Book.
5. Redick LF: Anesthesia for twin delivery, *Clin Perinatol* 1988; 15:107.
6. Chitkara U, Berkowitz RL: *Multiple gestations.* In Gabbe SG, Niebyl JR, Simpson JL, editors: Obstetrics: normal and problem pregnancies, New York, 1991, Churchill Livingstone.
7. Alvarez M, Berkowitz RL: Multifetal gestation, *Clin Obstet Gynecol* 1990; 33:79.
8. Cetrulo CL: The controversy of mode of delivery in twins: the intrapartum management of twin gestation (part I), *Semin Perinatol* 1986; 10:39.
9. Chervenak FA: The controversy of mode of delivery in twins: the intrapartum management of twin gestation (part II), *Semin Perinatol* 1986; 10:44.
10. Adams DM, Chervenak FA: Intrapartum management of twin gestation, *Clin Obstet Gynecol* 1990; 33:52.
11. Holcberg G, Biale Y, Lewenthal H, et al: Outcome of pregnancy in 31 triplet gestations, *Obstet Gynecol* 1982; 59:472.
12. James FM, Crawford JS, Davies P, et al: Lumbar epidural analgesia for labor and delivery of twins, *Am J Obstet Gynecol* 1977; 127:176.
13. Tindall VR, Beard RW, Sykes MK, et al: Report on confidential enquiry into maternal deaths in the United Kingdom 1985-87, London, 1991, Her Majesty's Stationery Office.
14. Mayer DC, Weeks SK: Antepartum uterine relaxation with nitroglycerin at Caesarean delivery, *Can J Anaesth* 1992; 39:166.
15. Unpublished data.
16. Craft JB, Levinson G, Shnider SM: Anaesthetic considerations in Caesarean section for quadruplets, *Can Anaesth Soc J* 1978; 25:236.
17. Crawford JS, Weaver JB: Anaesthetic management of twin and breech deliveries, *Clin Obstet Gynecol* 1982; 9:291.
18. Crawford JS: An appraisal of lumbar epidural blockade in labour in patients with multiple pregnancy, *J Obstet Gynaecol Br Commonw* 1975; 82:929.

27

Breech Presentation

A 29-year-old multigravida comes to the hospital for prenatal care for the first time when she is 36 weeks' pregnant. On examination the membranes rupture; the baby is found to be in the breech presentation. Contractions begin. Discuss the obstetric and anesthetic management.

Recommendations by Barry C. Corke, M.D.

Breech Presentation

A breech presentation occurs in 3% to 4% of all labors, but may be as common as 7% at the thirty-second week of pregnancy. Before the twenty-eighth week of pregnancy, a breech presentation occurs as frequently as 25%.

The cause of breech presentation generally is unknown. However, there are factors which make it more likely:

1. Prematurity
2. Abnormal uterine development
3. Fetal malformations
4. Abnormal placentation.

Breech presentations are subdivided into three categories that have some bearing on outcome, and therefore are important in the decision regarding mode of delivery:

1. *Frank breech* has fully flexed hips, but extended knees.
2. *Complete breech* has fully flexed hips and knees.
3. *Incomplete breech* has one or both hips extended; this constitutes the footling breech since one or both feet may be the presenting part.

A wide variation exists in the reported perinatal mortality associated with delivery from a breech presentation: 9% to 25%. Since prematurity and fetal malformations are more common in breech presentations, much of the increased mortality may be attributed to these factors. When these factors are excluded, it seems that the mortality rate is not much different from that for cephalic presentations at term.

The potential dangers associated with delivery from a breech presentation include (1) prolapsed umbilical cord, which is more common with an incomplete breech; (2) trapping of the after-coming head by an incompletely dilated cervix; and (3) trauma from excessive neck extension and rapid delivery of the head, which leads to injury of both the spinal cord and the brain.

Because of these potential risks, a significant increase has occurred in the use of cesarean section for delivery. This is one of several factors that has led to the marked increase in the overall incidence of cesarean section. Studies with conflicting results have been conducted to determine whether the mode of delivery has a major influence on neonatal outcome. The benefit of cesarean section to the fetus presenting by the breech is still far from clear.

There are some situations in which little controversy exists regarding the value of cesarean section. Regarding *prematurity,* there is good evidence to support that outcome improves for infants in the 1000- to 1500-g weight range. This is less certain when the range from 1500 to 2000 g is considered. Much of the value of operative delivery is related to the reduction in intraventricular hemorrhage. *Flexion of the head* is a prerequisite for safe delivery from the breech presentation. If the neck is extended, there is a markedly increased risk of spinal cord damage. When the *estimated fetal weight exceeds 4000 g* or the mother is judged to have an *inadequate pelvis,* there is little dispute that cesarean section is indicated.

Using these criteria, 65% to 75% of patients with a breech presentation require a cesarean section. It should be remembered, however, that although cesarean section may decrease morbidity for the neonate, potential exists for an increase in maternal morbidity. Therefore defining criteria for the selection of mode of delivery should continue to be utilized. A move to the elimination of all vaginal deliveries in breech presentation has been resisted, which makes economic as well as medical sense. It is likely in today's political and legal climate that further intense scrutiny will be given to this problem.

External Version

The use of this technique is receiving a resurgence of interest. Success rates vary considerably. Rates as high as 60% to 75% have been reported with a similar percentage remaining as vertex presentations until labor commenced.

The majority of versions are attempted after the thirty-fourth week of gestation since a significant proportion of breech presentations will turn spontaneously before this time.

In general, the technique has proved safe and the incidence of complications is low. Since there is a potential for complications that may require immediate delivery, version usually is attempted in the labor and delivery suite. It is expedient for the procedure to be undertaken when emergency personnel are available, including anesthesiologists. Also, the patient should be encouraged to take nothing by mouth for 8 hours before the procedure.[1]

Anesthetic Considerations

Cesarean Section

When a decision is made to effect a cesarean delivery, the choice of anesthesia will be governed by the usual factors related to this procedure. An overriding factor may be the degree of urgency. If the procedure is undertaken as an emergency, there may be insufficient time to obtain satisfactory regional anesthesia, and general anesthesia will become necessary. This long-standing viewpoint re cently has been challenged by several authorities[2]: (1) It is often possible to place a subarachnoid block very rapidly, and to provide adequate anesthesia as quickly as would be possible with general anesthesia. (2) Maternal morbidity may be reduced, especially if the mother has a full stomach, compromised airway, or respiratory complications including bronchial asthma. (3) The neonatal outcome has been shown to be much the same, provided a significant period of hypotension is avoided.[3,4] (4) Recent studies have suggested that prehydration may not be as important as was previously considered.[5]

The following should be included in the decision-making process: (1) the decision of the patient after a thorough, if possible, explanation of the advantages and disadvantages of each technique (this is obviously a problem in the emergency situation); and (2) the skills and experience of the anesthesiologist (the anesthesiologist should not attempt to use a procedure if he or she is not fully familiarized with it).

Overall, the chosen technique should be one that is considered safe and provides comfort for the mother; is the least depressant to the fetus, allowing it to be delivered in optimum condition; and provides the obstetrician with conditions suitable to undertake the surgery.

Vaginal Delivery

When a decision is made to attempt vaginal delivery, it is still important that an anesthesiologist continue to be involved in the patient's management. Progress to cesarean section may occur at any stage and this is best accomplished if adequate preparation has been made. The management of analgesia for labor should be integrated into the over all plan for the patient's management.

In the particular case under discussion, the patient comes to the hospital when she is 36 weeks' pregnant. The diagnosis of breech presentation is made at this time, precluding any opportunity for the patient to discuss her anesthetic management before the start of labor. The patient therefore may be unprepared for what she will encounter. In the ideal situation, the patient would be counseled before the onset of labor so that she can be given the fullest possible explanation of the anesthetic alternatives. Her ability to understand the problems involved will be greatly increased if she is not in labor at the time.

When the patient has been admitted and assessed, a decision will be made as to how delivery should be effected. The obstetrician should inform the anesthesiologist of this decision so that the anesthesiologist can be involved as fully as possible in the subsequent management.

If the patient is to be allowed to progress in labor and deliver vaginally, a plan to provide analgesia is required. It is assumed that since the membranes have ruptured, the patient will be delivered within a 24-hour period. Therefore the agreed plan for analgesia can be expedited.

The pain of labor with a breech presentation can be particularly intense. Also, there is frequently a desire to push before full dilation, which may lead to cervical edema and impede delivery. For these reasons, analgesia is likely to be required at an early stage of labor.

In the past it was considered that regional analgesia was contraindicated with a breech presentation. It was believed that regional analgesia would diminish the patient's ability to push during the second stage. This, it was thought, would increase the number of deliveries requiring breech extraction, which is known to have significantly increased morbidity and mortality for the fetus. The recommended regime for analgesia was, at that time, systemic analgesia consisting of a strong narcotic such as meperidine, either intravenously or intramuscularly, with or without the addition of a phenothiazide. At the time of delivery, this may be supplemented by inhalation analgesia with nitrous oxide or methoxyflurane, pudendal block or local infiltration.[6]

Independent studies comparing the outcome for infants delivered from a breech presentation to mothers receiving epidural analgesia to those born to mothers receiving other forms of analgesia have been conducted. The important finding was that infants born to mothers receiving epidural analgesia had a better outcome when judged by both Apgar scores and biochemical evaluations. Consequently the use of epidural analgesia in the management of breech presentation in labor and delivery has markedly increased. The advantages include the following: (1) The urge to push before complete dilation is abolished (early pushing leads to cervical edema and may delay progress of labor). (2) The necessity for excessive doses of depressant maternal medication is avoided.[7] (3) During the delivery process, an assisted breech delivery can be accomplished under optimum conditions. The patient will be able to fully cooperate with the obstetrician and the perineum will be relaxed. Should forceps be needed to deliver the after-coming head, this can be achieved more easily in a relaxed, comfortable patient.

In this patient's case the suggested plan of management of labor would include the use of epidural analgesia provided that (1) the patient consents, (2) no other contraindications are present, and (3) sufficient time is available.

The epidural should be inserted as soon as labor becomes fully established. A sensory block to a level of T-10 bilaterally should be maintained until delivery. To minimize the degree of motor blockade, dilute solutions of local anesthetics should be administered.

The block should be established with appropriate doses of 0.25% bupivacaine and maybe supplemented with a short-acting narcotic administered epidurally if necessary.

The block then is maintained with either incremental doses of the same solution or preferably with a more dilute solution administered as an infusion (0.075% bupivacaine, 2 μg/ml fentanyl) at 10 to 12 ml/hr. The use of such dilute solutions will allow adequate analgesia with a minimum of motor block.[8] Throughout labor, care must be taken to prevent any interference with uteroplacental perfusion. This is likely to occur if the patient is allowed to remain supine at any time. One must remember that changes in uteroplacental perfusion may occur in the absence of any changes in maternal blood pressure. Careful monitoring of the patient must be maintained (1) to treat any episodes of hypotension with intravenous (IV) fluids, change of position, and IV ephedrine, if necessary; and (2) to assess the level of block at regular intervals to ensure that an abnormally high block does not occur; since this might suggest a migration of the catheter.

To obtain the maximum advantage of the epidural analgesia, the extent of the block should be ascertained. In particular, the degree of perineal analgesia should be assessed and if inadequate, further increments of local anesthetic should be administered.

Delivery must always be attended by an anesthesiologist or anesthetist and should take place in a delivery suite that is adequately equipped to perform an immediate cesarean section, should this become necessary. All necessary drugs and equipment required to administer general anesthesia must be immediately available, having been checked to ascertain normal functioning.

One of the true emergencies in obstetric practice is trapping of the after-coming head during a vaginal delivery from the breech presentation. The trapping may be caused by the once fully dilated cervix beginning to contract. Should this occur, the neonate is not able to maintain ventilation via the lungs, and the umbilical cord is likely to be compressed. Should this problem arise, the obstetrician must immediately alert the anesthesiologist. General anesthesia then being induced using a rapid-sequence technique with cricoid pressure maintained until endotracheal intubation is attained. The induction should be accomplished with a single bolus of sodium thiopental followed immediately by succinylcholine. A mixture of 50% nitrous oxide in oxygen should be used for maintenance. An increasing concentration of volatile agent then is administered until cervical relaxation is achieved. This may require a concentration of 3% to 4% halothane. Although this concentration of a volatile agent may be depressant to the neonate, the exposure time is likely to be short. In the presence of adequate regional anesthesia and in the absence of fetal distress, nitroglycerine in small doses (100 to 200 μg) can be used intravenously to relax the uterus.

The delivery must be attended by a pediatrician fully trained in newborn resuscitation. For reasons previously discussed, there is an increased likelyhood of neonatal problems. Pediatricians should be made aware of the anesthetic management of the mother so that they will be able to determine whether neonatal depression, if it exists, maybe drug related.

At all times during the management of analgesia for labor, the anesthesiologist should be aware that a cesarean section may become necessary. If this occurs as an emergency, there may be insufficient time to provide adequate regional analgesia. Recently this traditional thinking has been challenged. The use of spinal anesthesia in the face of fetal distress has become increasingly accepted. This is the result of work that has shown that prehydration in the laboring pain is not as critical as was once thought.[5] Also, an increased use of spinal analgesia for cesarean section has resulted in a familiarity with the technique. It is now believed to be a valuable technique when fetal distress is present, providing that the onset of surgery is not delayed by the use of regional analgesia.

If a decision is made to administer general anesthesia, a rapid-sequence induction should be undertaken to minimize the risks of pulmonary aspiration of stomach contents. A technique such as the one described below should be followed:

1. Preanesthetic dose of a nonparticulate antacid, for example, 30 ml 0.3 M sodium citrate
2. Patient positioned on the table with a 15° left-lateral tilt
3. Preinduction oxygen with 100% oxygen by face mask
4. Induction with a precalculated dose of thiopental, 3 to 4 mg/kg pregnant body weight (PBW), and succinylcholine, 1.5 mg/kg (PBW)
5. Cricoid pressure applied before administration of thiopental and maintained until the airway is secured
6. Avoidance of mask ventilation before intubation
7. Protocol for failed intubation (firmly established by the anesthesiologist)
8. Inspired mixture of 50% oxygen and about 0.5 minimum alveolar concentration of a volatile agent, until the umbilical cord is clamped.

If there is sufficient time, a regional anesthetic technique may be selected. Either epidural or spinal analgesia would be appropriate. If an epidural catheter is already in place, an appropriate dose of local anesthetic can be administered to raise the dermatome level of the block to T-4. Alternatively, spinal analgesia may be administered. A dermatome level of T-4 again should be the goal to ensure optimum operating conditions.

Whether epidural or spinal analgesia is chosen, the following should be observed:

1. The patient should receive the same preanesthetic antacid as for general anesthesia.

2. If time allows, volume loading should be done with 1500 to 2000 ml of a nondextrose-containing crystalloid (e.g., lactated Ringer's)
3. The patient should be maintained in a supine position with a 15° left-lateral tilt
4. The systolic blood pressure should be maintained by use of IV fluid or, if necessary, incremental administration of ephedrine 5 to 10 mg intravenously.

If a decision is made from the onset to proceed with a cesarean section, the same principles will apply. A decision regarding the choice of anesthesia needs to be made and administered in the manner described above.

Summary

The major principle regarding the anesthetic management of this case is to be prepared for all eventualities, which includes the following:

1. Discussion of the management of the obstetric problems with the obstetrician and being aware of the plan for delivery
2. Discussion of alternatives of management with the patient
3. Maintaining facilities to do an immediate cesarean section at all times
4. Maintaining a satisfactory IV infusion
5. Having the ability to obtain blood should it become necessary.
6. Being present during vaginal delivery.

If the clinician strictly adheres to these principles, the outcome is likely to be optimum for both mother and infant.

References

1. Gabbe SG, Niebyl JR, Simpson JL, editors: *Obstetrics: normal and problem pregnancies, ed 2,* 1991, Churchill Livingston.
2. Marx GF, Loykx WM, Cohens S: Fetal-neonatal status following cesarian section for fetal distress, *Br J Anaesth* 1984; 56:1009.
3. Corke BC, Datta S, Alper MH, et al: Spinal anaesthesia for cesarean section: the influence of hypotension on neonatal outcome, *Anaesthesia* 1982; 37:658.
4. Hollmen AL, Jouppilla R, Kojvisto M, et al: Neurologic activity of infants following anesthesia for cesarean section, *Anesthesiology* 1978; 48:350.
5. Root CC, Rocke DA, Levin J, et al: A re-evaluation of the role of crystalloid pre-load in the prevention of hypotension associated with spinal anesthesia for elective cesarean section, *Anesthesiology* 1993; 79:262.
6. Crawford JS: *Principles and practice of obstetric anesthesia,* ed 3, Boston, 1972, Blackwell Scientific Publications.
7. Crawford JS: *Principles and practice of obstetric anesthesia,* ed 5, Boston, 1984, Blackwell Scientific Publications.
8. Shnider SM, Levinson G: *Anesthesia for obstetrics, ed 3,* 1993, Williams and Wilkins.

28

Preterm Labor

A 28-year-old primigravida with a breech presentation at 29 weeks' gestation is admitted to the hospital in premature labor. The obstetrician decides to try to inhibit her labor with a tocolytic agent. Tocolysis was successful for only 12 hours. Discuss the anesthetic management.

Recommendations by Stuart Bramwell, M.D.

Preterm birth is defined as delivery before 37 weeks' gestation. In 1980, the year that the Food and Drug Administration (FDA) approved the first tocolytic agent, preterm delivery accounted for 8.9% of births in the United States.[1] When delivery takes place in a center with appropriate resuscitative services, 90% of 29- to 30-week gestations will survive.[2] In the intervening years, it has been estimated that as many as 100,000 women per year are given ritodrine for preterm labor.[3] Recently a large multicenter trial came to the conclusion that although ritodrine prolonged pregnancy by 24 to 48 hours, its overall effects on perinatal mortality and morbidity were indistinguishable from those of placebo.[4] These sobering facts have prompted some to suggest a reappraisal of our management of preterm labor.[5]

The leading cause of morbidity in the preterm birth is periventricular and intraventricular hemorrhage rather than respiratory problems, and is accounted for by the higher incidence rate of breech presentation (more than 25%), birth trauma, and infection.

Respiratory maturity is estimated by assessing the lecithin/sphyngomyelin ratio via amniocentesis. A ratio of less than 1.5 suggests the probability of respiratory distress syndrome, although the incidence and severity can be ameliorated with lung surfactant treatment (Exosurf),[6] where trials have shown a reduction in mortality from 23% to 11%.

A new, more rapid measure of lung maturity is the TDx assay, evaluating surfactant and amniotic albumin. Rapid (30 minutes) results from this study can accelerate the decision-making process regarding delivery.[7]

Despite a study evaluating treatment with β-agonist tocolytics, which showed no beneficial effect on perinatal mortality or severe neonatal respiratory depression,[8] we remain ignorant of the precise mechanism that initiates labor, although a multifactorial origin seems likely. Uterine distension by multiple pregnancy, polyhydramnios, or macrosomia may be one mechanism. Infection—either generalized systemic as in pyelonephritis, or localized vaginal or cervical, with weakening or rupture of the membranes—may be another. Localized infection is associated with one third of preterm deliveries; the timing of the start of the infection process is not always clear, but it has been shown that many of the organisms responsible for the infections have phospholipase A activity. This enzyme could lead to increased release of arachidonic acid from preformed glycerophospholipids in the fetal membranes, followed by prostaglandin biosynthesis and labor.

One of the keys to uterine contraction is calcium in the uterine muscle. The oscillation of calcium during contractions originates intracellularly, where it is sequestered in the cell plasma membrane, sarcoplasmic reticulum, and mitochondria. Calcium is released before contraction, to interact with actin myosin and adenosine triphosphate before being released again into the cytoplasm, and then returned to the storage sites during relaxation.

Most drugs that have influence on uterine contractions do so through calcium regulation. Prostaglandins inhibit calcium binding within the uterine muscle cell, leading to release of calcium and contraction. Oxytocin inhibits calcium binding at the sarcoplasmic reticulum, leading to an increase of free calcium, hence muscle contraction. The calcium originates from both extracellular and intracellular sources. The calcium concentration outside the cell is 10^{-3} M or 10,000-fold higher than intracellular. Calcium can enter the cell through either a voltage- or hormone-controlled channel. Intracellularly, calcium is found in the sarcoplasmic reticulum.

The effect of oxytocin is mediated via receptors on the cell membrane, probably controlling one of the hormonal calcium channels. An increase in the number of receptors occurs as pregnancy progresses, regulated by the levels of estrogen and progesterone. The step between hormone binding and cellular action is mediated by second messengers.[9]

Prostaglandins are detected by radioimmunoassay in the amniotic fluid from mid pregnancy, and their concentration rises from that point to the onset of labor. The stimulus for increased prostaglandin formation in the fetal membranes at the onset of parturition may be estrogens. Overwhelming evidence in the literature implies that there is an interaction between prostaglandins and oxytocin, so that the presence of prostaglandins is obligatory for maximal oxytocin response. Hence the conclusion can be drawn that the physiologic changes that lead to human parturition are related to changes in the number of receptors and increased biosynthesis of prostaglandins. These hormones also appear to be important in the development of gap junctions, which are areas of low resistance between muscle cells, thus promoting the synchronized muscle contraction necessary to develop the expulsive force of labor.[10]

Tocolytic Agents

β-sympathomimetic agents act by increasing intracellular cyclic adenosine monophosphate, which increases sarcoplasmic reticular binding of calcium and inhibits myosin light chain kinase by dissociating calmodulin. Ritodrine, the only β2-sympathetic agent approved by the FDA, does have some β1 activity leading to profound maternal side effects:

1. Metabolic effects
   A. Hypokalemia
   B. Hyperglycemia
   C. Metabolic acidosis
2. Cardiac effects
   A. Tachycardia and arrhythmia
   B. Decreased peripheral resistance
   C. Increased cardiac output
   D. Cardiomyopathy[11]
   E. Pulmonary edema.

Magnesium sulfate is a direct antagonist of calcium and competes for the sites of action. The therapeutic range for tocolysis is a blood level of 6 to 8 mEq/L. Treatment is initiated with a loading dose of 4 to 6 g followed by an infusion of 1 to 3 g/hr, with little accommodation for maternal weight. Blood levels may be drawn every 6 to 12 hours.

Calcium channel blockers inhibit transmembrane movement and buildup of intracellular calcium. Nifedipine may be administered by the oral or sublingual route at a dose of 10 to 20 mg every 6 to 8 hours. The side effects of nifedipine are as follows:

1. Peripheral vasodilation and myocardial depression leading to hypotension
2. Nausea and vomiting
3. Hyperglycemia in the mother with secondary hypoglycemia in the newborn
4. Anesthetic potentiation of nondepolarizing muscle relaxants, and the cardiac effects of the inhalational agents and local anesthetics.[12]

Combining nifedipine with magnesium will lead to enhanced cardiac toxicity.[13]

Prostaglandin inhibitors, exemplified by indomethacin, are administered initially by the rectal route, 100 to 200 mg, then given 25 mg orally every 6 hours for up to 72 hours. The side effects are minor, with local effects such as proctitis or gastric ulcer, thrombocytopenia, nausea, vertigo, and hypothermia.

All tocolytic agents have multisystem actions with many side effects. Since inception of this treatment modality in 1980, at least 95 cases of pulmonary edema have been reported, with an incidence rate of 3% to 9%.[5] The cause of pulmonary edema is related to many factors associated with the use of β-2-adrenergic agents:

1. They have potent renal effects leading to sodium and water retention as well as decreased colloidal oncotic pressure
2. They are associated with increased capillary permeability, especially in presence of infection
3. They are associated with tachycardia and cardiac arrhythmias
4. They are associated with electrocardiogram evidence of myocardial ischemia
5. Excessive intravenous hydration may occur.

If pulmonary edema occurs, treatment includes reduction of fluid input, cessation of all tocolytic therapy, oxygenation, diuresis, elevating the head of the patient, oxygen saturation, and necessary invasive monitoring. The pulmonary artery catheter frequently reveals normal pressures, indicating that the cause of pulmonary edema is a fall in plasma oncotic pressure and an increase in capillary permeability, accompanying mild fluid overload.[14] The length of tocolytic therapy was thought to be important in predicting pulmonary edema, but this is not supported by experience, and there is no reliable way to predict which patient will develop this side effect.

Anesthetic Management

With the decision to allow the preterm labor to progress the anesthesiologist should be guided by various objectives:

1. Maintain the optimal milieux for the fetus. Avoid aortocaval compression by maintaining the patient on her side. Provide oxygen prophylactically to reduce the incidence of fetal asphyxia. Encourage relaxation techniques to avoid hyperventilation. Maintain hydration with glucose-free solutions to reduce hyperglycemia. Monitor the fetal heart rate.
2. Avoid the use of depressant medications in the mother, which may have an exaggerated and prolonged effect on the immature fetus with poorly developed liver function.
3. Provide early complete analgesia with a lumbar epidural, with perineal anesthesia to inhibit involuntary pushing.
4. Prepare for an operative delivery or cesarean section.

Many of the ideals of management are achieved by a lumbar epidural. The patient should be given 30 ml of Bicitra solution (sodium citrate dihydrate) as a prophylaxis against acid aspiration, in case a complication occurs during epidural placement. Routine fluid preload should be modified since the mother will have received fluids during her tocolytic therapy, and will have retained fluids if β-sympathetic agents were employed. If vasodilation was achieved by magnesium, β-sympathetic agents, or calcium channel blockers, it will not be exaggerated by lumbar epidural sympathectomy. The epidural should be inserted with the patient in the lateral position to avoid compression of the immature head, prolapse of the umbilical cord, or precipitous delivery.

The patient should be carefully monitored and the epidural incrementally dosed with 3- to 4-mL boluses, separated by 2- to 3-minute intervals, so that falls in blood pressure may be avoided, since the preterm fetus is very intolerant of asphyxia. Solid anesthesia should be established to the thoracic 10 dermatome, with the level maintained via an infusion of 0.25% bupivacaine with epinephrine 1:4000,000.

Rapidly progressing labor may justify the use of *low spinal anesthesia* (T-10 to S-5), either alone or by a combination spinal and epidural to enable expansion of the anesthesia if cesarean section becomes necessary. Hyperbaric bupivacaine 7.5 mg (1 ml), will provide 2 hours of good analgesia.

If regional anesthesia is contraindicated or rejected by the mother, inhalational analgesia with 40% nitrous oxide in oxygen can provide some pain relief to supplement a pudendal block with perineal infiltration.

Cesarean Section

The preterm neonate has a higher incidence of breech presentation and prolapsed cord. For these reasons and other indications, it may be necessary to deliver the baby abdominally. If the urgency allows, extension of the epidural anesthesia may be achieved with 2-chloroprocaine 3%, or lidocaine 2% with fresh epinephrine 1:400,000, and 50 μg of fentanyl to increase the speed of onset. Establishing an epidural *de novo* in the emergency situation needs to be attended by the same caution with fluid loading, as previously described, if tocolytic therapy has been used. Sipes et al. have shown that in the gravid hypertensive ewe, ephedrine remains the best agent to treat hypotension if it occurs while the effects of magnesium still are present.[15] With fetal distress, or breech presentation with or without ruptured membranes, it is preferable to use the lateral position for epidural or spinal insertion to avoid prolapse of the umbilical cord, or an exacerbation of the fetal distress. Subarachnoid anesthesia may be the appropriate technique if an epidural was not used during labor. Opioids may be added to the local anesthetic to speed the onset and enhance the intraoperative analgesia, as well as to provide good analgesia into the postoperative period. General anesthesia may be induced with either thiopentone 2 to 4 mg/kg or ketamine 0.75 to 1.0 mg/kg. Using standard preoxygenation, antacid, and cricoid pressure, with 60%/40% oxygen/nitrous oxide and isoflurane 0.75%, the preterm infant will not be depressed by the anesthetic. Magnesium potentiates the effects of both depolarizing and nondepolarizing muscle relaxants; a defasciculating dose of curare is unnecessary. It is preferable to avoid the use of nondepolarizing agents.

Summary

Many obstetricians still use tocolytic therapy to arrest preterm labor.

1. All of the tocolytic agents have widespread effects that impose greater risk on the mother and necessitate her transfer to a tertiary care center.
2. Fastideous attention to detail with strict monitoring of fluid balance, electrolytes, and physical signs is obligatory.
3. Careful hydration and cautious epidural dosing can provide the optimal conditions for controlled vaginal delivery as well as cesarean section.

References

1. U.S. Dept of Health and Human Services, Public Health Service, National Center for Health Statistics: *Vital Statistics of the United States 1980*. Hyattsville, Md, 1984, U.S. Department of Health and Human Services.
2. Man DM, Man EK. *Management of preterm delivery*. In Gabbe SG, Niebyl JR, Simpson JL, editors: *Obstetrics: normal and abnormal problem pregnancies,* New York 1986, Churchill Livingstone.
3. Leveno KJ, Little BB, Cunningham FG: The national impact of ritodrine hydrochloride for inhibition of preterm labor, *Obstet Gynecol* 1990; 76:12.
4. The Canadian Preterm Labor Investigators Group: Treatment of preterm labor with the beta-adrenergic agonist ritodrine, *N Engl J Med* 1992; 327:308.
5. Leveno KJ, Cunningham FG: Beta-adrenergic agonists for preterm labor, *N Engl J Med* 1992; 327:349.
6. Long W, Thompson T, Sundell H, et al: Effects of two rescue doses of a synthetic surfactant on mortality rate and survival without bronchopulmonary dysplasia in 700-1350 gram infants with respiratory distress syndrome, *J Pediatr* 1991; 118:595.
7. Russell JC, Cooper CM, Ketchum CH, et al: Multicenter evaluation of TDx test for assessing fetal lung maturity, *Clin Chem* 1989; 35:1005.
8. King JF, Grant A, Keirse MJN, Chalmers I: Beta-mimetics in preterm labour: an overview of the randomized controlled trials, *Br J Obstet Gynaecol* 1988; 95:211.
9. Carsten ME, Miller JD: A new look at uterine muscle contraction, *Am J Obstet Gynecol* 1987; 157:1003.
10. Huddleston JF: Preterm labor, *Clin Obstet Gynecol* 1982; 25:123.
11. Eggleston MK: Management of preterm labor and delivery, *Clin Obstet Gynecol* 1986; 29:232.
12. Edouard AR, Berdeaux A, Rnmad R, Samii K: Cardiovascular interactions of local anesthetics and calcium entry blockers in conscious dogs, *Reg Anesth* 1991; 16:95.
13. Thorp JM, Spielman FJ, Valea FA, et al: Nifedipine enhances the cardiac toxicity of magnesium sulfate in the isolated perfused Sprague-Dawley rat heart, *Am J Obstet Gynecol* 1990; 163:655.
14. Pisani RJ, Rosenow EC III: Pulmonary edema associated with tocolytic therapy, *Ann Intern Med* 1989; 100:714
15. Sipes SL, Chestnut DH, Vincent RD, et al: Which vasopressor should be used to treat hypotension during magnesium sulfate infusion and epidural anesthesia, *Anesthesiology* 1992; 77:101.

29

Respiratory Problems in Pregnancy

A 29-year-old primigravida with a history of severe chronic bronchitis and asthma visits her obstetrician when she is 29 weeks' pregnant because of her increasing dyspnea on walking up one flight of stairs. Her electrocardiogram and echocardiogram are within normal limits. Her obstetrician decides on an anesthetic consult in view of her poor respiratory status. How would a clinician manage this patient, either for a vaginal delivery or cesarean delivery (elective or emergent)?

Recommendations by Marcia A. Procopio, M.D.

Respiratory symptoms are common in pregnancy with at least 60% to 70% of normal pregnant patients experiencing dyspnea in the first and second trimesters.[1] Normal physiologic changes of pregnancy will account for the majority of respiratory complaints. In the upper airway, mucosal edema, hyperemia, and hypersecretion occur. There is a change to predominantly diaphragmatic breathing due to the elevation of the diaphragm by the enlarging uterus. Also, the sensation of normal breathing may be altered.[2] However, severe shortness of breath and wheezing are abnormal and need to be evaluated. The case presented deals with asthma and pregnancy; however, other diseases such as cystic fibrosis and tuberculosis may complicate pregnancy. Both cystic fibrosis and asthma are discussed in this chapter.

Respiratory Changes in Normal Pregnancy

Normal respiratory physiologic changes during pregnancy include a decrease of 15% to 25% in both functional residual capacity and residual volume,[3] whereas the total lung capacity remains essentially unchanged due to an increased inspiratory capacity.[4] Spirometric measures of air flow such as forced expiratory volume in 1 second and forced vital capacity remain unchanged in pregnancy.[3] Due to the decrease in functional residual capacity, the closing volume may exceed the residual volume in parts of the lung fields, leading to ventilation-perfusion mismatch. An increase in tidal volume results in a rise in minute ventilation out of proportion to the increase in oxygen consumption that occurs during pregnancy.[3] This is presumably a response to increased circulating levels of progesterone.[5] Progesterone has also been implicated in the improvement of airway responsiveness seen in pregnancy. Although this improvement is significant, progesterone does not appear to be the sole contributor.[6]

Arterial blood gas evaluation during pregnancy shows a higher oxygen pressure (Po_2) of 90 to 106 mm Hg and a lower carbon dioxide pressure (Pco_2) of 25 to 32 mm Hg than in the nonpregnant patient. The respiratory alkalosis is compensated for by renal excretion of bicarbonate, resulting in a pH of 7.40 to 7.47. A Pco_2 greater than 35 mm Hg or a Po_2 less than 70 mm Hg indicates respiratory compromise in the gravid woman.[5,7]

Throughout gestation the fetus lives in an environment of poor oxygen reserve. Fetal umbilical vein blood has a Po_2 of 32 mm Hg when the mother is breathing room air. After the mother inspires 100% oxygen, the fetal Po_2 increases to only 40 mm Hg due to the large shunt in the placenta. To compensate for this low oxygen tension, the fetus redistributes circulation to vital organs, decreases bodily movements, and increases tissue oxygen extraction. Also, fetal hemoglobin is less responsive to 2,3-diphosphoglycerate than is adult hemoglobin, so the high oxygen affinity of fetal hemoglobin is maintained.[8]

Cystic Fibrosis and Pregnancy

Cystic fibrosis (CF), an autosomal recessive disorder, is no longer unheard of among pregnant patients. The median survival for CF patients has increased from 1 year in the 1940s to 29 years today. This increase in life expectancy is due in large part to advances in antibiotic therapy, nutritional support, and early detection and intervention.[9]

Pathophysiology

Cystic fibrosis is a disease of the exocrine glands which alters the viscosity of secretions. Manifestations of the disease include obstructive pulmonary disease of varying severity, chronic pulmonary infections, pulmonary hypertension, cor pulmonale, malabsorption, diabetes mellitis, biliary disease, and diminished fertility. Although women with CF have normal reproductive tracts, it is believed that fertility is reduced due to an alteration of the physiochemical properties of the cervical mucous.[10] However, in 1990, the CF patient registry reported 111 pregnancies in patients with CF. Pregnancy will stress the pulmonary, cardiovascular, and nutritional reserves of the patient with CF.

Although the alterations of pulmonary function during pregnancy are well tolerated in normal women, the marginal pulmonary reserve in the CF patient may contribute to pulmonary decompensation and hypoxemia, putting both mother and fetus at risk. Patients with CF who have advanced lung disease resulting in pulmonary hypertension and cor pulmonale may be unable to tolerate the increased blood volume and cardiac output which occurs with pregnancy, and is later augmented during labor and delivery.[9] These patients are at risk for right ventricular failure, particularly during and immediately after delivery. Also, chronic uterine blood flow insufficiency may result from the inability to increase cardiac output during pregnancy in these patients.[9]

The nutritional status of the patient with CF is

compromised by the effects of malabsorption, excessive caloric requirements due to chronic infection, and increased respiratory work. The patient with CF may be unable to augment her caloric intake enough to meet the metabolic demands of pregnancy.[9]

It is generally believed that the course of pregnancy in the patient with CF is determined by the severity of disease before pregnancy. However if there was a decline of maternal health, it was difficult to distinguish from the natural history of the disease. A recent study by Canny and colleagues[11] further documents the ability of women with mild disease to tolerate pregnancy. Patients were considered to have mild disease if they exhibited the following characteristics: (1) late age at diagnosis (mean age 12 years), (2) high prevalence for pancreatic sufficiency (48% versus 15% in the general CF population), (3) excellent pregravid nutritional status, and (4) relatively mild pulmonary function impairment (mean forced expiratory volume in 1 second [FEV_1] of 66% predicted and mean arterial Po_2 of 75 mm Hg). None of the patients in this study had a history of right ventricular failure before pregnancy. Twenty-five women had a total of 38 pregnancies. Of these pregnancies, only two required therapeutic abortion because of declining health of the mother. None of the patients developed right ventricular failure. However, about one third of pregnancies were complicated by pulmonary exacerbations requiring intravenous antibiotics and chest physiotherapy.[11]

Anesthetic Management

The management of labor and delivery in the patient with CF may be a challenge for the anesthesiologist. As noted, this is a particularly stressful period for the cardiovascular system, particularly for the patient with previous right heart failure. Medical management may be assisted by the placement of a pulmonary artery catheter to monitor right-sided and left-sided filling pressures. Continuous monitoring of oxygen saturation with a pulse oximeter is necessary. Supplemental oxygen will reverse the component of pulmonary vasoconstriction due to hypoxemia. However, since some patients with severe pulmonary disease rely on hypoxic ventilatory drive to maintain respiratory, these patients should be watched closely if supplemental oxygen is administered.[12] Narcotics should be administered carefully because of their respiratory depressant effects. Diuretics are used to treat right ventricular failure. Anticholinergic agents should be avoided because they cause inspissation of airway secretions.

During labor, placement of an epidural catheter will provide analgesia, decrease preload to the right heart, and provide a route for the administration of anesthesia should cesarean delivery become necessary. Intrathecal opioids also will provide effective pain relief for these patients.

For cesarean delivery, both regional and general anesthetic techniques are suitable. Some patients with severe pulmonary disease may be unable to tolerate the supine position making a regional technique unacceptable. If general anesthesia is administered, the uptake of inhalation anesthetics may be delayed because of ventilation-perfusion abnormalities. The viscous bronchial secretions in these patients may cause intraoperative bronchospasm, and can obstruct the endotracheal tube. Humidification of inspired gases is necessary to decrease viscosity of secretions. The patient must be aggressively suctioned and well oxygenated before extubation. If a regional technique is chosen for cesarean delivery, an epidural anesthetic will allow careful titration of the level of anesthesia.

Asthma and Pregnancy

The American Thoracic Society's Joint Committee on Pulmonary Nomenclature has defined asthma as "a disease characterized by an increased responsiveness of the airways to various stimuli, manifested by slowing of forced expiration which changes in severity either spontaneously or as a result of therapy."[13] The incidence of asthma in the United States is 4% to 8%,[14] and results in 4000 deaths annually.[15] Seven percent of women of childbearing age have asthma,[5] and this disease complicates 0.4% to 1.5% of pregnancies.[15] Adolescent girls are particularly prone to this disease with an incidence of 6.6%.[16] The goals for management of the pregnant asthmatic patient should be to prevent episodes of status asthmaticus, endotracheal intubations, and hospitalizations, and to prevent significant wheezing and episodes of hypoxemia using appropriate medications.

In acute asthma, oxygen delivery to the fetus may be jeopardized. Maternal hypoxemia due to ventilation-perfusion abnormalities reduces the oxygen supply to the fetus. If maternal hypocarbia is severe, uterine artery vasoconstriction may occur. If the increase in intrathoracic pressure during expiration is significant, a decrease in venous return will cause maternal cardiac output to fall, thus decreasing oxygen delivery to the fetus.[5] Also, hyperventilation will cause a left shift in the maternal oxyhemoglobin dissociation curve. If fetal hypoxemia becomes chronic due to poor maternal asthma control, growth of the fetus is deferred in favor of vital functions. The result may be a fetus that is small for gestational age.[5]

Several early studies suggested that asthma may threaten the life of both mother and fetus. Bahna and Bjerkedal reported a statistically significant increase in low birth weight, increased neonatal mortality and hypoxia in asthmatic compared with nonasthmatic pregnant women. They also reported increased frequency of hyperemesis, vaginal bleeding, and toxemia.[17] In a more recent study, asthma was carefully managed in pregnant women and perinatal mortality was not increased.[18] However, preeclampsia in mothers and hypoglycemia in infants occurred more frequently in mothers with severe asthma. There was no increase in congenital malformations in infants born to asthmatic mothers. With the maternal asthma carefully controlled, there was no significant difference with regard to length of gestation, birth weight, or congenital malformations. In asthmatic mothers requiring the chronic use of steroids, the incidence of prematurity is increased.[19] Severe gestational asthma during pregnancy may also cause maternal mortality. Gordon et al. reported two maternal deaths due to asthma in their study of 277 pregnant asthmatic women,[20] and Schaefer and Silverman reported one maternal death due to asthma among their 293 pregnant asthmatic patients.[21]

The severity of asthma may change during pregnancy as is suggested by several studies. However, there is a large inconsistency between the results of these studies. Deterioration of asthma symptoms was reported in 4% to 43% of patients, whereas improvement occurred in 3% to 69% and no change was reported in 20% to 93%. The reasons for this variability may be the method by which the asthma course during pregnancy was assessed or variations in the severity of disease in the population being studied.[22]

There are several characteristics of the natural history of asthma during pregnancy. Asthma often returns to the prepregnancy course within 3 months postpartum.[23] Also, a woman can expect the course of her asthma during one pregnancy to be repeated in subsequent pregnancies. For patients with severe asthma, the symptoms are likely to worsen between the twenty-eighth to thirty-sixth week whereas the asthma tends to improve during the last 4 weeks of gestation, regardless of the prior course.[23] Fortunately, severe asthma during labor and delivery is rare. Of 360 patients in one study, 90% had no asthma symptoms during labor and delivery.[23]

Management of Asthma During Pregnancy

The goal for the management of asthma during pregnancy is to prevent maternal and fetal hypoxemia. The gravida needs to be educated about possible triggering agents such as cigarette smoke, some forms of exercise, or cold weather. Drugs such as aspirin, nonsteroidal antiinflammatory drugs, and β-blockers may precipitate asthma. Reflux esophagitis can initiate or exacerbate an acute asthma attack, and antacids will be helpful in decreasing the acid reflux.[3] Any sign of an upper respiratory infection should be evaluated and treated promptly. If a patient is on antiasthma medication before becoming pregnant, it should be continued. If symptoms improve during gestation, doses may be tapered slowly.

The decision to initiate antiasthma therapy should be made in conjunction with the patient, the obstetrician, and the physician managing the asthma. The goal of therapy is to prevent maternal and fetal hypoxia while limiting fetal drug exposure. If antiasthma therapy is initiated, the route of administration should be considered. The inhaled route of administration is considered to have the least systemic side effects and the least fetal exposure.[3] Unfortunately, there is a paucity of data regarding the fetal effects of antiasthma drugs. Whereas there should be an attempt to minimize fetal drug exposure, particularly during the first trimester, this should not come at the expense of poor maternal asthma control. The fetus is likely to be at higher risk from chronic bouts of hypoxia than from exposure to small amounts of antiasthma medications. It is preferable to recommend drugs that have been used widely in pregnancy with a long safety record rather than to initiate newer agents.[7]

The most commonly used drugs to treat asthma are β-sympathomimetics, corticosteroids, methylxanthines, cromolyn sodium, and anticholinergics. β-Agonists were previously considered to be the first drug of choice for chronic asthma in pregnancy. However, recent studies indicate that asthma may be a primary inflammatory process with reactive bronchospasm. This has lead many physicians to begin therapy with corticosteroids,[24] although β-agonists continue to be efficacious in the acute setting.

Schatz et al.[25] studied the effect of inhaled β-agonist therapy in pregnant and nonpregnant women. They found no significant difference in perinatal mortality, birth weight, congenital malformations, preterm births, or Apgar scores between the two groups. Also, there was no significant association between the use of inhaled bronchodilators and the increased incidence of chronic maternal hypertension, pregnancy-induced hypertension, and transient tachypnea of the neonate.[25] Some studies have suggested that inhaled β-agonists should be used for acute attacks, not for maintenance, and that these drugs may worsen asthma when used frequently.[26,27] Epinephrine, a nonselective β-agonist is recommended by some authors as a first-line therapy during acute severe asthma.[8] Opponents site the observation from the Collaborative Perinatal Project that exposure to epinephrine during the first trimester is associated with an increase in congenital malformations.[28] This conclusion has been challenged, and when observer judgment was controlled, no association was found.

Theophylline and aminophylline have been used extensively in pregnant asthmatic patients with minimal adverse effects. The effect of pregnancy on theophylline pharmacokinetics is unclear with studies showing both higher and lower blood levels.[29-31] Since the fetal theophylline level is similar to that of the mother, blood levels must be followed. In patients who have not received theophylline, a loading dose of 6 mg per kg of body weight in 100 ml of dextrose is given over 20 to 30 minutes, followed by an infusion of 0.7 mg · kg · hr for 12 hours. The infusion is then decreased to 0.5 mg · kg · hr. Serum theophylline levels should be checked after 12 hours and the therapeutic range is 10 to 20 μg per milliliter of serum.

Recent clinical trials using corticosteroids to manage acute asthma during pregnancy have not demonstrated an increased risk of congenital malformations. The oral corticosteroids prednisone and prednisolone are slowly transported across the placenta,[4] which may explain the low incidence of abnormal fetal adrenal function after birth. Of the inhaled corticosteroids, beclomethasone dipropionate has been studied the most and found to be safe during pregnancy.[3] In acute severe asthma, parenteral administration of corticosteroids is indicated. Any patient receiving corticosteroids regularly or who has been treated with frequent courses of steroids during pregnancy should receive prophylactic steroids during labor and delivery or any other surgical or medical stress.[5,32] The recommended dose is hydrocortisone 100 mg intravenously, then every 8 hours through labor and for 24 hours after delivery.

Cromolyn sodium is useful as a prophylactic agent and has been used without adverse effect in pregnancy.[33] Anticholinergic agents such as ipratropium bromide are not as effective a bronchodilator as β_2-agonists in most patients. These medications may have an additive effect when used with β_2-agonists and they may increase the duration of action of inhaled β_2-agonist therapy.[34] There have been no congenital malformations associated with the use of atropine or ipratropium.[33,34] Food and Drug Administration classification and animal and human data on the safety of asthma medications during pregnancy are summarized in Tables 29-1 and 29-2.

Allergic immunotherapy is considered safe during pregnancy if the treatment was begun before pregnancy. The injections should continue during the pregnancy and may decrease medication requirements. Many clinicians advise against beginning immunotherapy during pregnancy because of the small risk of anaphylaxis.[5]

Pregnant patients with mild intermittent asthma

TABLE 29-1

FOOD AND DRUG ADMINISTRATION PREGNANCY RISK CLASSIFICATION

Category A:	Controlled studies in women fail to demonstrate a risk to the fetus in the first trimester (and there is no evidence of a risk in later trimesters), and the possibility of fetal harm appears remote.
Category B:	Animal-reproduction studies have not demonstrated a fetal risk, but there are no controlled studies in pregnant women, or animal reproduction studies have shown an adverse effect (other than a decrease in fertility) that was not confirmed in controlled studies in controlled studies in women in the first trimester (and there is no evidence of a risk in later trimesters).
Category C:	Studies in animals have revealed adverse effects on the fetus (teratogenic or embryocidal effects or other), and there are no controlled studies in women, or studies in women and animals are not available. Drugs should be given only if the potential benefit justifies the potential risk to the fetus.
Category D:	There is positive evidence of human fetal risk, but the benefits from use in pregnant women may be acceptable despite the risk (e.g., if the drug is needed in life-threatening situation, or for a serious disease for which safer drugs cannot be used or are ineffective). There will be an appropriate statement in the *warnings* section of the labeling
Category X:	Studies in animals or humans have demonstrated fetal abnormalities, or there is evidence of fetal risk based on human experience or both, and the risk of using the drug in pregnant women clearly outweighs any possible benefit. The drug is contraindicated in women who are or who may become pregnant. There will be an appropriate statement in the *contraindications* section of the labeling

may be treated symptomatically. Table 29-3 gives an example of a pharmacologic protocol for the treatment of asthma during pregnancy.[5]

Acute Asthma During Pregnancy

Symptoms of an acute asthma attack include inspiratory and expiratory wheezing, use of accessory muscles of respiration, respiratory rate greater than 30 breaths per minute, FEV_1 less than 1 L, and a heart rate greater than 120 beats/min. Patients are considered to have potentially fatal asthma if they have experienced at least one major criterion such as (1) acute respiratory acidosis, (2) respiratory arrest or intubation from asthma, (3) two or more hospitalizations for status asthmaticus despite use of chronic oral corticosteroids, or (4) two or more

TABLE 29-2

HUMAN AND ANIMAL DATA REGARDING THE USE OF ASTHMA MEDICATIONS DURING PREGNANCY

	Teratogenicity			
Drug	**Animal Studies***	**Human Congenital Malformation†**	**Other**	**FDA Class**
Inhaled β_2-agonists	—	No association [259]	No increase in perinatal mortality, prematurity, growth retardation, gestational hypertension in 259 women	—
Metaproterenol	Positive (P)	—	May inhibit labor‡	C
Albuterol	Positive (P)	—	May inhibit labor‡	C
Pirbuterol	Negative (P) Positive (M)	—	—	C
Terbutaline	Negative (M)	—	May inhibit labor‡ Preserves or increases uteroplacental blood flow in humans	B
Epinephrine	Positive (P)	Positive association [189]	Reduced uteroplacental blood flow in animals; may inhibit labor‡	—
Isoproterenol	Positive (P)	No association [31]	—	—
Isoetharine	—	—		
Bitolterol	Positive (M)	—	—	C
Ephedrine	Positive (P)	No association [373]	Reduction in uterine blood flow reported in animals but not in humans	—
Theophylline	Positive (P)	No association [193] No association [cardiovascular, case control] 3 cases of infants with cardiac congenital malformations	Newborns exposed to theophylline in utero may show signs of theophylline intoxication may inhibit labor no increased risk of stillbirth in 410 women	C
Atropine	Negative (P)	No association [401]	Alteration of fetal heart rate and fetal breathing reported after maternal IV atropine	—

TABLE 29-2—cont'd.

HUMAN AND ANIMAL DATA REGARDING THE USE OF ASTHMA MEDICATIONS DURING PREGNANCY

Drug	Teratogenicity		Other	FDA Class
	Animal Studies*	Human Congenital Malformation†		
Ipratropium	Negative (P)	—	—	—
Cromolyn	Negative (P)	No association [296]	No increase in perinatal mortality or prematurity in 296 women	B
Systemic corticosteroids	Positive (P)	No association [154] No association (261 in combined series)	Decreased birth weight in 119 women treated with 10 mg/day prednisone but not in 152 women treated only during the first trimester No increase in perinatal mortality in 261 women Association with preeclampsia in 67 women	—
Beclomethasone	Positive (injection) (P) Negative (inhalation) (P)	No association [45]	Increased incidence of low birth weight infants in 45 women§	C
Triamcinolone	Positive (P)	—	Fetal growth retardation in patient using 40 mg/day topical triamcinolone from 12-19 week's gestation	D
Flunisolide	Positive (M)	—	—	C

FDA, Food and Drug Administration.

*Positive, positive for teratogenicity in at least one species; negative, negative for teratogenicity in all species tested; P, published study; M, reported by the manufacturer.[33]

†Listing in brackets indicates no. of exposed women. All studies are cohort studies and report total congenital malformation except as indicated.

‡When administered systemically.

§82% of patients also received oral corticosteroids.

Modified from Schatz M: Pulmonary pharmacology in pregnancy in asthma during pregnancy: interrelationships and management, *Ann Allergy* 1992; 68:128.

episodes of pneumothorax or pneumomediastinum associated with status asthmaticus. The fatality rate is greater in this subset of patients than in other patients with asthma.[7]

Therapy for the pregnant patient with an acute asthma attack should begin with the administration of supplemental oxygen adjusted to maintain the Po_2 greater than 70 mm Hg and the O_2 saturation greater than 95%. Intravenous hydration with a balanced salt solution also is important at this stage, initially running at approximately 100 ml/hr. If the patient is not hyperglycemic, dextrose may be added to the intravenous fluid. The pharmacologic protocol in Table 29-4 is an example of a reasonable approach to the treatment of acute asthma during pregnancy.

In late pregnancy, terbutaline should be used cautiously because of the risk of maternal pulmonary

TABLE 29-3

Outpatient Management of Gestational Asthma

Prophylactic therapy (medications generally are considered sequentially as indicated)
Inhaled cromolyn (2 puffs tid to qid)*
Inhaled beclomethasone (2-4 puffs bid to qid)*
Regular oral theophylline (general long-acting preparations bid)
Oral prednisone at lowest effective dose, preferably on alternate days
Therapy for increased symptoms
Inhaled terbutaline (up to 3 puffs every 3 hr)
Oral theophylline
Oral prednisone course
Antibiotics (generally amoxicillin, erythromycin, or cefaclor) for documented or suspected bacterial sinusitis, bronchitis, or pneumonia

tid, three times daily; qid, four times daily.
*May be initially preceded by regular inhaled terbutaline (2 puffs qid).
Modified from Schatz M: *Management of asthma during pregnancy.* In Schatz M, Zeiger RS, editors: *Asthma and allergy in pregnancy and early infancy,* New York, Marcel Dekker; and Schatz M: Pulmonary pharmacology in pregnancy in asthma during pregnancy: interrelationships and management, *Ann Allergy* 1992; 68:129.

TABLE 29-4

Pharmacologic Management of Acute Asthma during Pregnancy

Nebulized terbutaline (2-4 mg + 2 ml saline)
May be repeated every 20-30 minutes, monitoring pulse rate, until respiratory distress corrected, $Po_2 \geq 70$, $Pco_2 < 35$
Then taper to q 4-hr maintenance
Intravenous methylprednisolone (with initial therapy in patients on regular corticosteroids and for those with poor response during first hour of treatment)
125 mg q 6 hr initially
Taper as patient improves
Consider anticholinergics for patients responding poorly; nebulized atropine (0.025-0.050 mg/kg) or metered dose ipratropium (2-4 puffs with spacer device) every 6 hr
Consider intravenous aminophylline. If it is to be used:
For patient not receiving oral theophylline: 5 mg/kg over 20-30 min, then maintenance dose
For patients receiving oral theophylline: Stat theosphylline level (< 5 µg/ml: 2.5 mg/kg over 20-30 min, then maintenance dose; ≥ 5 µg/ml: proceed to maintenance dose)
Maintenance dose (initially) 0.5 mg/kg/hr after response, side effects, and serum theophylline levels
Subcutaneous terbutaline 0.25 mg if not responding to the above therapy

Po_2, oxygen pressure; Pco_2, carbon dioxide pressure; q, every; Stat, immediate.
Reprinted from Schatz M: *Management of asthma during pregnancy:* In Schatz M, Zeiger RS, editors: *Asthma and allergy in pregnancy and early infancy,* New York, Marcel Dekker.

edema.[35] Since the onset of action of corticosteroids is 6 hours, their use should be considered early in the course of treatment. The fetal heart rate should be monitored continuously, and maternal blood gases should be monitored frequently. If maternal respiratory status continues to decline despite aggressive therapy, indications for endotracheal intubation include Po_2 less than 60 mm Hg despite supplemental oxygen, Pco_2 greater than 40 mm Hg, or evidence of maternal exhaustion.

Management of Labor and Delivery

The anesthetic management of the pregnant patient with asthma begins with a history and physical exam. Previous anesthetic history, allergies, medications, including any use of steroids, and recent respiratory symptoms should be noted. A physical examination of the lungs and heart are essential. A forced expiration may reveal wheezing. Further tests including FEV_1, forced vital capacity, electrocardiogram, and arterial blood gas may be indicated in the patient with severe asthma. As stated above, if the patient has a history of prolonged steroid use within the previous year, hydrocortisone 100 mg intravenously should be given on admission, then every 8 hours for 24 hours.[5,35] For all patients with a history of asthma, continuous monitoring of oxygen saturation with a pulse oximeter is indicated.

Pitocin is considered safe for the induction of labor. Intravenous or intraamniotic prostaglandin F2α has been reported to cause airway obstruction.[36] Although prostaglandin E2 is thought to have bronchodilating properties, it has been shown to cause increased airway resistance and bronchospasm in women receiving transcervical, intraamniotic, or intravenous prostaglandin E2. A recent report suggests that prostaglandin E2 suppositories or gel have not caused bronchospasm.[37] In the case of postpartum hemorrhage, ergonovine and prostaglandin F2α should be avoided. If their use is necessary, pretreatment with methylprednisolone is recommended. Alternatives to ergonovine include oxytocin and prostaglandin E2, although specific data are unavailable.[5]

During labor, supplemental oxygen is recommended and adequate hydration will help minimize the retention of thickened secretions. If asthma becomes symptomatic during labor, treatment should begin with aminophylline intravenously since this will not interfere with uterine contractions. If this initial therapy is unsuccessful, then β2-agonists should be added in order to control the bronchospasm.

For the pregnant patient with mild asthma desiring a vaginal delivery, natural childbirth can be safe. Narcotics can provide supplemental analgesia. However, since morphine releases histamine, fentanyl and meperidine are preferred.

For the pregnant patient with a history of moderate to severe asthma, consideration should be given to the early placement of an epidural catheter. The analgesia obtained with a properly placed epidural catheter should prevent maternal hyperventilation due to pain. A continuous infusion of a low concentration of local anesthetic such as bupivacaine 0.125% with the addition of fentanyl will provide analgesia with minimal maternal sedation and minimal effect on respiratory status. The epidural analgesia continues through second and third stages of labor and is discontinued after delivery. Placement of an epidural catheter for analgesia during labor in a patient with asthma also provides a mode of administering an anesthetic should a cesarean delivery become necessary.

For the pregnant asthmatic patient requiring an elective cesarean delivery, the types of anesthesia available include spinal, epidural, and general anesthesia. In all cases the patient is considered to have a full stomach and a nonparticulate antacid should be administered. All types of anesthesia may be administered safely to asthmatic patients; however, there are some advantages of regional anesthesia in these patients. Regional anesthesia blocks the maternal stress response to surgery and delivery whereas the fetal response to the stress of birth remains intact.[38] Most importantly, regional anesthesia avoids airway instrumentation, which is a powerful stimulus for bronchospasm.

The epidural technique allows a gradual onset and controlled level of blockade, thus avoiding respiratory compromise. Since blockade of the intercostal muscles may lead to difficulty with effective coughing and clearing of secretions, the level of anesthesia must be carefully monitored in the asthmatic patient. With epidural anesthesia, there is a greater difference between sensory level and level of motor blockade when compared to spinal anesthesia, which minimizes the respiratory compromise due to blockade of intercostal muscles.[39] An epidural technique allows the ability to extend the duration of the block intraoperatively and the catheter may then be used for postoperative analgesia.

During surgery, supplemental oxygen should be administered with routine monitors, including continuous oxygen saturation. An inhaler should be readily available in the operating room.

For the pregnant patient with asthma requiring a general anesthetic the anesthesiologist has several considerations. As stated earlier in this section, each patient is considered to have a full stomach and a nonparticulate antacid should be administered preoperatively. Cimetidine and ranitidine, H_2-receptor blockers, should be avoided since they could unmask unopposed bronchoconstriction. After preoxygenation for 3 minutes, rapid-sequence induction and intubation followed by awake extubation are indicated because of the full-stomach status of the pregnant patient. Intravenous induction of anesthesia is achieved with ketamine, which has been shown to decrease airway resistance in patients with pulmonary dysfunction.[10] Thiopental may not protect against bronchospasm in doses used clinically.[41] Emergence delirium associated with the use of ketamine may be attenuated with the administration of a benzodiazepine.[42] Endotracheal intubation is facilitated by succinylcholine.

Anesthesia is maintained with inhalational agents. Halothane, enflurane, and isoflurane depress airway reflexes and have a direct effect on airway smooth muscle.[43] If a patient is receiving aminophylline, halothane should be avoided since the combination of intravenous aminophylline and halothane has been associated with ventricular dysrhythmias in patients.[44] After delivery of the baby, narcotics and benzodiazepines are added to maintain an adequate anesthetic depth while the concentration of inhalational agent is decreased to avoid uterine relaxation.

Anesthetic considerations for an emergency cesarean delivery vary from the previous routine. If epidural analgesia was used for labor, the catheter may be injected with a rapidly acting local anesthetic such as chloroprocaine, and a surgical level of anesthesia will be obtained in minutes. If no previous block is in place, either spinal or general anesthesia are available. For the severe asthmatic patient requiring emergency surgery, a spinal anesthetic may be preferable to general anesthesia if it can be performed efficiently. For an emergency general anesthetic for cesarean delivery, preoxygenation is sufficient after four deep breaths of 100% oxygen.[45] Induction, intubation, maintenance, and emergence proceed as for the nonemergent surgery.

As with any patient with reactive airways and potential for air trapping, a slow respiratory rate with adequate expiratory time should be maintained. Inspired oxygen concentration of at least 50% during surgery is recommended.

Muscle relaxants such as curare or atracurium are associated with histamine release and should be avoided in the patient with asthma. Vecuronium and pancuronium can be used safely in these patients. Reversal of neuromuscular blockade can be achieved with neostigmine or edrophonium. However, since the muscarinic action of these drugs may precipitate bronchospasm, an antimuscarinic drug such as atropine or glycopyrrolate should precede their use.

Should an intraoperative episode of asthma occur it may be treated by temporarily deepening the inhalational anesthetic. If the bronchospasm continues, β_2-agonists should be given through the breathing circuit. The respiratory status should be stabilized before attempting extubation.

Since the risk of aspiration is high in pregnant patients and is particularly dangerous for asthmatic patients, extubation should be attempted only after reversal of muscle relaxant and after the patient is awake enough to protect her airway. The presence of the endotracheal tube in the patient emerging from anesthesia is a strong stimulus for bronchospasm, but coughing on the endotracheal tube can be decreased by small doses of narcotics or the use of intravenous lidocaine. Postoperative ventilation is indicated if there is any possibility that adequate ventilation will not be maintained due to ongoing bronchospasm. Continued therapy includes inhaled bronchodilators and humidified oxygen.

Summary

1. Since fetal and maternal outcomes are optimal when maternal symptoms are controlled and pulmonary function is maximized, pregnancy is an indication for maximally effective therapy, including bronchodilator and antiinflammatory medications.
2. For vaginal delivery in a patient with asthma, epidural anesthesia has the advantage of controlling maternal hyperventilation while providing a route for the administration of anesthesia for a cesarean delivery if this becomes necessary.
3. For cesarean delivery in a patient with asthma, epidural anesthesia has the advantages as stated above. The maternal stress response to surgery is attenuated with epidural anesthesia. In addition, the airway manipulation required by general anesthesia and intubation is avoided. Also, the level of epidural anesthesia is more easily controlled than with a spinal anesthetic, thus limiting respiratory compromise due to intercostal muscle paralysis.
4. Ketamine is useful for induction of general anesthesia for cesarean section in patients with asthma because it decreases airway resistance. Inhalational agents will cause uterine relaxation. After delivery of the baby, benzodiazepines and narcotics are given to maintain the depth of anesthesia while the concentration of inhalation agent is decreased. Intraoperative bronchospasm is treated initially by increasing the concentration of inhalation agent. If this is unsuccessful in breaking the bronchospasm, inhaled β-agonists are administered via the endotracheal tube. Respiratory status must be stabilized before attempting extubation.

References

1. Tenholder MF, South-Paul JE: Dyspnea in pregnancy, *Chest* 1989; 96:381.
2. Elkus R, Popovich J: Respiratory physiology in pregnancy, *Clin Chest Med* 1992; 13:555.
3. D'Alonzo GE: The pregnant asthmatic patient, *Semin Perinatol* 1990; 14(2):119.
4. DiMarco AF: Asthma in the pregnant patient: a review, *Ann Allergy* 1989; 62:527.
5. Schatz M: Asthma during pregnancy: interrelationships and management, *Ann Allergy* 1992; 68:123.
6. Juniper EF, Daniel EE, Roberts RA, et al: Effect of airway on airway responsiveness and asthma severity, *Am Rev Respir* 1991; 143:S78.
7. Greenberger PA: Asthma during pregnancy, *J Asthma* 1990; 27:341.
8. Greenberger PA, Patterson R: Management of asthma during pregnancy, *N Engl J Med* 1985; 312:897.
9. Kotloff RM, Fitzsimmons SC, Fiel SB: Fertility and pregnancy in patients with cystic fibrosis, *Clin Chest Med* 1992; 13(4):623.
10. Kopito LE, Kosasky HJ, Schwachman H: Water and electrolytes in cervical mucous from patients with cystic fibrosis, *Fertil Steril* 1973; 24:512.
11. Canny GJ, Corey M, Livingstone RA, et al: Pregnancy and cystic fibrosis, *Obstet Gynecol* 1991; 77:850.
12. Norris MD, Chan L: *Respiratory changes during pregnancy.* In Datta S, editor: *Anesthetic and obstetric management of high risk pregnancy,* Chicago, 1991, Mosby-Year Book.
13. Burrows B, Huang N, Huthes R, et al: Pulmonary terms and symbols: a report of the ACCP-ATS Joint Committee on Pulmonary Nomenelative, *Chest* 1975; 67:583.
14. McColgin SW, Glee L, Brian BA: Pulmonary disorders complicating pregnancy, *Obstet Gynecol Clin North Am* 1992; 19:697.
15. Barth WH, Hankins GDV: *Severe acute asthma in pregnancy.* In Clark SL, Phelan JP, Cotton DB, Hankins GDV, editors: *Critical care obstetrics, ed 2,* Blackwell Scientific Publications.
16. Apter AJ, Greenbuger PA, Patterson R: Outcomes of pregnancy in adolescents with severe asthma, *Arch Intern Med* 1989; 149:2571.

17. Bahna SL, Bjerkdal T: The course and outcome of pregnancy in women with bronchial asthma, *Acta Allergol* 1972; 27:397.
18. Stenius-Aarniala B, Pirila P, Teramo K: Asthma and pregnancy: a prospective study of 198 pregnancies, *Thorax* 1988; 43:12.
19. Fitzsimmons R, Greenberger PA, Patterson R: Outcome of pregnancy in women requiring corticosteroids for severe asthma, *J Allergy Clin Immunol* 1986; 78:349.
20. Gordon M, Niswander KR, Berendes H, et al: Fetal morbidity following potentially anoxigenic obstetric conditions: VII bronchial asthma, *Am J Obstet Gynecol* 1970; 106:4231.
21. Schaefer G, Silverman F: Pregnancy complicated by asthma, *Am J Obstet Gynecol* 1961; 82:182.
22. Coutts II, White RJ: Asthma in pregnancy, *J Asthma* 1991; 28(6):433.
23. Schatz M, Harden K, Forsythe A, et al: The course of asthma during pregnancy, postpartum, and with successive pregnancies: a prospective analysis, *J Allergy Clin Immunol* 1988; 81:509.
24. Barnes PJ: New concepts in the pathogenesis of bronchial hyperresponsiveness and asthma, *J Allergy Clin Immunol* 1989; 83:1013.
25. Schatz M, Zeiger RS, Harden KM, et al: The safety of inhaled β-agonist bronchodilators during pregnancy, *J Allergy Clin Immunol* 1988; 82:686.
26. Burrows B, Lebowitz MD: The beta agonist dilemma, *N Engl J Med* 1992; 326:560.
27. Spitzer WO, Suissa S, Ernst D, et al: The use of beta agonists and the risk of death and near death from asthma, *N Engl J Med* 1992; 326:501.
28. Heinonen OP, Soane D, Shapiro S: *Birth defects and drugs in pregnancy.* Littleton, CA, 1977, Publishing Sciences Group.
29. Gardner MJ, Schatz M, Cousins L, et al: Longitudinal effects of pregnancy on the pharmacokinetics of theophylline, *Eur J Clin Pharmacol* 1987; 32:289.
30. Carter BL, Driscoll CF, Smith GD: Theophylline clearance during pregnancy, *Obstet Gynecol* 1986; 68:555.
31. Frederikson MC, Ruo TL, Chow MJ, et al: Theophylline pharmacokinetics in pregnancy, *Clin Pharmacol Ther* 1986; 40:321.
32. Montella KR: Pulmonary pharmacology in pregnancy, *Clin Chest Med* 1992; 13(4):587.
33. Wilson J: Use of cromoglycate during pregnancy, *J Pharmacol Med* 1982; 8:45.
34. Gross NJ, Skorodin MS: Anticholinergic, antimuscarinic bronchodilators, *Am Rev Respir Dis* 1984; 129:856.
35. Benedetti TJ: Maternal complications of parenteral β-sympathomimetic therapy for premature labor, *Am J Obstet Gynecol* 1983; 145:1.
36. Fishburne JI, Brenner WE, Braaksam JT, et al: Bronchospasm complicating intravenous prostaglandin F_{22} for therapeutic abortion, *Obstet Gynecol* 1972; 39:892.
37. Towers CV, Rojas JA, Lewis DF, et al: Usage of prostaglandin E_2 (PGE_2) in patients with asthma, *Am J Obstet Gynecol* 1991; 164(suppl):295 (abstract).
38. Namba Y, Smith JB, Fox GS, et al: Plasma cortisol concentrations during cesarean section, *Br J Anaesth* 1980; 52:1027.
39. Freund FG, Bonica JJ, Ward RJ: Ventilatory reserve and level of motor block during high spinal and epidural anesthesia, *Anesthesiology* 1967; 28:834.
40. Corssen G, Gutierrez J, Reves JG, et al: Ketamine in the anesthetic management of asthmatic patients, *Anesth Analg* 1972; 51:588.
41. Kingston HG, Hirshman CA: Perioperative management of the patient with asthma, *Anesth Analg* 1984; 63:844.
42. White PF, Way WL, Trevor AJ: Ketamine: its pharmacology and therapeutic uses, *Anesthesiology* 1985; 63:827.
43. Hirshman CA, Edelstein G, Peetz S, et al: Mechanisms of action of inhalational anesthesia on airways, *Anesthesiology* 1982; 56:107.
44. Stirt JA, Sullivan SF: Aminophylline, *Anesth Analg* 1981; 60:587.
45. Norris M, Dewan DM: Preoxygenation for cesarean section: a comparison of two techniques, *Anesthesiology* 1985; 62:827.

30

Cardiac Problems

A 35 year old woman, gravida 3 para 0, with known severe aortic stenosis, is admitted to the hospital at 39 weeks' gestation for induction of labor. The electrocardiogram shows left ventricular hypertrophy and left bundle branch block. Aortic valve orifice is less than 1 cm^2. Discuss the anesthetic management of labor and delivery, as well as for cesarean section.

Recommendations by Philip M. Hartigan, M.D.

Maternal heart disease affects an estimated 0.2% to 0.3% of pregnancies, and is the leading nonobstetric cause of maternal mortality.[1] Overall mortality has declined to less than 2%,[1] but the projected risk is highly lesion dependent (Table 30-1).[2] Within a given lesion, the maternal risk generally correlates to the degree of cardiovascular functional reserve, as reflected by the New York Heart Association (NYHA) functional classification (Table 30-2).[3] The anesthesiologist plays a critical role in minimizing the risk of an expectant mother with cardiac disease. Optimal anesthetic care requires early evaluation of the patient and collaboration with obstetric and cardiology caregivers. Because of their rarity, controlled outcome studies directed to guide anesthetic decisions do not exist for parturients with cardiovascular disease. Therefore decisions regarding monitoring and anesthetic choice must be derived from an integration of existing information about the following:

1. Pathophysiology of the specific cardiac lesion
2. Cardiovascular effects of pregnancy, labor, and delivery
3. Hemodynamic effects of the anesthetic options

Although the incidence is declining, rheumatic heart disease (RHD) remains the most common source of cardiac problems during pregnancy.[4]

TABLE 30-1
PROJECTED MATERNAL MORTALITY RISK ASSOCIATED WITH HEART DISEASE

Cardiac Lesion	Maternal Mortality (%)
Mitral stenosis	
Class I and II	0-1
Class III and IV	4-5
Atrial fibrillation	14-17
S/P valvotomy	4-6
Mitral insufficiency	1-5
Aortic insufficiency	2-7
Aortic stenosis	6-7
Prosthetic valves	2
Coarctation of the aorta	3-18
Tetralogy of Fallot	4-12
Eisenmenger's syndrome	10-30
Primary pulmonary hypertension	Up to 53
Marfan's syndrome	Up to 50
Peripartum cardiomyopathy	15-60

From Bogard TD: *Pregnancy and cardiovascular diseases.* In Hood DD, editor: *Problems in anesthesia,* Philadelphia, 1989, JB Lippincott.

TABLE 30-2
NYHA FUNCTIONAL CLASSIFICATION OF CARDIAC DISEASE

Class I
- No functional limitation of activity
- No symptoms of cardiac decompensation with activity

Class II
- Mild amount of functional limitation
- Patients are asymptomatic at rest
- Ordinary physical activity results in symptoms

Class III
- Limitation of most physical activity
- Asymptomatic at rest
- Minimal physical activity results in symptoms

Class IV
- Severe limitation of physical activity
- Patients may be symptomatic at rest
- Any physical activity results in cardiac symptoms

NYHA, New York Heart Association.
From Gianopoulos JG: Cardiac disease in pregnancy, *Med Clin North Am* 1989; 73(3):639.[97]

Therefore this chapter limits itself to valvular lesions of rheumatic origin, with a brief discussion of Eisenmenger's syndrome as an important example of congenital cardiac lesions in pregnancy, before addressing the case at hand.

Cardiovascular Effects of Pregnancy, Labor, and Delivery

The cardiovascular adaptations to pregnancy have been reviewed (see Chapter 1) and are summarized in Table 30-3 and Fig. 30-1.[5-7] Pregnancy essentially stresses the heart on two fronts. First, the heart must accommodate and circulate a larger intravascular volume of blood. Second, the heart must increase the rate of circulation (i.e., the cardiac output [CO]) to meet the increased metabolic demands of the mother and the developing fetus.

Intravascular Volume

Blood volume steadily increases to about 35% (1000 to 1500 ml) above prepregnant levels, peaking at about 36 weeks' gestation.[8] This gradual increase is normally accommodated by *(overfill hypothesis),* or perhaps triggered by *(underfill hypothesis)* an expansion of the intravascular space through generalized vasodilation, left atrial (and possibly left ventricular [LV]) enlargement, and development of the low-resistance placental and uterine vascular beds.[9,10] As a result, central venous pressure (CVP) and pulmonary capillary wedge pressure (PCWP) normally remain unchanged.[5] A *physiologic anemia of pregnancy* results from the increase in plasma volume exceeding the increase in red cell mass.[11] Colloid oncotic pressure (COP) decreases by 14%, and this decrease in COP relative to PCWP predisposes parturients to pulmonary edema.[5]

TABLE 30-3

Central Hemodynamic Changes in 10 Normal Nulliparous Women between 35 and 38 Weeks' Gestation and Again When 11 to 13 Weeks' Postpartum

	Pregnant*	Postpartum	Change
Mean arterial pressure (mm Hg)	90 ± 6	86 ± 8	No change
Cardiac output (L/min)	6.2 ± 1.0	4.3 ± 0.9	+43%
Heart rate (beats/min)	83 ± 10	71 ± 10	+17%
Central venous pressure (mm Hg)	4 ± 3	4 ± 3	No change
Pulmonary capillary wedge pressure (mm Hg)	8 ± 2	6 ± 2	No change
Systemic vascular resistance (dyne . sec . cm^{-5})	1210 ± 266	1530 ± 520	−21%
Serum colloid osmotic pressure (mm Hg)	18.0 ± 1.5	20.8 ± 1.0	−14%
COP-PCPW gradient (mm Hg)	10.5 ± 2.7	14.5 ± 2.5	−28%
Left ventricular stroke work index (g . min . m^{-3})	48 ± 6	41 ± 8	No change

COP, Colloid osmotic pressure; PCWP, pulmonary capillary wedge pressure.

*Made in lateral recumbent position.

Adapted from Clark SL, Cotton DB, Pivarnik JM, et al: Position change and central hemodynamic profile during normal third trimester pregnancy and post-partum, *Am J Obstet Gynecol* 1991; 164:883; and Clark SL, Cotton DB, Lee W, et al: Central hemodynamic assessment of normal term pregnancy, *Am J Obstet Gynecol* 1989; 161:1439.

Increased Cardiac Output

A 40% to 45% rise in CO gradually begins as early as 5 weeks and reaches a plateau at about 24 weeks (Fig. 30-1).[6,7,12] Increases in both heart rate (HR) and SV contribute asynchronously to the rise in CO (Fig. 30-1). The increase in SV is thought to be the result of increased preload and decreased afterload. Contractility appears to remain within a normal range.[5,13] The increased preload from expansion of intravascular volume is reflected by echocardiographically demonstrated increases in left atrial and left ventricular end-diastolic dimensions.[7,12] The decrease in afterload is reflected by a significant decrease in total peripheral vascular resistance,[14] which is thought to be caused by hormonally mediated vasodilation, development of the uteroplacental vascular bed, and possibly by an enhancement of endothelium-derived relaxing factor activity.[15] In addition, uterine arteries, and possibly other resistance vessels, display a decreased responsiveness to vasopressors (norepinephrine, epinephrine, and phenylephrine).[16] Mean arterial pressure remains essentially unchanged despite the above perturbations, although the diastolic blood pressure (BP) may decrease slightly during the second trimester.

Because the rate of increase in CO levels off between 24 and 28 weeks, and because about 80% of the *volume stress* has occurred by 28 weeks, it is often the case that the compromised heart, which is destined to decompensate in pregnancy, will have declared itself by this time with the development of symptoms.

Morphologic Changes in the Heart During Pregnancy

The cardiac adaptations to pregnancy have been likened to the mild dilation that occurs in the hearts of athletes involved in isotonic exercises (e.g., running or swimming).[7,17] The cardiovascular response

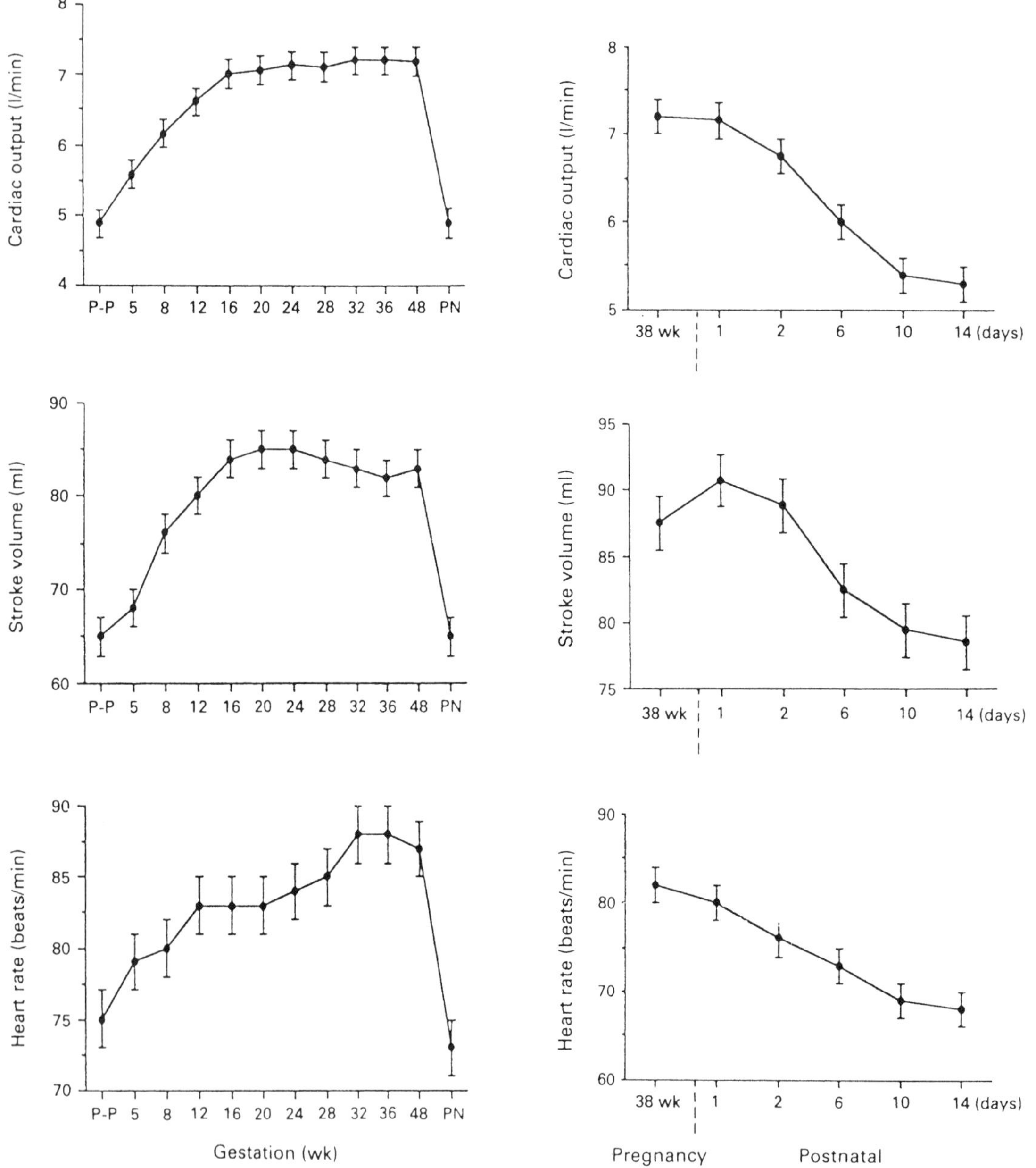

Fig. 30-1.

Hemodynamic changes of pregnancy. Serial measurements of cardiac output, stroke volume, and heart rate during normal gestation and the postpartum period in healthy women assessed by echo Doppler techniques. From Hunter S, Robson SC: Adaptation of the maternal heart in pregnancy, *Br J Med* 1992; 68:540.[6]

to exercise is augmented during the third trimester compared with the nonpregnant state, and this change requires up to 7 months after delivery to revert to baseline.[18] Serial echocardiographic studies have documented increases in left atrial and left ventricular dimensions, wall thickness, and mass, primarily during the first two trimesters.[7,13] Vered et al.[12] found that the increase in left ventricular cavity was primarily limited to the left ventricular outflow tract. Others have found no change in left ventricular cavity size,[19] but most studies agree on a 15% to 20% increase in left atrial area, which is consistent with a chronic adaptation to a relative volume overloaded state. Alternatively, it has been proposed that cardiac morphologic changes during pregnancy are the result of a possibly hormonally induced remodeling process, the results of which (increased left ventricular end diastolic volume [LVEDVP] and SV) may be enduring.[20] Aortic, pulmonic, and mitral valve orifice sizes also may increase during the course of pregnancy.[7] The effect of this on valvular lesions, independent of loading conditions, has not been studied. A benign pericardial effusion was found to be present in 43% of normal pregnancies,[21] which may further contribute to an enlarged cardiac silhouette on radiographic examination.

Aortocaval Compression

The imperative of avoiding aortocaval compression (see Chapter 1) assumes increased importance in parturients with cardiovascular disease. The decreased venous return from caval compression and the increased afterload from partial compression of the distal aorta may be poorly tolerated by the compromised heart (depending on the extent of collaterals). Clark et al. recently provided invasive hemodynamic evidence that either right or left lateral decubitus positions were equivalent in relieving the depression of CO from aortocaval compression compared with the supine position in 36- to 38-week parturients.[22]

Cardiovascular Effects of Labor and Delivery

Labor, delivery, and the immediate postpartum period is a time when the profound and incompletely understood acute cardiovascular changes place the parturient with cardiac disease at greatest jeopardy. Two thirds of all maternal deaths recorded in patients with heart disease occur around the time of delivery.[23]

The net effect of labor is an acute additional volume stress and workload stress on the heart, superimposed on the chronic cardiovascular changes of gestation. CO has been reported to increase by 30% in the first stage, 45% in the second stage, and up to 80% in the immediate postpartum period.[24] Each uterine contraction may shift or *autotransfuse* up to 500 ml of blood to the central circulation.[25] Both SV and CO increase with each uterine contraction by an additional 10% to 20%.[26-28] Pain and apprehension are known to increase maternal catecholamine levels during labor[29,30] which may increase HR and contractility. Exaggerated respiratory patterns during labor may, in theory, affect venous return and CO, but this has not been rigorously studied. The net effect of labor on BP usually is an increase by 5% to 25%.[31] HR may increase or reflexively decrease.

The cardiovascular effects of the second stage of labor are an extension of those described above, complicated considerably by intermittent Valsalva maneuvers, and the increased workload imposed by the aerobic demands of pushing. In nonpregnant patients, the Valsalva maneuver initially increases BP and intrathoracic pressure, which decreases (or delays) venous return to the heart, resulting in a decrease in CO and, eventually, BP. The surge in venous return after release of the Valsalva maneuver, together with residual reflex vasoconstriction, often leads to an overshoot phenomenon with increased CO and BP.[32] In the full and pushing gravida, these events are superimposed on intense uterine contractions, with associated autotransfusion and partial or complete aortic or caval obstruction.[26]

The immediate postdelivery period is a time of even more profound and difficult-to-predict cardiovascular changes. CO may increase by as much as 80% after vaginal delivery.[24] Many events impact on the net hemodynamic effect at this time. Caval compression is acutely relieved. Uterine contractions vigorously augment preload. Acute blood loss occurs, averaging 500 ml for vaginal deliveries and 1000 to 1500 ml for cesarean sections. Relief of aortic compression and the peripheral vasodilating effects of oxytocin conspire to acutely decrease peripheral resistance. Profound emotions may trigger maternal humoral changes. One to three liters of crystalloid are commonly administered intravenously, particularly after operative deliveries. The cardiovascularly compromised parturient is at high risk for decompensation during this period.

Cardiovascular Effects of Regional Anesthesia

The cardiovascular effects of spinal and epidural anesthesia in nonpregnant patients without heart disease have been well reviewed.[33-35] The net hemodynamic effects of central neuraxial blockade superimposed on the cardiovascular changes of pregnancy have been much less thoroughly studied, and prediction about these effects in the setting of maternal heart disease remains largely the product of anecdotal reports and extrapolation.

In healthy, nonpregnant patients, the hemodynamic effects of spinal or epidural anesthesia are attributable to preganglionic sympathetic blockade and may be summarized as follows. *Preload* decreases due to dilation of venous capacitance vessels. This usually is the most important cause of the commonly seen decrease in SV, CO, and mean arterial pressure (MAP).[34] Impediments to venous return such as caval compression, hypovolemia, or reverse trendelenberg position may profoundly amplify the decrease in preload and its cardiovascular consequences. *Afterload,* or SVR, generally decreases, but only to a limited extent (<20%).[33] Unlike veins, arteries retain a considerable degree of tone despite sympathetic blockade.[34] On average, *HR* tends to decrease slightly (5% to 20%)[33] after sympathetic blocks in nonpregnant patients. This may be a result of decreased venous return, as well as decreased sympathetic traffic to the heart with high-level blocks.[33,34] However, considerable variability exists in the response of HR to regional anesthetics, and a recent study found no correlation between sensory block height and degree of bradycardia after spinal anesthesia in nonpregnant patients.[36] *Contractility* also declines after epidural or spinal anesthesia in which sympathetic blockade extends to the cardiac sympathetic nerves (T-1-4). Convincing evidence for such a decrease in contractility has only recently been provided by Goertz and colleagues who employed a relatively load-independent technique to measure contractility.[37]

The magnitude of the above changes depends roughly on the extent of the sympathetic block. The level of sympathetic blockade is imperfectly related to the level of sensory blockade.[38,39] Despite this, T-10 level sensory blocks may be anticipated to have only a mild hemodynamic impact. Vasoconstriction in sympathetically intact regions above the level of the block may partially compensate for vasodilation in the lower extremities. A sensory level of T-4, however, as is used for cesarean section, may be associated with a sympathetic level affecting the cardiac accelerator nerves, resulting in significant decreases in MAP, CO, preload, afterload, contractility, and HR.

Epidural analgesia during labor has several salutary hemodynamic effects. Alleviation of pain leads to decreased maternal catecholamines, which would be expected to moderate the increases in HR and CO associated with labor. Epidural-induced venodilation may alleviate the volume (preload) stress of pregnancy, labor, and delivery. Indeed, Ueland and Hansen found that caudal analgesia significantly blunted the increases in CO and HR associated with labor and delivery, including the substantial surge in CO normally seen after delivery.[24] The acute changes associated with uterine contractions, however, were unaffected by the caudal analgesia. By blocking the urge to push and allowing painless forceps delivery, epidurals can prevent the acute cardiovascular stresses of the Valsalva maneuver.

Epidural or spinal anesthetics at the T-4 level for cesarean section are associated with a higher incidence of hypotension. This may be minimized by prior intravascular volume expansion (fluid preloading) and gradual imposition of the sympathectomy (epidural or continuous spinal technique). Single-shot spinals for cesarean section are associated with a high incidence of hypotension, which is only partially preventable by fluid preloading with 10 ml/kg of crystalloid.[40] This may reflect the fact that decreased preload is only part of the mechanism of spinal hypotension. The abrupt decline in peripheral vascular resistance, contractility and, in some cases, HR, also contribute to spinal hypotension. In contrast, the gradual, controlled titration of an epidural block for cesarean section may be accomplished with minimal hemodynamic disruption if performed with attention to maintain preload, afterload, and contractility with fluids, vasopressors, and intropes as needed.

The addition of epinephrine to epidural local anesthetics results in greater arterial dilation and possibly augmented venous return and CO.[41] In effect, the degree of intravascular absorption results in the equivalent of a low-level intravascular infusion of epinephrine such that the β-adrenergic effects of epinephrine are the dominant hemodynamic result. Therefore epinephrine is better avoided in patients with cardiac disease who would tolerate tachycardia and exaggerated vasodilation poorly.

Pregnant patients with coexisting cardiac disease generally benefit from epidural anesthesia for labor and delivery since the benefits described above outweigh the hemodynamic risks. For cesarean section, there is little consensus whether gradually induced epidural anesthesia affords greater hemodynamic stability than general anesthesia. High-dose, narcotic-based general anesthetics, as used for cardiac surgery, are associated with good hemodynamic stability, but require compromise of the usual rapid-sequence induction to prevent aspiration, and may necessitate postoperative ventilatory support for both mother and newborn. Reducing the narcotic dose requires supplementation with other anesthetic agents (all of which have their own hemodynamic impact) to achieve adequate depth and to blunt the cardiovascular effects of laryngoscopy and intubation. Ultimately, the choice of anesthetic for cesarean section will depend on the specific cardiac lesion and the experience and ability of the anesthesiologist with epidural versus general anesthesia. Within limits, the hemodynamic impact of the anesthetic depends less on the choice of anesthetic than on the manner with which it is administered.

Rheumatic Heart Disease in Pregnancy

Rheumatic fever is a diffuse inflammatory disease that occurs as a delayed sequela of group A β-hemolytic streptococcal infection, usually of the oropharynx. A subset of those with rheumatic fever may manifest rheumatic carditis, which may lead to RHD. The natural history of RHD is one of gradual, progressive, structural deterioration of affected heart valves over several asymptomatic decades until the appearance of symptoms of congestive heart failure, syncope, or angina herald impending death in the ensuing 3 to 5 years.

Ninety percent of cardiac disease in pregnancy was of rheumatic origin before 1960.[2] The incidence rate of RHD in pregnancy has declined from

3.5% in the 1940s to less than 0.7%.[42] This decline has been attributed to changes in the virulence and rheumatogenicity of the streptococcus organism as well as to improvements in medical therapy. Despite the declining incidence, RHD still remains the most common and important cause of maternal heart disease complicating pregnancy.

The relative incidence rate of valvular lesions from RHD includes mitral stenosis (MS) (90%), mitral regurgitation (MR) (6.6%), aortic insufficiency (2.5%), and aortic stenosis (AS) (1%).[42] Major complications of rheumatic valvular disease include pulmonary edema, congestive heart failure, atrial fibrillation, systemic embolization, and endocarditis. The cardiovascular changes of pregnancy and the stress of delivery may precipitate such complications in previously asymptomatic patients with apparently well-compensated valvular disease. Long-term follow-up of patients with rheumatic cardiac disease, however, reveals that life expectancy of such patients is not shortened by pregnancy, provided that the patient survives gestation.[43]

Mitral Stenosis

Mitral stenosis is the most common rheumatic valvular lesion seen in pregnancy. Scarring, contractures of chordae tendinae, and commissural fusion of leaflets results in a characteristic funnel-shaped mitral valve (MV) with a progressively stenotic opening. The normal mitral valve area is 4 to 6 cm^2. MV areas less than 1.5 cm^2 are associated with symptoms, and areas under 1 cm^2 are considered critical and may be associated with symptoms at rest.[44]

Pathophysiology

The stenotic MV obstructs LV filling and, thus limits CO while volume and pressure overloading the left atrium (LA). Elevated left atrial pressures reflect backstream to increase pulmonary venous and PCWPs and favor transudation of fluid into pulmonary interstitial spaces. Eventually, pulmonary edema and the increased work of breathing due to decreased pulmonary compliance, results in symptoms of dyspnea on exertion, orthopnea, and paroxysmal nocturnal dyspnea. The elevated pulmonary vascular resistance eventually leads to right ventricular hypertrophy, tricuspid regurgitation, and biventricular failure. Left atrial distension may lead to atrial fibrillation, thrombus formation, and systemic thromboembolization. The rheumatically deformed valves are vulnerable to endocarditis.

Pregnancy and Mitral Stenosis

Parturients with mild asymptomatic MS generally tolerate pregnancy well and are at minimally increased risk.[4] However, the increase in intravascular volume and HR, as well as the imperative for increased CO during pregnancy, may precipitate pulmonary congestion, pulmonary edema, or frank congestive heart failure in patients with moderate to severe MS. Atrial fibrillation is more likely to occur during pregnancy and may precipitate decompensation in patients with MS.[42] Left atrial unloading and left ventricular filling is impaired by atrial fibrillation or tachycardia, which disproportionately shortens diastolic filling time. Severe MS has been reported to be associated with a 5% maternal mortality.[45] Atrial fibrillation increases that risk to 14% to 17%.[46] The time of greatest risk is during the acute hemodynamic changes of labor, delivery, and the puerperium.[47] The surge in preload immediately after delivery has been shown to result in an 8- to 15-mm Hg rise in PCWP in patients with NYHA class III-IV mitral stenosis.[47] Thus patients with MS complicated by pulmonary hypertension are at extremely high risk.

Anesthetic Considerations for Mitral Stenosis in Pregnancy

The physiologic goals of MS are summarized in Table 30-4. *Tachycardia* must be avoided because it

TABLE 30-4

HEMODYNAMIC EFFECTS OF PREGNANCY, LABOR, AND T-4 LEVEL REGIONAL ANESTHESIA COMPARED TO HU HEMODYNAMIC GOALS OF VARIOUS VALVULAR LESIONS

	Hemodynamic Effects			Hemodynamic Goals			
	Pregnancy	**Labor**	**T-4 Epidural**	**AS**	**MS**	**AI**	**MR**
Preload	↑	↑↑	↓	↑	(↑)	↑	↑
HR	↑	↑↑	(↓)	↓	↓	↑	↑
SVR	↓	(↑)	↓	↑	—	↓	↓
Contractility	—	—	↓	—	—	—	—
PVR	↓	(↑)	(↓)	—	↓	—	↓
CO	↑	↑↑	↓	—	—	—	—

↑, Increase; ↓, decrease; —, maintain unchanged; (↑), increase slightly; (↓), decrease slightly; HR, heart rate; CO, cardiac output; AS, aortic stenosis; MS, mitral stenosis; MR, mitral regurgitation; AI, aortic insufficiency.

will impair ventricular filling, increase the transmitral valvular gradient, and exacerbate pulmonary congestion and pulmonary hypertension. In this regard, adequate analgesia during labor and delivery to control pain and anxiety is essential and may best be provided by epidural narcotics and low concentrations of local anesthetics. Abrupt declines in SVR from rapid or extensive sympathetic blockade, however, may cause hypotension and reflex tachycardia. In deference to avoiding tachycardia, epinephrine should be excluded from the epidural mix and phenylephrine would be a better choice than ephedrine to treat hypotension. In addition, some advocate aggressive use of β-blockers to control HR during the peripartum period.[48] Maternally administered esmolol has been associated with fetal bradycardia[49]; therefore it should be used cautiously and only when necessary. Should atrial fibrillation occur, precipitating pulmonary edema, immediate cardioversion is indicated.[4] Cardioversion during pregnancy has been demonstrated to be safe for the fetus[50,51] and should begin with 25 watt-seconds. In the absence of pulmonary edema, hemodynamic instability, or fetal distress, atrial fibrillation may be treated medically with digoxin or β-blockers.

Preload of the left ventricle must be preserved in order to maintain CO. In addition to a sinus rhythm and a slow HR, preload depends on adequate central blood volumes. Sudden decreases in venous return, as a result of anesthesia, caval compression, or blood loss at delivery will thus compromise CO. On the other hand, sudden increases in central blood volume may precipitate pulmonary edema. The more severe the mitral stenosis, the more delicate intravascular volume management becomes. Most authors recommend invasive hemodynamic monitoring with pulmonary artery catheters in patients with severe or symptomatic MS. A pulmonary artery catheter will provide accurate information about the extent of pulmonary hypertension and the effect of volume manipulations on pulmonary artery pressures. Although the PCWP will falsely overestimate the LV filling pressures, the trends in PCWP ought to reliably track trends in LV preload, barring significant tachycardia. In addition, pressures at the proximal port (CVP) will reflect the right ventricle's response to the changes in volume and pulmonary pressure.

Clark et al. noted a mean peripartum increase of 10 mm Hg in the PCWP of eight parturients with severe MS.[47] Since frank pulmonary edema often is observed with a PCWP of 28 to 30 mm Hg, he advocated cautious *preload reduction* to a PCWP of 14 mm Hg or less in anticipation of postpartum volume shifts. Fluid restriction was used to achieve preload reduction. Epidural analgesia also may be used to gradually reduce preload, control the urge to Valsalva, and blunt the intrapartum and postpartum volume shifts. However, preload reduction must be performed with close attention to CO, BP, and fetal HR patterns, since CO is highly dependent on preload in such patients. Parturients with pulmonary hypertension complicating MS may be so critically dependent on a high preload to maintain an adequate CO that preload reduction should be avoided, even at the possible expense of pulmonary edema.[47] Such patients may benefit from inotropic support. Caution should be exercised in the interpretation of PCWP during tachycardia. Reflex tachycardia resulting from sudden blood loss could cause an increase in the transmitral pressure gradient, and thus an increase in PCWP despite intravascular hypovolemia.

Factors which elevate *pulmonary vascular resistance (PVR)* should also be avoided, particularly in those with pulmonary hypertension. Supplemental oxygen and pulse oximetry should be used to prevent or signal hypoxemia. Excess sedation runs the risk of maternal hypoventilation, hypercarbia, and acidosis, which also would increase PVR. Prostaglandins (PG F2-α) used to treat uterine atony also may exacerbate pulmonary hypertension with the risk of precipitating right-sided heart failure.

The vaginal route usually is preferred for delivery and carefully titrated epidural opioids and low concentrations of local anesthetics have distinct advantages for this, as discussed earlier in the chapter. When cesarean section is required for obstetric reasons, gradual extension of the epidural anesthesia is an acceptable technique, provided that preload and intravascular volume are maintained, guided, if necessary, by invasive monitors. If general anesthesia is required, use of preinduction β-blockade will help prevent tachycardia during laryngoscopy and intubation. Patients with severe MS may not tolerate the vasodilation of sodium thiopental and inhalational agents. Such patients would likely benefit from the greater hemodynamic stability of an etomidate induction or a high-dose, narcotic-based general anesthetic. This may avoid cardiovascular collapse on induction at the marginal cost of compromising strict rapid-sequence protocol and committing both mother and newborn to a period of ventilation after delivery. Control of pain and tachycardia is as essential after delivery as during delivery. If an epidural was used for delivery or cesarean section, the block should be allowed to wear off gradually, and should be replaced by epidural opioids, as needed.

Patients with severe MS who decompensate hemodynamically during pregnancy may now be relatively safely palliated by percutaneous transeptal balloon mitral valvotomy. Experience is accumulating to suggest that this technique in selected patients is effective in relieving MS with less risk to mother and fetus than mitral commissurotomy or mitral valve replacement.[52-54] Appropriate candidates are those with tight, pliable MS, NYHA functional class III or IV without significant mitral regurgitation or left atrial thrombi.[54] Because the process involves fluoroscopy and radiation exposure, gestational age of more than 20 weeks is preferred. In the most recent series, 19 pregnant patients with tight MS achieved an average decrease in MV gradient from 17.9 to 5.9 mm Hg, an increase in MV area of 0.8 to 1.7 cm^2, and an average decrease in systolic PA pressures from 52 to 37 mm Hg.[54] All patients enjoyed an improvement in functional class by at least one NYHA grade, and all but one completed their pregnancies without complications.

Aortic Stenosis

Aortic stenosis rarely is the sole or dominant valvular lesion in RHD. The most common nonrheumatic cause of AS is a congenitally bicupid aortic valve. The normal aortic valve area is 2.6 to 3.5 cm^2. Aortic valve areas 1.0 cm^2 or less are considered hemodynamically significant, and those 0.7 cm^2 or less are considered severely stenotic.

Pathophysiology

The obstruction to LV outflow imposes a chronic pressure overload which stimulates parallel replication of sarcomeres and concentric left ventricular hypertrophy (LVH). The mural thickening is initially a palliative adaptation inasmuch as it serves to reduce LV wall tension according to the law of Laplace.[44] Such compensatory changes may provide several symptom-free decades until eventually, concentric LVH reaches a point of diminishing returns. The severely hypertrophic left ventricle becomes less compliant and vulnerable to ischemia. Symptoms of congestive heart failure, syncope, or angina are ominous as signals of minimal residual reserve, and indicate a life expectancy of less than 5 years.

Ischemia may occur in such patients even in the absence of coronary artery disease for several reasons. The increased myocardial mass and the increased afterload imposed by the stenotic aortic valve dramatically increases myocardial oxygen demand. Oxygen supply is reduced because severe mural thickening tends to outpace the growth of coronary microvasculature.[55] In addition, the increased pressure generated in the left ventricle may increase the resistance to coronary flow, particularly to the subendocardium. Adequate coronary perfusion becomes critically dependent on aortic diastolic pressure which, in turn, depends on adequate intravascular volume, CO, and particularly arterial tone (SVR). Tachycardia further tips the balance toward ischemia by further increasing myocardial oxygen consumption and decreasing the time for diastolic coronary perfusion, as well as ventricular filling and LV ejection. Systemic hypotension may trigger a vicious cycle leading to decreased coronary perfusion pressure, ischemia, decreased CO, and further hypotension and ischemia.

Left ventricular compliance decreases with advanced concentric LVH. It has been postulated that repeated episodes of subendocardial ischemia and/or infarctions (or microinfarctions) may further contribute to diminished ventricular compliance and diastolic dysfunction.[44] The consequence of LVH and decreased compliance is a fixed SV and critical dependence on preload. Because SV is relatively fixed, CO becomes dependent on HR, and thus bradycardia may be as dangerous as tachycardia. Adequate preload depends on an adequate intravascular volume, venous tone, venous return, and a sinus rhythm. Up to 40% of ventricular filling may depend on atrial systole.[44]

Pregnancy and Aortic Stenosis

The physiologic changes of pregnancy are largely counter to the hemodynamic goals of AS (Table 30-3). The decrease in SVR tends to increase the pressure gradient across the aortic valve and decrease coronary perfusion pressure as previously discussed. Because stroke volume is relatively fixed, the requisite increase in CO must be largely accomplished by an increase in HR. As previously discussed, however, tachycardia may precipitate ischemia and compromise LV filling and ejection. The elevated intravascular volume and preload generally is desirable in such patients, but may precipitate LV failure and pulmonary edema in patients with severe AS and limited reserve.

Despite this, women with mild to moderate AS generally tolerate pregnancy well. Severe or symptomatic AS (NYHA class III-IV) is associated with a prohibitive maternal and fetal mortality. The literature contains insufficient numbers of cases to establish meaningful prognostic statistics in this regard. The most widely quoted review reported a maternal mortality rate of 17% with a perinatal mortality of 31%, without stratifying for severity of AS.[56] These figures have been questioned recently by Lao and colleagues,[57] who reported no maternal or fetal deaths in their series of 25 pregnancies with congenital AS. However, only three of Lao's patients had severe AS. Of those three, one underwent balloon valvuloplasty at 16 weeks, another terminated her pregnancy at 13 weeks due to development of symptoms, and the third remained asymptomatic throughout. Therefore the contention that people with symptomatic or severe AS are at high risk of death remains unchallenged. Termination of pregnancy also has been associated with high mortality, but these statistics have a selection bias.[56] Aortic valve replacement during pregnancy is well tolerated by the mother but has been associated with a 50% fetal loss.[56]

Despite the more favorable statistics, even asymptomatic patients with mild to moderate AS may display abnormal hemodynamic responses to exertion. Clyne et al.[58] recently demonstrated that nonpregnant, asymptomatic patients with AS responded to treadmill exercise with a reduction in SV and CO, in contrast to normal controls who displayed an increase in SV and CO during exertion. Lao and colleagues[57] found that one third of initially asymptomatic patients with AS deteriorated at least one NYHA functional classification during the course of their pregnancy. Clearly, ventricular dysfunction and reduced cardiac reserve precede the appearance of symptoms. Therefore some respect for the preferred physiology of AS should be applied to even the apparently well-compensated, asymptomatic patient with AS.

Anesthetic Considerations for Aortic Stenosis in Pregnancy

The anesthetic considerations and management of a parturient with AS is discussed at the end of this chapter in the context of the test case presented.

Mitral Regurgitation

Mitral regurgitation ranks as the second most common rheumatic valvular lesion in pregnancy. MR of rheumatic origin rarely stands alone and usually is accompanied by MS. Nonrheumatic causes of MR include mitral valve prolapse, ischemic papillary muscle dysfunction, ruptured chordae tendineae, bacterial endocarditis, LV dilatation (e.g., cardiomyopathy), and connective tissue diseases. Rheumatic MR has an indolent natural history similar to other rheumatic valvular lesions. After the onset of symptoms (fatigability or dyspnea), usually in the third or fourth decade of life, the 5-year mortality approaches 50%. Complications of MR include pulmonary edema, atrial arrhythmias, embolization, and infectious endocarditis. As with MS, terminal complications of MR include pulmonary hypertension, right ventricular hypertrophy, and biventricular failure.

Pathophysiology

Mitral regurgitation volume overloads the LA and left ventricle with compromise of "forward" CO in proportion to the regurgitant fraction. The LA initially accommodates the regurgitant volume by increasing in size and compliance. As such, it buffers the pulmonary vasculature against backstream transmission of pressure. Thus, pulmonary vascular hypertension and pulmonary edema tend not to occur until late in the progression of chronic MR. This differs from acute MR (e.g., ruptured chordae tendineae) in which sudden regurgitant volume overloading of the normally sized and normally compliant left atrium results in acute pulmonary edema. In chronic MR, enlargement of the LA often leads to atrial fibrillation and left atrial thrombus formation.

The increased volume transmitted to the left ventricle from the dilated LA during diastole leads to primarily eccentric left ventricular hypertrophy. The increased compliance of the left ventricle tends to maintain relatively normal end-diastolic pressures, despite markedly increased end-diastolic volumes. The increased stroke volume tends to maintain relatively normal forward CO during the asymptomatic phase. Increasing regurgitant fraction and insidious deterioration of LV function eventually contributes to inadequate forward CO and symptoms of fatigability and weakness. Dilation of left-sided cardiac chambers may exacerbate MR over time by enlarging the mitral annulus and regurgitant orifice size. The amount of regurgitant flow is related to the size of the regurgitant mitral orifice and the difference in systolic pressures between the LA and left ventricle. Afterload, or SVR, is an important determinant of systolic LV pressures, and thus, regurgitant fraction.

Pregnancy and Mitral Regurgitation

Patients with mild or asymptomatic MR tolerate pregnancy well. The increased intravascular volume is accommodated by the compliant enlarged LA without pulmonary congestion. The decrease in SVR decreases the regurgitant fraction. This, together with the increase in HR associated with pregnancy, favors forward CO. The murmur of MR may actually decrease during pregnancy.[59] Patients with severe or symptomatic MR with associated LV compromise, however, may develop pulmonary congestion in response to the volume stress of pregnancy, labor, or delivery.[60] In addition, elevations in SVR as a result of pain, apprehension, aortic compression, or uterine contractions may exacerbate MR at the expense of forward CO. The risks of atrial fibrillation, systemic thromboembolic phenomena, or infective endocarditis are enhanced by pregnancy in patients with MR.

Anesthetic Considerations for Mitral Regurgitation in Pregnancy

The physiologic goals of MR are outlined in Table 30-4. The principle challenge during labor and delivery usually is to defend an adequate forward CO rather than to avoid pulmonary edema. To this end, *preload* should be maintained at an appropriately elevated state. Sudden withdrawal of venous return from blood loss, rapid sympathetic blockade, or caval compression can lead to decreased LA pressure and a reflex increase in SVR, which favors MR at the expense of forward CO. The balance between adequate and excessive preload tends to be much less delicate in patients with MR compared with those with MS, and pulmonary artery monitoring seldom is warranted, except in severe symptomatic cases of MR. If used, the size of the V-wave may correlate to the degree of MR.[4] An elevated *HR* and decreased *afterload,* as mentioned earlier, help to maintain forward flow. Epidural analgesia for labor and delivery has the advantages of decreasing SVR and blunting maternal pain and catecholamine release. For these reasons, epidural anesthesia is an excellent choice for cesarean section as well, with the caveat that the sympathetic block should not be imposed or allowed to wear off too abruptly. Volume loading before the epidural may be performed empirically for patients with mild MR or guided by invasive central hemodynamic monitoring in patients with severe MR or symptoms of dyspnea.

Hypotension should be treated with ephedrine because of its chronotropic and inotropic effects in addition to its effects on venous return. Positive inotropes decrease MR by decreasing ventricular size, and thus, annular and regurgitant orifice size.[44] Only when hypotension is accompanied by marked tachycardia is it likely that an alpha adrenergic agonist would be of greater benefit than harm. A useful approach in such a scenario is to use a combination of ephedrine and phenylephrine, adjusting the ratio as indicated by the hemodynamic response. If general anesthesia is required, standard thiopental/succinylcholine rapid-sequence induction techniques are generally well tolerated. Isoflurane would be a good choice for maintenance due to its effects of decreasing SVR and increasing HR. Only patients with severe MR and LV compromise may not tolerate the myocardial depression of potent inhalational agents. In deference to this possibility and uterine tone, a useful combination for maintenance is 50% nitrous oxide/50% oxygen and 0.5 minimum alveolar concentration (MAC) isoflurane supplemented by narcotics after the clamping of the umbilical cord. Further reductions in SVR may be accomplished with sodium nitroprusside, if necessary. Infusion rates below 10 μg · kg · min are thought to be safe for both mother and fetus.[61] Postpartum oxytocin infusion also may have physiologic benefits for the mother through decreased SVR. In theory, patients with severe MR might be expected to be at risk after surgery if SVR is allowed to increase from the weaning off of the epidural anesthetic combined with pain- and possibly cold-induced vasoconstriction. Such patients may benefit from a gradual weaning of an epidural local anesthetic infusion with replacement by epidural or parenteral narcotics.

Aortic Regurgitation

Rheumatic aortic regurgitation (AR) results from fibrous infiltration of the cusps with retraction and failure of apposition during diastole. Nonrheumatic causes of chronic AR include any processes which produce dilation of the aortic root or annulus (aortic aneurysm, dissection, syphilitic aortitis, connective tissue disorders, etc.) and congenital valvular defects. Acute causes of AR include infectious endocarditis and trauma. Rheumatic AR displays a slowly progressive course during which the degree of valvular incompetence and LV enlargement increases in severity. Initial symptoms are usually those of congestive heart failure, although syncope and angina may also occur. Life expectancy after onset of symptoms tends to be longer with AR than with other rheumatic valvular lesions, averaging 9 years.[62] Thus, with the exception of angina, symptoms associated with AR tend to be less ominous, and there is a poor correlation between symptom severity and degree of contractile dysfunction.[44]

Pathophysiology

The retrograde regurgitation of blood across the incompetent aortic valve during diastole imposes a chronic volume overload stress on the left ventricle, which stimulates serial replication of sarcomeres and eccentric hypertrophy. In contrast to MR, however, the left ventricle in AR must eject its entire stroke volume into the relatively high-resistance arterial system. This, together with the increased wall tension which accompanies ventricular dilation (in accordance with the law of Laplace), leads to significant concentric hypertrophy, as well. Left ventricular dysfunction is suggested by an LVEDP greater than 20 mm Hg, a regurgitant fraction in excess of 60% of SV, or elevated end-systolic dimensions.

The degree of regurgitation is related to the size of the aortic orifice, the aortoventricular pressure gradient, and the diastolic time interval. Thus regurgitation is alleviated by relative tachycardia and afterload reduction. An elevated preload is desirable to optimally fill the dilated left ventricle. Forward CO is optimized by a fast HR, low SVR, elevated preload, and maintenance of cardiac contractility.

There is some increased risk for ischemia in patients with AR, although it is a rare but ominous occurrence among parturients. The derangement in myocardial oxygen supply and demand imposed by concentric LVH has been described previously (see the discussion on the Pathophysiology of Aortic Stenosis). The degree of concentric LVH is generally far less than in patients with AS; however, aortic diastolic pressure, and thus the coronary perfusion pressure, is reduced in AR.[63]

Pregnancy and Aortic Regurgitation

As with MR, the increased intravascular volume of pregnancy is generally well tolerated by patients with all but severe AR. The decreased SVR and tachycardia of pregnancy are desirable physiologic changes. Patients with AR advanced to the point of contractile dysfunction, however, may respond to the imperative increases in CO and the volume stresses of pregnancy, labor, and delivery with congestive heart failure, pulmonary edema, or myocardial ischemia. Because symptoms correlate poorly with degree of contractile dysfunction, it may be difficult to predict which patients are likely to decompensate during delivery, the time of greatest stress and risk.

Anesthetic Considerations for Aortic Regurgitation in Pregnancy

The physiologic goals for AR are summarized in Table 30-4, and have been discussed above. As with MR, the balance between adequate and excessive preload is more forgiving than for stenotic valvular lesions, and therefore the threshold for pulmonary artery catheterization should be higher. In the absence of signs of ischemia or contractile dysfunction, patients with AR may be managed as discussed above for patients with MR. Lumbar epidural anesthesia for labor and delivery with vacuum or forceps extraction, or for cesarean section if indicated for obstetrical reasons, imparts all of the advantages previously described for MR. General anesthesia, if indicated, should also be conducted as described for MR. Although patients with AR have an increased risk of myocardial ischemia, a relative tachycardia is usually preferable to bradycardia, since a longer diastolic interval leads to an increased regurgitant fraction and elevated LVEDP.

Because it is more true with AR than with the other rheumatic valvular lesions discussed—that significant contractile dysfunction may exist despite the absence of symptoms—thorough noninvasive cardiologic evaluation is even more important to evaluate the degree of reserve before embarking on the potentially perilous road of labor and delivery.

Congenital Heart Disease

Congenital heart disease (CHD) encompasses a vast spectrum of anomalies, a comprehensive discussion of which is beyond the scope of this chapter. The more commonly occurring lesions may generally be classified as *left-to-right shunts* (atrial septal defects [ASD], ventricular septal defects [VSD], patent ductus arteriosus [PDA]), *right-to-left shunts* (Eisenmenger's syndrome, tetralogy of Fallot), valvular lesions (aortic stenosis, pulmonary stenosis, tricuspid atresia, etc.), or *other* defects (coarctation of the aorta, single ventricle, etc.). The incidence of CHD in pregnancy is increasing both relatively (compared with the declining incidence of RHD) and absolutely.[4] The increase in the absolute incidence is a consequence of improved medical and surgical therapy, which allows increasing numbers of women with CHD to survive to childbearing age. Maternal outcome depends on the individual lesion and the extent of reserve due to compensation or repair. Patients with acyanotic CHD who are NYHA functional class I or II are generally at minimally increased risk during pregnancy.[64] In contrast, NYHA class III and IV acyanotic CHD, cyanotic CHD, or primary pulmonary hypertension are associated with such high maternal and fetal mortality that pregnancy is contraindicated and inadvertent pregnancies should be terminated as early as possible.[64] Maternal complications of CHD during pregnancy most often include congestive heart failure, arrhythmias, hypertension, hypotension, infective endocarditis, and pulmonary or systemic (paradoxical) embolism. The incidence of pregnancy-induced hypertension is more common among women with CHD.[64] Prematurity, low birth weight, and fetal death are frequent fetal complications of cyanotic CHD. In addition, CHD is fourfold more common in the offspring of mothers with CHD.[65]

Eisenmenger's Syndrome

Eisenmenger's syndrome and pulmonary hypertension deserve special mention because they have the highest maternal mortality rates of any CHD (in excess of 50%).[66] Currently Eisenmenger's syndrome is defined as pulmonary hypertension with bidirectional or right-to-left shunting of blood through an intracardiac or aortopulmonary communication.[67] It generally represents the preterminal physiology of a chronic left-to-right shunt from an ASD, VSD, or PDA. The chronic volume overload to the right side of the heart and pulmonary vasculature eventually stimulates right ventricular hypertrophy and medial and intimal hyperplasia of pulmonary arteries, with fibrotic occlusions leading to an increased and relatively fixed PVR.[68] This results in pulmonary hypertension, often approaching systemic levels, and a bidirectional, largely resistance-dependent shunt with variable degrees of cyanosis. A reactive polycythemia may increase blood viscosity, increase cardiac workload, and further impair blood flow when hematocrit levels exceed 60%.[66] Surgical correction is not an option since the right ventricle will be unable to eject blood against the fixed, elevated PVR.

Eisenmenger's Syndrome in Pregnancy

The cardiovascular changes of pregnancy may be particularly devastating to patients with Eisenmenger's syndrome. Whereas the anemia of pregnancy may alleviate the increased blood viscosity, the volume stress and decreased SVR exacerbate the degree of right-to-left shunting. Patients may succumb to cyanosis, heart failure, thromboembolic events, or arrhythmias at any stage of gestation, but are at greatest risk during the acute hemodynamic stresses of labor, delivery, and the postpartum period. A large percentage of the maternal deaths occur during the first postpartum week.[64] The etiology of postpartum sudden death is poorly understood, but thromboembolic phenomena have been implicated. On theoretical grounds, some authors recommend anticoagulation with heparin from 20 weeks' gestation through 1 month postpartum, with only a brief interruption during labor and delivery.[64,69,70] Other reports have suggested that heparinization contributed to maternal mortality in patients with Eisenmenger's syndrome.[71,72]

The goals of management are to minimize right-to-left shunt (maintain SVR and minimize PVR), and to avoid abrupt hemodynamic perturbations in any direction. These patients poorly tolerate a decrease in preload, yet abrupt increases in intravascular volume or venous return to the right heart may precipitate right-sided heart failure or increased right-to-left shunt. Decreased afterload or increased PVR from hypoxia, hypercarbia, or acidosis will exacerbate right-to-left shunting. Maintenance of adequate CO requires avoiding decreases in contractility, ischemia, bradycardia, or a nonsinus rhythm. Tachycardia may precipitate right ventricular ischemia and shorten ventricular filling time.

The safest mode of delivery is controversial. Some authors prefer cesarean section,[73,74] which avoids the maternal pain, Valsalva, and fatigue associated with labor. Elective operative delivery also affords greater control over the timing of delivery, which is desirable in a multidisciplinary coordinated management plan. Others,[67,69,75,76] including this author, believe that cesarean section should be reserved for obstetric indications only, since it is accompanied by greater and less predictable blood loss, and because it requires either general or extensive regional anesthesia. A central premise is the bias that maternal pain, Valsalva, and fatigue of labor can be well controlled by appropriate, limited regional techniques, so that net hemodynamic perturbations during vaginal delivery will be less than those accompanying a cesarean section. With skillful anesthetic management of labor and delivery, adequate cephalopelvic proportions, and the use of forceps or vacuum extraction to shorten the second stage, this premise is likely valid.

Anesthetic Considerations for Eisenmenger's Syndrome in Pregnancy

Various combinations of analgesia have been used with success for vaginal delivery in the presence of Eisenmenger's syndrome. Mangano[4] has recommended systemic narcotics, inhalation analgesia, and paracervical or pudendal blockade in preference to epidural analgesia for labor on the compelling theoretical concern for the effects of a sympathetic blockade on SVR and thus, shunt direction. Pollack and colleagues[67] successfully used single-shot subarachnoid morphine (1.5 mg) for 14 hours of labor supplemented by a pudendal block for stage 2 in a woman with PDA and Eisenmenger's syndrome. By using a double-pulse oximeter setup, they were able to detect increases in right-to-left shunt by the difference in saturation between the right hand (preductal) and left foot (postductal). Pain just before the placement of the pudendal block resulted in a decrease in left foot saturation (77%), whereas the right hand remained 100% saturated. While perineal anesthesia was established, postductal saturation returned to baseline (90%), emphasizing the critical importance of adequate pain control in these patients.

Several authors have successfully employed epidural analgesia supplemented by epidural, subarachnoid, or intravenous narcotics for vaginal delivery and even cesarean section.[75,77-80] Midwall et al. determined that the ratio of systemic to pulmonary blood flow (Qp/Qs) and thus, shunt direction, was unaffected by gradual imposition of an epidural block.[80] In general, SVR tends to remain unchanged with T-10–level sympathetic blocks, while vasodilation in the legs is compensated by reflex vasoconstriction in the sympathetically intact upper body.[34] Moreover, supplementation with narcotics and/or a pudendal block makes adequate analgesia for vaginal delivery possible with low concentrations of local anesthetics. This author favors such an approach for several reasons. Epidural anesthetics not only provide reliable, titratable pain control for labor, but may be gradually extended toward the ends of stage 1 to blunt the urge to Valsalva and to allow painless application of forceps. If the sympathetic block is poorly tolerated, phenylephrine should restore peripheral tone, and the epidural can be altered to a lower level with greater supplementations as needed by epidural, intravenous, or intramuscular narcotics, or a pudendal block. If it is well tolerated, the epidural level should be maintained at a T-6 to T-8 level, so that it may be gradually extended without excessive delay to achieve a level adequate for a cesarean section, should the need arise. This potential of epidural analgesia to obviate the need for general anesthesia is regarded as a significant advantage, since it is this author's bias that the hemodynamic perturbations of positive pressure ventilation (increased PVR), laryngoscopy, intubation, and extubation are likely greater than those imposed by a gradually applied epidural. The excellent postoperative pain control afforded by an epidural anesthetic is an additional advantage. Ultimately, the magnitude of anesthetic-related hemodynamic fluctuations may depend more on the skill and experience of the anesthesiologist than the specific technique used.

If an epidural is employed, epinephrine should not be used, and loss of resistance to saline rather than air will avoid the possibility of a pulmonary or paradoxical embolus, either of which could be catastrophic. Since many of these patients are on heparin, coagulation status must be considered before epidural catheter placement. Notice also that patients with a right-to-left shunt may experience faster and more potent cerebral and cardiovascular side effects from intravenously absorbed local anesthetics or narcotics from the epidural space.[66] Whatever method is employed, supplemental oxygen should be provided to optimize any reversible component of pulmonary hypertension. It has been suggested that the margin of safety provided by oxygen-mediated reduction of PVR may be responsible for the ability of patients to tolerate epidural anesthesia in case reports in which that technique was successfully employed.[67] Currently it is unclear whether epidural anesthesia would be tolerated in severe cases of Eisenmenger's syndrome in which PVR is absolutely fixed.

Monitoring recommendations for patients with Eisenmenger's syndrome also are a source of controversy, for which insufficient literature exists to settle the issue. Most clinicians would agree that electrocardiogram (ECG), pulse oximetry, and arterial pressure monitoring are essential. When a PDA is present, the right hand, left foot double oximetry described by Pollack et al. may suggest information regarding the degree of right-to-left shunt.[67] Because right-sided heart failure is a constant threat, most would agree that CVP monitoring justifies its attendant risks of hematoma, pneumothorax, infection, arrhythmias, thrombus formation, and air embolus. On the other hand, pulmonary artery catheterization—which carries a greater risk of arrhythmias and the additional risk of pulmonary artery perforation, malpositioning through an intracardiac shunt, and balloon occlusion of a PDA—may not be justified by the additional information provided.[67,81,82,83] Pulmonary artery pressure monitoring may be useful if the catheter is properly positioned, and indeed there is a reversible component of the pulmonary hypertension. Thermodilutional CO determinations (and thus, calculated SVR), however, may be uninterpretable in the presence of a variable shunt. Moreover, measurements of oxygen saturation form the distal port do not represent true mixed venous oxygen saturation in the presence of an intracardiac shunt.[66] A risk-benefits analysis for the use of a pulmonary artery catheter must be carefully applied to each case of Eisenmenger's syndrome on an individual basis. Transesophageal echocardiography would likely be extremely useful for detecting changes in the magnitude of right-to-left intracardiac shunting, preload, and ventricular dysfunction, but this would require general anesthesia.

Anesthetic Management of the Case Presented

The case at hand is that of a term, gravida 3 para 0, 35-year-old woman with severe AS admitted to the hospital for induction of labor. Anesthetic management should be based on the aforementioned pathophysiologic principles and physiologic goals (Table 30-4). Maintenance of adequate preload and avoidance of systemic hypotension, ischemia, myocardial depression, and extremes of bradycardia or tachycardia will minimize her risk. Throughout her labor and delivery, a posture which prevents caval compression should be assured at all times and supplemental oxygen should be provided to decrease the probability of ischemia. Several forms of analgesia for labor and vaginal delivery have been suggested, including combinations of inhalational, intravenous, and pudendal blocks,[4] or epidural or subarachnoid opioids[83] or local anesthetics.[57] The specific choice of analgesia is of less importance than is strict attention to the physiologic goals.

Monitors

In view of the high maternal mortality, the narrow margin of cardiovascular reserve, and the potential for significant, sudden, and unpredictable hemodynamic changes during labor, delivery, and the postpartum period. This author and others[76] believe that the benefits of aggressive hemodynamic monitoring outweigh the risks. In addition to a five-lead ECG and pulse oximeter, this patient should receive a radial arterial line and pulmonary artery catheter. If anxiety and tachycardia occur despite local infiltration for these lines, the patient may be cautiously sedated with judicious dosages of intravenous fentanyl, diazepam, or butorphanol. The minimal risk of an arterial line placement is justified by the potentially life-saving early detection of hypotension which, as discussed earlier, may precipitate ischemia, increase the transvalvular gradient, and lead to rapid cardiovascular collapse. Moreover, resuscitation of patients with severe AS is particularly difficult because closed-chest cardiac massage may not create enough intraventricular pressure to overcome the outflow obstruction.

The risks of inserting a pulmonary artery catheter are more significant, but are outweighed by the benefits. Maintenance of appropriately elevated LV filling pressures is essential to insure adequate CO during labor, delivery, and the postpartum period when the demand for CO may increase by as much as 80%. However, excess fluid can easily lead to pulmonary edema, hypoxemia, and ischemia in this setting. Therefore the margin for error in managing intravascular volume is narrow. In patients with reduced left ventricular compliance, CVP is a particularly unreliable estimate of preload. Although PCWP also may overestimate LV filling pressures when ventricular compliance is reduced, it remains the best indicator of preload practically available. In addition, it allows measurement of thermodilution derived CO and SVR, as well as mixed venous oxygen saturation. It also provides access for rapidly establishing transvenous pacing. Finally, the sudden appearance of V-waves on the pulmonary artery occlusion tracing may provide an early indication of myocardial ischemia. Otherwise it would be exceedingly difficult to monitor for ischemia, given the left bundle branch pattern on her ECG. In addition, many such patients with LV hypertrophy display *strain* patterns on their ECG that make ischemia difficult to detect, even in the absence of a left bundle branch block. The most significant risk of this monitor is that of catheter-induced arrhythmias during insertion. Catheter insertion may theoretically cause a transient right bundle branch block which, in this patient, may result in a complete heart block.

Analgesia for Labor and Delivery

At the Brigham and Women's Hospital, Boston, labor analgesia would be provided by subarachnoid or epidural narcotics plus, as necessary, cautiously titrated dilute solutions of local anesthetic. The combined technique of injecting a single dose of subarachnoid opioid (e.g., 10 μg sufentanil) via a long spinal needle passed through the epidural needle before threading the epidural catheter would have the advantage of providing up to 2 hours of stage 1 labor analgesia with no significant hemodynamic impact. Alternatively, subarachnoid morphine (0.5 mg) will provide longer lasting analgesia. Since this patient will receive postpartum intensive care unit attention, concerns regarding delayed respiratory depression will not become a management issue. If and when more analgesia is needed for stage 2 or before, the epidural catheter is already in place without subjecting the patient to a second procedure.[84]

Confirmation of epidural catheter placement is controversial. The use of an epinephrine-containing test dose should be avoided because (1) it may be unreliable in laboring parturients[85], and (2) intravascular absorption may lead to catastrophic vasodilation, tachycardia, or hypotension in these patients.[86] For supplemental epidural narcotics, no test dose is indicated. For epidural local anesthetics, each injection should be its own test dose. This author would choose serial injections of 0.25% bupivacaine (2 ml at a time) injected every 10 to 20 minutes with close attention to hemodynamic parameters until comfort or a T-10 level is obtained. Once comfort is established, a continuous epidural drip of bupivacaine (0.125%) plus opioid may be employed. If well-tolerated hemodynamically, raising the level to T-6 to T-8 has the advantage of shortening the time required to gradually extend the level for cesarean section, should fetal distress occur. Bupivacaine has the advantage of gradual onset. The theoretical risk of cardiotoxicity should be considered, but given the low dosages, careful titration, and close hemodynamic monitoring, it seems exceedingly unlikely that significant cardiovascular depression would inadvertently occur without early detection. Later, in stage 2, when a more dense sensory block is desirable to block the urge to push and allow vacuum or outlet forceps delivery, lidocaine or higher concentrations of bupivacaine may be substituted. Lidocaine 2% has a more rapid onset of sympathetic block, however, and must be titrated slowly. Easterling et al. have published a dramatic polygraph strip showing an abrupt decrease in BP and pulmonary artery pressures in a patient with severe AS after epidural injection of just 3 ml of 3% 2-chloroprocaine.[87] However, with care to avoid rapid sympathetic blockade and maintain preload, epidural blockade may safely provide analgesia for labor, delivery, and even cesarean section.[57,87,88]

Also controversial is the issue of intravascular volume expansion before initiation of an epidural block. The prevention of systemic hypotension (and its attendant decrease in cardiac preload and coronary perfusion pressure) is probably a greater risk than pulmonary edema.[83] On the other hand, the efficacy of a fluid bolus in preventing hypotension before sympathetic blockade recently has been challenged.[40] A reasonable approach is to cautiously administer a conservative fluid bolus (250 to 500 ml) guided by PCWP while slowly titrating the epidural catheter with the aim of maintaining high normal filling pressures.

Hypotension, from whatever cause, should be immediately treated to restore coronary perfusion pressure and interrupt the cycle of hypotension and ischemia. A presumption here is that caval compression has been avoided throughout by uterine displacement or lateral decubitus positioning. Barring bradycardia, phenylephrine would be this author's choice of vasopressor. As an α-adrenergic agonist, it increases SVR (and thus, coronary perfusion pressure) while reversing the trend of reflex tachycardia. The increase in afterload, which may be an issue in patients with ischemia from coronary artery disease, is not an issue in patients with severe AS, because peripheral vascular tone makes only a trivial contribution to afterload compared with the stenotic aortic valve. Therefore, the net effect is to restore BP and improve the myocardial oxygen supply demand balance by slowing HR and increasing coronary perfusion pressure, at no cost in terms of afterload. After the BP has been restored, the cause of the hypotension (hypovolemia, sympathetic block, arrhythmia) may be addressed, but fluid infusions or cardioversion should not delay the administration of a vasoconstrictor. Ephedrine would be an acceptable alternative or adjunct to phenylephrine when HR is low, but care should be exercised to avoid overshoot tachycardia, which can exacerbate ischemia and compromise diastolic LV filling and systolic ejection in these patients. Concern for the effects of an α-adrenergic agonist on uterine perfusion[89] should take a back seat to optimal treatment of the critically threatened parturient. When used in judicious dosages to promptly correct spinal anesthetic—induced hypotension during cesarean section, phenylephrine has been shown to be free of adverse effects on the fetus, as determined by Apgar scores and acid-base profiles.[90,91]

The expulsive phase and immediate postpartum period are the times of the greatest hemodynamic changes (see the discussion on Cardiovascular Effects of Pregnancy, Labor, and Delivery) and the greatest risk to this patient. Epidural analgesia may lessen some of these changes.[92] Effective epidural analgesia alleviates the pain, anxiety, and attendant tachycardia, and can block the reflex urge to push. This prevents the hemodynamic perturbations of the Valsalva maneuver and would be expected to reduce workload, oxygen consumption, and hyperventilation. Nevertheless, SV and CO rise by 60% to 80% immediately after delivery.[92] Although preload generally is well maintained by autotransfusion from the involuted uterus, many variables make this an unpredictable time. Blood loss significantly in excess of the usual 500 ml should be recognized early and replaced by crystalloid or colloid, guided by MAP and PCWP. Ischemia may result from the increased CO coupled with decreased coronary perfusion pressure. Pulmonary edema may occur if CO cannot match the venous return augmented by uterine autotransfusions. Thus causes of hypotension during the immediate postpartum period may be difficult to sort out. One must remember that patients with AS are not immune from other obstetric causes of cardiovascular collapse, such as blood loss or amniotic fluid embolism. Because the cardiovascular effects of labor and delivery dissipate gradually after delivery, such high-risk patients should be maintained under close invasive hemodynamic surveillance for at least 24 hours.

In the event of fetal distress, anesthesia for an emergent cesarean section is best accomplished with general endotracheal anesthesia. Although case reports are accumulating of cesarean sections under epidural anesthesia in patients with even severe AS,[57,87,88] this should only be considered a viable option when enough time exists to permit very gradual titration of the sympathetic block. General anesthesia may be induced in traditional rapid sequence fashion using etomidate and succinylcholine with minimal hemodynamic trespass.[93] Because etomidate lacks analgesic properties, it should be accompanied by or preceded by a dose of opioid sufficient to blunt the hemodynamic response to laryngoscopy and intubation. Alternatively, a traditional *cardiac anesthetic* may be employed using high-dose nonhistamine releasing narcotics such as fentanyl, sufentanil, or alfentanil. This has the disadvantage of compromising the speed of induction (slightly increased aspiration risk) and committing both mother and newborn to ventilatory support for some postoperative period. In patients with virtually no cardiovascular reserve due to critically severe AS, it may be argued that this is the safest course. Narcotic based general anesthesia has been reported with extubation at the end of surgery using the shorter acting alfentanil for cesarean section in a women with stenotic valvular disease.[94] Even with a pure narcotic induction, some hypotension may occur, possibly due to withdrawal of endogenous catecholamine support. Phenylephrine, for reasons cited earlier, should be available to promptly reverse this trend. In patients less severely compromised by AS, general anesthesia may be accomplished with a lower dose of opioid supplemented by other hemodynamically stable agents such as etomidate, nitrous oxide, or even a bolus of epidural narcotic. In either case, the pediatric receiving team should be made aware of the probability of a narcotized infant, and arrangements should be made for intensive care level vigilance and continued invasive hemodynamic monitoring of the mother for a minimum of 24 hours after surgery. A surge in CO of 60% to 80% also is seen after cesarean delivery, and blood loss frequently is twofold to threefold greater than that seen after vaginal delivery. Therefore greater intravascular fluid requirements should be anticipated, guided by PCWP and the total hemodynamic picture. The obstetricians, intent on delivering the baby, may need to be reminded of the crucial importance of avoiding caval compression with their hands or retractors. If hypertension is encountered, it often is tolerated reasonably well (compared with hypotension), and should be treated cautiously by deepening anesthetic depth with care to avoid an overshoot. Intravenous vasodilators should be avoided because of their effect on SVR, and thus coronary perfusion pressure and aortic valve gradient. Similarly, volatile agents should be employed with great caution to prevent decreases in SVR and myocardial contractility.

Rapid administration of oxytocin or bolus doses in excess of 2 U intravenously also have been associated with decreases in peripheral vascular resistance and hypotension.[66] One case report attributed ventricular fibrillation and cardiovascular collapse to the administration of 5 U followed by 10 U of oxytocin to a 23-year-old woman with severe AS (aortic valve area [AVA] of 0.3 cm^2) for therapeutic abortion.[95] Therefore if uterine atony occurs despite a slow or dilute infusion of oxytocin, it may be safer to employ a trial of methyl ergometrine rather than speeding up the oxytocin infusion. In one study, 0.2 mg of methyl ergometrine (intravascularly) were found to produce an increase in femoral artery pressure (11%), pulmonary artery pressure (27%), and PCWP (31%),[96] all of which would likely be better tolerated than a decrease in SVR in a parturient with severe AS.

Finally, it deserves reemphasizing that the hemodynamic changes in the intrapartum and immediate postpartum period may be profound and unpredictable. Close attention must be paid to the total hemodynamic picture, including uterine tone and blood loss, in addition to invasive hemodynamic indices or signs of ischemia to promptly reverse trends that are at odds with the physiologic goals for aortic stenosis.

Summary

1. The risk associated with maternal heart disease in pregnancy depends on the specific cardiac lesion and the degree of functional reserve.
2. Anesthetic management requires an integrated understanding of the hemodynamic requirements of the specific cardiac lesion together with the cardiovascular effects of pregnancy, labor and delivery, and the various anesthetic options.
3. Pregnancy gradually and progressively stresses the heart with increases in intravascular volume, CO, SV, and HR, whereas SVR decreases. Labor and delivery superimpose an additional acute and less predictable volume and workload stress on the heart, and this represents the time of greatest risk.
4. The hemodynamic effects of epidural analgesia or anesthesia include primarily decreased preload, and to a lesser extent, decreased afterload, contractility, and possibly HR with higher level sympathetic blocks.
5. Rheumatic valvular disease is the most common type of cardiac lesion. Women with NYHA class I and II generally tolerate pregnancy well. Those with NYHA class III and IV generally require invasive hemodynamic monitoring and tighter adherence to the optimal hemodynamics for the specific valvular lesion.
6. Congenital heart disease is increasingly common in pregnancy. Eisenmenger's syndrome with pulmonary hypertension is discussed as an example of a congenital cardiac lesion associated with high maternal mortality regardless of the functional classification, the anesthetic management of which is highly controversial.

7. In general, the advantages of an epidural for labor and delivery outweigh the risks. The hemodynamic effects of a low (T-8 to T-10), gradually imposed labor epidural are minimal, provided that preload is preserved through positioning and volume expansion, guided by invasive hemodynamic monitoring in the high-risk parturient. Supplementation with epidural or subarachnoid narcotics or a pudendal block allows for lighter local anesthetic dosages and even greater hemodynamic stability.
8. For cesarean section, gradual extension of the epidural, as described earlier, has been successfully employed in patients with Eisenmenger's syndrome and severe valvular lesions. Alternatively, a *hemodynamically stable* (i.e., etomidate versus high-dose narcotic-based) general anesthetic may be employed in the very high-risk patient.
9. Optimization of the hemodynamic parameters for the specific cardiac lesion is of greater importance than the specific anesthetic choice.

References

1. Kaunitz AM, Hughes JM, Grimes DA, et al: Causes of maternal mortality in the United States, *Obstet Gynecol* 1985; 65:605.
2. Bogard TD: *Pregnancy and cardiovascular diseases.* In Hood DD, editor: *Problems in anesthesia,* Philadelphia, 1989, JB Lippincott.
3. Hess DB, Hess WL: Cardiovascular disease in pregnancy, *Obstet Gynecol Clin North Am* 1992; 19(4):679.
4. Mangano DT: *Anesthesia for the pregnant cardiac patient.* In Shnider SM, Levinson G, editors: *Anesthesia for obstetrics, ed 3,* Baltimore, 1993, Williams and Wilkins.
5. Clark SL, Cotton DB, Lee W, et al: Central hemodynamic assessment of normal term pregnancy, *Am J Obstet Gynecol* 1989; 161:1439.
6. Hunter S, Robson SC: Adaptation of the maternal heart in pregnancy, *Br Heart J* 1992; 68(6):540.
7. Robson SC, Hunter S, Boys RJ: Serial study of factors influencing changes in cardiac output during human pregnancy, *Am J Physiol* 1989; 256:(H)1060.
8. Ueland K: Maternal cardiovascular hemodynamics. VII: intrapartum blood volume changes, *Am J Obstet Gynecol* 1976; 126:671.
9. Schrier RW: Pathogenesis of sodium and water retention in high-output and low-output cardiac failure, nephrotic syndrome, cirrhosis, and pregnancy, *N Engl J Med* 1988; 319:1127.
10. Schrier RW, Durr JA: Pregnancy: an overfill or underfill state, *Am J Kidney Dis* 1987; 9:284.
11. Assali NS, Brinkman CR III: *Disorders of maternal circulatory and respiratory adjustments.* In Assali NS, Brinkman CR III, editors: *Pathophysiology of gestation: maternal disorders,* New York, 1972, Academic Press.
12. Vered Z, Poler SM, Gibson P, et al: Noninvasive detection of the morphologic and hemodynamic changes during normal pregnancy, *Clin Cardiol* 1991; 14:327.
13. Katz R, Karliner JS, Resnik R: Effects of a natural volume overload state (pregnancy) on left ventricular performance in normal human subjects, *Circulation* 1978; 58:434.
14. Metcalf J, Ueland K: Maternal cardiovascular adjustment to pregnancy, *Prog Carovasc Dis* 1974; 16:363.
15. Weiner C, Martinez E, Zhu LK, et al: In vitro release of endothelium-derived relaxing factor by acetylcholine is increased during the guinea pig pregnancy, *Am J Obstet Gynecol* 1989; 161:1599.
16. Weiner CP, Martinez E, Chestnut D, et al: Effect of pregnancy on uterine and carotid artery response to norepinephrine, epinephrine, and phenylephrine in vessels with documented functional endothelium, *Am J Obstet Gynecol* 1989; 161:1605.
17. Lusiani L, Rousisvalle G, Bonanome E, et al: Echocardiographic evaluation of the dimensions and systolic properties of the left ventricle in freshman athletes during physical training, *Eur Heart J* 1986, 7:196.
18. Sady MA, Haydon BB, Sady SP, et al: Cardiovascular response to maximal cycle exercise during pregnancy and at two and seven months post-partum, *Am J Obstet Gynecol* 1990; 162:1181.

19. Sadaniantz A, Kocheril AG, Emaus SP, et al: Cardiovascular changes in pregnancy evaluated by two-dimensional and doppler echocardiography, *J Am Soc Echocardiogr* 1992; 5(3):253.
20. Capeless EL, Clapp JF: When do cardiovascular parameters return to their preconception values? *Am J Obstet Gynecol* 1991; 165:883.
21. Enein M, Zina AA, Kassem M, et al: Echocardiography of the pericardium in pregnancy, *Obstet Gynecol* 1987; 69:851.
22. Clark SL, Cotton DB, Pivarnik JM, et al: Position change and central hemodynamic profile during normal third trimester pregnancy and post-partum, *Am J Obstet Gynecol* 1991; 164:883.
23. Jalauvka V: Heart disease and maternal mortality, *Gynaekol Rundsch* 1970; 10:209.
24. Ueland K, Hansen JM: Maternal cardiovascular dynamics. III: labor and delivery under local and caudal analgesia, *Am J Obstet Gynecol* 1969; 103:8.
25. Burlew BS: Managing the pregnant patient with heart disease, *Clin Cardiol* 1990; 13:757.
26. Ueland K, Hansen JM: Maternal cardiovascular dynamics. II: posture and uterine contractions, *Am J Obstet Gynecol* 1969; 103:1.
27. Lee W, Rokey R, Miller J, et al: Maternal hemodynamic effects of uterine contractions by M-mode and pulsed Doppler echocardiography, *Am J Obstet Gynecol* 1989; 161:974.
28. Robson SC, Dunlop W, Boys RJ, et al: Cardiac output during labor, *Br Med J* 1987; 295(7):1169.
29. Shnider SM, Wright RG, Levinson G, et al: Uterine blood flow and plasma norepinephrine changes during maternal stress in the pregnant ewe, *Anesthesiology* 1979; 50:524.
30. Shnider SM, Abboud TK, Artal R, et al: Maternal catecholamines decrease during labor after lumbar epidural analgesia, *Am J Obstet Gynecol* 1983; 147:13.
31. Hendricks CH: Hemodynamics of uterine contractions, *Am J Obstet Gynecol* 1958; 76:968.
32. Nunn JF: *Nunn's applied respiratory physiology,* ed 4, Oxford, 1993, Butterworth-Heinmann.
33. Mark JB, Steele SM: Cardiovascular effects of spinal anesthesia, *Int Anesth Clin* 1989; 27(1):31.
34. Greene NM, Brull SJ: *Physiology of spinal anesthesia, ed 4,* Baltimore, 1993, Williams and Wilkins.
35. Covino BG: Cardiovascular effects of spinal and epidural anesthesia, *Reg Anesth* 1978; 1:23.
36. Carpenter RL, Caplan RA, Brown DL, et al: Incidence and risk factors for side effects of spinal anesthesia, *Anesthesiology* 1992; 76(6):906.
37. Goertz AW, Seeling W, Heinrich H, et al: Influence of high thoracic epidural anesthesia on left ventricular contractility assessed using the end-systolic pressure-length relationship, *Acta Anaesth Scand* 1993; 37:38.
38. Bengtsson M, Löfström, Malmquist LA: Skin conductance responses during spinal analgesia, *Acta Anaesth Scand* 1985; 29:67.
39. Chamberlain DP, Chamberlain BDL: Changes in the skin temperature of the trunk and their relationship to sympathetic blockade during spinal anesthesia, *Anesthesiology* 1986; 65:139.
40. Route CC, Rocke DA, Levin J, et al: A reevaluation of the role of crystalloid preload in the prevention of hypotension associated with spinal anesthesia for elective cesarean section, *Anesthesiology* 1993; 79:262.
41. Kerkkamp HEM, Gielen MJM: Hemodynamic monitoring in epidural blockade: cardiovascular effects of 20 ml 0.5% bupivacaine with and without epinephrine, *Reg Anesth* 1990; 15:137.
42. Szekely P, Snaith L: *Heart disease and pregnancy.* London, 1974, Churchill Livingston.
43. Chesley LC: Severe rheumatic heart disease in pregnancy: the ultimate prognosis, *Am J Obstet Gynecol* 1980; 136:552.
44. Jackson JM, Thomas SJ: *Valvular heart disease.* In Kaplan JA, editor: *Cardiac anesthesia, ed 3,* Philadelphia, 1993, WB Saunders.
45. Ueland K: *Rheumatic heart disease and pregnancy.* In Elkayam U, Gleicher N, editors: *Cardiac problems in pregnancy,* New York, 1982, Alan R. Liss.
46. Sullivan JM, Ramanathan KB: Management of medical problems in pregnancy—severe cardiac disease, *N Engl J Med* 1985; 313(5):304.
47. Clark SL, Phelan JP, Greenspoon J, et al: Labor and delivery in the presence of mitral stenosis: central hemodynamic observations, *Am J Obstet Gynecol* 1985; 152:984.
48. Kasab SM, Sabag T, Zeibag M: Beta adrenergic blockade in the management of pregnant women with mitral stenosis, *Am J Obstet Gynecol* 1990; 165:37.
49. Larson CP, Shuer LM, Cohen SE: Maternally administered

esmolol decreases fetal as well as maternal heart rate, *J Clin Anesth* 1990; 2:427.
50. Vogel JHK, Pryor R, Blount SG, Jr: Direct-current defibrillation during pregnancy, *JAMA* 1965; 193:970.
51. Schroeder JS, Harrison DC: Repeated cardioversion during pregnancy: treatment of refractory paroxysmal atrial tachycardia during three successive pregnancies, *Am J Cardiol* 1971; 27:445.
52. Esteves CA, Ramos AIO, Braga SLN, et al: Effectiveness of percutaneous balloon mitral valvotomy during pregnancy, *Am J Cardiol* 1991; 68:930.
53. Smith R, Brender D, McCredie M: Percutaneous transluminal dilation of the mitral valve in pregnancy, *Br Heart J* 1989; 61:551.
54. Patel JJ, Mitha AS, Hassen F, et al: Percutaneous balloon mitral valvotomy in pregnant patients with tight pliable mitral stenosis, *Am Heart J* 1993; 125:1106.
55. Rakusan K: Quantitative morphology of capillaries of the heart: number of capillaries in animal and human hearts under normal and pathological conditions, *Methods Achieve Exp Pathol* 1971; 5:272.
56. Arias F, Pineda J: Aortic stenosis and pregnancy, *J Reprod Med* 1978; 20(4):229.
57. Lao TT, Sermer M, MaGee L, et al: Congenital aortic stenosis and pregnancy: a reappraisal, *Am J Obstet Gynecol* 1993; 169:540.
58. Clyne CA, Arrigh JA, Maron BJ, et al: Systemic and left ventricular responses to exercise stress in asymptomatic patients with valvular aortic stenosis, *Am J Cardiol* 1991; 68:1469.
59. Goodman DJ, Rossen RM, Holloway EL, et al: Effect of nitroprusside on left ventricular dynamics in mitral regurgitation, *Circulation* 1974; 50:1025.
60. Baxley WA, Kennedy JW, Field B, et al: Hemodynamics in ruptured chordae tendinae and chronic rheumatic mitral regurgitation, *Circulation* 1973; 48:1288.
61. Shoemaker CT, Meyers M: Sodium nitroprusside for control of severe hypertensive disease of pregnancy: a case report and discussion of potential toxicity, *Am J Obstet Gynecol* 1984; 149(2):171.
62. Smith HJ, Neutze JM, Roche AHG, et al: The natural history of rheumatic aortic regurgitation and the indications for surgery, *Br Heart J* 1976; 38:147.
63. Brady K, Duff P: Rheumatic heart disease in pregnancy, *Clin Obstet Gynecol* 1989; 32(1):21.
64. Elkayam U, Gleicher N: Congenital heart disease in pregnancy, *Heart Failure* 1993; 9(2):46.
65. Allen LD, Crawford DC, Chita SK, et al: Familial recurrence of congenital heart disease in a prospective series of mothers referred for fetal echocardiography, *Am J Cardiol* 1986; 58:334.
66. Weiss BM, Atanasoff PG: Cyanotic congenital heart disease and pregnancy: natural selection, pulmonary hypertension, and anesthesia, *J Clin Anesth* 1993; 5:332.
67. Pollack KL, Chestnut DH, Wenstrom KD: Anesthetic management of a parturient with Eisenmenger's syndrome, *Anesth Analg* 1990; 70:212.
68. Heath D, Edwards JE: The pathology of hypertensive pulmonary vascular disease: a description of six grades of structural changes in the pulmonary arteries with special reference to congenital cardiac septal defects, *Circulation* 1958; 18:533.
69. Elkayam U, Cobb T, Gleicher N: *Congenital heart disease in pregnancy.* In Elkayam U, Gleicher N, editors: *Cardiac problems in pregnancy, ed 2,* New York, 1990, Alan R. Liss.
70. Elkayam U: *Pregnancy and cardiovascular disease.* In Braunwald E, editor: *Heart Disease, ed 4,* Philadelphia, 1992, WB Saunders.
71. Pitts JA, Crosby WM, Basta LL: Eisenmenger's syndrome in pregnancy: does heparin prophylaxis improve the maternal mortality rate? *Am Heart J* 1977; 93:321.
72. Heytens L, Alexander JP: Maternal and neonatal death associated with Eisenmenger's syndrome, *Acta Anaesthesiol Belg* 1986; 37:45.
73. Lumley J, Whitwam JG, Morgan M: General anesthesia in the presence of Eisenmenger's syndrome, *Anesth Analg* 1977; 56(4):543.
74. Atanasoff P, Alon E, Schmid ER, et al: Epidural anesthesia for cesarean section in a patient with severe pulmonary hypertension, *Acta Anaesthesiol Scand* 1989; 33:75.
75. Lui P, Silway G, Palop R, et al: Eisenmenger's syndrome: anesthetic management for labour and delivery. A case report, *Mt Sinai J Med* 1978; 45(3):441.
76. Johnson MD, Saltzman D: *Cardiac disease.* In Datta S, editor: *Anesthetic and obstetric management of high risk pregnancy,* St. Louis, 1991, Mosby–Year Book.

77. Spinnato JA, Kraynack BJ, Cooper MW: Eisenmenger's syndrome in pregnancy: epidural anesthesia for elective cesarean section, *N Engl J Med* 1981; 304(20):1215.
78. McMurray TJ, Kenny NT: Extradural anaesthesia in parturients with severe cardiovascular disease: two case reports, *Anaesthesia* 1982; 37:442.
79. Lieber S, DeWilde PH, Huyghens L, et al: Eisenmenger's syndrome in pregnancy, *Acta Cardiol* 1985; 4:421.
80. Midwall J, Jaffin H, Herman MV, et al: Shunt flow and pulmonary hemodynamics during labor and delivery in the Eisenmenger's syndrome, *Am J Cardiology* 1978; 42(2):299.
81. Robinson S: Pulmonary artery catheters in Eisenmenger's syndrome: many risks, few benefits, *Anesthesiology* 1983; 58:588.
82. Devitt JW, Noble WH, Byrick BJ: A Swan-Ganz catheter related complication in a patient with Eisenmenger's syndrome, *Anesthesiology* 1982; 57:335.
83. Thornhill ML, Camann WR: *Cardiovascular disease during pregnancy.* In Chestnut D, editor: *Obstetric anesthesia: principles and practice,* St. Louis, 1994, Mosby–Year Book.
84. Stacey RGW, Watt S, Kadim MY, et al: Single space combined spinal-extradural technique for analgesia in labour, *Br J Anaesth* 1993; 71:499.
85. Biehl DR: The dilemma of the epidural test dose, *Can J Anaesth* 1987; 34(6):545.
86. Bonica JJ, Akamatsu TJ, Berges PU, et al: Circulatory effects of peridural blocks. II: effects of epinephrine, *Anesthesiology* 1971; 34:514.
87. Easterling TR, Chadwick HS, Otto CM, et al: Aortic stenosis in pregnancy, *Obstet Gynecol* 1988; 72:113.
88. Brian JE, Seifen AB, Clark RB, et al: Aortic stenosis, cesarean delivery, and epidural analgesia, *J Clin Anesth* 1993; 5:154.
89. Shnider SM, DeLorimer AA, Asling JH, et al: Vasopressors in obstetrics. II: fetal hazards of methoxamine administration during obstetric spinal anesthesia, *Am J Obstet Gynecol* 1965; 106:680.
90. Ramanathan S, Grant GJ: Vasopressor therapy for hypotension due to epidural anesthesia for cesarean section, *Acta Anaesth Scand* 1988; 32:559.
91. Moran DH, Perillo M, Laporta RF, et al: Phenylephrine in the prevention of hypotension following spinal anesthesia for cesarean delivery, *J Clin Anesth* 1991; 3(4):301.
92. Hansen JM, Ueland K: The influence of caudal analgesia on cardiovascular dynamics during labor and delivery, *Acta Anaesth Scand Suppl* 1966; 23:449.
93. Gooding JM, Weng J, Smith RA, et al: Cardiovascular and pulmonary responses following etomidate induction of anesthesia in patients with demonstrated cardiac disease, *Anesth Analg* 1979; 58:40.
94. Batson MA, Longmire S, Csontos E: Alfentanil for urgent cesarean section in a patient with severe mitral stenosis and pulmonary hypertension, *Can J Anaesth* 1990; 37(6):685.
95. Robinson M, Newman N, Creevy DC, et al: Congenital aortic stenosis in pregnancy: ventricular fibrillation induced by oxytocin, *JAMA* 1967; 200:378.
96. Secher NJ, Arnsbo P, Wallin L: Haemodynamic effects of oxytocin (Syntocinon®) and methyl ergometrine (Methergin®) on the systemic and pulmonary circulation of pregnant anaesthetised women, *Acta Obstet Gynecol Scand* 1978; 57:97.
97. Gianopoulos JG: Cardiac disease in pregnancy, *Med Clin North Am* 1989; 73(3):639.

31

Anesthetic Concerns in Severe Pregnancy-Induced Hypertension

A 29-year-old primigravida is admitted to the hospital at 28 weeks of pregnancy with a blood pressure of 170/115 mm Hg and proteinuria (3+). A diagnosis of pregnancy-induced hypertension (PIH) is made. Discuss the pathophysiology of PIH and the anesthetic management.

Recommendations by Stephen P. Gatt, M.D., F.A.N.Z.C.A.

Preoperative Considerations

Anesthesia for cesarean section (CS) for the parturient with severe pregnancy-induced hypertension (PIH) is fraught with a number of problems and dilemmas. The administration of an anesthetic, be it regional major conduction blockade or general anesthesia, represents a period of grave danger to an already compromised patient. Each time an anesthetic is given to a patient with severe PIH, the anesthesiologist must ask:

- Is the diagnosis of PIH correct? Is there any underlying pathology?
- Does the mother require stabilization before the anesthetic is started? Is the systemic arterial pressure controlled? Is eclampsia prophylaxis necessary? Has it been started?
- Is kidney or liver failure present, and, if so, can anesthetic agents with minimal renal and hepatic effect be selected?
- Has volume/blood loss been corrected? Is the urine output (u.o.) being measured? Is it adequate?
- Is coagulopathy present? Is it severe? Is the patient on aspirin? Can the coagulopathy be reversed or improved?
- Are there any poor prognostic features in the symptoms complex which make the anes-

thetic an unacceptably high risk undertaking? Can any of these be improved preoperatively?

- Will institution of an epidural block help control the arterial pressure (BP)?
- Is there any evidence of head and neck edema? If yes, does the patient require tracheostomy prior to CS? Has the airway been assessed with regard to intubation difficulty?[1,2]
- If a CS is to be performed? is this best managed with LEA or GA? If a GA is necessary, how can the intubation and laryngoscopy pressor responses be attenuated?
- Is the hemodynamic monitoring adequate? Is invasive monitoring needed? Which agents will be used to treat hypertensive crises?
- Is there any evidence of recent bleeding (e.g., from placental abruption) causing hemodynamic instability?
- Is the mother on magnesium, β-blocker, α-blocker, or calcium channel blocker?
- Is the fetus compromised by PIH or its complications (intrauterine growth limitation, abruptio placentae, hypovolemia)?

Attenuation of Pressor Responses to Airway Manipulation and Intubation

If the systemic arterial pressure (BP) is not well controlled or if there are clinical signs of raised intracranial pressure (ICP), laryngoscopy and intubation can precipitate pulmonary edema or intracranial hemorrhage.[3] A multitude of techniques have been used to modify or abolish the pressor responses to tracheal intubation and laryngoscopy.

Agents used include vasodilators (including α-adrenoreceptor blockers), increased or additional doses of induction agent, narcotics, β-adrenoreceptor antagonists (e.g., esmolol), magnesium, and (topical and intravenous) local anesthetics. Some of these agents have limited use because they can produce significant hypotension, appreciable falls in uteroplacental blood flow, or detrimental effects on the fetus (e.g., fetal hypoglycemia, respiratory depression, or hypotension). The pressor responses include rises in heart rate (HR), systolic, mean, and diastolic pressure (SAP, MAP, and DAP), pulmonary artery pressure (PAP), pulmonary capillary wedge pressure (PCWP), and rate pressure product (RPP). The responses occur in many patients receiving anesthesia but are exaggerated in those with PIH.[4] These pressor responses can be severe and are responsible for rises in ICP. They can cause severe morbidity from intracerebral hemorrhage and heart failure.[5] Although it is important to control these pressor responses, none of the methods mentioned above is completely effective in blocking the SAP, DAP, or RPP changes.

The gold standard against which all other agents have traditionally been assessed in pressor response attenuation is intravenous lidocaine. Even when lidocaine is used, RPPs can be very high. It has been suggested that magnesium and alfentanil are better than lidocaine in attenuating the mean cardiovascular responses to intubation.[6] Alfentanil is not as satisfactory as magnesium in that it fails to control SAP to less than 180 mm Hg in about 25% of mothers with PIH. Magnesium has the added advantage that it has the least detrimental effect on the fetus and does not produce significant hypotension (because it produces a concomitant increase in cardiac output).[6]

Misdiagnosis in Hemolysis–Elevated Liver Enzymes–Low Platelet Count Syndrome and PIH

A generation ago, PIH often was misdiagnosed as a medical or surgical disease unrelated to pregnancy. Currently the opposite is the more common error, that is, medical or surgical conditions unrelated to pregnancy are misdiagnosed as hemolysis–elevated liver enzymes–low platelet count syndrome (HELLP syndrome or PIH), so that appropriate therapy is delayed.[7] Goodlin [7] reports cases of essential hypertension and renal disease (14 cases), immune thrombocytopenia purpura (4), gangrenous or ruptured gall bladder (4), lupus erythematosus (3), acute fatty liver of pregnancy (3), pheochromocytoma (2), cocaine abuse (2), cardiomyopathy (2), dissecting aortic aneurysm (2), glomerulonephritis (2), and ruptured bile duct (1 case) masquerading as PIH. This is especially so in those with HELLP syndrome where CS rates can reach 61.5% to 94%.[8,9] Keeping this in mind, it becomes very important that the anesthesiologist review the diagnosis before proceeding to anesthetize the patient.

Is There an "Ideal" Anesthetic?

In those with no contraindication to major regional block, lumbar epidural anesthesia (LEA) would seem to be the *best* anesthetic for severe PIH for both vaginal delivery and CS. Indeed, epidural sympathetic blockade has become one of the mainstays of BP management during labor and delivery for PIH. From 1990 to 1991, 6.1% of over 1800 epidural procedures at the Royal Hospital for Women, Sydney, Australia (Fig. 31-1) were undertaken not for pain relief, but for control of BP.

Epidural analgesia (LEA) produces control of systemic arterial pressure (BP) by reducing the arteriolar vasospasm, which is at the center of this dis-

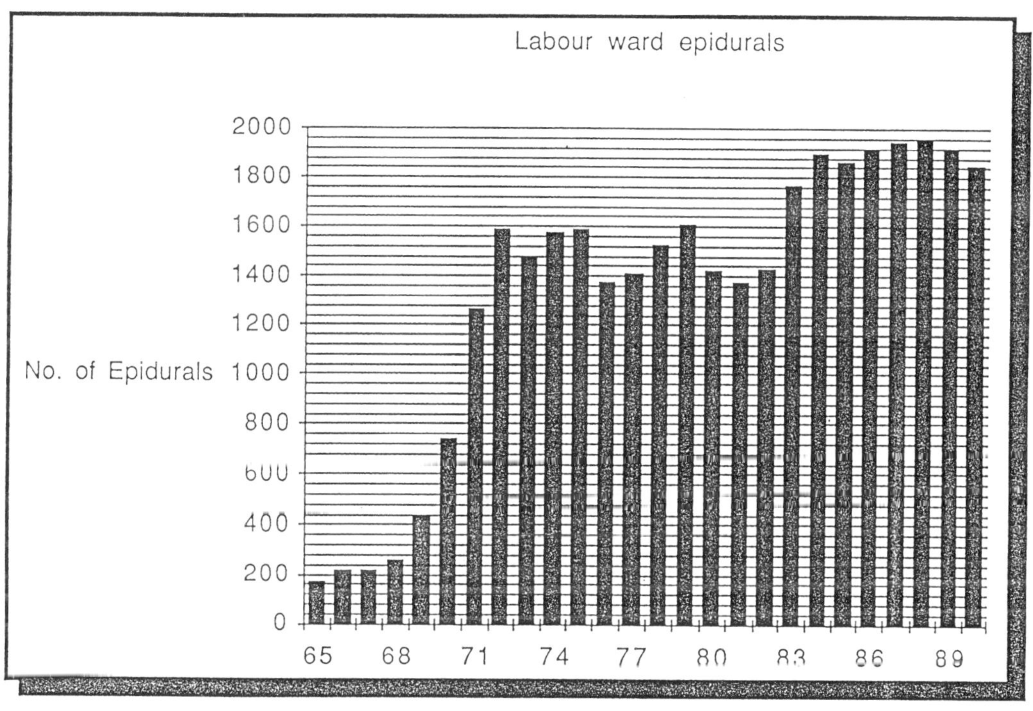

Fig. 31-1.

Total number of epidurals performed in the labor and delivery suite of the Royal Hospital for Women, Sydney, Australia, between 1965 and 1991. Epidurals performed in the operating rooms and other areas of the hospital (e.g., Obstetric Acute Care Center) have been excluded.

ease. Provided LEA is preceded by either crystalloid or colloid fluid preloading to maintain PCWP between 8 and 12 mm Hg, LEA will reduce MAP and systemic vascular resistance (SVR) without altering cardiac index (CI), pulmonary vascular resistance (PVR), central venous pressure (CVP), or PCWP.[10,11] LEA confers some specific advantages or PIH patients: it increases intervillous blood flow, improves cardiovascular stability, and decreases SVR and levels of circulating catecholamines.[12] Indeed, in some recent studies[13-15] most of the maternal hemodynamic changes occurred after preloading and not during insertion and establishment of the LEA. The changes included 11% increase in HR, 10% increase in stroke volume (SV), and 20% increase in cardiac output (CO). The HR remained elevated and the SVR was low (and SV and CO returned to normal) after establishment of LEA. Uterine blood flow was not compromised by bupivacaine 0.25% epidural anesthesia to the T-9 level.[13] Provided maternal hypotension is avoided with rapid prehydration using 2000 ml of electrolyte solution, LEA with plain bupivacaine in normal parturients having elective CS did not have detrimental effects on uteroplacental (maternal uterine, placental arcuate, and fetal umbilical arteries) or fetal (fetal renal and middle cerebral arteries) circulations.[14] Whereas mean uterine artery systolic:diastolic ratios on uterine artery velocimetry do not change after LEA in chronic hypertensives or normal parturients, they actually fall in PIH parturients. LEA reduces uterine artery vasospasm and improves intrapartum fetal well-being.[15] Epinephrine-containing solutions and pressor agents should be used with caution in severe PIH. These mothers are exquisitely sensitive to exogenous pressors. The LEA should be placed without an epinephrine-containing test dose and the block should be raised gradually to reduce the need for ephedrine or other pressors. In the postpartum period, especially once the LEA is ceased, fluid intake should be restricted; loop diuretics (e.g., furoemide) also may be needed.[16]

Unfortunately, epidural blockade may be contraindicated, for instance, if there is severe fetal distress requiring immediate delivery or hemodynamic compromise from abruptio placentae, which is common in PIH or thrombocytopenia (see the discussion later in this chapter). This is especially so in HELLP syndrome where optimum management consists of (1) stabilization of the clinical condition of the mother, followed by (2) expeditious delivery of the fetus, usually by CS.

Maternal resuscitation before delivery includes seizure prophylaxis, control of BP, correction of overt hypovolemia *or* judicious intravascular volume repletion, as appropriate, and institution of hemodynamic monitoring. A short period of resuscitation and preparation before instituting general anesthesia (GA) for CS is time well spent and should include (1) acid aspiration (Mendelson's) syndrome prophylaxis with clear antacid, ranitidine, and metoclopramide; (2) blood grouping, antibody screening, and blood crossmatch; (3) left uterine displacement on a wedge to minimize the supine hypotensive syndrome from inferior vena cava (IVC) compression; (4) preoxygenation; and (5) pretreatment of the pressor responses to airway manipulation and intubation.

Ketamine is best avoided in the rapid-sequence induction regimen. In those with renal or hepatic impairment, agents exhibiting diminished biotransformation (e.g., isoflurane), minimal renal excretion (e.g., atracurium), and short half-life (e.g., propofol) are preferable. The action of depolarizing and nondepolarizing neuromuscular blockers is prolonged by magnesium sulphate (see Chapter 14).

Poor-Risk Anesthetic Status

There are some clinical signs, laboratory studies, and patient symptoms for which the anesthesiologist should watch because they are indicators of poor outcome from anesthesia. These are as follows:

1. More than 2+ proteinuria, which suggests that considerable disruption of the glomerular basement membrane already has occurred;[17] severe hypoproteinemia is associated with poor perinatal outcome; the current patient with a blood pressure of 170/115 and 3+ proteinuria should have her blood pressure stabilized immediately before anesthesia is contemplated
2. HELLP syndrome with severe thrombocytopenia, which preclude the use of regional techniques
3. Elevated serum uric acid, which suggests that there could be a combination of decreased plasma volume, hemoconcentration, and decreased plasma flow[18]
4. Presence of lupus anticoagulant (anticardiolipin antibody), which often is associated with platelet damage, interference with procoagulant cascade clotting, and high perinatal wastage[19]
5. Low platelet count, which correlates with severity of PIH[20]
6. Haemoconcentration, especially if associated with hypoproteinemia
7. Disseminated intravascular coagulation (DIC) or neurologic or hepatic symptoms
8. PIH superimposed on chronic hypertension or associated with insulin-dependent diabetes[21] (see Chapter 33).

How Does the Coagulation Disorder of PIH Affect the Conduct of Anesthesia?

In-depth investigation of the coagulation disorder produced by severe PIH and HELLP syndrome can be laborious, expensive, and time consuming (Table 31-1). In most situations, initial screening with a platelet count is all that is required before placement of the epidural block.[19,22] Coagulation screening is not necessary in *all* PIH patients because (1) coagulation abnormalities (prolonged kaolin cephalin clotting time, thrombin clotting time, and one-stage prothrombin time) are invariably associated with thrombocytopenia; and (2) thrombocytopenia of less than 100 × 10^9/L only occurs in *severe* PIH (DAP > 100 mm Hg *and* proteinuria 2+ or greater)[20,23] (Fig. 31-2). Platelet count can be used as the single first-line test for screening.[23] Unnecessary delays in provision of adequate analgesia in labor can be avoided by limiting screening to those with severe PIH and by reducing to a minimum the number of investigations required. In the current case of BP 170/115 and proteinuria (3+), a platelet count would be all that is required before insertion of the LEA. Only if the platelet count were less than 100 × 10^9/L would bleeding time be necessary.[19]

It can be argued that in HELLP syndrome, whereas the signs of PIH can be mild, the platelet count may be low. If platelet count testing is restricted to those with severe PIH, cases of thrombocytopenia secondary to HELLP syndrome may be missed.[23] Although this may indeed occur, it is uncommon in HELLP syndrome to see decompensated DIC.[22] Using more sensitive and specific coagulation assays (antithrombin III, protein C, thrombin–antithrombin III complex) compensated DIC (activated coagulation) is seen in *all* HELLP syndrome pregnancies.[22]

Thrombocytopenia occurs in up to 15% to 50% of gravide women with PIH.[24,25] Although it is usually mild in degree, the 15% of PIH patients who go on to develop the HELLP syndrome have markedly decreased platelet counts.[9] Platelet counts rise above 100 × 10^9/L within 95 hours after delivery.[26] The nadir of the platelet count occurs at a mean of 29 hours after delivery.[26]

Extradural hematoma after LEA is rare. On the

TABLE 31-1

INVESTIGATIONS WHICH MAY BE REQUIRED TO INVESTIGATE THE PLATELET, TISSUE/VASCULAR, AND PROCOAGULANT PHASES OF BLEEDING DISORDERS

Vascular & Tissue Phase Investigations		
Bleeding time (BT):	Mielke template	2-10 min
	Duke	1-3 min
	Ivy	5-7 min
Capillary fragility tests:	Hess venoocclusion	
	Rumpel Leede	
Inspection of bleeding site & surgical field		
Platelet Phase Investigations		
Platelet count		140,000-440,000/mm^3
Bleeding time (BT)		Above
Platelet Antibody tests (e.g., anti-IgG consumption test)		
ADP/adrenalin/collagen platelet aggregation		
Clot retraction		
Megathrombocyte count		
Release tests (e.g., ^{51}Cr, serotonin)		
Rumpel Leede test		
Whole blood prothrombin activation rate		
Bone marrow: megakaryocyte count		
Procoagulant Phase Investigations		
Intrinsic pathway		
Partial thromboplastin time (PTT)	II V VIII IX X XI	24-36 sec
	Fletcher Fitzgerald	
PTT with kaolin (PTTK)		35-52 sec
Activated PTT (aPTT)	All except VII XIII	25-35 sec
Whole blood clotting time Heparin		4-8 min
Activated clotting time (ACT)	Heparin	2 min
Extrinsic Pathway		
Prothrombin time (PT)	V VII X when level <0.2 U/ml	11-12 sec
	II <0.1	
	I <100 mg/dl	
Prothrombin index	Oral anticoagulation	
Common Pathway		
Activated PTT (aPTT)	All except VII XIII	25-35 sec
Thrombin time (TT)	I & II split products	12-20 sec
	Heparin	
Fibrinogen	I	160-400 mg/100 ml
		400-600 (pregnancy)
Fibrinolysis		
Fibrin degradation products (FDPs) by Latex agglutination	Fibrin split products	<4 μg/ml
Euglobulin clot lysis		
Fibrinogen	I	Above

ADP, Adenosine diphosphate.

From Gatt S: Haematological disorders responsible for bleeding in late pregnancy, *Anaesth Intensive Care* 1990;18:337.

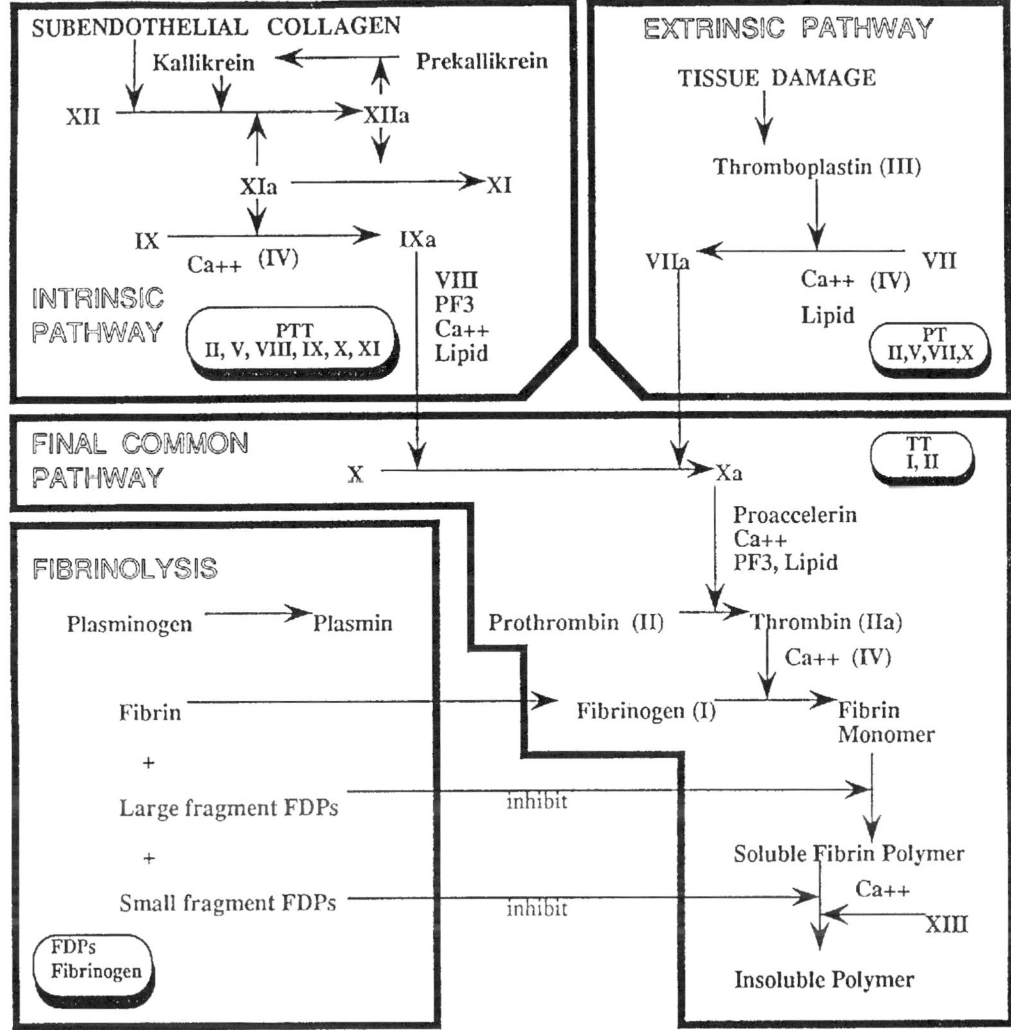

Fig. 31-2.

Coagulation and fibrinolytic cascades. The appropriate hematologic investigations for each segment of the cascade are shown in the inset box. (From Gatt S: Haematological disorders responsible for bleeding in late pregnancy, *Anaesth Intensive Care* 1990;18:338.)

other hand, a large hematoma can be responsible for serious neurologic aftermath. In parturients with severe PIH the threat is even more severe because of the cumulative effect of thrombocytopenia, aspirin intake, and platelet function defect. Those with a proven coagulopathy, prolonged bleeding time, or platelet count 50×10^9/L or higher should not receive an epidural block.[27] Aspirin should be discontinued 7 to 10 days before delivery. A platelet transfusion of 6 U should be given to those with platelet count less than 50×10^9/L presenting for CS and less than 20×10^9/L for vaginal delivery. Fresh whole blood transfusion may be necessary when hemoglobin concentration drops to less than 9 g/dl.

When GA poses considerable risk and epidural analgesia is relatively contraindicated, the technique of choice is the narrow-gauge needle, incremental LA narcotic spinal anesthesia or continuous microcatheter subarachnoid block (not currently available in the United States but available in many other countries).[28] Even these techniques, however, carry increased risk in those with a low platelet count or platelet functional defects. Conventional single-shot spinal anesthesia should be avoided in severe PIH because of the risk of profound, sudden hypotension.[29] Close postoperative follow-up of these patients is vital for early diagnosis of epidural hematoma.

In our current patient, the presence (or lack) of coagulopathy needs to be investigated. If the patient has been receiving low-dose aspirin or if the platelet count is 50×10^9/L or higher but 100×10^9/L or lower, a bleeding time (BT) is indicated. If no thrombocytopenia is present and BT is normal the anesthesiologist can proceed with LEA.[19]

Hemodynamic Changes in Severe Gestational Proteinuric Hypertension

Before delivery the untreated gravida with severe gestational proteinuric hypertension may have a classic hemodynamic picture consisting of the following:

- CO even higher than the 50% rise normally expected of a term pregnancy[30]
- Hyperdynamic ventricular function (higher left ventricular stroke work index per unit PCWP than in normal pregnant controls[31]
- High SVR and MAP[32]
- Low or normal CVP
- 10% to 40% reduction in plasma volume with low colloid osmotic pressure (COP) and blood viscosity increased by 30%[33,34]
- *No* pulmonary hypertension[35]
- Oliguria

Traditionally it has been assumed that PIH is a disease state in which the SVR is elevated. This SVR rise is responsible for the hypertension and the hypoperfusion state which ensues. PIH has classically been described as a condition in which increased systemic arterial vascular resistance is the *main* element responsible for hypertension. Recently this dogma has been brought into question.[36] A new hypothesis has emerged in which an elevated CO is presented as the central feature of PIH. This elevated CO occurs as early as the first trimester of pregnancy, precedes the development of hypertension, and persists into the postpartum period. These concepts could revolutionize the way clinicians think about the hemodynamic pathophysiology of PIH. It shifts the emphasis away from an elevated SVR and hypoperfusion as the cause of PIH. It postulates that the hemodynamic abnormalities may well antedate the pregnancy.[36]

In severe PIH and HELLP syndrome, Wasserstrum and Cotton, on the basis of pulmonary artery (PA) catheter studies, define six subsets (Table 31-2) of patients.[35] This work is particularly interesting because each subset requires radically different treatment, ranging from vasodilatation to β-blocker (in left ventricular failure), and from inotropic support to preload reduction. In Table 31-2 subset 1 is the commonest and subset 6, the least common.

Hypertensive crises in pregnancy (even in normokalemic patients) are associated with a very high incidence (62%) of ventricular tachycardia.[37] This may explain the reason for the sudden pulmonary edema and sudden and unexpected death of these

TABLE 31-2

Six Subsets of Parturients with Severe PIH with Swanz-Ganz PA Catheters In Situ

Subset	Profile	Treatment	Therapeutic Aim
1	Low PCWP Low CO High SVR	Volume expansion, then, Vasodilators	Raise PCWP Raise CO Lower SVR
2	Low PCWP High CO Low SVR	Cautious fluid therapy	Modest rise in PCWP
3	Normal PCWP Low CO Raised SVR	Vasodilatation (e.g., hydralazine), and if PCWP falls, administer Fluids	Lower SVR
4	Normal PCWP	? β-blockade	(Unknown)
5	High PCWP High SVR Low CO	Arterial vasodilator, and if CO drops & PCWP rises Inotrope (e.g., dopamine, dobutamine)	Drop SVR Lower MAP Raise CO Lower PCWP
6	High PCWP High CO Low SVR	Preload reduction (e.g., frusemide, TNG, SNP)	Reduce PCWP

PCWP, Pulmonary capillary wedge pressure; CO, cardiac output; SVR, systemic vascular resistance; MAP, mean arterial systemic pressure; TNG, glyceryl trinitrate; SNP, sodium nitroprusside.
From Wasserstrum N, Cotton DB: Hemodynamic monitoring in severe pregnancy-induced hypertension, *Clin Perinatol* 1986;13(4):781.

patients. These serious ventricular dysrhythmias subside when the BP is controlled.[37]

In our primigravida with PIH, the hypertension (170/115 mm Hg) needs to be controlled immediately. There is general agreement that the BP must be lowered (to prevent intracerebral hemorrhage) once the BP rises above 170 mm Hg systolic and/or 110 mm Hg diastolic pressure.[2] Parenteral hydralazine, minibolus diazoxide, and labetalol and sublingual or oral nifedipine generally are safe, provided care is taken not to reduce the BP precipitiously.[2]

Management of Hypertensive Crises

The agents most commonly used to control hypertension in pregnancy are seldom appropriate to control rapidly a hypertensive crisis. Table 31-3 shows the common antihypertensives and gives some indication of their relative usage in institutions in Australia. Agents such as captopril, prazosin, and methyldopa, which are the main agents employed in most centers for outpatient hypertension control, are hardly ever used in severe hypertensive crises (see Table 31-3).

The antihypertensive agents usually employed in the Obstetric Intensive Care Unit (Royal Hospital for Women, Paddington) to control severe hypertension caused by hypertensive disorders of pregnancy are labetalol, nitroprusside, bolus hydralazine, nifedipine, minibolus diazoxide, and trimetaphan as well as intravenous β- or α-adrenoreceptor blockers (e.g., labetalol) or β-blocker (e.g., esmolol, metoprolol).[3]

Since SAP, MAP, and DAP are maximal immedi-

TABLE 31-3
COMMON ANTIHYPERTENSIVE AGENTS

Antihypertensive Agent		Management of Hypertension in Pregnancy	Management of Acute Hypertensive Emergency
Diuretic	Thiazide	0	0
	Frusemide	0	+++
β-blocker	Atenolol, metoprolol	++	++
	Esmolol	0	+++
β/α-blocker	Labetalol	+++	++
Adrenergic blocker	Methyldopa	++++	++
	Clonidine	+/0	0
α-blocker	Phenoxybenzamine	0	0
Postsynaptic α-blocker	Prazosin	++	0
Sympathetic postganglionic transmission blocker	Reserpine	+	0
Ganglion blocker	Trimetaphan	0	++
Vasodilator	Hydalazine	+	++++
	Diazoxide	+/0	+++
	Nitroprusside	0	++++
	Minoxidil	0	0
	Magnesium	0/+	0/+
	Nitroglycerin	0	+++
Serotonin II antagonist	Ketanserin	+/0	0
Sedative	Barbiturate	+	0
Calcium channel blocker	Nifedipine	++	++
Angiotensin converting enzyme inhibitor	Captopril	+/0	0

ately before and during delivery, antihypertensive agents are commonly required either in the labor and delivery suite or in the operating rooms before and during lower segmental cesarean section[20] (Fig. 31-3).

Sodium nitroprusside (SNP) by infusion is used to produce controlled BP reduction. Remember that SNP is a cerebral arterial vasodilator so that it can increase cerebral blood flow. It should be used in conjunction with appropriate ICP reduction measures (e.g., posture, hypocarbia, mannitol) in patients with severe cerebral edema. It can also cause fetal cyanide and thiocyanate toxicity and, since fetal blood levels may be higher than those in the mother, if SNP is to be used for a prolonged period, it should be monitored carefully.[38] Regular checking of maternal serum pH, plasma and erythrocyte cyanide and methemoglobin should alert clinicians to the possibility of fetal toxicity. SNP also can cause transient fetal bradycardia.

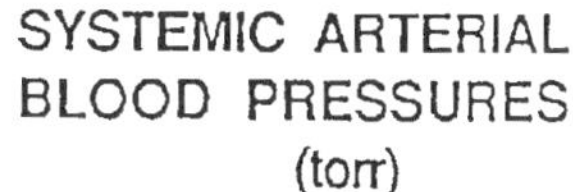

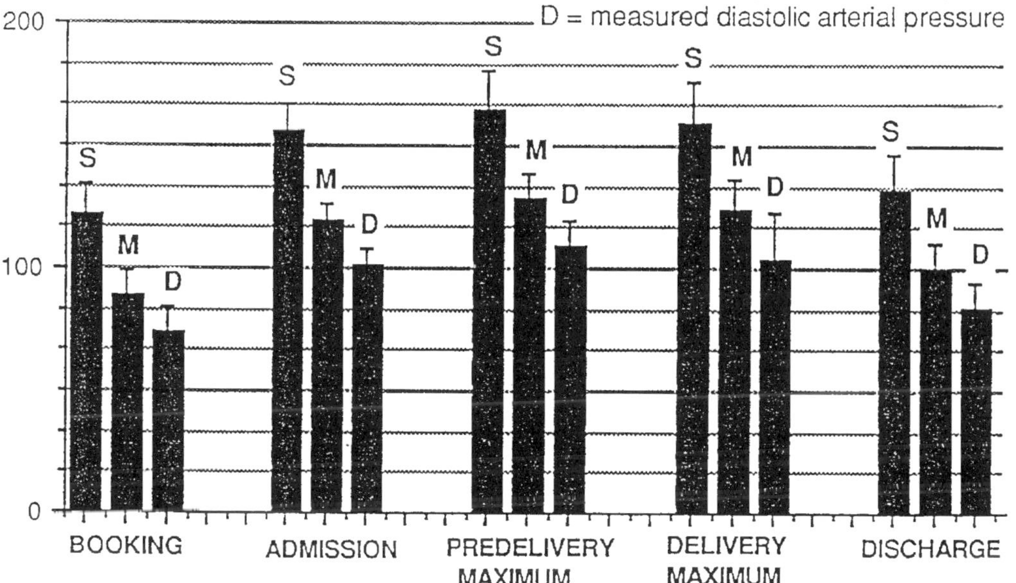

Fig. 31-3.
Systolic, mean, and diastolic systemic arterial pressure in a group of parturients with severe gestational proteinuric hypertension at Royal Hospital for Women, Sydney, Australia, showing the blood pressure at booking, admission into hospital, maximum before delivery and at delivery, and on discharge. (From Schindler M, Gatt S, et al: Thrombocytopenia and platelet functional defects in pre-eclampsia: implications for regional anaesthiesa, *Anaesth Intensive Care* 1990;18:169.)

Trimetaphan (Arfonad) is one of the best agents to use in pregnancy because it has limited placental transfer and some added margin to safety conferred by its ability to be hydrolyzed by fetal pseudocholinesterase. Unfortunately its sympathetic ganglionic blockade is unreliable in pregnancy so that it is not always effective in hypertensive control in PIH. It can also cause papillary dilation.

Glyceryl trinitrate, or nitroglycerine (Nipride), acts by reduction of preload so that it can be unreliable in a gravida. It crosses the placenta and can cause fetal hypotension.

In the current case, the BP initially would b\e controlled with an α- or β-blocker (labetalol) and an antihypertensive (hydralazine, nifedipine, or methyldopa) if necessary, and the patient would be admitted to hospital for observation, monitoring of the fetus, and full clinical and laboratory assessment.[2] If the disease process were found to be easy to control, the pregnancy would be allowed to proceed.

Invasive Monitoring

Whereas many patients with severe PIH (DAP more than 100 mm Hg and proteinuria 2 + or neurologic or abdominal signs) require monitoring of volume status with a CVP line, only a very small proportion of PIH patients require PA catheterization.

Even when considerable disease is present, a considerable degree of misadventure will be tolerated, even if management is conducted in an empirical *trial and error* method. Whatever the mode of delivery, the peripartum period always is associated with considerable hemodynamic fluctuations. This is especially so in the postpartum period when autotransfusion of 65% of CO compounds the difficulties of assessing vascular dynamics.

The wisdom of reserving invasive monitoring for a few selected cases is based on the overall experience that

1. Management of severe PIH using noninvasive protocols has, in general, been very satisfactory[39]
2. Left ventricular failure is an uncommon feature of PIH
3. Insertion and subsequent management of the PA catheter is associated with hazards to the patient[40,41]
4. Acute volume expansion in severe PIH does not raise MAP;[42] somewhat counter-intuitively, it usually produces a *fall* in MAP and SVR and a rise in CO[35,43]

Such rationale recently has been questioned. Although the CVP alone is sometimes inadequate in dealing with the rapidly evolving pathologic process, several studies of severe PIH parturients show

1. There is poor correlation between CVP and PCWP[44]
2. It is often impossible to estimate whether CVP will underestimate or overestimate PCWP
3. The PA catheter often gives new insights and additional (sometimes unexpected) information[32,45,46]
4. With the exception of ventricular ectopy, the incidence of complications from initial insertion of a PA (Swan Ganz) catheter is no different from the problems associated with placement of the CVP line[40,41]

The main indications for insertion of a PA catheter are as follows:

1. Hypertensives who remain *oliguric in spite of volume expansion* (an initial fluid challenge of 500 ml 5% Hartmann's lactated Ringer's bolus would be reasonable) and diuretics as dictated by volume status measurements *especially if oliguria occurs postpartum.* In PIH, oliguria can occur secondary to elevated SVR, selective renal arteriospasm, or inadequate CO.[45] On the basis of PA catheter measurements Clark et al.[45] divided oliguric hypertensives who fail to respond to volume expansion with a diuresis into three subsets (Table 31-4). Each group required a different form of treatment depending on the PCWP, SVR, and CI value.
2. Development of *pulmonary edema resistant to fluid restriction and standard diuretic therapy.* In PIH, pulmonary edema usually is secondary to iatrogenic fluid overload, but it also can be caused by disrupted pulmonary capillary architecture, decreased COP or left ventricular dysfunction secondary to grossly increased afterload.[35]
3. *Hypertension that fails to respond* to aggressive management with conventional doses of standard antihypertensives (e.g., labetalol plus nifedipine or hydralazine) *in a patient with demonstrated hypovolemia.* Although hypertension usually is due to elevated SVR, it also may be due to elevated CO.[39,46] If hypovolemia is suspected, rapid diagnosis and treatment of unresponsive hypertension becomes especially important.

TABLE 31-4

THREE SUBSETS OF OLIGURIC HYPERTENSIVE PARTURIENTS WHO FAILED TO RESPOND TO A FLUID CHALLENGE

Group	Hemodynamic Profile	Typical Values	Management
1	Low LVEDP Hyperdynamic LV Moderate SVR elevation	PCWP 4 mm Hg SVR 1330 $dyne \cdot sec \cdot cm^{-5}$	Volume replacement
2	Normal/elevated PCWP Normal/elevated CI Normal SVR	PCWP 12 mm Hg CI 5.4 $L/min/m^2$ SVR 1019 $dyne \cdot sec \cdot cm^{-5}$	Vasodilator therapy
3	Markedly elevated PCWP Markedly elevated SVR Decreased CI	PCWP 18 mm Hg SVR 2790 $dyne \cdot sec \cdot cm^{-5}$ CI 2.61 $L/min/m^2$	Volume restriction + Afterload reduction

LVEDP, Left ventricular end-diastolic pressure; LV, left ventricle; SVR, systemic vascular resistance; PCWP, pulmonary capillary wedge pressure; CI, cardiac index.

From Clark SL, Greenspoon JS, Aldahl D, et al: Severe preeclampsia with persistent oliguria: management of hemodynamic subsets. *Am J Obstet Gynecol* 1986;154(3):490.

Summary

In conclusion, the PA catheter allows the clinician to

1. Define the etiology and monitor the treatment of pulmonary edema
2. Measure the left ventricular filling pressure
3. Draw modified Frank-Starling curves to define contractile status
4. Monitor the progress of hydrostatic pulmonary edema
5. Calculate SVR to quantitate the degree of vasospasm[35,46]

In the current case (severe, untreated PIH at 28 weeks' gestation) invasive monitoring would not be necessary unless complications supervened after the institution of appropriate therapy.

References

1. Mallampati RS, Gatt SP, Gugino LD, et al: Clinical sign to predict difficult tracheal intubation: a prospective study, *Can Anaesth Soc J* 1985;32:429.
2. Brown MA, Gallery EDM, Gatt SP, et al: *Management of hypertension in pregnancy: consensus statement of the Australasian Society for the Study of Hypertension in Pregnancy,* Sydney, Australia, 1993, New Era Printing Pty Ltd.
3. Barton JR, Sibai BM: Acute life-threatening emergencies in preeclampsia-eclampsia, *Clin Obstet Gynecol* 1992; 35:402.
4. Liu P, Gatt S, Gugino LD, et al: Esmolol for control of increases in heart rate and blood pressure during tracheal intubation after thiopental and succinylcholine, *Can Anaesth Soc J* 1986; 33:556.
5. Gatt SP: Gestational proteinuria hypertension, *Curr Opinion Anesthesiol* 1992; 5:354.
6. Allen RW, James MF, et al: Attenuation of the pressor response to tracheal intubation in hypertensive proteinuric pregnant patients by lignocaine, alfentanil and magnesium sulphate, *Br J Anaesth* 1991; 66:216.
7. Goodlin RC: Preeclampsia as the great impostor, *Am J Obstet Gynecol* 1991; 6(1):1577.
8. Patterson KW, O'Toole: HELLP syndrome: a case report with guidelines for diagnosis and management, *Br J Anaesth* 1991; 66:513.
9. Crosby ET: Obstetrical anesthesia for patients with the syndrome of haemolysis, elevated liver enzymes and low platelets, *Can J Anaesth* 1991; 38(2):227.

10. Newsome LR, Bramwell RS, Cunling PC: Severe preeclampsia: hemodynamic effects of lumber epidural anesthesia, *Anesth Analg* 1976; 65:31.
11. Brown MA: Pregnancy-induced hypertension: pathogenesis and management, *Aust NZ J Med* 1991; 21:257.
12. Albright GA, Cohen H, Forster RM, et al: Anesthesia for patients with preeclampsia, *JAMA* 1991; 265(12):1587 (letter).
13. Patton DE, Lee W, Miller J, et al: Maternal, uteroplacental, and fetoplacental hemodynamic and doppler velocimetric changes during epidural anesthesia in normal labor, *Obstet Gynecol* 1991; 77(1):17.
14. Alahuhta S, Räsänen J, Joupilla R, et al: Uteroplacental and fetal haemodynamics during extradural anaesthesia for caesarean section, *Br J Anaesth* 1991; 66:319.
15. Ramos-Santos E, Devoe LD, Wakefield ML, et al: The effects of epidural anesthesia on the Doppler velocimetry of umbilical and uterine arteries in normal and hypertensive patients during active term labor, *Obstet Gynecol* 1991; 77(1):20.
16. Pearson JF: Fluid balance in severe preeclampsia, *Br J Hosp Med* 1992; 48:47.
17. Chesley LC: Diagnosis of preeclampsia, *Obstet Gynecol* 1985; 65:423.
18. Gabert HA, Miller JM: Renal disease in pregnancy, *Obstet Gynecol Surv* 1985; 40:449.
19. Schindler M, Gatt S, Isert P, et al: Thrombocytopenia and platelet functional defects in pre-eclampsia: implications for regional anaesthesia, *Anaesth Intensive Care* 1990; 18:169.
20. Redman CW, Bonnar J, Beilin L: Early platelet consumption in preeclampsia, *Br Med J* 1978; 1:467.
21. Siddiqi T, Rosenn B, Mimounl F: Hypertension during pregnancy in insulin-dependent diabetic women, *Obstet Gynecol* 1991; 77(4):514.
22. de Boer K, Büller HR, Tencate JW, et al: Coagulation studies in the syndrome of hemolysis, elevated liver enzymes and low platelets, *Br J Obstet Gynaecol* 1991; 98:42.
23. Barker P, Callander CC: Coagulation screening before epidural analgesia in pre-eclampsia, *Anaesthesia* 1991; 46:67.
24. Janes SL: Thrombocytopenia in pregnancy, *Postgrad Med J* 1992; 68:321.
25. Macdonald R: Aspirin and extradural blocks, *Br J Anaesth* 1991; 66:1.
26. Neiger R, Contag SA, Coustan DR, et al: The resolution of preeclampsia-related thrombocytopenia, *Obstet Gynecol* 1991; 77(5):692.
27. Gatt SP: Gestational proteinuric hypertension, *Curr Opin Anaesthesiol* 1991; 5:354.
28. Perry KG, Martin JN: Abnormal hemostasis and coagulopathy in preeclampsia and eclampsia, *Clin Obstet Gynecol* 1992; 35:338.
29. Chadwick HS, Easterling T: Anesthetic concerns in the patient with preeclampsia, *Semin Perinatol* 1991; 15:397.
30. Gallery ED, Huynor SN, Gyory AZ: Plasma volume contraction: a significant factor in both pregnant associated hypertension (pre-eclampsia) and chronic hypertension in pregnancy, *Q J Med* 1979; 48:593.
31. Buchan PC: Pre-eclampsia: a hyperviscosity syndrome, *Am J Obstet Gynecol* 1982; 142:111.
32. Hankins GD, Wendel GD, Cunningham FG, et al: Longitudinal evaluation of hemodynamic changes in eclampsia, *Am J Obstet Gynecol* 1984; 150:506.
33. Clark SL, Horenstein JM, Phelan JP, et al: Experience with the pulmonary artery catheter in obstetrics and gynecology, *Am J Obstet Gynecol* 1985; 152:374.
34. Writer WDR: Anaesthetic considerations in high-risk pregnancy, *Can Anaesth Soc J* 1986; 33:S16.
35. Wasserstrum N, Cotton DB: Hemodynamic monitoring in severe pregnancy-induced hypertension, *Clin Perinatol* 1986; 13:781.
36. Easterling TR, Benedetti TJ, Shumucker BC, et al: Maternal hemodynamics in normal and preeclamptic pregnancies: a longitudinal study, *Obstet Gynecol* 1990; 76(6):1061.
37. Naidoo DP, Bhorat I, Moodley J, et al: Continuous electrocardiographic monitoring in hypertensive crises in pregnancy, *Am J Obstet Gynecol* 1991; 164(2):530.
38. Naulty S, Cefalo RC, Lewis PE: Fetal toxicity of nitroprusside in the pregnant ewe, *Am J Obstet Gynecol* 1981; 139:708.
39. Pritchard JA, Cunningham FG, Pritchard SE: The Parkland Memorial Hospital protocol for the treatment of eclampsia: evaluation of 245 cases, *Am J Obstet Gynecol* 1984; 148:951.
40. Sise MJ, Hollingworth P, Brimm JE, et al: Complications of the flow-directed pulmonary artery catheter, *Crit Care Med* 1981; 9:315.
41. Elliott CG, Zimmerman GA, Clemmer TP: Complications of pulmonary artery catheterisation in the care of critically ill patients, *Chest* 1979; 76:647.
42. Groenendijk R, Trembos MJ, Wallenburg HC: Hemodynamic measurements in pre-eclampsia: preliminary observations, *Am J Obstet Gynecol* 1984; 150:232.

43. Gallery ED, Delprado W, Gyory AZ: Antihypertensive effect of plasma volume expansion in pregnancy-associated hypertension, *Aust NZ Med J* 1981; 11:20.
44. Cotton DB, Gonik B, Dorman K, et al: Cardiovascular alterations in severe pregnancy induced hypertension: relationship of central venous pressure to pulmonary capillary wedge pressure, *Am J Obstet Gynecol* 1985; 151:762.
45. Clark SL, Greenspoon JS, Alctahl D, et al: Severe pre-eclampsia with persistent oliguria: management of hemodynamic subsets, *Am J Obstet Gynecol* 1986; 154:490.
46. Clark SL, Cotton DB: Clinical indications for pulmonary artery catheterization in the patient with severe pre-eclampsia, *Am J Obstet Gynecol* 1988; 158:453.

32

Disseminated Intravascular Coagulation

A 32-year-old woman, gravida 3 para 1, with a 35 weeks' gestation is admitted to the obstetric unit with a blood pressure of 240/140 mm Hg. Initial laboratory values include the following: hematocrit 37%; fibrinogen 120 mg/dl; fibrin split products, more than 40 mg/dl; platelets 75,000/mm^3; and partial thromboplastin time 52.7 seconds. A diagnosis of disseminated intravascular coagulation is made. The obstetrician decides to perform a cesarean section. Discuss the anesthetic management.

Recommendations by Lisa Wollman, M.D.

Disseminated intravascular coagulation (DIC) represents a common pathologic pathway, which can result from a variety of clinical conditions and can range from mild to life threatening in its presentation. A number of obstetrical complications are associated with such a coagulopathy. Therefore, a high index of suspicion and an understanding of the mechanism of this disorder and its treatment are crucial in the care of these patients. The obstetric anesthesiologist must be ready to provide rational anesthetic management of these parturients as well as urgent, aggressive resuscitation when it is necessary.

Definition

Disseminated intravascular coagulation is a state where consumption of procoagulant proteins and platelets occurs diffusely throughout the vascular system, incited by a triggering event. The clotting in turn activates the fibrinolytic proteins, which is the body's normal physiologic response. In this diseased state these processes lose both their localization of activity and normal balance, which provides homeostasis in the circulation. As a result, either bleeding or thrombosis can predominate. Simultaneously, the kinin and complement cascades are initiated, leading to extreme vascular permeability and vasodilation. The development and progression of these events can be acute or chronic, mild, or severe. Extensive deposition of fibrin within the microvasculature, known as the generalized Schwartzman reaction, is the likely cause of end-organ damage and necrosis seen in the most severe clinical picture.

Pathophysiology

The abnormal coagulation can be triggered by endothelial cell disruption, endotoxin released by bacteria, or by fetal-placental thromboplastic material that has entered into the maternal circulation. Either via the extrinsic or intrinsic clotting pathways, factor X activates factor V, which initiates the conversion of prothrombin to thrombin. Thrombin then enzymatically cleaves fibrinogen to create fibrin or stable clot. Thrombin at the same time induces the cleavage of plasminogen to form plasmin, which serves as the checks and balances in the system since plasmin results in the degradation of the clot and prevents its further propagation (Fig. 32-1). In addition, the fibrin degradation products (FDPs) created from fibrinolysis directly inhibit the conversion of fibrinogen to fibrin by thrombin, as well as platelet-mediated coagulation.[1] Antithrombin III is a glycoprotein that binds irreversibly to several clotting factors, most importantly, factor X, the crucial factor for both the extrinsic and intrinsic pathways. It also slowly inactivates thrombin. Via these two mechanisms, antithrombin III is the principal physiologic inhibitor of coagulation in the nondiseased state. These cascades, or substrate-enzyme reactions, normally occur at the site of damaged tissue. However, DIC represents the generalized activation and amplification of such pathways with loss of regulation and feedback inhibition. Excess free plasmin degrades fibrinogen as well as factors V, VIII, IX, and XI; corticotropin; growth hormone; insulin; complement; and other plasma proteins.[1] Fibrin is deposited in the microvasculature and coats circulating platelets. Thrombocytopenia results from both the irreversible entrapment of platelets by the fibrin deposits and the increased clearance of fibrin-coated platelets by the reticuloendothelial system.

Pregnancy-Associated Trigger Mechanisms

Pregnancy is characterized by coagulation activation, as evidenced by the increased levels of all factors of the clotting cascade (except factor XIII) and increased levels of fibrinogen and FDPs. Also, the circulating levels of antithrombin III are reduced. In fact, some authors argue that normal pregnancy is a state of low-grade self-limited DIC, or at least that parturients have an increased susceptibility to its development (Fig. 32-2).

Several triggers, indeed, are unique to pregnancy.

1. The preeclampsia-eclampsia syndrome is the most common cause of DIC in parturients. Many of these women have been found to have a chronic, subclinical coagulopathy, although it is exceedingly rare for these patients to have symptomatic bleeding problems. Parturients with preeclampsia have been shown to have increased fibrin deposits in glomerular, hepatic, and placental microvasculature.[1] This finding is consistent with increased levels of FDPs and decreased activity of antithrombin III seen in the same patients.[2] Women at risk for preeclampsia currently are being placed on low-dose aspirin with increased frequency since it has been shown that such therapy can prevent both the development of symptoms of pre-

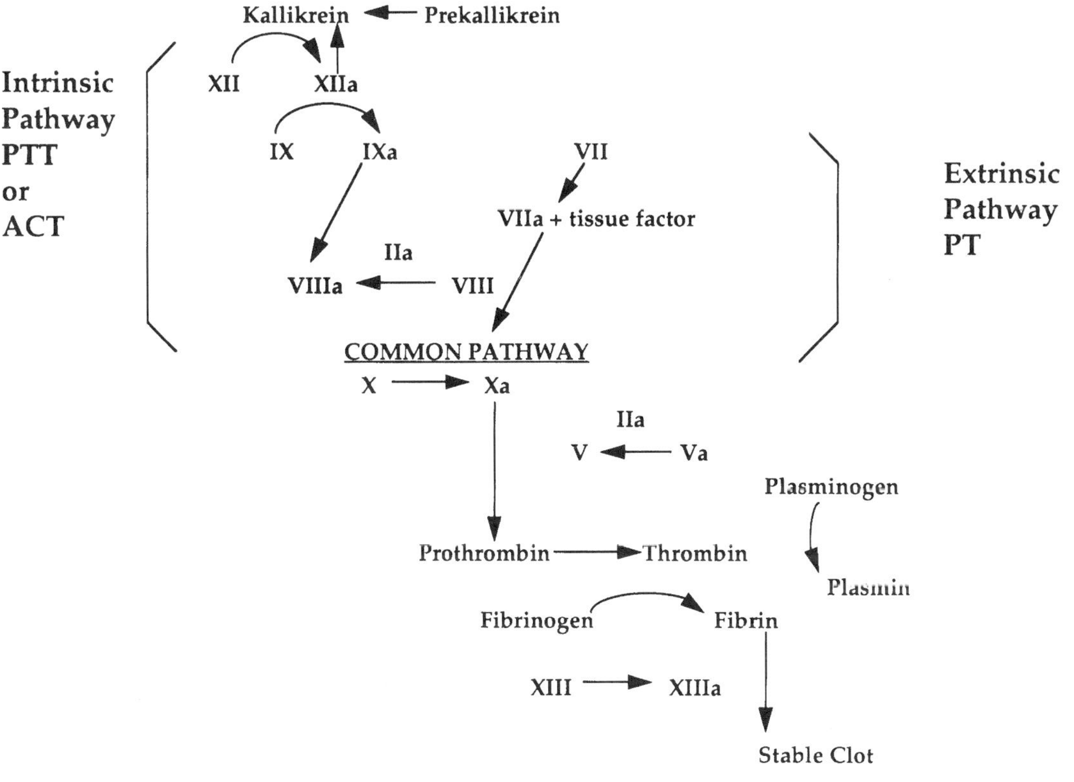

Fig. 32-1.
Blood coagulation cascade.

COAGULATION FACTOR	LATE PREGNANCY	DIC
I-Fibrinogen	150-200%	↓
V	100-150%	↓
VII	200-500%	↓
XIII	35-75%	↓
Antithrombin III	75-100%	↓

Fig. 32-2.
Coagulation factor levels with respect to normal, nonpregnant controls.

eclampsia and the coagulation complications. It is not known what triggers DIC in this syndrome or why the coagulopathy rarely is clinically apparent. Thrombocytopenia may be the only detected hematologic abnormality in the otherwise asymptomatic patient.

2. Placental abruption is probably the most common cause of acute DIC in obstetric patients. The coagulopathy results not only from the local, extravascular consumption of clotting proteins, but also from the systemic activation of fibrin synthesis and degradation by the release of thromboplastin into the maternal circulation. The clinical severity of hemostatic abnormalities usually correlates well with the degree of placental separation. Common findings in these patients include increased FDPs, thrombocytopenia, and hypofibrinogenemia. This DIC state usually is self-limited in that these parameters tend to normalize as the release of thromboplastin ceases with delivery. These patients are, however, at increased risk of postpartum hemorrhage.
3. Intrauterine fetal death can be associated with a consumptive coagulopathy, presumably secondary to release of fetal thromboplastin, which gains access to the maternal circulation. The onset of DIC is gradual and rarely begins unless the dead fetus has been retained for days to weeks.[1] Rapid delivery is the usual management, which eliminates much of the concern of the development of this syndrome. In the rare scenario of an intrauterine fetal death in a multiple gestation, there is a significant morbidity and mortality risk for the surviving fetus, presumably from the ensuing coagulopathy.
4. Amniotic fluid embolism is a fulminant life-threatening crisis that is likely to result in hemodynamic collapse. Maternal mortality is extremely high, usually within hours of the event. Patients who survive the initial cardiopulmonary insult have been frequently noted to go on to develop DIC. Amniotic fluid has a procoagulant effect: it stimulates the conversion of fibrinogen to fibrin and activates platelets.
5. Another cause of DIC is gram-negative sepsis; the syndrome is triggered by the presence of endotoxin in the circulation. Some authors believe that pregnancy actually enhances the sensitivity to endotoxin and its effects.[1] The ensuing coagulopathy complicates and worsens the shock state by causing the release of kinins, histamine, serotonin, and prostaglandins. Fibrinogen production increases initially because it is an acute-phase reactant, but with the development of uncontrolled consumption, hypofibrinogenemia results. Thrombocytopenia also can be marked.

Diagnosis

Acute fulminant DIC rarely requires any laboratory studies to diagnose. Bleeding usually occurs from venipuncture sites, surgical incisions, and mucous membranes. Patients often have hypotension that is out of proportion to the amount of blood loss as a result of the release of vasoactive substances. Aggressive resuscitation is necessary to prevent end-organ damage. Renal failure is the most frequently observed sequela; however, adrenal, cerebral, and pulmonary hemorrhage and/or microthrombi are common.

Chronic low-grade DIC is the more likely clinical scenario in obstetric patients. These parturients may report bruising easily, gingival bleeding, or epistaxis, but often there is no pertinent history. Laboratory studies are necessary to confirm the diagnosis. The initial screening test should be a platelet count, since 90% of patients with some degree of consumptive coagulopathy will have thrombocytopenia.[2] In severe preeclamptic patients, platelet counts have been shown to be strongly correlated with the severity of disease and risk of bleeding. In fact, it is exceedingly rare for abnormalities in prothrombin time (PT), partial thromboplastin time (PTT), or fibrinogen levels to occur in the setting of a normal, stable platelet count.[3] For this reason many clinicians now support using the platelet count as a sole screening test of coagulation status in parturients, except those with severe preeclampsia or evidence of bleeding. Serial platelet counts are indicated, however, to reveal a possible downward trend. The PT and PTT results, which are slightly shorter than controls in normal pregnancy, are prolonged in the acute DIC picture and variable in the chronic, compensated syndrome. In the early stages of the coagulopathy the PT is prolonged and the PTT often is normal. Fibrinogen levels, which are increased in the pregnant state, are depressed in proportion to the severity of the consumptive process. The hallmark laboratory finding in DIC is the elevated plasma levels of FDPs (or D dimer); this abnormality is present in 95% to 100% of cases of DIC.[2] Fibrin degradation products have half lives of 5 to 72 hours, and therefore help to detect recent fibrinolytic processes, but may not accurately reflect current coagulation status.

There are many other known laboratory aberrations that occur in DIC that are reliable, sensitive determinants of its severity, such as decreased antithrombin III levels or increased concentrations of fibrinopeptide A. Although these two tests are referred to throughout the literature as *the gold standards* in the diagnosis, it is clear that they are not mandatory. Because of the short half lives of both antithrombin III and FPA (seconds to minutes), the complex assays required for the studies, and the prohibitive expense, these tests are not practical. Bleeding times are no longer indicated in the workup of a patient with a suspected coagulopathy, since studies have repeatedly illustrated a lack of standardization and reliability in the test.[4] Also, no current evidence exists that bleeding from a cut in the skin reflects the risk of bleeding elsewhere in the body.[5] Bleeding times, presumed to assess platelet function, do not correlate well with platelet aggregation in vitro and become extremely difficult to interpret in patients on aspirin therapy.[6] A possible alternative method to estimate the patient's ability to produce clot is thromboelastography. The test measures changes in elasticity sensed by a pin bathed in blood in an oscillating tube. As fibrin is deposited on the pin and clot is created, the movement of the pin is altered and a pattern is recorded. Whether this device will aid in the diagnosis of DIC remains to be seen.[13]

Of course, routine laboratory studies such as hemoglobin levels, hematocrit, creatinine, serum glutamic oxaloacetic transaminase, serum glutamic pyruvic transaminase, alkaline phosphatase, and arterial blood gas values, as well as urine output, are indicated to follow and manage the possible complications of this disorder once the diagnosis has been made.

Treatment

In low-grade DIC the primary management is to remove the underlying triggering mechanism, which is most often accomplished by prompt delivery of the fetus and placenta. Patients require close monitoring of their clinical status and serial coagulation studies, but rarely need any therapy beyond adequate fluid replacement and/or antibiotics. In the cases of parturients with acute, fulminant DIC, it is crucial that resuscitation of the mother by the priority for both maternal survival and fetal salvageability. The initial management of the gravida is the same as that of any patient presenting with hemorrhage. Multiple large-bore intravenous (IV) access is necessary and fluid resuscitation should begin immediately, either with blood if it is available, or crystalloid and colloid solutions until blood can be obtained. Large quantities of dextran-containing colloids should not be infused since they can worsen bleeding by lowering fibrinogen levels. Crossmatched packed red blood cells or fresh whole blood is of course preferred, but in the case of life-threatening hemorrhage, O-negative blood should be transfused.

The parturient must be positioned with left uterine displacement to avoid limiting venous return, which would further contribute to hypotension. Vasopressors or inotropes often are necessary, despite adequate volume infusion, secondary to the circulating vasoactive substances, which include prostaglandins, serotonin, kinins, and histamine. High-flow oxygen by face mask is sufficient until a surgical plan has been established, unless the patient's blood pressure is not sufficient to maintain consciousness. If the patient's level of consciousness is altered or if there is any question as to whether she can protect her airway, intubation and mechanical ventilation with 100% oxygen are indicated.

Transfusion of blood components is warranted in the case of DIC that is severe enough to produce hemorrhage; the goal of this therapy is to correct each of the coagulation defects. Fresh frozen plasma (FFP) is a source of fibrinogen, each unit containing roughly 200 to 400 mg. Plasma fibrinogen levels should rise 10 to 20 mg/dl for each unit of FFP administered; a level of greater than a 100 mg/dl is an appropriate target. If the patient's volume status needs to be tightly managed due to oliguria or prior sufficient volume replacement with respect to blood loss, cryoprecipitate can be substituted since it is a concentrated source of fibrinogen. Each unit of cryoprecipitate also contains 200 to 400 mg of fibrinogen in a 20- to 30-ml volume, and it is therefore rapidly infused without difficulty. Platelet transfusion is indicated as well to provide a count greater than 50,000/mm^3; each unit is expected to raise the number of circulating platelets by 5000/mm^3 to 10,000/mm^3. Red blood cells can be given, either as packed cells or as whole blood, to maintain a hematocrit of roughly 30%. Every 3 to 4 U of packed blood cells should be accompanied by a unit of FFP, if it has not already been given for the fibrinogen defect. This will correct various factor deficiencies, namely, deficiencies of factors V, VIII, and XIII. Progress of resuscitation and blood component therapy must be monitored by serial examinations of hemoglobin levels, hematocrit, platelet count, PT, PTT, and fibrinogen levels. The FDPs will remain positive for 1 to 2 days but general trends can be followed.

Many treatment alternatives other than the previously mentioned supportive measures have been used in DIC but remain controversial. In patients having hemorrhage from this coagulopathy, the use of epsilon-amino caproic acid (EACA) or aprotinin (Trasylol) may theoretically be beneficial. The former is a synthetic plasmin inhibitor that prevents fibrinolysis and can be thought of as a clot stabilizer. There is a risk of uncontrollable thrombosis throughout the body, so its use has been avoided. Aprotinin is a naturally occurring serine protease inhibitor that is thought to inactivate plasmin. Its actual mechanism of action remains unclear, so although it is effective at bringing bleeding to a halt, the same fear of thrombosis exists. Although thrombosis has not been seen, further studies are needed to elucidate the exact means by which aprotinin provides hemostasis.

Heparin therapy for DIC is still controversial; however, in patients with widespread thrombosis, heparin is clearly indicated. It serves to block the formation of thrombin by stimulating the formation of and accelerating the activity of antithrombin III. Antithrombin III forms a complex with activated thrombin, which prevents the conversion of fibrinogen to fibrin; it also prevents factor X from inducing the conversion of prothrombin to thrombin.[8] As previously mentioned, the quantity and activity of this protein are greatly reduced in DIC. Despite this, heparin therapy can easily cause severe hemorrhage by removing any ability the patient has to form a clot, thereby increasing the risk of exsanguination. As a result, its use currently is limited to patients with low-grade DIC where delivery is not imminently planned or has already occurred, and patients with evidence of thrombosis either peripherally or involving vital organs. It remains to be seen whether there is a role for combination therapy of heparin and a plasmin inhibitor such as EACA or aprotinin in cases of DIC presenting with hemorrhage.

Anesthetic Implications

The parturient with DIC can pose a significant management challenge to even the most prepared anesthesiologist. In the case scenario described at the beginning of this chapter the woman presents with a documented coagulopathy secondary to severe preeclampsia, and therefore the only acceptable anesthesia for this patient is general anesthesia. No mention of bleeding or fetal distress was made, so the cesarean section may be necessary but is not yet an emergency; controlling maternal blood pressure is the most crucial issue. Pharmacologic intervention should begin as soon as IV access is obtained and hydration has begun. (The hematocrit of 37% reflects a volume-contracted state.) The coagulation profile is consistent with DIC, so a cesarean section should be done only if otherwise indicated and only once blood products are in the room. In the case of a gravida presenting with hemorrhage, rapid interventions are needed to prevent or treat severe fetal distress and maternal exsanguination. General anesthesia is the only appropriate means of providing prompt and safe analgesia and anesthesia for delivery. Any available personnel should be immediately delegated the responsibility of notifying the blood bank of the need for several units of blood products to be in the operating room, initiating fluid resuscitation after adequate IV access is obtained, and assisting with the induction of anesthesia. A separate team skilled in neonatal resuscitation should be on hand to evaluate the baby while the anesthesiologist addresses the needs of the mother. A rapid-sequence induction is indicated for the parturient; in light of the hypovolemic status, either a reduced dose of barbiturate or ketamine are the drugs of choice. Both agents, however, are myocardial depressants in an already maximally stressed patient. The dose of succinylcholine should remain unchanged at 1.5 mg/kg. In a parturient with a significant coagulopathy, intubation of the trachea must be rapid yet careful to prevent trauma which may result in hemorrhage or subsequent hematoma of the airway. Maintenance of anesthesia should include a minimal amount of volatile agent because of both the risk of hemodynamic instability of the mother as well as that of increased bleeding from vascular and muscular relaxation of the uterus. Once the baby has been delivered, narcotics and/or benzodiazepines can be administered as desired. None of the anesthetic agents currently available have been shown to have any effect on coagulation or pose any increased risks to the patient with DIC. In cases of impaired hepatic or renal function, from either thrombosis or hemorrhage, doses of anesthetic agents and muscle relaxants need to be adjusted accordingly.

The coagulopathy and fluid administration should be treated as outlined previously. A strong attempt must be made to keep the patient's temperature up by delivering warmed fluids; this will avoid any further coagulopathy from platelet dysfunction, which is thought to occur below 34° C.[9] Continuous clinical assessments and serial laboratory studies are necessary throughout the perioperative period to evaluate the adequacy of therapy. Therefore if an arterial catheter has not been placed to help guide the care of this predictably labile patient, one is frequently placed for the ease of drawing serial blood samples. In addition to the standard routine monitoring, a

Foley catheter must be placed so that urine output can be followed during rapid fluid losses and replacement. Invasive hemodynamic monitoring such as a central venous pressure or Swan-Ganz catheter is rarely needed to manage patients with DIC from abruption or intrauterine fetal demise (IUFD). Patients with DIC as a complication of severe preeclampsia, sepsis, or amniotic fluid embolism, on the other hand, usually are critically ill and such measures are indicated based on the underlying pathologic process.

Regional anesthesia clearly is contraindicated in the patient with a known coagulopathy because of the obvious risk of epidural hematoma and spinal cord compression. However, most parturients do not have any history or clinical evidence of altered hemostasis. Patients with some of the diagnoses associated with the risk of DIC, such as preeclampsia or IUFD, would benefit greatly from a regional technique for labor. As described earlier, coagulation aberrations are known to be an integral part of the syndrome of preeclampsia and are likely to correlate well with the severity of the disease process. Clinically it is extremely common to have a preeclamptic parturient who has a reduced platelet count, (less than $150,000/mm^3$); however, it is exceedingly rare to have a patient with an abnormal PT, PTT, fibrinogen levels, or other tests of clotting ability. In fact, significant coagulation abnormalities are almost without exception, only found in patients with severe preeclampsia in association with a markedly reduced platelet count (less than 100,000/mm).[3] Isolated platelet dysfunction with a normal count also is rare in preeclampsia, perhaps no more common than in normal nonparturients.[3] Based on these facts, most authors support the position that if a patient has a platelet count greater than $150,000/mm^3$, then a regional anesthetic can be placed without any additional laboratory studies and without any increased morbidity. Furthermore, epidural catheters can be safely placed in the laboring preeclamptic patient with a platelet count in the $100,000/mm^3$ to $150,000/mm^3$ range, but these patients probably should have initial PT and PTT studies, as well as follow-up platelet counts to reveal any possible downward trend. Some clinicians support the position that regional anesthesia is safe in patients, provided that the platelet count is greater than $75,000/mm^3$ and that coagulation studies are within the normal limits of control.

The laboring patient with preeclampsia usually is best managed with early placement of an epidural for reasons of improved uterine perfusion, reduced plasma catecholamines, and improved control of hypertension. Progressive thrombocytopenia can be an indication in and of itself; the catheter should be placed before any deterioration of coagulation status. The risk of epidural hematoma is exceedingly rare even in this group of patients. There must, however, be extra diligent follow-up of these parturients since they are at an increased, ongoing risk of developing a consumptive coagulopathy. Routine physical evaluations are imperative and the patients must be informed to notify staff of any symptoms of prolonged neurologic deficit or any *recurrence of anesthesia* once the initial level has resolved. Rapid diagnosis and intervention are mandatory if an epidural hematoma is suspected.

In the rare case scenario where the patient goes on to develop DIC or severe thrombocytopenia, the appropriate time and conditions for epidural catheter removal remain controversial. Most clinicians would advocate leaving the catheter in place until coagulation studies normalize and the platelet count is greater than $75,000/mm^3$. A minority believe that if placement was uneventful the catheter should be pulled, provided the platelet count is greater than 50,000/mm; the argument for this position is that the risks of catheter migration and/or infection are possibly more likely than that of significant bleeding in a patient without clinical evidence of altered hemostasis.

Summary

In review, when a patient with suspected DIC presents to labor and delivery the following management guidelines should be followed:

1. A routine medical/obstetric/anesthetic history should be taken to illicit any recent alteration in clotting ability.
2. A platelet count is necessary; initial PT, PTT, and hematocrit can be simultaneously ordered.
3. If a delivery is planned and the platelet count is greater than $100{,}000/mm^3$ a regional anesthetic technique may be used. If the platelet count is lower, regional anesthesia is not recommended. Therefore if a cesarean section becomes necessary a general anesthetic is indicated. However, risk versus benefit regarding the outcome of the anesthetic management should be weighed before making the final decision.
4. Before inducing anesthesia the blood bank must be notified and blood products made available.
5. Large-bore IV access should be placed.
6. Serial laboratory studies are needed to evaluate coagulation status and direct blood product replacement therapy.
7. The definitive treatment of DIC is removal of the triggering mechanism which usually is accomplished by delivery of the fetus.
8. Any patient at risk for DIC given a regional anesthetic warrants meticulous follow-up care, including serial hematologic profiles and observation for any symptoms of an epidural hematoma.

References

1. Weiner C: The obstetric patient and disseminated intravascular coagulation, *Clin Perinatol* 1986; 13:705.
2. Finley B: Acute coagulopathy in pregnancy, *Med Clin of North Am* 1989; 73:723.
3. Voulgaropoulos DS, Palmer CM: Coagulation studies in the pre-eclamptic parturient: a survey. *J Clin Anesth* 1993; 5:99.
4. Rodgers RPC, Levin J: A critical reappraisal of the bleeding time, *Semin Thromb Hemost* 1990; 16:1.
5. Lind SE: The bleeding time does not predict surgical bleeding, *Blood* 1991; 77:2547.
6. Amrein PC, Ellman L, Harris WH: Aspirin induced prolongation of bleeding time and perioperative blood loss, *JAMA* 1981; 245:1825.
7. Lui S, Wong C, Glassenberg R: Comparison of thromboelastography with common coagulation tests in preeclamptic and normal parturients, *Reg Anesth* 1991; 17(1s):34 (abstract).
8. Stoelting R: *Pharmacology and physiology in anesthesia practice, ed 2,* Philadelphia, 1991, JB Lippincott.
9. Barker P, et al: Coagulation screening before epidural analgesia in preeclampsia, *Anesthesia* 1991; 46:64.
10. Leduc L, Wheeler JM, Kirshon B, et al: Coagulation profile in severe preeclampsia, *Obstet Gynecol* 1992; 79:14.
11. Pearlman M, Faro S: Obstetric septic shock: a pathophysiologic basis for management, *Clin Obstet Gynecol* 1990; 33:482.
12. Pritchard JA, Cunningham FG, Mason RA: Coagulation changes in eclampsia: their frequeny and pathogenesis, *Am J Obstet Gynecol* 1976; 124:855.
13. Remaley AT, Kennedy JM, Laposata M: Evaluation of the clinical utility of platelet aggregation, *Am J Hematol* 1989; 31:188.

33

Diabetes Mellitus

A 32-year-old primigravida (class F-R diabetic) is admitted in active labor at 39 weeks' gestation. Discuss the anesthetic management

Recommendations by Sanjay Datta, M.D., F.F.A.R.C.S. (Eng.)

Diabetes is the most common medical problem of pregnancy, occurring once in every 700 to 1000 gestations.[1] However, advances in the obstetric and anesthetic management in diabetic parturients have considerably decreased perinatal mortality for insulin-dependent diabetic mothers.[2] This chapter reviews the metabolic and hormonal adjustments in normal and diabetic pregnancy; the maternal, fetal, and neonatal complications of diabetes during pregnancy; and modern modes of treatment.

Fuel-Hormone Balance During Pregnancy

Pregnancy is associated with hyperplasia of the β cells of the maternal islets of Langerhans. Islets from pregnant animals secrete more insulin and are more sensitive to a lower dose of glucose than islets from nonpregnant animals.[3] These morphologic and secretory changes can be induced by treating animals with gestational hormones such as estrogen, progesterone, and human placental lactogen. Compared with nonpregnancy controls, humans in the second half of pregnancy have higher basal plasma concentrations of immunoreactive insulin; therefore, any glucose load produces a faster increase in insulin to a higher peak plasma concentrations. Insulin requirement in nonpregnant patients and diabetic parturients in different gestations is shown in Fig. 33-1.

Pregnancy produces major changes in the homeostasis of all metabolic fuels. Plasma concentrations of glucose in the postabsorptive state decline as pregnancy advances, owing to increasing placental uptake of glucose and a probable limitation on

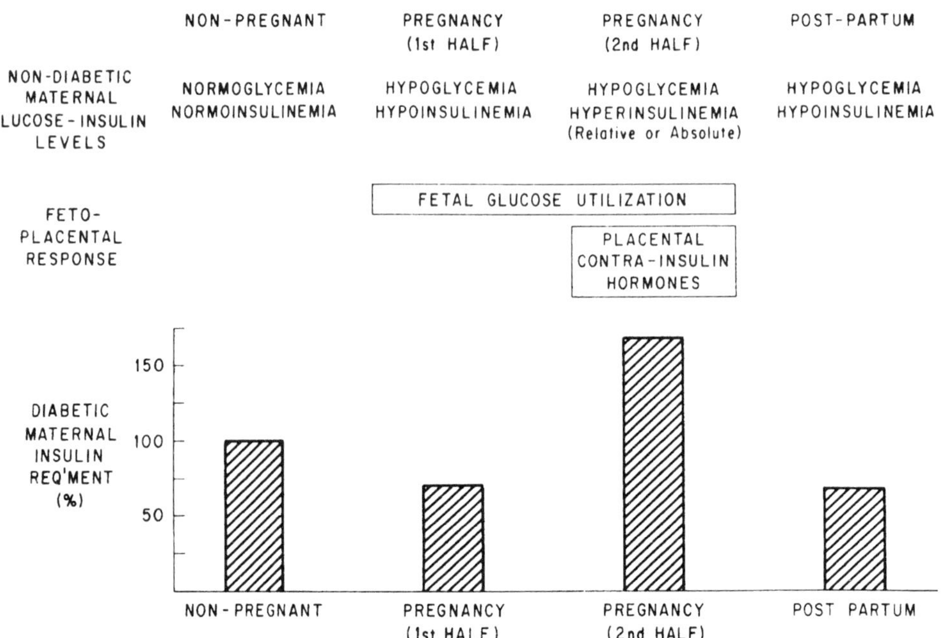

Fig. 33-1.

Relation of maternal insulin requirements to altered carbohydrate homeostasis in pregnancy. Maternal insulin requirements (in diabetics) are presented as a percent of the usual prepregnancy dose, which is arbitrarily defined as 100%. (From Tyson JE, Felig P: Medical aspects of diabetes in pregnancy and the diabetogenic effects of oral contraceptives, *Med Clin North Am* 1971; 55:947.)

hepatic output of glucose. Gluconeogenesis could be limited by a relative lack of the major substrate alanine.

Although fat deposition is accentuated in early pregnancy, later in gestation lipolysis is enhanced, and in the postabsorptive state more glycerol and free fatty acids are released. The lipolytic effects of human placental lactogen override the antilipolytic influence of insulin. Ketogenesis also is accentuated in the postabsorptive state during pregnancy.

The balance of metabolic fuels also differs for the fed state during pregnancy. Despite associated hyperinsulinism, the disposal of glucose is impaired, producing somewhat higher maternal blood levels, perhaps to ensure maximal "feeding" of the conceptus. The antiinsulin effects of gestation have been attributed to interference of human placental lactogen, progesterone, and cortisol.[4] The decay of administered insulin in plasma is not greater during pregnancy, despite the presence of placental insulin receptors and degrading enzymes. Glucagon is well suppressed by glucose during pregnancy, and the secretory response of glucagon to amino acids is not higher than levels during nonpregnancy.

Metabolic Disorders in Parturients

Deficient secretion of insulin in type I insulin-dependent parturients increases glucose concentrations in the blood after meals. In the postabsorptive state, the liver manufactures more glucose by breakdown of glycogen secondary to lack of inhibition by insulin. Concentrations of insulin-sensitive branched-chain amino acids such as leucine, isoleucine, and valine are higher in diabetic subjects having fasting hyperglycemic (i.e., having glucose levels higher than 105 mg/dl during fasting).[5] Gluconeogenesis mainly takes place from the mobilization of amino acids and glycerol from the muscle and fat stores, respectively. Some of the free fatty acids released from adipose cells can be converted in the liver to triglycerides, cholesterol, and phospholipids.[6] Knopp and colleagues[5] found elevated plasma triglyceride levels in obese pregnant women having gestational or adult-onset diabetes. In contrast, when compared with normal parturients, patients having juvenile-onset diabetes did not differ in plasma triglyceride levels. Because of lack of insulin in diabetic patients, increased amounts of free fatty acids are converted to ketone bodies, acetoacetate, and β-hydroxybutyric acid. During pregnancy the physiologic changes of insulin resistance, increased lipolysis, and ketogenesis increase metabolic disturbances in diabetic women.

Diabetic Ketoacidosis

Diabetic ketoacidosis is a major cause of perinatal morbidity. Fetal death rate can reach as high as 90%. Without careful and rigorous treatment, diabetic pregnant women are at increased risk of severe hyperglycemia and ketoacidosis.[7] Four factors are mainly responsible for ketoacidosis in diabetics: a relative insulin deficiency, an excess of stress hormone, lack of food, and dehydration. Glucose accumulates in extracellular fluid because of relative insulin deficiency and excessive stress hormone. Because of lack of effect of insulin on adipose cells and because of elevated catecholamine and glucagon levels, and excessive amount of free fatty acid is released. These increased free fatty acids provide increased substrate for hepatic ketogenesis. Water loss from osmotic diuresis secondary to glucosuria is excessive. Despite dehydration and hyperosmolarity, most patient with ketoacidosis can be hyponatremic. Insulin deficiency and glucagon excess exacerbate the loss of sodium in urine. Another major factor in hyponatremia is the shift of intracellular water to the extracellular space, because without adequate insulin cells are impermeable to glucose. Urinary and gastrointestinal losses produce a marked deficit in total body potassium. The potential for hyponatremia and hypokalemia must be a major consideration when treatment is formulated.

Hypertension

The incidence of hypertension and preeclampsia are higher in diabetic parturients than in the normal population. Diabetic pregnant patients associated with nephropathy (Class F) and hypertension may be more prone to pulmonary edema; this is related to both low colloidal oncotic pressure as well as left ventricular dysfunction.[8]

Stiff Joint Syndrome

Stiff joint syndrome (SJS) usually is associated with juvenile-onset diabetes, nonfamilial short stature, and joint contractures. Involvement of the atlantooccipital joint may prohibit proper extension of the neck and one might encounter difficult intubation in such a situation.[9]

White's Classification of Pregnant Diabetic Women

White[10] classified diabetic pregnant women on the basis of duration and severity of diabetes (Table 33-1). This system which was used worldwide, was originally designed to predict perinatal outcome and to define arbitrary management goals. Because perinatal mortality has declined dramatically in all of White's classes, this system is no longer used to describe and compare populations of pregnant diabetic women. However, certain characteristics of patients of the different White classes still are pertinent. The risk of complications is minimal in gestational diabetic patients (glucose intolerance of

TABLE 33-1
MODIFIED WHITE'S CLASSIFICATION OF DIABETES IN PREGNANCY

Gestational Diabetes Melitus Noninsulin Requiring (GDMNI): Abnormal carbohydrate tolerance during pregnancy only not requiring insulin	
Gestational Diabetes Mellitus Insulin Requiring (GDM): Abnormal carbohydrate tolerance during pregnancy only requiring insulin	
Class A:	Abnormal carbohydrate tolerance in the nonpregnant state identified before the present pregnancy that does not require insulin either before or during the pregnancy
Class B:	Onset of insulin-requiring diabetes after 20 years of age, with duration of less than 10 yr
Class C:	Onset of insulin-requiring diabetes between 10 and 20 years of age with duration of less than 20 yr, or duration 10-20 yr regardless of age of onset
Class D:	Onset of insulin-requiring diabetes before 10 years of age, or duration greater than 20 yr regardless of age of onset, or insulin-requiring diabetes with chronic hypertension, or insulin-requiring diabetes with benign retinopathy
Class F:	Insulin-requiring diabetes with diabetic nephropathy (proteinuria of greater than 500 mg in a 24-hr urine collection)
Class R:	Insulin-requiring diabetes with proliferative retinopathy
Class T:	Insulin-requiring diabetes with renal transplant
Class H:	Insulin-requiring diabetes with coronary artery disease

pregnancy) or in a class A patients whose diabetes is well controlled by diet alone; such patients may be otherwise managed as normal pregnant women. If insulin is required to keep fasting plasma glucose levels at less than 105 mg/dl or postprandial plasma glucose levels at less than 120 mg/dl, the patient should be managed as in class B. Class B women whose insulin dependence is of recent onset will probably have residual islet β-cell function; although control of hyperglycemia may be easier than in class C or D patients, fetal and neonatal risks generally are equivalent. Finally, the most complicated and difficult pregnancies occur in women with renal, retinal, or coronary vascular disease.

Perinatal Morbidity

Even with substantial advances in the treatment of diabetes, maternal mortality is slightly higher in diabetic parturients.[11] Associated vascular disease such as myocardial infarction, hypertension, and preeclampsia or renal disease can bring about major complications. Polyhydramnios still is common in diabetic parturients. Maternal convulsions after hypoglycemia can occur in early pregnancy in insulin-treated patients. Ketoacidosis may develop during the second and third trimesters.

The leading causes of morbidity in neonates of diabetic mothers are major congenital anomalies, intrauterine fetal distress, prematurity, respiratory distress syndrome (RDS), macrosomia, birth trauma, and neonatal hypoglycemia.[12,13] Congenital anomalies currently are the most frequent cause of perinatal mortality and morbidity in diabetic parturients. The incidence of congenital anomalies is as high as three times greater in infants of diabetic mothers. Poor metabolic control during 4 to 8 weeks of pregnancy appears to be related to a higher incidence of such anomalies.[14] In addition to increased perinatal mortality, morbidity also is greater among these infants: hypoglycemia, hyperbilirubinemia, and hyperglycemia occur much more frequently in infants of diabetic mothers.

Management

Diet and Insulin Therapy

The diet of a diabetic parturient should consist of 30 to 35 kcal/kg of ideal body weight. Carbohydrates should comprise 40% to 50% of the total calories, the remaining calories being divided between fat and protein. Lewis et al.[15] suggested that more protein be included in the diet to keep glucose concentrations at a constant level.

The ultimate goal of insulin therapy during pregnancy should be to avoid not only hyperglycemia, but also hypoglycemic reactions. It has been shown that the percentage of hemoglobin A_{1c} (Hb A_{1c}), correlates well with mean daily capillary blood glucose levels over a few weeks during pregnancy.[12] A sequential measurement of Hb A_{1c} (range 5% to 10%) will provide the physician with another indicator of long-term control. However, since insulin dosage frequently must be adjusted during the metabolically dynamic state of pregnancy, glucose levels (in capillary blood or urine) must be ascertained several times each day. Self-monitoring of capillary blood glucose levels at home with glucose oxidase strips and portable reflectance colorimeters has proved reliable in the hands of almost all patients and provides excellent end points of therapy.[16] At Brigham and Women's Hospital, Boston, the obstetrician's goal is to keep the average capillary blood glucose level at 100 mg/dl or less during fasting, and at less than 140 mg/dl at 2 hours after eating.

Most insulin-dependent parturients require at least two injections of a 1 : 2 mixture of regular and intermediate-acting insulin each day to prevent fasting and postprandial hyperglycemia. Usually, two thirds of the insulin is given before breakfast and one third before supper. Occasionally, to manage patients whose blood glucose level is difficult to control, regular insulin is given three or four times each day with one or two injections of intermediate-acting insulin. Small portable pumps for continuous infusions of regular insulin are used at a few perinatal centers.

Monitoring of the Fetus

In the last decade the incidence of sudden intrauterine death in the third trimester of pregnancies complicated by diabetes was about 5% to 10%. Poor control of diabetes accompanied by ketoacidosis, preeclampsia, and diabetes-induced nephropathy were the major causes. Other factors included a combination of relative fetal hypoxia and hyperglycemia, severe hypoglycemia, or fetal myocardial dysfunction.

Recent technologic advances have allowed earlier detection of fetal distress and have facilitated prevention of stillbirth. For example, ultrasound quantitates fetal activity patterns. Also, measurement of estriol levels in maternal urine and serum is an important diagnostic tool because estriol is produced by the placenta from aromatization of dehydroepiandrosterone sulfate manufactured by the fetal adrenals and further hydroxylated in the fetal liver. Hence, most estriol in the maternal compartment is a product of fetal placental function. Chronically low maternal levels (below 95% confidence limits for stage of gestation) or a rapid fall below 40% from the mean estriol level of the previous 3 days may indicate fetal distress. Estriol assays must be performed daily to be of value in preventing stillbirths in high-risk pregnancies.

In such pregnancies, fetal heart rate also should be monitored routinely. The oxytocin challenge test (OCT) was the first test to be used to establish the adequacy of placental perfusion. Deceleration of the fetal heart rate after uterine contractions signifies transient fetal hypoxia and deranged uteroplacental function. Recently nonstress tests have become popular for the same purpose. With good long-term variability of the fetal heart rate and accelerations greater than 15 beats/min with fetal movements, fetal well-being can be predicted. If the fetus is nonreactive even with stimulation, a full OCT is performed. Diabetic parturients should be hospitalized early if control of diabetes is poor, if hypertension is significant, or if fetal well-being is suspected of being in jeopardy. In the hospital, estriol levels should be measured daily and nonstress tests performed at least twice a week. If results of the estriol and fetal heart rate tests remain normal, the pregnancies should continue until term. Diagnostic specificity is increased by using both tests.

Experience at the Brigham and Women's Hospital indicates that diabetic gravidas in whom capillary blood glucose levels can be extremely well controlled in the third trimester are at very low risk of antepartum fetal distress. Therefore such patients are not admitted to the hospital until the thirty-eighth or thirty-ninth week of gestation. After 36 weeks they are seen biweekly to assess results of home blood glucose monitoring and nonstress tests.

Timing and Route of Delivery

To reduce neonatal morbidity from preterm deliveries, and unless risks to the mother and fetus make it impossible, pregnancy should not be terminated until the thirty-eighth week of gestation. Before delivery the lecithin-sphingomyelin (L-S) ratio should be obtained by amniocentesis. According to the experience at Brigham and Women's Hospital, the incidence of severe RDS when the L-S ratio is 2:3 is 12%. Therefore fetal lung is considered mature when the L-S ratio is 3:5. Other amniotic fluid assays such as desaturated phosphatidylcholine, phosphatidylglycerol, or the so-called foam test are being evaluated for greater diagnostic specificity. The presence of phosphatidylglycerol (PG) of greater than 1000 ng/ml is an extremely reliable indicator of fetal lung maturity. However, only 50% of fetuses may be associated with fetal lung immaturity if the phosphatidylglycerol amount is less than 1000 ng/ml. At Brigham and Women's Hospital both the L-S ratio and PG level are used for observation of fetal lung maturity.

Route of delivery is determined by several factors. If the ultrasonic examination confirms that the fetus is large (4300 g or 9.5 pounds), cesarean section should be performed because of the possibility of shoulder dystocia. Otherwise, provided that the cervix and pelvis are favorably positioned, labor should be induced since fewer risks are associated with vaginal delivery. If the cervix is unfavorable for induction of labor, an attempt is made to "ripen" the cervix by inserting laminaria overnight. Continuous monitoring of fetal heart rate and scalp pH values should be used routinely during labor, since the incidence of intrapartum fetal distress (i.e., persistent late decelerations and scalp pH of less than 7.25) is high in pregnancies complicated by diabetes. At the Brigham and Women's Hospital, if progress of cervical effacement and dilatation is minimal on the first day, a *staged induction* is performed.

β-Adrenergic drugs like salbutamol,[17] terbutaline, and ritodrine[18] are used to arrest premature labor. These drugs can cause hyperglycemia and, subsequently, metabolic acidosis as a result of increased lactate and ketones. Corticosteroids also are used to accelerate lung maturation in premature babies. In diabetic subjects, these drugs also possess a potent hyperglycemic effect.[19] As a result, severely uncontrolled diabetes can occur within a few hours of starting treatment, thus leading to a substantial increase in insulin requirement. Such an increase is best prevented by continuously infusing low doses of regular insulin intravenously.

Glucose and Insulin Therapy During Labor or Before Cesarean Section

Tight control of diabetes in the intrapartum period is essential. Maternal hypoglycemia may interfere with the progress of labor, whereas hyperglycemia may increase fetal distress.

Glucose crosses the placenta by facilitated diffusion. Oakley et al.[20] reported that when maternal blood glucose levels were within the physiologic range, the difference in maternal and fetal blood glucose levels was about 20 mg/dl or less. In hyperglycemia, when the maternal level was over 300 mg/dl, the fetal blood glucose level reached a plateau at 150 to 200 mg/dl. At the Brigham and Women's Hospital, glucose levels in umbilical cord blood at delivery correlated well with the somewhat higher maternal levels. Also, there did not seem to be an upper limit on placental transfer of glucose. Umbilical vein glucose concentrations were very high (> 300 mg/dl) after acute maternal volume expansion with solutions containing dextrose.

Disturbed glucose homeostasis during labor can result in neonatal hypoglycemia. Light et al.[21] observed a direct correlation between the rate of disappearance of glucose in infants of diabetic mothers (and ultimate neonatal hypoglycemia) and the concentration of glucose in umbilical cord blood. This relationship has been attributed to maternal hyperglycemia, producing fetal hyperglycemia and consequently fetal hyperinsulinemia.

Lactate concentrations increase in the plasma of the fetus when glucose or fructose levels are high in humans[22] or animals.[23] Shelley[24] observed an increased accumulation of lactate in fetal lambs during hyperglycemia and hypoxia. Bassett and Madill[25] confirmed these results. However, hyperglycemia did not appear to be harmful to well-oxygenated fetuses. Robillard et al.[26] compared fetal blood gases, pH, and plasma lactate concentrations at different levels of hyperglycemia in well-oxygenated sheep fetuses. Plasma lactate concentration increased, pH decreased (from 7.38 to 7.32), and blood gases were stable in the fetus when fetal plasma glucose concentrations were over 150 mg/dl. However, severe metabolic acidosis and concomitant decreases in blood gases and pH from 7.38 to 7.18) occurred when fetal plasma glucose concentrations were over 300 mg/dl. Preliminary studies in primates by this author and others[27] showed that acute hyperglycemia accentuated metabolic acidosis secondary to acute hypoxia.

A well-recognized plan for insulin management for labor and delivery consists of administering one third to one half the pregnancy dose in the morning. Because the diabetic parturient is sensitive to insulin after delivery, insulin shock is possible if delivery is earlier than anticipated. West and Lowy[28] described low-dose intravenous infusion of insulin and glucose during labor. Patients were given a normal dose of insulin the day before delivery; thereafter food was withheld after 10 PM. The next morning the patients were given 1 L of 5% dextrose every 6 hours together with Actrapid insulin, usually 1 to 2 U/hr. The insulin infusion was adjusted to keep the blood glucose concentrations between 90 and 125 mg/dl. None of the neonates became hypoglycemic.

On the other hand, Soler and Malins[29] also achieved good metabolic control of diabetic mothers and their babies by administering a standard dose of intermediate-acting insulin (i.e., 24 U for those requiring more than 60 U/day in the third trimester, and 16 U for those requiring less). During labor, Soler and Malins infused 200 ml of 5% dextrose (10 g glucose) hourly. This regimen was very successful if the blood glucose level during fasting on the day of induction of labor was less than 110 mg/dl. If the blood glucose level was higher, they recommended an intravenous infusion of insulin during labor.

Brudenell[30] reported a higher incidence of fetal distress when mothers were given a subcutaneous injection of insulin instead of an intravenous infusion of insulin (21% versus 4%). Jovanovic and coworkers[31] studied glucose and insulin requirements during induction of labor in 10 insulin-dependent women having previously well-controlled diabetes. All patients received their usual subcutaneous dose of insulin in the morning (26 U PZI and 40 U NPH before breakfast) and before supper (10 U PZI). All had small amounts of food at 9 PM and no food after midnight. In the morning the patients were transferred to the labor and delivery floor, where they had an external fetal monitor placed and connected to a Biostator to keep blood glucose concentrations between 70 and 90 mg/dl. (This machine maintains a constant glucose blood level using a continuous sensing device.) Glucose (5% dextrose with Ringer's lactate) was infused at a rate of 150 ml/hr. Blood glucose levels were kept normal during the administration of 7.5 mg of dextrose/hr, despite the fact that none of these patients required insulin in the intrapartum period.

Our protocol for administering insulin during labor varies according to the fasting blood glucose level. If such levels are less than 120 mg/dl, intermediate-acting insulin is administered in one third the daily dose given during pregnancy and capillary blood glucose levels are measured every 1 to 2 hours during labor. If capillary blood glucose levels then exceed 120 mg/dl during labor, an intravenous infusion of 0.5 to 2.0 U of regular insulin per hour is added. If the original fasting blood glucose levels are higher than 120 mg/dl, an intravenous infusion of insulin is used from the very beginning. In diabetic parturients, surprisingly little insulin is required to keep blood glucose levels almost normal during labor. If cesarean section is scheduled early in the morning, no insulin is given until after surgery. However, if abdominal delivery is planned later in the day, we follow the protocol for labor.

Anesthetic Considerations

Optimal anesthetic management of diabetic parturients requires an understanding of a few special pathophysiologic changes that occur in such patients.

Deranged Uteroplacental Blood Flow

Placental abnormalities are associated with even mild, well-controlled gestational diabetes in the mother.[32] Nylund et al.[33] compared the uteroplacental blood flow index in the last trimester of pregnancy for 26 women having diabetes mellitus with that for 41 healthy control parturients. After injecting indium 113m intravenously, these investigators recorded the radiation over the placenta with a computer-linked gamma camera. Uteroplacental blood flow decreased 35% to 45% in diabetic parturients. Also, the index tended to be further impaired in those having higher blood glucose values. However, the reduction in the blood flow index in gestational diabetes did not differ statistically from that in severe diabetes. This result substantiated the ultrastructural study of the placenta by Jones and Fox,[32] who observed identical placental abnormalities in women having well-controlled diabetes and in parturients having long-standing, moderately controlled disease. Bjork and Persson[34] observed that the placenta of diabetic patients was denser because the villi were enlarged. These enlarged villi can reduce the uteroplacental blood flow by reducing the intervillous space. Such changes in placental perfusion make the infants of diabetic parturients more vulnerable to reduced placental blood flow.

Impairment of Oxygen Transport

Hemoglobin A_{1c} is two to three times higher in insulin-treated diabetes than in control subjects.[35] In Hb A_{1c}, glucose has entered the internal cavity of hemoglobin, and as glucose becomes covalently bound to the two β-chains, the approximation of the H helices to each other is prevented. This movement is a normal allosteric response of the hemoglobin molecule for oxygen (O_2) loading. In contrast to hemoglobin A, the oxygen affinity of Hb A_{1c} is little affected by the in vitro addition of 2,3-diphosphoglycerate (2,3-DPG). No effect occurs because the binding of 2,3-DPG to hemoglobin is impaired by the presence of a hexose on the amino-terminal residues of Hb A_{1c}.[36] Madsen and Ditzel[37] observed that red blood cell oxygen transport, saturation, and O_2 tension are impaired in insulin-dependent diabetic subjects. In poorly regulated patients, in whom concentrations of Hb A_{1c} are higher and concentrations of 2,3-DPG tend to be lower,

O_2 release at the tissue level may be more impaired.

Another disadvantage of poor control of maternal diabetes is chronic fluctuation of fetal blood glucose. Maternal hypoglycemia will be associated with fetal hyperglycemia and subsequently may lead to fetal hypoxemia as well as acidosis.[38]

Deranged Buffering Capacity in Infants of Diabetic Mothers

In 1981 Brouillard et al.[39] observed that the infants of diabetic mothers may have a decreased buffering capacity and a different response to an increased acid load. In these infants, the affinity of hemoglobin to O_2 increased. Values for the partial pressure of O_2 at a hemoglobin saturation of 50% (P_{50}) were significantly lower in infants of diabetic mothers than in control infants (17.9 versus 22.6 torr). Normally, while carbon dioxide (CO_2) or fixed acid increases in the blood, oxyhemoglobin affinity decreases and O_2 is released, thereby increasing the amount of reduced hemoglobin. This reduced hemoglobin thus is available for buffering. This principle is the *Bohr effect*. When CO_2 or fixed acid is decreased in the blood, oxyhemoglobin affinity increases. Thus more hemoglobin is available for binding with O_2 because of its release of hydrogen ion. This is called the *Haldane effect*. The higher intracellular pH values in infants of diabetic mothers is consistent with the fact that oxyhemoglobin affinity was also higher.

This multiplicity of problems makes the infants of diabetic mothers more vulnerable to hypoxia; hence, careful anesthetic management is mandatory.

Anesthetic Management

For labor and vaginal delivery, moderate pain relief can be obtained by administering small doses of narcotics in the early part of the first stage of labor. Lumbar epidural block can provide excellent pain relief for both labor and delivery. Pearson[40] noted that the fetus commenced the second stage in a less acidotic state when mothers were given epidural anesthesia than when mothers were given no anesthesia. Acidosis was metabolic in origin and was related to high lactate concentration. In 1980 Shnider et al.[41] showed that epidural anesthesia reduced the maternal endogenous catecholamines during labor, a reduction that might benefit placental perfusion. Such a benefit might be more important in diabetic parturients.

Spinal anesthesia also can be used if required at the time of delivery. If rapid infusion of a dextrose-free solution is necessary to treat hypotension while avoiding hyperglycemia, a separate intravenous catheter should be used. Also, it is important to realize that the fetus of a diabetic mother might be susceptible to hypoxia secondary to maternal hypotension.

Anesthesia for cesarean section requires special attention for diabetic parturients. The incidence of cardiovascular depression is higher during regional anesthesia for cesarean section and is related to higher sympathetic blockade accentuated by compression of the inferior vena cava and aorta by the uterus.

In 1977 Datta and Brown[42] compared spinal and general anesthesia for abdominal delivery in healthy mothers and diabetic parturients. Infants of diabetic mothers given spinal anesthesia were more acidotic than infants of diabetic mothers given general anesthesia. Acidosis appeared to be related to both maternal diabetes and maternal hypotension. Subsequently, maternal and neonatal acid-base values also were examined after epidural anesthesia was administered in this special group of parturients.[43] The incidence of neonatal acidosis (i.e., an umbilical artery pH value of 7.20 or less) during epidural anesthesia was 60%. Fetal acidosis was related to both the degree of maternal diabetes and to the presence of maternal hypotension. The umbilical artery pH value was always greater than 7.20 when the mother was not hypotensive. In both studies 5%

dextrose with lactated Ringer's solution was used for acute volume expansion.

The genesis of fetal acidosis in diabetic parturients appears to be complex. The human placenta produces lactate in vitro, especially during hypoxia[44] or increased glycogen deposition, as occurs in maternal diabetes.[10] The placenta of the ewe also can produce lactic acid.[45] In sheep, such lactate accounts for 25% of fetal oxygen consumption, compared with 50% attributable to glucose utilization. Glycogen-rich placentas of diabetic parturients might contribute lactate to fetal blood during conditions of relative hypoxia, such as decreased uterine blood flow, which may happen during hypotension.

In human pregnancies, elevated fetal blood glucose levels have been associated with acidosis at birth. Swanstrom and Bratteby[46] observed a significant correlation between blood glucose concentration and base deficit in infants having low 1-minute Apgar scores. In a randomized controlled study of maternal intravenous fluid administration (with or without dextrose) in healthy patients having cesarean delivery, Kenepp et al.[47] found significantly lower umbilical artery pH values in glucose-loaded infants. Fetal lactic acidemia might occur due to hypoxia (secondary to maternal hypotension) in the presence of hyperglycemia after acute volume loading with solutions containing dextrose. To test this hypothesis Kitzmiller and co-workers[27] noticed the effect of acute hyperglycemia in monkey fetuses in response to acute maternal hypoxia. Hyperglycemic fetuses had (1) a greater reduction in arterial O_2 tension and content than did normoglycemic controls, despite similar values for maternal arterial O_2 partial pressure in each group; and (2) severe metabolic acidosis, compared with a modest reduction of arterial pH in normoglycemic fetuses. However, hyperglycemic monkey fetuses exposed to moderate maternal hypoxia did not have greater increases in blood lactate levels than did normoglycemic fetuses. Further investigation is necessary to determine the full nature of the interrelationship between blood glucose levels, O_2 content, and pH in pregnancies complicated by hyperglycemia. An additional risk of maternal and fetal hyperglycemia that accompanies acute volume expansion with dextrose-containing solutions before cesarean section in diabetic parturients is the occurrence of neonatal hypoglycemia. Soler and Mallins[29] reported an incidence of more than 40% in their series when the mean maternal blood glucose level at delivery was more than 130 mg/dl.

Finally, Carson et al.[48] observed that chronic infusion of insulin directly into the sheep fetus increased fetal glucose uptake and oxidative utilization of glucose by the fetus, and, surprisingly, reduced fetal arterial oxygen content. They speculated that hyperinsulinemia may increase oxygen consumption and that fetal hyperglycemia and hyperinsulinemia might result in reduced fetal oxygenation in pregnancies complicated by uncontrolled diabetes.[38]

Myself and colleagues[49] recently reevaluated acid-base status in 10 rigidly controlled insulin-dependent diabetic mothers and 10 healthy nondiabetic control women having spinal anesthesia for cesarean section. Dextrose-free intravenous solutions were used for volume expansion before induction of anesthesia, and hypotension was prevented in all cases by prompt treatment with ephedrine. No significant differences occurred in acid-base values between diabetic and nondiabetic mothers and between infants of diabetic mothers and infants of control subjects. Therefore if maternal diabetes is well controlled, if dextrose-containing solutions are not used for maternal intravascular volume expansion before delivery, and if maternal hypotension is avoided spinal anesthesia appears to be a safe technique for diabetic mothers having cesarean section (Table 33-2).

TABLE 33-2

EFFECT OF STRICT CONTROL OF MATERNAL BLOOD GLUCOSE, NONDEXTROSE SOLUTION FOR VOLUME EXPANSION, AND PREVENTION OF MATERNAL HYPOTENSION ON NEONATAL ACID BASE STATUS IN DIABETIC PARTURIENTS*

Umbilical Artery (n = 20)	No Hypotension (Diabetic) (n = 10)	No Hypotension (Control) (n = 10)
pH	7.27 ± 0.01	7.30 ± 0.01
Po_2 (mm Hg)	20 ± 2	22 ± 2
Pco_2 (mm Hg)	56 ± 2	50 ± 2.5
Base deficit (mEq/L)	4 ± 1	3 ± 0.7

Po_2, oxygen pressure; Pco_2, carbon dioxide pressure.
*Values represent mean ± standard error.
From Datta S, Kitzmiller JL, Naulty JS, et al: Acid-base status of diabetic mothers and their infants following spinal anesthesia for cesarean section, *Anesth Analg* 1982; 61:662.

Summary

In summary, the following criteria should be considered in the use of anesthesia for cesarean section in diabetic parturients:

1. Acute hydration should be provided with dextrose-free solution before induction of anesthesia; a separate intravenous catheter should be used. Solutions containing dextrose should be administered by constant infusion pump at the rate of 7.5 g/hr.
2. Routine left uterine displacement should be provided from the beginning of induction of anesthesia until delivery.
3. Hypotension should be treated promptly with intravenous injection of 10 to 30 mg of ephedrine.
4. An ester-type local anesthetic such as 2-chloroprocaine, which is rapidly hydrolyzed in both maternal and fetal plasma by pseudocholinesterase, might be considered.
5. Amide local anesthetics having a long half-life, such as mepivacaine, should be avoided.
6. Well-conducted general anesthesia can be used, if necessary, with good neonatal outcome. One should be aware of SJS and the possibility of difficult intubation in such a situation.

After the procedure, regular insulin can be administered as needed in small doses. Lev-Ran[50] noted a drop of insulin requirement to zero for 1 or 2 days in 11 of 12 patients undergoing cesarean section; in 3 of these 11, hypoglycemia appeared. This temporary drop in insulin requirement was followed by a steep rise in blood glucose levels. Thus judicious use of insulin is essential at this stage.

References

1. White P: Pregnancy and diabetes: medical aspects, *Med Clin North Am* 1965; 49:1015.
2. Kitzmiller JL, Cloherty JP, Younger MD, et al: Diabetic pregnancy and perinatal morbidity, *Am J Obstet Gynecol* 1978; 1312:560.
3. Kitzmiller JL: *The endocrine pancreas and maternal metabolism.* In Tulchinski DT, Ryan RJ, editors: *Maternal-fetal endocrinology,* Philadelphia, 1980, WB Saunders.
4. Malaisse WJ, Malaisse-Lagae F, Picard C, Effects of pregnancy and chorionic growth hormone upon insulin secretion, *Endocrinology* 1969; 84:41.
5. Knopp RH, Montes A, Childs M, et al: Metabolic adjustments in normal and diabetic pregnancy, *Clin Obstet Gynecol* 1981; 24:21.
6. Kalkhoff RK, Jacobson M, Lemper D: Relative effects of progesterone, pregnancy and the augmented insulin response, *J Clin Endocrinol* 1970; 31:24.
7. Kitzmiller JL: Diabetic ketoacidosis, *Contemp obstet Gynecol* 1982; 20:141.
8. Datta S, Greene MF: *The diabetic parturient.* In Datta S, editor: *Anesthetic and obstetric management of high risk pregnancy,* Chicago, 1991, Mosby-Year Book.
9. Hogan K, Rusy D, Springman SR: Difficult laryngoscopy and diabetes mellitus, *Anesth Analg* 1988; 67:1162.

10. White P: Diabetes mellitus in pregnancy, *Clin Perinatol* 1974; 1:331.

11. Gabbe SG, Mestman JG, Freeman RK, et al: Management and outcome of pregnancy in diabetes mellitus, classes B to R, *Am J Obstet Gynecol* 1977; 129:723.

12. Datta S, Kitzmiller JL: Anesthetic and obstetric management of diabetic pregnant women, *Clin Perinatol* 1982; 9:153.

13. Robert MF, Neff NK, Hubbell JP, et al: Maternal diabetes and the respiratory distress syndrome, *N Engl J Med* 1976; 294:354.

14. Gabbe SG: Congenital malformations in infants of diabetic mothers, *Obstet Gynecol Surv* 1977; 32:125.

15. Lewis SB, Murrary WK, Wallin JD, et al: Improved glucose control in non hospitalized pregnant diabetic patients, *Obstet Gynecol* 1976; 48:260.

16. Constan DR: Recent advances in the management of diabetic pregnant women, *Clin Perinatol* 1980; 7:299.

17. Fredholm BB, Lunell NO, Persson B, Wager J: Actions of salbutamol in late pregnancy: plasma cyclic AMP, insulin and C-peptide, carbohydrate and lipid metabolites in diabetic and nondiabetic women, *Diabetologia* 1978; 14:235.

18. Steel JM, Parboosingh J: Insulin requirements in pregnant diabetics with premature labour controlled by ritodrine, *Br Med J* 1977; 1:880.

19. Watkins PJ: Diabetic control in pregnancy and labour, *JR Soc Med* 1978; 71:202.

20. Oakley NW, Beard RW, Turner RC: Effect of sustained maternal hyperglycemia in normal and diabetic pregnancies, *Br Med J* 1972; 1:466.

21. Light IJ, Keenan WJ, Sutherland JM: Maternal intravenous glucose administration as a cause of hypoglycemia in the infant of the diabetic mother, *Am J Obstet Gynecol* 1972; 113:345.

22. Pearson JF, Shuttleworth R: The metabolic effects of a hypertonic fructose infusion on the mother and fetus during labor, *Am J Obstet Gynecol* 1971; 111:259.

23. Ames AC, Cobbolds, Maddock J: Lactick acidosis complicating treatment of ketosis in labour, *Br Med J* 1975; 4:611.

24. Shelley HJ: *The use of chronically catheterized foetal lambs for the foetal metabolism in combine.* In Gross RS, Dawes KW, Nathanielsz PW, editors: *Foetal and neonatal physiology*, London, 1973, Cambridge University Press.

25. Bassett JM, Madill D: Influence of prolonged glucose infusions on plasma insulin and growth hormone concentrations of foetal lambs, *J Endocrinol* 1974; 62:299.

26. Robillard JE, Sessions C, Kennedy RL, Smith FG Jr: Metabolic effects of constant hypertonic glucose infusion in well-oxygenated fetuses, *Am J Obstet Gynecol* 1978; 130:199.

27. Kitzmiller JL, Phillipe M, VonOeyen P, et al: Hyperglycemia, hypoxia and fetal acidosis in rhesus monkey, *Proc Soc Gynecol Invest* 1981; 50:98 (abstract).

28. West TET, Lowy C: Control of blood glucose during labor in diabetic women with combined glucose and low dose insulin infusion, *Br Med J* 1977; 1:1252.

29. Soler NG, Malins JM: Diabetic pregnancy: management of diabetes on the day of delivery, *Diabetologica* 1978; 15:441.

30. Brundenell JM: Delivering the baby of the diabetic mother, *JR Soc Med* 1978; 71:207.

31. Jovanovic L, Peterson CM, Saxena BB, et al: Feasibility of maintaining normal glucose profiles in insulin-dependent pregnant diabetic women, *Am J Med* 1980; 68:105.

32. Jones CJP, Fox H: Placental changes in gestational diabetes: an ultrastructural study, *Obstet Gynecol* 1976; 48:274.

33. Nylund L, Lunell N-O, Lewander R, et al: Uteroplacental blood flow in diabetic pregnancy: measurements with indium 113m and a computer-linked gamma camera, *Am J Obstet Gynecol* 1976; 144:298.

34. Bjork O, Persson B: Placental changes in relation to the degree of metabolic control in diabetes mellitus, *Placenta* 1983; 3:367.

35. Trivelli LA, Ranney HM, Lai H-T: Hemoglobin components in patients with diabetes mellitus, *N Engl J Med* 1971; 284:353.

36. Bunn HF, Briehl RW: The interaction of 2,3-diphosphoglycerate with various human hemoglobin, *J Clin Invest* 1970; 49:1088.

37. Madsen H, Ditzel J: Changes in red blood cell oxygen transport in diabetic pregnancy, *Am J Obstet Gynecol* 1982; 143:421.

38. Milley JR, Rosenberg AA, Philipps AF, et al: The effect of insulin on ovine fetal oxygen extraction, *Am J Obstet Gynecol* 1984; 149:673.

39. Brouillard RG, Kitzmiller JL, Datta S: Buffering capacity and oxyhemoglobin affinity in infants of diabetic mothers, *Anesthesiology* 1981; 55:A318.

40. Pearson JF: *The effect of continuous lumbar epidural block on maternal and fetal acid-base balance during labor and at delivery.* In

Doughty A, editor: *Proceedings of the Symposium on Epidural Analgesia in Obstetrics,* London, 1972, Lewis and Co.

41. Shnider SM, Abboud T, Artal R, et al: Maternal endogenous catecholamine decrease during labor after lumbar epidural anesthesia, *Am J Obstet Gynecol* 1983; 147:13.
42. Datta S, Brown WU: Acid-base status in diabetic mothers and their infants following general or spinal anesthesia for cesarean section, *Anesthesiology* 1977; 47:272.
43. Datta S, Brown WU, Ostheimer GW, et al: Epidural anesthesia for cesarean section in diabetic parturients: maternal and neonatal acid base status and bupivacaine concentration, *Anesth Analg* 1981; 60:574.
44. Gabbe SG, Demer SLM, Greep RO, Villee AC: The effects of hypoxia on placental glycogen metabolism, *Am J Obstet Gynecol* 1972; 114:540.
45. Shelley JH, Bassett JM, Milner RDG: Control of carbohydrate metabolism in the fetus and newborn, *Br Med Bull* 1975; 31:37.
46. Swanstrom S, Bratteby LE: Metabolic effects of obstetric regional analgesia and of asphyxia in the newborn infant during the first two hours after birth, *Acta Paediatr Scand* 1981; 70:791.
47. Kenepp NB, Shelley WC, Kuman S, et al: Effects on newborn of hydration with glucose in patients undergoing caesarean section with regional anaesthesia, *Lancet* 1980; 1:645.
48. Carson BS, Phillips AF, Simmon MA, et al: Effects of a sustained insulin infusion upon glucose uptake and oxygenation of the ovine fetus, *Pediatr Res* 1980; 13:147.
49. Datta S, Kitzmiller JL, Naulty JS, et al: Acid-base status of diabetic mothers and their infants following spinal anesthesia for cesarean section, *Anesth Analg* 1982; 61:662.
50. Lev-Ran A: Sharp temporary drop in insulin requirement after cesarean section in diabetic patients, *Am J Obstet Gynecol* 1974; 120:905.

34

Neurologic Problems

A 25-year-old paraplegic (T-6 level) woman comes for an antenatal visit while she is 10 weeks' pregnant. She has a normal antenatal course and is admitted to the hospital at 36 weeks' gestation. Labor began at 38 weeks' gestation.

Recommendations by Angela M. Bader, M.D.

Patients with a variety of neurologic conditions will present for management of labor and delivery. The goal in these patients is to provide a safe delivery without worsening of the neurologic condition in the peripartum period. Proper clinical decision making should be based on knowledge of the pathophysiologic features of the particular condition involved and of any controversies regarding obstetric and anesthetic management. Antepartum consultation is important to provide accurate documentation of the extent of neurologic involvement, as well as to allow formulation of an appropriate obstetric and anesthetic plan. This chapter first describes the appropriate management of the paraplegic parturient described in the case above. Several other specific neurologic conditions seen in the parturient are then discussed. These conditions include myasthenia gravis, multiple sclerosis, epilepsy, myotonia and myotonic dystrophy, and polio.

Spinal Cord Injury

The parturient with spinal cord injury, as presented in the case above, has a number of significant clinical problems which will require careful management in the peripartum period. As listed in Table 34-1, many of the medical conditions accompanying spinal cord injury will be aggravated by pregnancy.[1] Pulmonary reserve is further decreased and deep venous thrombosis becomes more common. Renal and bladder problems may be aggravated.

TABLE 34-1
MEDICAL COMPLICATIONS IN SPINAL CORD–INJURED WOMEN AGGRAVATED BY PREGNANCY

Pulmonary
- Decreased respiratory reserve
- Atalectasis and pneumonia
- Impaired cough

Hematologic
- Anemia
- Thromboembolic phenomena
- Deep vein thrombosis

Urogenital
- Chronic urinary tract infections
- Urinary tract calculi
- Proteinuria
- Renal insufficiency

Dermatologic
- Decibitus ulcers

Cardiovascular
- Hypotension
- Autonomic hyperreflexia

From Crosby E, St. Jean B, Reid D, et al: Obstetric anaesthesia and analgesia in chronic spinal cord injured women, *Can J Anaesth* 1992; 39:489.

Obstetric Implications

The extent of disability will obviously depend on the exact location of the lesion in the spinal cord.[2] Injury to the sacral cord will result in minimal disability, with relaxed perineal musculature and abnormalities of bladder and bowel function. If the spinal cord injury is below the level of T-10, labor pain will be present. Preterm labor is seen more frequently in women with a lesion above T-11.[3] Since these women will not experience labor pain, weekly cervical exams usually will be done during the third trimester. Because of weakened perineal musculature, the use of forceps may be necessary for vaginal delivery.[4] Most concerning are the patients with injuries above the level of T-6, who will be at risk during the peripartum period for the syndrome of autonomic hyperreflexia.

Autonomic Hyperreflexia

Autonomic hyperreflexia is a syndrome which may be experienced by about 85% of patients with chronic spinal cord injuries at the level of T-6 or above.[5] In the absence of central inhibition on the sympathetic neurons in the cord below the injury, noxious stimuli result in extreme sympathetic hyperactivity. Vasoconstriction below the level of the lesion results in severe systemic hypertension. In response, the reflex arcs involving the baroreceptors of the aortic and carotid bodies lead to bradycardia and vasodilation above the level of the lesion. These compensatory mechanisms usually are not sufficient to prevent the severe hypertension, which in extreme cases may result in intracranial hemorrhage. Medical management (Fig. 34-1) usually is necessary for control of hypertension, and a variety of methods have been used.[6] Epidural analgesia has been shown to be extremely effective for the prevention or treatment of autonomic hyperreflexia during labor and delivery. Bupivacaine in concentrations of 0.25% or 0.5% has been successful in this regard.[7,8] Although epidural meperidine alone also has been shown to successfully control autonomic hyperreflexia,[9] epidural fentanyl alone did not.[10] Spinal anesthesia also has been shown to effectively control blood pressure in paraplegic patients undergoing general surgical procedures.[11] Theoretically, distortion of the vertebral column might make it more difficult to predict and control the level of the anesthesia, although in clinical practice spinal anesthesia has been used safely and effectively in these patients.[11-13] The use of a continuous spinal technique would circumvent these concerns.

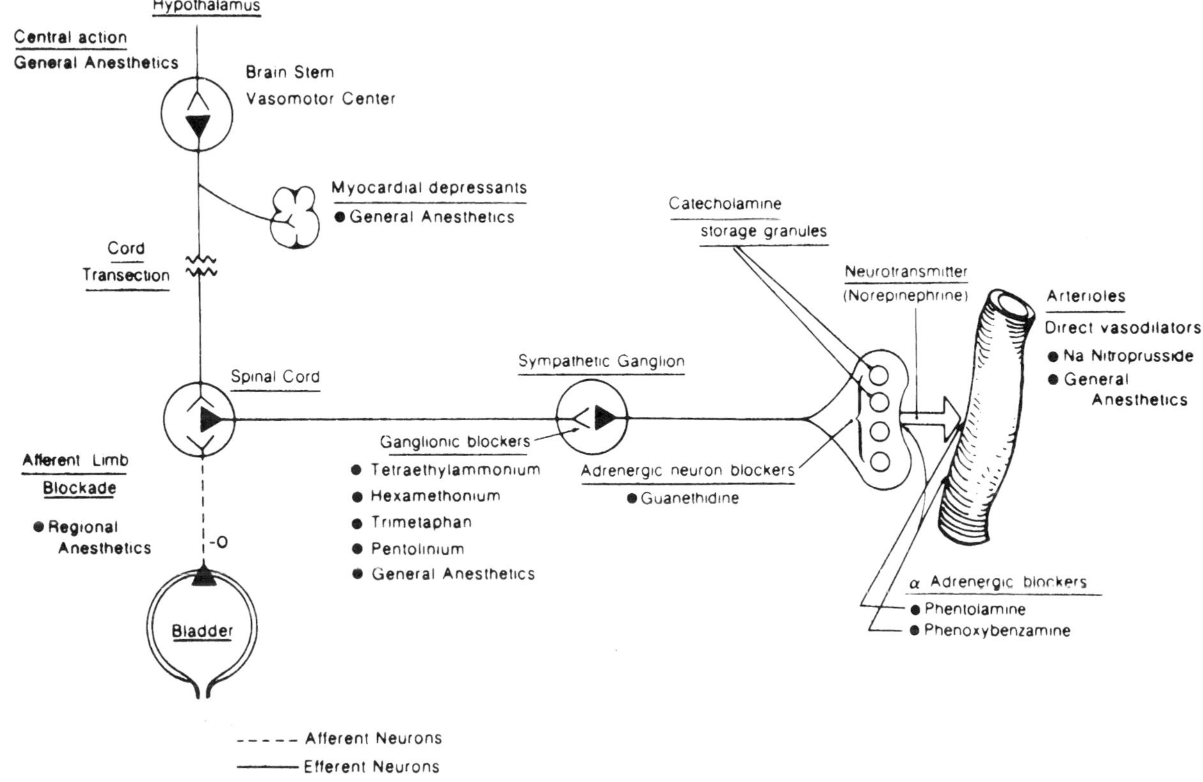

Fig. 34-1.

The sites of action of the agents used for control of the hypertension of autonomic hyperreflexia are shown. (From Schonwald G, Fish K, Perkash I: Cardiovascular complications during anesthesia in chronic spinal cord injured patients, *Anesthesiology* 1981; 55:552.)

Anesthetic Management of the Paraplegic Parturient

The parturient as described in the case presented has a spinal cord injury at the T 6 level. This patient should be referred to anesthetic consultation early in her pregnancy. At the time of the anesthetic consultation, information should be obtained regarding her previous medical and obstetrical history, with particular attention paid to the extent of respiratory involvement and any history of frequent respiratory or urinary infections. The patient's neurologic examination should be documented in the chart. Examination of the back should also be performed since these patients may have some distortion of the vertebral column. The patient should be informed at the time of the consultation that although she will not experience labor pain, epidural anesthesia is recommended because of the risk of autonomic hyperreflexia.

When performing the epidural anesthetic, the usual test dose will not identify accidental subarachnoid injection. Cautious administration of local anesthetic is necessary. Segmental reflexes such as the abdominal muscle reflex can be evaluated to assess anesthetic level below the level of the spinal cord lesion. The anesthesiologist can lightly stroke each side of the abdomen above and below the umbilicus, looking for contraction of the abdominal muscles and deviation of the umbilicus toward the stimulus. Below the level of the block, these reflexes will be absent.

Either epidural or spinal anesthesia can be used if cesarean delivery is necessary. If general anesthesia is required, depolarizing agents should not be used during the period of denervation injury to avoid hyperkalemia. This period can conservatively be defined as lasting up to 1 year after the injury.

Myasthenia Gravis

Myasthenia gravis is an autoimmune disorder which is characterized by episodes of increasing muscle fatigability with activity. A wide range of severity exists. Symptoms can range from ocular myasthenia to acute, rapidly progressive myasthenia with respiratory crises and poor drug response.[14]

The pathophysiology in this disorder is believed to result from an autoimmune mechanism. In 85% to 90% of patients, an antibody to the acetylcholine receptor can be demonstrated.[15] These antibodies result in a decrease in acetylcholine receptors at the neuromuscular junction. Smooth and cardiac muscle are not affected. Associations exist between myasthenia gravis and other autoimmune disorders such as rheumatoid arthritis and polymyositis. Thymic tumors occur in about 10% of patients.

A variety of therapeutic modalities may result in an improvement in symptoms.[15,16] The primary therapy includes the administration of anticholinesterase medications. Pyridostigmine generally is the preferred drug for long-term therapy because it has less severe muscarinic side effects.[17] Edrophonium is administered as a diagnostic test; improvement in symptoms after an intravenous dose confirms the diagnosis of myasthenia. Immunosuppressive agents such as corticosteroids and plasmapheresis have been used with some success. More than 90% of patients develop complete remission or improvement in symptoms after thymectomy. The outcome of pregnancy has been shown to be favorably influenced by thymectomy, with decreased maternal and perinatal morbidity, as well as a decrease in symptom frequency.[18]

Two types of crises can be seen with this disorder. A myasthenic crisis consists of muscle weakness due to worsening of the disease. A cholinergic crises results from an excess of the muscarinic effects of anticholinesterase medication in combination with a poor response to anticholinesterase therapy. The administration of edrophonium will result in improvement of symptoms if a myasthenic crises is present and indicates the need for a higher dose of anticholinesterase medication.

The anesthesiologist needs to be aware of the numerous drugs that can cause a worsening of myasthenic symptoms. In general, any drug that potentiates muscle weakness can worsen symptoms. These agents include neuromucular blocking agents, quinidine, propranolol, and aminoglycoside antibiotics. Drugs frequently administered to the parturient which have been reported to worsen myasthenic symptoms include magnesium sulfate and terbutaline.[19-21]

Obstetric Management

The course of myasthenia during pregnancy is variable; about one third of patients improve, one third worsen, and one third show no change.[15] There is an increase in the spontaneous abortion rate, incidence of preterm labor, and maternal morbidity and mortality.[22] Symptoms worsen postpartum in about 30% of patients.

The parturient needs to be monitored carefully throughout pregnancy and the postpartum period since adjustment of anticholinesterase dosage may be required. As the diaphragm elevates during pregnancy, respiratory compromise may increase. Although the uterus consists of smooth muscle and therefore is not affected by the disorder, the perineal muscles are striated, and muscle weakness in this area may result in a need for forceps delivery.[23] Anticholinesterase agents have known oxytocic effects.[24]

Neonatal myasthenia gravis is a syndrome reported to occur in 12% to 19% of infants of myasthenic mothers.[22,25] This syndrome occurs because the maternal antibody to the acetylcholine receptor is transferred across the placenta. The infant presents with symptoms of myasthenia (feeding problems, hypotonia, respiratory difficulty) within the first few days of life. Symptoms resolve as the antibodies are metabolized during the first few weeks of life.

Anesthetic Management

Antepartum consultation should include an assessment of the degree of bulbar and respiratory involvement. In more severely affected cases, baseline pulmonary function testing and arterial blood gas values may be helpful.

Narcotics should be used cautiously in patients with some degree of respiratory compromise. Regional analgesia generally is the preferred method for pain relief during labor and vaginal delivery.[26] Since plasma cholinesterase activity is decreased in patients taking anticholinesterase drugs, ester local anesthetics may have a prolonged half-life. Unless the patient has a significant degree of respiratory compromise or bulbar involvement, regional anesthesia is preferred for cesarean delivery.[27]

If general anesthesia is necessary, sodium thiopental, ketamine, and propofol all can be used successfully as induction agents.[26,28,29] Muscle relaxants should be used cautiously since they have an unpredictable effect in these patients. Muscles affected by the disease generally are more sensitive to depolarizing agents and unaffected muscles are more resistant.[30] Although any muscle relaxant can be used for intubation, in the obstetric patient concerns about optimizing visualization for intubation should be paramount. Therefore, since the response to muscle relaxants is unpredictable, using a full dose of muscle relaxant (either succinylcholine or a short-acting nondepolarizing agent) will optimize intubating conditions. The metabolism of succinylcholine will be decreased in patients taking an anticholinesterase medication. The anesthesiologist should be aware that prolonged effects of succinylcholine may occur in some of these patients and careful neuromuscular monitoring is essential. Myasthenic patients are extremely sensitive to the effects of nondepolarizing muscle relaxants and shorter acting agents should be used.[16] Small doses of neostigmine can be given for reversal of neuromuscular blockade.

Some patients who require general anesthesia for cesarean delivery will need postoperative ventilation. In general surgical patients, four factors have been identified that are predictive of the need for postoperative ventilation. These include duration of myasthenia of longer than 6 years, history of chronic respiratory disease, pyridostigmine dose greater than 750 mg/day, and vital capacity less than 2.9 L.[31]

Multiple Sclerosis

Multiple sclerosis is characterized by altered patterns of neurologic disability over years. Most relapses reproduce previous neurologic deficits. The course of the disease may be either exacerbating-remitting, in which attacks appear and resolve over several months; or chronic progressive.[32] The etiology is unknown; early exposure to a viral agent may later trigger an autoimmune response with resultant inflammation and loss of myelin in the central nervous system.[33] Patients may experience motor weakness, visual changes, bladder and bowel dysfunction, and emotional lability.

Immunosuppressive therapies may hasten recovery from a relapse but have not been definitively shown to influence the eventual progression of the disease. Relapses may be provoked by such factors as stress, infection, and increased body temperature, and deficits tend to become more debilitating over time.[34]

Obstetric Management

Pregnancy does not appear to be affected by multiple sclerosis. There is no increase in the incidence of preterm labor or stillbirth.[35] Although the relapse rate during the 9 months of pregnancy is similar or slightly less than that in the nonpregnant patient, about 40% of women will have a relapse during the first 6 postpartum months.[36-38] The loss of antenatal immunosuppression and the postpartum decline in maternal concentrations of reproductive hormones may in part be responsible for this. Stress, exhaustion, infection, and hyperpyrexia in the postpartum period may all contribute to this increase in relapse rate.

Anesthetic Management

Antepartum consultation should include an assessment of the patient's degree of respiratory compromise and documentation of existing deficits. Great controversy has existed regarding the use of anesthesia in patients with multiple sclerosis. Some anesthesiologists have been reluctant to administer spinal or epidural anesthesia to these patients because of theoretical concerns that regional anesthesia will expose demyelinated areas of the spinal cord to any potential neurotoxic effects of local anesthetics.

The relapse rate of multiple sclerosis is not affected by diagnostic lumbar puncture.[39] The reports by Bamford et al.[40] and Stenuit and Marchand,[41] which have implicated spinal anesthesia in the exacerbation of multiple sclerosis, have included only a small number of patients. Bamford et al. described one postoperative relapse after nine spinal anesthetics and Stenuit and Marchand reported 2 relapses after 19 spinal anesthetics. The presence of other postoperative factors known to increase the relapse rate of multiple sclerosis was not discussed in either study.

A small number of studies describe the use of regional anesthesia in patients with multiple sclerosis. Crawford et al. reported 1 postoperative relapse in 50 nonobstetric and 7 obstetric patients who received epidural anesthesia.[42] Warren and coworkers reported minor exacerbations after two separate epidural anesthetics for vaginal deliveries in the same patient.[42] In a retrospective study of 32 pregnancies in women with multiple sclerosis, those who received epidural analgesia did not have a higher incidence of relapse.[44] The data suggest that the concentration of local anesthetic used for epidural anesthesia should be minimized, since all patients in the relapse group in this study had received higher concentrations of bupivacaine or lidocaine. Narcotics should be added to the local anesthetic solutions used for epidural analgesia in these patients, since the addition of opioid will reduce the concentration of local anesthetic required. The successful use of intrathecal diamorphine has been reported in these patients[45]; no data currently exist on the use of epidural or intrathecal fentanyl in patients with this disease. In conclusion, current data do not contraindicate the use of regional anesthesia for the parturient with multiple sclerosis. The patient should be aware of the increased relapse rate in the postpartum period that exists, regardless of her choice of anesthetic.

Epilepsy

Epilepsy is one of the more common neurologic disorders seen in the parturient. About 0.5% of all parturients have a chronic seizure disorder.[46] A number of forms of recurrent seizure activity can be seen. A variety of anticonvulsant therapeutic agents are used.[47] Familiarity with the therapeutic ranges and side effects of these agents is essential when dealing with these patients.

Obstetric Management

Pregnancy has a variable effect on the course of epilepsy, with about one third of women demonstrating an increase in seizure frequency during pregnancy.[48] Theories proposed as causes for the increase in seizure frequency during this period include increased estrogen concentrations,[49] increased sodium and water retention, sleep deprivation, and alkalosis secondary to hyperventilation.[50] Dose requirements for anticonvulsants often increase during pregnancy, perhaps due to increased drug clearance.[51] Serum levels of anticonvulsant agents should be monitored throughout pregnancy and the postpartum period to ensure therapeutic levels.

Prevention of the occurrence of seizures in the parturient is extremely important, since maternal seizures have been reported to have devastating consequences. Fetal distress and even intrauterine fetal death can result from the hypoxia and acidosis that can occur during a generalized seizure. In one report of 29 cases, 14 of the infants and 9 of the mothers died shortly after the episode.[52]

A higher incidence of congenital malformations is seen in infants of mothers treated with anticonvulsants during pregnancy.[53] No anticonvulsant drug can be considered absolutely safe in pregnancy.

Anesthetic Management

Should a seizure occur during labor and delivery, the anesthesiologist will be required to provide airway protection and support of ventilation. The seizure may be self-limited or may require a small dose of sodium thiopental or diazepam. The fetal heart rate should be monitored since hypoxia and acidosis may result in fetal distress and the need for urgent delivery.

Regional anesthesia has been safely used in these patients. The systemic concentrations of local anesthetics seen after epidural analgesia may have an anticonvulsant effect.[54]

If general anesthesia is needed, drugs known to lower the seizure threshold should be avoided. These agents include ketamine, enflurane, and meperidine.[55] Some recommend avoidance of meperidine for postoperative analgesia as well. One report states that patients receiving phenytoin are resistant to vecuronium but not to atracurium.[56]

Myotonia and Myotonic Dystrophy

Myotonia is a symptom associated with several disorders and describes prolonged contraction of muscles followed by a delay in relaxation.[14]

The most frequently seen disorder of this group is called myotonic dystrophy, which is inherited in an autosomal dominant pattern. Progressive muscle wasting occurs over time. Characteristically the hand, facial, masseter, and pretibial muscles are involved. Involvement of the pharyngeal muscles, laryngeal muscles, diaphragm proximal limb muscles, and uterine smooth muscle can occur. Cardiac conduction abnormalities may be present. There is a wide range in severity of symptoms. The most severe type of myotonic dystrophy is called congenital myotonia, which appears early in infancy.[14]

The symptom of myotonia also is seen in the disorder myotonia congenita.[14] This disorder differs from myotonic dystrophy in that cardiac abnormalities are not present, smooth muscle is not affected, and the inheritance pattern can be dominant or recessive.

To relieve myotonic symptoms, a variety of agents including quinine, procainamide, corticosteroids and phenytoin have been used.

Obstetric Management

The incidence of spontaneous abortion and preterm labor increases in patients with myotonic dystrophy.[57] In cases involving severe muscle weakness, instrumental delivery may be required. There have been reports of increasing myotonic symptoms after ritodrine tocolysis.[58] In myotonic dystrophy with uterine smooth muscle involvement, uterine atony and obstetric hemorrhage can result.[59]

Anesthetic Management

Since these patients may be extremely sensitive to the respiratory depressant effects of narcotics, regional anesthesia is preferred for labor and delivery.[60] Since myotonia is an intrinsic symptom of muscle, regional anesthesia will not relieve the symptoms; only infiltration with local anesthetic will relieve the myotonia. Triggers of myotonic crises such as cold and shivering should be avoided; intrathecal or epidural narcotics therefore may be helpful.[61]

Since fasciculations may trigger myotonia, depolarizing muscle relaxants such as succinylcholine should be avoided in these patients.[62] The response to nondepolarizing muscle relaxants seems to be normal. In any case, careful neuromuscular monitoring is essential.

Polio

Although most cases of polio are asymptomatic or accompanied by only mild systemic symptoms, in about 1% of patients, motor neuron involvement occurs and asymmetric flaccid paralysis develops.[14] In 20% of these cases the bulbar musculature is affected. Pathologic features are consistent with a viral meningitis, which is caused by a picornavirus that is spread via the fecal-oral route. Most patients will recover over 1 to 2 months, but residual deficits can persist.

Postpoliomyelitis muscular atrophy is a slowly progressive syndrome of neurologic deficits that can appear as long as 40 years after the initial illness. Several theories for the appearance of this disorder have been postulated. Some believe that this syndrome results from reactivation of the initial viral infection.[63] Others speculate that the increased functional demands slowly result in late death of the remaining neurons.[64]

Obstetric Management

Today concern about polio is largely confined to countries in which vaccination programs are not in force. Evidence suggests that vaccination during pregnancy does not threaten either mother or fetus.[65] Patients with residual deficits that result in ineffective ability to push during the second stage of labor may require instrumental delivery.[66]

Anesthetic Management

Because of the theoretical concern that postpoliomyelitis syndrome may result from reactivation of the virus, some anesthesiologists are reluctant to administer regional anesthesia to patients with a previous history of polio. No data in the literature supports this association. There are reports of the successful use of epidural analgesia in parturient with a history of poliomyelitis,[42] and this is the current practice at Brigham and Women's Hospital, Boston, MA.

Summary

1. Patients with spinal cord lesions above the level of T-10 are subject to the syndrome of autonomic hyperreflexia and will require anesthesia for labor and delivery, even though they may not experience labor pain.
2. Regional anesthesia is the preferred method for prevention or treatment of autonomic hyperreflexia during labor and delivery.
3. Patients with myasthenia gravis may experience increasing fatigue during labor and may require adjustment of anticholinesterase dosage.
4. Patients with epilepsy are not more sensitive to the convulsant effects of local anesthetics.

5. Patients with myotonic dystrophy should not receive depolarizing muscle relaxants.
6. Myotonic symptoms will not be relieved by regional anesthesia since myotonia involves an intrinsic characteristic of muscle.
7. There is no association in the literature between the use of regional anesthesia and the occurrence of postpoliomyelitis syndrome.

References

1. Crosby E, St Jean B, Reid D, et al: Obstetric anaesthesia and analgesia in chronic spinal cord injured women, *Can J Anaesth* 1992; 39:487.
2. Donaldson JO: *Neurology of pregnancy,* London, 1989, WB Saunders.
3. Catanzarite VA, Ferguson JE, Weinstein C, et al: Preterm labor in the quadriplegic parturient, *Am J Perinatol* 1986; 3:115.
4. Greenspoon JS, Paul RH: Paraplegia and quadraplegia: special considerations during pregnancy and labor and delivery, *Am J Obstet Gynecol* 1986; 155:738.
5. Kurnick NB: Autonomic hyperreflexia and its control in patients with spinal cord lesions, *Ann Intern Med* 1956; 44:678.
6. Schonwald G, Fish KJ, Perkash I: Cardiovascular complications during anesthesia in chronic spinal cord injured patients, *Anesthesiology* 1981; 55:550.
7. Stirt JA, Marco A, Conklin KA: Obstetric anesthesia for a quadraplegic patient with autonomic hyperreflexia, *Anesthesiology* 1979; 51:560.
8. Watson DW, Downey GO: Epidural anesthesia for labor and delivery of twins of a paraplegic mother, *Anesthesiology* 1980; 52:259.
9. Baraka A: Epidural meperidine for control of autonomic hyperreflexia in a paraplegic parturient, *Anesthesiology* 1985; 62:688.
10. Abouleish EI, Hanley ES, Palmer SM: Can epidural fentanyl control autonomic hyperreflexia in a quadriplegic parturient? *Anesth Analg* 1989; 68:523.
11. Lambert DH, Deane RS, Mazuzan JE: Anesthesia and the control of blood pressure in patients with spinal cord injury, *Anesth Analg* 1982; 61:344.
12. Ciliberti BJ, Goldfein J, Rovenstine EA: Hypertension during anesthesia in patients with spinal cord injuries, *Anesthesiology* 1954; 15:273.
13. Thorn-Alquist AM: Prevention of hypertensive crises in patients with high spinal lesions during cystoscopy and lithostripsy, *Acta Anaesthesiol Scan Suppl* 1975; 57:79.
14. Adams RD, Victor M: *Principles of neurology,* ed 4, New York, 1989, McGraw-Hill.
15. Plauche WC: Myasthenia gravis, *Clin Obstet Gynecol* 1983; 26:592.
16. Baraka A: Anesthesia and myasthenia gravis, *Can J Anaesth* 1992; 39:476.
17. Donaldson JO: *Neurology of pregnancy,* London, 1989, WB Saunders.
18. Eden RD, Gall SA: Myasthenia gravis and pregnancy: a reappraisal of thymectomy, *Obstet Gynecol* 1983; 62:328.
19. Cohen BA, London RS, Goldstein PJ: Myasthenia gravis and pre-eclampsia, *Obstet Gynecol* 1976; 48s:35s.
20. Bashuk RG, Krendal DA: Myasthenia gravis presenting as weakness after magnesium administration, *Muscle Nerve* 1990; 13:708.
21. Catanzarite VA, McHargue AM, Sandberg EC, et al: Respiratory arrest during therapy for premature labor in a patient with myasthenia gravis, *Obstet Gynecol* 1984; 654:819.
22. Plauche WC: Myasthenia gravis in mothers and their newborns, *Clin Obstet Gynecol* 1991; 34:82.
23. Giwa-Osagie OF, Newton JR, Larcher V: Obstetric performance of patients with myasthenia gravis, *Int J Gynaecol Obstet* 1981; 19:267.
24. McNall PG, Jafarnia MR: Management of myasthenia gravis in the obstetrical patient, *Am J Obstet Gynecol* 1965; 92:518.
25. Namba T, Brown SB, Grob D: Neonatal myasthenia gravis: report of two cases and a review of the literature, *Pediatrics* 1970; 45:488.
26. Rolbin WH, Levinson G, Shnider SM, et al: Anesthetic considerations for myasthenia gravis and pregnancy, *Anesth Analg* 1978; 57:441.
27. Mitchell PJ, Bebbington M: Myasthenia gravis in pregnancy, *Obstet Gynecol* 1992; 80:178.
28. Riegler R, Lischka A, Neumark J: Problems of anesthesia for cesarean section in myasthenia gravis, *Anaesthetist* 1983; 32:403.

29. O'Flaherty D, Pennant JH, Rao K, Giesecke AH: Total intravenous anesthesia with propofol for transternalthymectomy in myasthenia gravis, *J Clin Anesth* 1992; 4:241.
30. Foldes FF, McNall PG: Myasthenia gravis: a guide for anesthesiologists, *Anesthesiology* 1962; 23:837.
31. Leventhal SR, Orkin FK, Hirsh RA: Prediction of the need for postoperative mechanical ventilation in myasthenia gravis, *Anesthesiology* 1980; 53:26.
32. Kurtzke JF: Patterns of neurologic involvement in multiple sclerosis, *Neurology* 1989; 39:1235.
33. McDonald WI: The mystery of the origin of multiple sclerosis, *J Neurol Neurosurg Psych* 1986; 49:113.
34. Watson CW: Effect of lowering of body temperature on the symptoms and signs of multiple sclerosis, *N Engl J Med* 1959; 261:1253.
35. Sweeney WJ: Pregnancy and multiple sclerosis, *Am J Obstet Gynecol* 1953; 66:124.
36. Birk K, Smeltzer SC, Rudick R: Pregnancy and multiple sclerosis, *Semin Neurol* 1988; 8:205.
37. Nelson LM, Franklin GM, Jones MC: Risk of multiple sclerosis exacerbation during pregnancy and breast feeding, *JAMA* 1988; 259:3441.
38. Korn-Lubetski I, Kahana E, Cooper G, et al: Activity of multiple sclerosis during pregnancy and puerperium, *Ann Neurol* 1984; 16:229.
39. Shapira K: Is lumbar puncture harmful in multiple sclerosis? *J Neurol Neurosurg Psych* 1959; 22:238.
40. Bamford C, Sibley W, Laguna J: Anesthesia in multiple sclerosis, *Can J Neurol Sci* 1978; 5:41.
41. Stenuit J, Marchand P: Les sequelles de rachi-anaesthesie, *Acta Neurol Psychiatr Belg* 1968; 68:626.
42. Crawford JS, James FM, Nolte H, et al: Regional analgesia for patients with chronic neurologic disease and similar conditions, *Anaesthesia* 1981; 36:821.
43. Warren TM, Datta S, Ostheimer GW: Lumbar epidural anesthesia in a patient with multiple sclerosis, *Anesth Analg* 1982; 61:1022.
44. Bader AM, Hunt CO, Datta S, et al: Anesthesia for the obstetric patient with multiple sclerosis, *J Clin Anesth* 1988; 1:21.
45. Leigh J, Fearnley SJ, Lupprian KG: Intrathecal diamorphine during laparotomy in a patient with advanced multiple sclerosis, *Anaesthesia* 1990;43:640.
46. Dalessio DJ: Current concepts: seizure disorders and pregnancy, *N Engl J Med* 1985; 312:559.
47. Svigos JM: Epilepsy and pregnancy, *Aust NZ J Obstet Gynaecol* 1984; 24:182.
48. Schmidt D, Canger R, Avanzini G, et al: Change of seizure frequency in pregnant epileptic women, *J Neurol Neurosurg Psych* 1983; 46:751.
49. Ramsay RE: Effect of hormones on seizure activity during pregnancy, *J Clin Neurophysiol* 1987; 4:23.
50. Yerby MS: Pregnancy and epilepsy, *Epilepsia* 1991; 32(s6):s51.
51. Nau H, Kuhnz W, Egger HJ, et al: Anticonvulsants during pregnancy and lactation: transplacental, maternal and neonatal pharmacokinetics, *Clin Pharmacokinet* 1982; 7:508.
52. Teramo K, Hiilesmaa VK: *Pregnancy and fetal complications in epileptic pregnancies: review of the literature.* In Janz D, Boosi L, Dam M, et al., editors: *Epilepsy, pregnancy and the child,* New York, 1982, Raven Press.
53. Kelly TE: Teratogenicity of anticonvulsant drugs 1: review of the literature, *Am J Med Genet* 1984; 19:413.
54. Merrell DA, Koch MA: Epidural anaesthesia as an anticonvulsant in the management of hypertension and the eclamptic patient in labor, *S Afr Med J* 1980; 58:875.
55. Modica PA, Tempelhoff R, White PF: Pro- and anti-convulsant effect of anesthetics, *Anesth Analg* 1990; 70:303.
56. Ornstein E, Matteo RS, Schwartz AE, et al: The effect of phenytoin on the magnitude and duration of neuromuscular block following atracurium or vecuronium, *Anesthesiology* 1987; 67:191.
57. Shore RN, MacLachlan TB: Pregnancy with myotonic dystrophy: course, complications and management, *Obstet Gynecol* 1971; 38:448.
58. Sholl JS, Hughey MJ, Hirschmann RA: Myotonic muscular dystrophy associated with ritodrine tocolysis, *Am J Obstet Gynecol* 1985; 151:83.
59. Arulkumaran S, Rauff M, Ingemarsson I, et al: Uterine activity in myotonic dystrophy, *Br J Obstet Gynaecol* 1986; 93:634.
60. Ravin M, Newmark Z, Saviello G: Myotonia dystrophia, an anesthetic hazard: two case reports, *Anesth Analg* 1975; 54:216.
61. Camann WR, Johnson MD: Anesthetic management of a parturient with myotonia dystrophica: a case report, *Reg Anesth* 1990; 15:41.

62. Paterson IS: Generalized myotonia following suxamethonium: case report, *Br J Anaesth* 1962; 34:340.
63. Sharief MK, Hentges R, Chiardi M: Intrathecal immune response in patients with the post-polio syndrome, *N Engl J Med* 1991; 325:749.
64. Klingman J, Chui H, Corgiat M, et al: Functional recovery: a major risk factor for the development of postpoliomyelitis muscular dystrophy, *Arch Neurol* 1988; 45:645.
65. Harjulehto T, Aro T, Hovi T et al: Congenital malformations and oral poliovirus vaccination during pregnancy, *Lancet* 1989; i:771.
66. Daw E, Chandler G: Pregnancy following poliomyelitis, *Postgrad Med J* 1976; 52:492.

35

Malignant Hyperthermia

A 22-year-old primigravida at 39 weeks' gestation is admitted to the hospital in active labor. An anesthetic consultation is requested because of a family history of malignant hyperthermia. Discuss the anesthetic management.

Recommendations by Betty Lou Koffel, M.D.

Malignant hyperthermia (MH) terrifies both patients and their families. Most anesthesiologists see only a few cases in their careers so their *hands on* experience is limited. A plan for dealing with the MH-susceptible parturient is best developed in advance of the critical moment.

Incidence

Fulminant cases of MH occur in about 1 in 62,000 anesthetic procedures using a combination of potent inhalation agents and succinylcholine, or in 1 in 250,000 total anesthetic procedures. The incidence increases to 1 in 4200 when the diagnostic criteria are expanded to include cases of masseter muscle spasm and/or mild symptoms of MH.[1] Labor might be expected to trigger a MH crisis due to stress and pain, but this has not been documented.

Definition

Normal muscle contraction occurs when the free (unbound) ionized intracellular calcium concentration increases. Relaxation occurs while the calcium is pumped back into the sarcoplasmic reticulum. Both contraction and relaxation require energy. Malignant hyperthermia causes an acute loss in the intracellular control of calcium. The resultant release of free ionized calcium triggers an increased aerobic and anaerobic metabolism in an attempt to provide enough adenosine triphosphate to maintain calcium homeostasis via the calcium pumps.

TABLE 35-1

Specific Signs of Malignant Hyperthermia

Increased end-tidal carbon dioxide
Marked rapid temperature elevation
Muscular rigidity
Rhabdomyolysis
Increased oxygen consumption
Increased carbon dioxide production

Recognition

The specific signs and symptoms of MH are listed in Table 35-1. The temperature elevation may be as rapid as 1° C per 5 minutes. Recognition and suspicion of the nonspecific signs (Table 35-2) should alert one to look more specifically at the possibility of a MH crisis. Evaluation of an unexplained tachycardia (one should remember that hypotension and visible or concealed blood loss are common in parturients) should include central *venous* blood gas analysis. A carbon dioxide pressure (P_vCO_2) greater than 55 to 60 mm Hg and a base deficit greater than 5 mEq/L make the diagnosis of a MH crisis likely. Venous chemistry values are more indicative of the severity and progression of the crisis than are arterial chemistry values.

The familial nature of the disease supports an autosomal dominant pattern with variable penetrance pattern of inheritance. Thus family members of a patient with a documented MH crisis may wish to further evaluate their own susceptibility with further testing. Although elevated creatine phosphokinase (CPK) values suggest MH susceptibility in an *at risk* family member, normal CPK values (if obtained on three occasions) have no predictive value.[2] Muscle biopsy for contracture studies provides further information regarding susceptibility. Vigorous contracture to halothane and a reduced contracture threshold to caffeine identify the muscle specimen donor as MH susceptible.[3]

TABLE 35-2

Nonspecific Signs and Symptoms of Malignant Hyperthermia

Tachycardia
Tachypnea
Hyperkalemia
Disseminated intravascular coagulation
Mixed respiratory and metabolic acidosis
Arrhythmias

Therapy of an Acute Crisis

The anesthesiologist often requires additional personnel to optimally deal with a fulminant MH crisis. Dantrolene administration is the cornerstone of therapy for the acute MH crisis (Table 35-3). Supportive therapy with oxygen, hyperventilation, sodium bicarbonate, and cooling also plays an important role. Dysrhythmias usually improve with the treatment of hyperkalemia and acidosis. Urine output must be maintained. For additional information one may contact the Malignant Hyperthermia Association of the United States (MHAUS) via a 24-hour hotline at (209) 634-4917 (ask for Index Zero) or for nonemergency issues at (203) 847-0407.

Anesthesia for a Susceptible Patient

The avoidance of triggering agents (Table 35-4) appears to be of much more importance than the prophylactic administration of dantrolene. Anesthetic machines may be prepared by removing or sealing vaporizers, replacing the fresh gas outlet hose, and using a disposable circuit with a flush of 10 L/min for 10 minutes. Immediate availability of therapeutic doses of dantrolene is required whenever and wherever general anesthesia is administered.

Regional anesthesia, when appropriate for the surgical procedure, generally is preferred in MH-

TABLE 35-3

EMERGENCY THERAPY FOR MALIGNANT HYPERTHERMIA*,†

Acute-Phase Treatment

1. Immediately discontinue all volatile inhalation anesthetics and succinylcholine. Hyperventilate with 100% oxygen at high gas flows, at least 10L/min. The circle system and CO_2 absorbent need not be changed.
2. Administer dantrolene sodium 2-3 mg/kg initial bolus rapidly with increments up to 10 mg/kg total. Continue to administer dantrolene until signs of MH (e.g., tachycardia, rigidity, increased end-tidal CO_2, and temperature elevation) are controlled. Occasionally a total dose greater than 10 mg/kg may be needed. Each vial of dantrolene contains 20 mg of dantrolene and 3 g mannitol. Each vial should be mixed with 60 ml of sterile water for injection USP without a bacteriostatic agent.
3. Administer bicarbonate to correct metabolic acidosis as guided by blood gas analysis. In the absence of blood gas analysis, 1-2 mEq/kg should be administered.
4. Simultaneous with the above, actively cool the hyperthermic patient. Use IV iced saline (not Ringer's lactate) 15 ml/kg q 15 min × 3
   a. Lavage stomach bladder, rectum, and open cavities with iced saline as appropriate.
   b. Surface cool with ice and hypothermia blanket.
   c. Monitor closely since overvigorous treatment may lead to hypothermia.
5. Dysrhythmias will usually respond to treatment of acidosis and hyperkalemia. If they persist or are life threatening, standard antiarrhythmic agents may be used, with the exception of calcium channel blockers (may cause hyperkalemia and CV collapse).
6. Determine and monitor end-tidal CO_2; arterial, central, or femoral venous blood gases; serum potassium; calcium; clotting studies; and urine output.
7. Hyperkalemia is common and should be treated with hyperventilation, bicarbonate, IV glucose and insulin (10 U regular insulin in 50 ml 50% glucose titrated to potassium level). Life-threatening hyperkalemia may also be treated with calcium administration (e.g., 2-5 mg/kg of $CaCl_2$).
8. Ensure urine output of greater than 2 ml/kg/hr. Consider central venous or PA monitoring because of fluid shifts and hemodynamic instability that may occur.

Postacute Phase

1. Observe the patient in an ICU setting for at least 24 hr since recrudescence of MH may occur, particularly after a fulminant case resistant to treatment.
2. Administer IV dantrolene 1 mg/kg q 6 hr for 24-48 hr after episode. After that, oral dantrolene 1 mg/kg q 6 hr may be used for 24 hr as necessary.
3. Follow ABG, CPK, potassium calcium, urine and serum myoglobin, clotting studies, and core body temperature until they return to normal values (e.g., q 6 hr). Central temperature (e.g., rectal, esophageal) should be continuously monitored until stable.
4. Counsel the patient and family regarding MH and further precautions. Refer the patient to MHAUS. Fill out an Adverse Metabolic Reaction to Anesthesia (AMRA) report available through the North American Malignant Hyperthermia Registry (717) 531-6936.

CO_2, Carbon dioxide; MH, malignant hyperthermia; IV, intravenous; $CaCl_2$, calcium chloride; ICU, intensive care unit; ABG, arterial blood gases; CK, creatine phosphokinase; CV, cardiovascular collapse; USP, United States Pharmacopeia; q, every; PA, pulmonary artery; MHAUS, Malignant Hyperthermia Association of the United States.

*Revised 1993.

†This protocol may not apply to every patient and must of necessity be altered according to specific patient needs.

TABLE 35-4
Known Triggering Agents

Halothane
Enflurane
Isoflurane
Desflurane
Methoxyflurane
Cyclopropane
Sevoflurane
Ether
Succinylcholine

susceptible patients. Either ester or amide local anesthetics may be used safely.

Obstetric Anesthesia Management

Prepartum evaluation of parturients with any medical problem allows maximal preparation, discussion, and education for potentially difficult cases. The absence of prior consultation limits the ability to thoroughly evaluate the clinical characteristics of patients in this case. Despite this shortfall, preparations must occur quickly since any laboring patient may require anesthesia for an emergency abdominal delivery.

Triggering Agents

In addition to the agents listed in Table 35-4, it may be preferable to avoid some additional controversial drugs. Sympathomimetic (and parasympatholytic) drugs are considered partial triggers because of their tendency to decrease sweating and heat loss. Thus, in conjunction with other triggering agents, they may exacerbate a crisis. Meperidine, although it has been used safely, also decreases heat loss, which makes other opiates preferable in the MH-susceptible patients, particularly in the febrile parturient.

Oxytocin is considered safe. Ergot preparations may detrimentally decrease muscle perfusion through vasoconstriction. 15-Methyl F2-α prostaglandin may be preferable to other prostaglandins, which are associated with fever production.

Anesthesia for Labor

Since there have been no documented cases of MH in laboring patients, with or without anesthesia or analgesia, the prophylactic use of dantrolene is not encouraged. Dantrolene does cross the placenta[4] and may be associated with uterine atony.[5] Epidural anesthesia or combined spinal-epidural anesthesia provides the advantage of adaptability to changing obstetric and anesthetic needs while being safe for the MH susceptible parturient. In this patient one should administer routine aspiration prophylaxis.

Baseline laboratory evaluation in the MH-susceptible patient should include hemoglobin concentration, hematocrit, platelet count, serum electrolytes, and creatine phosphokinase. Intramuscular injections should be avoided to lessen confusion with subsequent measurements of creatine phosphokinase. Platelet dysfunction may exist in MH-susceptible patients[2] and a bleeding time or thromboelastogram may be considered.

Since sympathomimetic (and parasympatholytic drugs) are considered to be partial triggers of MH, one would prefer to avoid the need for a vasopressor if at all possible. However, ephedrine, or if indicated, neosynephrine, can be used to treat maternal hypotension. Thus meticulous attention to a generous acute intravenous fluid infusion before the institution of epidural anesthesia becomes necessary, as does the avoidance of aortocaval compression.

Continuous electronic fetal monitoring provides evidence of fetal well-being or the lack thereof. Continuous maternal electrocardiogram monitoring, frequent blood pressure and axillary temperature measurements, and assessment of urine for the red-brown color of myoglobinuria provide reasonable additional maternal safeguards.

Bupivacaine, lidocaine, or 2-chloroprocaine can be used *without epinephrine* in incremental doses. MH susceptibility does not contraindicate epidural narcotics. The sensory block can be maintained between T-6 and T-8 level. The advantage of such technique will be avoidance of general anesthesia if there is sudden fetal distress. Surgical anesthesia can be achieved quickly with the use of 2-chloroprocaine.

For spontaneous vaginal delivery or a forceps delivery, appropriate volumes and concentrations of local anesthetics should be administered. A "low" spinal anesthetic, avoiding hypotension as described above, will be useful in the patient with no prior anesthetic.

Anesthesia for Cesarean Delivery

A labor epidural may be extended for an abdominal delivery as in any other patient. Regional anesthesia provides significant advantages over general anesthesia for the MH-susceptible patient, but the choice must be made as it is for other parturients. Maternal intravascular volume status and presence of fetal stress or distress also must be considered. If time permits and regional anesthesia is planned, epidural anesthesia may be elected over spinal anesthesia for its lower incidence of hypotension and subsequent need for vasopressors. However, hypotension should be corrected either with small doses of ephedrine or neosynephrine when indicated.

General anesthesia with nontriggering agents, without need for dantrolene prophylaxis, can be used in the emergency situation. Induction of anesthesia with thiopental, intubation facilitated with a nondepolarizing muscle relaxant, and maintenance of anesthesia with nitrous oxide in oxygen will suffice until delivery. The addition of narcotics and benzodiazepines follow delivery in a nontriggering anesthetic. Careful postpartum observation for 4 to 6 hours will alert one to a postoperative MH crisis, which is treated as described in Table 35-3.

Summary

1. The anesthetic management of a MH-susceptible parturient challenges the obstetric anesthesiologist.
2. Triggering agents must be avoided.
3. Analgesia must be provided to minimize stress.
4. Appropriate monitoring and the ability to rapidly administer dantrolene when needed will optimize the outcome for mother and baby.

References

1. Ording H: Incidence of malignant hyperthermia in Denmark, *Anesth Analg* 1985; 64:700.
2. Gronert GA: Malignant hyperthermia, *Anesthesiology* 1980; 53:395.
3. Rosenberg H, Reed S: *In vitro* contracture tests for susceptibility to malignant hyperthermia, *Anesth Analg* 1983; 62:415.
4. Morison DH: Placental transfer of dantrolene, *Anesthesiology* 1983; 59:265.
5. Weingarten AE, Korsh JI, Neuman GG, et al: Postpartum uterine atony after intravenous dantrolene, *Anesth Analg* 1987; 66:269.

36

Thromboembolic Disease

A 41-year-old multiparous parturient is admitted to the hospital with a swollen and painful right lower leg. Additionally, she complains of dyspnea, which has persisted for several hours before admission. Discuss the management of the case, as if the gestation was 17 weeks and 31 weeks.

Recommendations by Christopher R. Swayze, M.D.
Jonathan H. Skerman, B.D.S., M.Sc.D., D.Sc.

Embolic events in pregnancy are a frequent cause of maternal morbidity and mortality.[1,2] Many types of emboli may present during gestation and include thrombotic, septic, air, and amniotic fluid. The clinical presentation and management will depend on the type and volume of material embolized.

Venous Air and Amniotic Fluid Emboli

Air and amniotic fluid emboli most often are observed during labor and delivery or during cesarean section.[3,4] Although air emboli may be common to both vaginal delivery and cesarean section,[5] air entrainment requires an open portal into the venous system, which is rarely observed before delivery. Likewise, embolization of amniotic fluid typically is associated with tumultuous labors and operative deliveries.[6]

Septic Emboli

Septic emboli generally originate from subacute bacterial endocarditis with bacterial vegetations on a damaged heart valve. The bacterial emboli seed to various parts of the arterial system with potentially disastrous effects.

Thrombotic Emboli

Emboli originating from thrombotic sources may be either venous or arterial in origin. Venous thrombosis in the deep veins of the leg or pelvis is the source of thrombotic emboli.[7] Dislodged portions of venous thrombus migrate to the right heart where they may be passed on to the pulmonary vasculature, creating a potentially fatal pulmonary embolism (PE).

Venous thrombosis occurs as a result of three etiologic factors: venous stasis, vessel wall trauma, and a hypercoagulable state.[7] All of these factors are present during pregnancy. The enlarged uterus causes a mechanical obstruction to the lower extremities, resulting in venous stasis in the legs, a common site for thrombosis in the parturient.[8]

Diagnosis of Venous Thromboembolism

The reported incidence of leg vein thrombi varies from 0.00052 to 0.018 per delivery.[9,10] Thrombosis of the deep veins of the leg may occur silently, making diagnosis difficult in some cases. Pain, tenderness, and swelling of the extremity may be noticed on physical examination. Homans' sign is present in about 35% of patients with deep venous thrombosis (DVT) but is not specific. Palpable cords may be present in the foot or calf and often are tender. *Sentinel veins,* which remain distended even with the legs elevated 45°, also may be noticed.[11] These physical signs are most reliable in detecting DVT in the lower leg; unfortunately, thrombi in the upper leg (in the large veins of the iliofemoral system) are much more likely to cause pulmonary embolism.[12] Detection of DVT in these sites is more challenging. They are often diagnosed after a suspected PE has occurred. Doppler ultrasound and impedance plethysmography (IPG) are noninvasive tests without known risk to mother or fetus, and may be used for detection of upper-leg DVT. Doppler studies of the iliofemoral and popliteal veins have a sensitivity of 90%; however, small thrombi may be missed and the sensitivity falls to 50% in the lower leg.[13] In the upper leg, IPG is both highly sensitive (95%) and highly specific (98%), but is less reliable in the lower venous system.[13,14] Uterine compression of the vena cava, as noticed during pregnancy, may cause false-positive results on IPG, which lowers the specificity of the otherwise excellent technique.[14]

Venography is the gold standard for detection of DVT. Intravenous contrast is injected into the distal veins of the foot and images of the venous system are taken radiographically. Filling defects often indicate DVT, but occasional false-positive results are noticed with external venous compression from popliteal cysts, muscle rupture, and hematoma. Venography yields excellent images of the lower venous system but is less useful for the femoral and pelvic veins.[15] Venography is not without risk, and fatal reactions to intravenous contrast do occur, although rarely. Other problematic side effects noted in one study[16] include local swelling, pain, and tenderness present in almost one fourth of patients having venography. Multiple radiographic images of the lower extremity are required, so appropriate shielding for the parturient and fetus are indicated. The risks of the required radiation exposure and potential contrast reactions must be considered when contemplating venography.

Technetium-99 radionuclide venography is reported to have low risk to the fetus and has over 90% accuracy in diagnosis of DVT in the upper leg.[13,17] Special gamma cameras required for this study unfortunately may not be available in some centers. Radionuclide scanning with iodine-125–labeled fibrinogen is sensitive and is widely available, but is contraindicated in the pregnant and lactating female.[18] Because the radionuclide crosses the placenta and appears in breast milk, the risk of damage to the fetal-neonatal thyroid is great. This technique is probably of most value in the postpartum patient who is not breast feeding.

Diagnosis of Pulmonary Embolism

The clinical presentation of PE is variable, and may even be silent. However, dyspnea, tachypnea, chest pain, and a feeling of impending doom are common complaints. Rales and wheezing usually are present on chest auscultation. Syncope also may occur. The PE that produces pulmonary infarction is frequently associated with pleuritic pain, cough, and hemoptysis. Large emboli produce acute pulmonary hypertension and right heart failure, manifested by venous distention of the head and neck, tachycardia, hypotension, and pulsus paradoxus. Shock may ensue and death is distressingly frequent after a large PE. Arterial blood gas measurement often reveals an increased alveolar-arterial oxygen gradient. Radiographic changes in chest films occur in some patients, but generally are nonspecific and may take several hours or days before they appear. Electrocardiography often is normal but may be useful to rule out other cardiac problems.[13]

Radiologic evaluation is the cornerstone of diagnosis for PE. Ventilation-perfusion (V/Q) radionuclide scanning often is recommended for the nonpregnant patient, since it has few risks and is sensitive. Specificity is lower, however, and patients can only be categorized as having a low, intermediate, or high probability for PE. Fetal effects of the radionuclides administered in V/Q scans are not truly known, and therefore the benefit must clearly outweigh the risks to mother and fetus if this study is to be performed.

Pulmonary arteriography affords the greatest sensitivity and specificity for the diagnosis of PE. Although risks of intravenous contrast reaction, hematoma, and bleeding are present, the exceptional accuracy in diagnosis may be worth the risk to the parturient facing long-term anticoagulation therapy.

Arterial Thromboembolism

Embolism from arterial thrombosis usually is associated with mechanical prosthetic heart valves. Thrombosis of artificial mitral or aortic valves may release emboli into the left heart with consequent systemic arterial occlusion.

The parturient with a prosthetic valve thus is at particularly high risk for thrombosis. Essentially all patients with mechanical valves require long-term anticoagulation[19] and the parturient attains a relative hypercoagulability as well,[20] which increases the likelihood for a thrombotic event. Thrombosis of the valve, limb weakness, and cerebral embolism with death have been reported in parturients who apparently received inadequate anticoagulation therapy.[21]

Treatment of Thromboembolic Disease in Pregnancy

Pulmonary embolism was the second most common cause of maternal death in *The Report on Confidential Enquiries in Maternal Death in England and Wales, 1979-81,* accounting for 9.4 deaths per million pregnancies.[2] Given the high mortality from PE, aggressive treatment generally is indicated. In the nonpregnant patient, immediate therapy is instituted with intravenous heparin, which may be converted to oral warfarin at a later date. Anticoagulation prevents the formation of additional thrombi and heparin inhibits release of vasoactive mediators in the lung, which may worsen vasospasm of the pulmonary arteries.

Experience with anticoagulation in parturients began with patients having mechanical prosthetic heart valves.[22] Unfortunately the administration of warfarin to parturients led to the discovery of the fetal warfarin syndrome. This syndrome consists of stippled epiphyses (chondrodysplasia punctata), hypoplastic nose, skeletal abnormalities (primarily involving the phalanges), and ocular abnormalities including blindness.[23,24] Other abnormalities were later attributed to the drug, including diaphragmatic hernia,[25] hydrocephalus and Dandy-Walker malformation,[26] and other assorted central nervous system abnormalities.[27]

Sodium warfarin, which acts as a competitive inhibitor of vitamin K in the liver, is a small molecule (molecular weight, 1000 daltons) that crosses the placenta readily. In fact, the oral anticoagulants appear to affect the fetus more profoundly than they do the mother because of immature liver enzyme systems. The use of warfarin agents during the first trimester is associated with significant teratogenic potential, as manifested in the congenital warfarin syndrome. Continued warfarin therapy in the late third trimester can cause fetal bleeding either before or after delivery. Other effects secondary to fetal hemorrhage have reportedly resulted from exposure to warfarin during the second and third trimesters. Warfarin embryopathy results when coumadin is administered in the first trimester in 15% to 25% of cases. Exposure in the second trimester results in a 3% or higher incidence of severe central nervous system anomalies.[27]

Hall et al.[28] reviewed 418 pregnancies involving the use of coumadin derivatives and concluded that one sixth of those terminated in stillbirth or spontaneous abortion, one sixth yielded abnormal liveborn babies, and two thirds produced normal offspring.[24] The critical period of exposure to warfarin in utero was at 6 to 9 weeks' gestation, which resulted in the most frequent and profound congenital warfarin syndromes.

Heparin is a large mucopolysaccharide molecule (molecular weight approximately 20,000 daltons). It acts by combining with antithrombin III, (heparin cofactor) to inhibit the formation of thrombin. The lack of thrombin prevents the conversion of fibrinogen to fibrin. Heparin also increases the level of activated factor X inhibitor, which again interferes with the production of thrombin from prothrombin. Heparin also inhibits the activation of factor IX (Christmas factor).

Heparin is not absorbed from the gastrointestinal tract and intramuscular injection is not advisable because of the risk of hematoma formation at the injection site. In fact, intramuscular injection of any drug should be avoided in a patient on heparin therapy. The greatest risk with heparin therapy is hemorrhage, which has been noted to have an incidence between 4% and 33%.[29] In addition, heparin can result in allergic reactions, alopecia, osteoporosis, and thrombocytopenia.

Hall et al.[28] examined 135 pregnancies involving the use of heparin; again, two thirds were normal neonates, whereas one eighth were stillborn and one fifth delivered prematurely. The use of both coumadin and heparin (in a fixed, low-dose regimen) was examined prospectively in patients with prosthetic valves,[30] but 25% to 30% of the liveborn offspring exhibited coumadin embryopathy; in addition, three patients in the heparin group developed valvular thrombosis (fatal in two of the three). Consequently these authors believed that heparin in such a regimen was ineffective and that coumadin should not be used from 6 to 12 weeks' gestation. In efforts to improve the outcome, other strategies have been examined, including a regimen of dipyridamole and aspirin,[31] but due to an extremely limited number of patients involved, it is difficult to draw conclusions from this study.

More recently a higher dose regimen of heparin has been studied.[32] In this investigation the authors administered subcutaneous heparin in doses sufficient to maintain the partial thromboplastin time (PTT) at 1.5 times the control value during the first trimester and during the last 3 weeks of gestation. Warfarin was used from gestational weeks 13 to 37. In the 18 pregnancies examined, there were neither congenital malformations nor thromboembolic complications. There were, however, spontaneous abortions in nine pregnancies. The authors believed this was likely due to warfarin ingestion early during the first trimester, before the patients realized they were pregnant. Since all 18 parturients in this study had mechanical heart valves and all but one had chronic atrial fibrillation, they were at very high risk for thromboembolic complications. The successful self-administration of heparin without thromboembolic sequelae is indeed encouraging in spite of a high rate of spontaneous abortion.

Opinions differ regarding the duration of anticoagulant therapy advisable after an acute episode of thromboembolic disease. DeSwiet[33] advocates continuing full anticoagulation until 6 weeks after delivery for all patients who had either DVT or PE during pregnancy. Laros and Alger[34] would also continue anticoagulation for the patient with pulmonary embolus.

Management of the Patient

In the case scenario previously presented, the patient appears to have a DVT of the leg with a possible PE. In a case such as this, initial management consists of rapid evaluation of vital signs and gas exchange as part of the physical examination, whereas arterial blood gas analysis, chest radiograph, and electrocardiography also are indicated. Although the chest film and the electrocardiogram may not make the diagnosis of PE or DVT, they are necessary to rule out other disorders that may present with a similar clinical picture. Oxygen and inotropic support may be necessary if the patient is hypoxic or hemodynamically compromised. The arterial oxygen pressure (PaO_2) levels should be maintained at 70 mm Hg or above to prevent fetal hypoxia. If the diagnosis is unclear but suspicion of PE remains, pulmonary arteriography may be used to rule out PE. If PE is unlikely, based on the examination and testing, but clinical suspicion for DVT remains, doppler ultrasonography or IPG are the first-line tests; if the findings of these studies are equivocal, venography is probably indicated. Although this might not be the case in the nonpregnant patient, this study is probably worthwhile in the parturient, since a negative result could prevent the exposure of the fetus to either coumadin or heparin. If negative, a search for other causes of the problem should ensue. If tests for either PE or DVT give positive results, full-dose intravenous heparin therapy should begin immediately. Continued monitoring for worsening of the clinical picture is essential.

Treatment of PE is designed to support cardiopulmonary function and to prevent extension or recurrence of the PE by institution of systemic anticoagulant therapy. Surgical intervention may be indicated in very few selected cases. Morphine sometimes is necessary to relieve pain and anxiety.

The cornerstone of therapy is anticoagulation.[33] Thrombolytic agents often used for the resolution of a thrombus currently are contraindicated and should be avoided during pregnancies.[35] After one thromboembolic event, there is a 12% risk of repeat thrombosis during the same pregnancy and a 5% to 10% risk of recurrent thromboembolism with subsequent pregnancies.[8,36] The initial anticoagulation should always be induced with intravenous heparin, since its effect is immediate. Serial measurements of the PTT should be performed to keep the result at 1.5 times the control value. After successful anticoagulation with intravenous heparin, a conversion to an equivalent self-administered dose of subcutaneous heparin is probably permissible with close outpatient monitoring of the PTT.[37]

Both patient scenarios here (17 weeks' and 34 weeks' gestation) could be satisfactorily treated with this regimen. The patient at 17 weeks' gestation could be converted to coumadin until 37 weeks' gestation, but unless there are specific reasons why a subcutaneous heparin regimen is not feasible, it seems prudent today to avoid exposure to coumadin altogether. At the onset of labor, the heparin should be stopped; the therapy may be resumed 4 to 8 hours after delivery if bleeding is not excessive.

If the patient is on heparin therapy at the time of labor and delivery, the situation is less complicated. First, the fetus is not affected by heparin, so fetal hemorrhage is not a risk factor. Second, the half-life of heparin is short; if delivery is anticipated more than 4 to 6 hours after the last heparin injection, there is no need to reverse the anticoagulant activity. The usual recommendation is simply to stop the heparin as soon as the patient goes into labor, or to omit the heparin dose on the morning of induction or elective cesarean section. If an emergency delivery or cesarean section is needed while the heparin is still active, protamine, a heparin antagonist, may be given. Protamine forms a stable salt in the presence of heparin, with the result that both drugs lose their intrinsic anticoagulant activity. Each milligram of protamine neutralizes 100 U of heparin. The calculated dose of protamine, up to 50 mg, should be administered intravenously over a 3-minute period. Regional anesthesia has been used after reversal of heparin by protamine. Protamine also can be used if the patient develops hemorrhagic complications from heparin therapy, but it must be used with care and caution as protamine sulfate excess may cause anticoagulation. Needless to say, strict attention to circulatory homeostasis during surgery or delivery is essential if anticoagulation is to be resumed in the postpartum period.

Summary

1. Parturients are at increased risk for thromboembolic disease.
2. Diagnosis of DVT of the leg often may be done noninvasively with doppler ultrasonography or IPG. Diagnosis of PE may require arteriography.
3. Whereas PE can be lethal, the drug therapy is associated with significant risk for the fetus as well.
4. Intravenous heparin therapy is the preferred drug regimen for the pregnant patient with an acute PE or DVT.
5. Self-administered subcutaneous heparin with close monitoring of the PTT to ensure adequate anticoagulation appears promising for longer term use.

References

1. Kaunitz AM, Hughes JM, Grimes DA, et al: Causes of maternal mortality in the United States, *Obstet Gynecol* 1985; 65:605.
2. Turnbull AC: Report on confidential enquiries into maternal deaths in England and Wales 1979-81, London, 1986, HMSO.
3. Malinow AM, Naulty JS, Hunt CO, et al: Precordial ultrasonic monitoring during cesarean delivery, *Anesthesiology* 1987; 66:816.
4. Morgan M: Amniotic fluid embolism, *Anaesthesia* 1979; 34:20.
5. Vartikar JV, Johnson MD, Datta S: Precordial Doppler monitoring and pulse oximetry during cesarean delivery: detection of venous air embolism, *Reg Anesth* 1989; 14:145.
6. Clark SL: New concepts of amniotic fluid embolism: a review, *Obstet Gynecol Surv* 1990; 45:360.
7. Sabiston DC: Pathophysiology, diagnosis and management of pulmonary embolism, *Am J Surgery* 1979; 138:384.
8. Ikard RW, Veland D, Folse R: Lower limb venous dynamics in pregnant women, *Surg Gynecol Obstet* 1979; 132:483.
9. Villasanta U: Thromboembolic disease in pregnancy, *Am J Obstet Gynecol* 1965; 93:142.
10. Aaro LA, Juergens JL: Thrombophlebitis associated with pregnancy, *Am J Obstet Gynecol* 1971; 109:1128.
11. DeGowin EL, DeGowin RL: *The thorax and cardiovascular system.* In DeGowin EL, DeGowin RL, editors: *Bedside diagnostic examination,* ed 4, New York, 1981, Macmillan.
12. Rubenstein E: Cardiovascular medicine: *thromboembolism.* In Rubenstein E, Federman DD, editors: *Scientific American Medicine,* New York, 1989, Scientific American.
13. Moser KM: Diagnosis and management of pulmonary embolism, *Hosp Pract* 1980; 15:57.
14. Morris GK, Mitchell JR: Clinical management of venous thromboembolism, *Br Med Bull* 1978; 34:169.
15. Skerman JH, Huckaby T, Walker EB, et al: *Perinatal management of maternal and fetal emergencies.* In Diaz JH, editor: *Peri-*

natal anesthesia and critical care, Philadelphia, 1991, WB Saunders.

16. Markisz JA: *Radiologic and nuclear medicine diagnosis.* In Goldhaber SZ, editor: *Pulmonary embolism and deep venous thrombosis,* Philadelphia, 1985, WB Saunders.
17. Bettman MA, Paulin S: Leg phlebography: the incidence, nature and modifications of undesirable side effects, *Radiology* 1977; 122:101.
18. Kakkar V: The diagnosis of deep vein thrombosis using the ^{125}I fibrinogen test, *Arch Surg* 1972; 104:152.
19. Edmunds LH: Thromboembolic complications of current cardiac vascular prosthesis, *Ann Thorac Surg* 1982; 34:96.
20. Schaffer AT: The hypercoagulable states, *Ann Intern Med* 1985; 102:814.
21. Chen WC, Chan CS, Lee PK, et al: Pregnancy in patients with prosthetic heart valves: an experience with 45 pregnancies, *QJ Med* 1982; 51:358.
22. DiSaia PJ: Pregnancy and delivery of a patient with a Starr-Edwards mitral valve prosthesis, *Obstet Gynecol* 1966; 28:469.
23. Baillie M, Allen Ed, Elkington AR: The congenital warfarin syndrome: a case report, *Br J Ophthalmol* 1980; 64:633.
24. Ruthnum P, Tolmie JL: Atypical malformations in an infant exposed to warfarin during the first trimester of pregnancy, *Teratology* 1987; 36:299.
25. Normann EK, Stray-Pedersen B: Warfarin-induced fetal diaphragmatic hernia: case report, *Br J Obstet Gynaecol* 1989; 96:729.
26. Kaplan LC, Anderson GG, Ring BA: Congenital hydrocephalus and Dandy-Walker malformation associated with warfarin use during pregnancy, *Birth Defects* 1982; 18:79.
27. LoSasso AM: *Pulmonary embolism.* In Stoelting RK, Dierdorf SF, editors: *Anesthesia and co-existing disease,* New York, 1992, Churchill-Livingstone.
28. Hall JG, Pauli RM, Wilson KM: Maternal and fetal sequelae of anticoagulation during pregnancy, *Am J Med* 1980; 68:122.
29. Salzman JG, Deykin K, Shapiro RM, et al: Management of heparin therapy: a controlled prospective trial, *N Engl J Med* 1975; 292:2046.
30. Iturbe-Alessio I, Fonseca MC, Mutchinik O, et al: Risks of anticoagulant therapy in pregnant women with artificial heart valves, *N Engl J Med* 1986; 315:1390.
31. Biale Y, Cantor A, Lewenthal H, et al: The course of pregnancy in patients with artificial heart valves treated with dipyridamole, *Int J Gynaecol Obstet* 1980; 18:128.
32. Lee PK, Wang RC, Chow JF, et al: Combined use of warfarin and adjusted subcutaneous heparin during pregnancy in patients with an artificial heart valve, *J Am Coll Cardiol* 1986; 8:221.
33. deSwiet M: Thromboembolism, *Clin Haematol* 1985; 14:643.
34. Laros RK, Alger LS: Thromboembolism and pregnancy, *Clin Obstet Gynecol* 1979; 22:871.
35. Bounameaux H, Vermylen J, Collen D: Thrombolytic treatment with recombinant tissue-type plasminogen activator in a patient with massive pulmonary embolism, *Ann Intern Med* 1985; 103:64.
36. Bolan JC: Thromboembolic complications of pregnancy, *Clin Obstet Gynecol* 1983; 26:913.

37

Newborn Resuscitation

A 25-year-old primigravida at 29 weeks' gestation is admitted in active labor. A course of terbutaline to stop the labor is tried with success. The perinatologist advises the patient to receive steroid therapy to help mature the fetal lungs. She agrees. Three days later she goes into labor, does not respond to terbutaline therapy, and ruptures her membranes. At this point she is fully dilated and delivers a small, premature baby with Apgar scores of 3 and 5 at 1 and 5 minutes, respectively. The neonatologist arrives to continue newborn care.

Recommendations by Stephen B. Corn, M.D.

The care of the newborn in the delivery room most often is a seemingly simple and pleasant aspect of medical care. However, the newborn care team must always be prepared to care for the severely depressed neonate. The care given to the newborn, in the first moments after birth, can have impact that extends and affects the individual's entire life. Often there may be clues that the fetus will be in need of rescusiatory efforts. These include a maternal history of coexisting disease or maternal drug use, a complicated course of pregnancy, prematurity, suspicion of fetal distress, meconium-stained amniotic fluid, multiple gestations, and diagnosis or suspicion of fetal anomalies. Occasionally, an otherwise normal pregnancy and labor may result in the delivery of a depressed infant requiring resuscitation. Therefore it is imperative that all facilities caring for the pregnant patient be prepared to resuscitate and stabilize the newborn.

This chapter addresses aspects, by way of a case discussion, of the immediate care of the premature newborn in need of resuscitation. Certain controversial areas of newborn care are highlighted, for example, care of the infant with passage of meconium, pharmacologic interventions, and the immediate treatment of respiratory distress syndrome (RDS). Also discussed are nonroutine treatment modalities and interventions that may reduce morbidity and mortality of the newborn, such as inhaled nitric oxide therapy and fetal-tracheal intubation. All individuals involved in newborn care should be cardiopulmonary resuscitation (CPR) and ACLS (Advanced Cardiac Life Support) certified. Therefore the focus is not on these fundamental skills. The reader is referred to the *Textbook of Neonatal Resuscitation* by the American Heart Association (AHA).[1]

Role of the Anesthesiologist in Neonatal Resuscitation

An important aspect in the immediate care of the newborn is to have the members of the newborn care team, and their specific roles, clearly defined so that this unit may respond swiftly and effectively. At the Brigham and Women's Hospital, Boston, for all high-risk births, the Neonatal Intensive Care Unit (NICU)/Pediatric Team is notified before delivery. On their arrival, the maternal history; course of the pregnancy, including gestational age, progress of the labor, and anesthetic management (including all epidural or subarachnoid anesthetics); and systemic drug administrations are discussed with the newborn team.

The American Society of Anesthesiologists' Guideline VII for Regional Anesthesia in Obstetrics states that

> Qualified personnel, other than the anesthesiologist attending the mother, should be immediately available to assume responsibility for resuscitation of the newborn. The primary responsibility of the anesthesiologist is to provide care to the mother. If the anesthesiologist is also requested to provide brief assistance in the care of the newborn, the benefit to the child must be compared to the risk to the mother.

At the Brigham and Women's Hospital, in accordance with the American Society of Anesthesiologists' Guidelines, the following is taught for newborns requiring resuscitation in the delivery room:

If you are the sole individual trained in the care of the newborn in the delivery room, you should request that the newborn be brought to you on the warming bassinet so that you can immediately begin the resuscitation without leaving your patient unattended. This is not a simple or easily performed task, but it must be remembered that the parturient is under your direct care and it is your responsibility to get her safely through the procedure. As soon as it becomes evident that the newborn may require special care, an assigned individual should call the NICU/Pediatric Team and the Anesthesia Code Team.

Universal Precautions

It is imperative that all members of the delivery room team adhere to universal precautions without exception.

General Principles of Neonatal Resuscitation

The birth process involves major physiologic adaptations for the neonate as the infant adjusts to extrauterine life. The routine care of the newborn involves clearance of secretions from the airway, maintenance of a neutral thermal environment, and monitoring of ventilation and perfusion. The care of the depressed neonate involves these basic principles, frequently in concert with establishment of an artificial airway for positive-pressure ventilation with 100% oxygen, chest compressions, and pharmacologic intervention.

Apgar Score

The Apgar score is a scoring system that assigns the newborn with a score from 0 to 10. This score has been used to objectively quantitate neonatal depression.[2] The clinical signs that are evaluated are heart rate, respiratory effort, reflex irritability, muscle tone, and color. Typically newborns achieving a score of 8 to 10 require only routine care. Infants with a score of 5 to 7 often require only tactile stimulation and high inspired oxygen concentration. The neonate with a score of 3 to 4 frequently requires immediate positive-pressure ventilation. The infant with an Apgar score of 0 to 2 requires immediate CPR.

Apgar scores are typically determined at 1 and 5 minutes after delivery. However, the decision to initiate newborn resuscitation should not be delayed until the 1-minute Apgar score is obtained. One must make an immediate assessment of the neonate's condition and begin appropriate measures. The American Heart Association recommends a decision tree, shown in Fig. 37-1, for the immediate care of the newborn.

Thermal Environment

The newborn is limited in its ability to maintain core temperature. Low birth weight infants are less able to maintain their thermal environment and may show the greatest drop in core temperature if measures are not employed to conserve heat.

The newborn has a large surface area to body mass ratio and thin skin. The premature infant has an even greater surface area to body mass ratio than the full-term infant and even thinner skin, making the preterm infant especially prone to excessive heat loss. Additionally, the thin skin of the preterm infant leads to excessive fluid losses.

In response to heat loss the infant employs cutaneous vasoconstriction and nonshivering thermogenesis. Nonshivering thermogenesis occurs in the brown adipose tissue. This process is adenosine triphosphate dependent and leads to a marked increase in the oxygen requirement, placing a further demand on the depressed neonate. The liberation of heat via this mechanism can lead to a metabolic acidosis, which may lead to an increase in pulmonary vascular resistance and subsequent revision to a transitional circulation.

The neonate should be immediately dried of amniotic fluid and placed under radiant warming lights. The lights should be servocontrolled to avoid burns to the infant. The infant should not be allowed to stay in contact with blankets wet with amniotic fluid since considerable heat loss can occur through the evaporative process.

Airway and Ventilation

The oropharynx should initially be suctioned at the time of delivery with a soft suction bulb device. Oropharyngeal suctioning and drying should be continued once the infant is placed under the radiant warming lights. After suctioning of the oropharynx the nares should be gently suctioned. Vigorous suctioning can lead to a delay in spontaneous respiration. Heart rate should be monitored since suctioning may lead to hypoxia or increased vagal tone, resulting in neonatal bradycardia.

If respiratory efforts remain ineffective or the heart rate remains less than 100 beats/min, positive-pressure ventilation with 100% oxygen should be initiated. Initially peak airway pressures may need to be as high as 25 to 50 cm H_2O to open the alveoli. If the infant does not begin regular respiration or maintains a heart rate less than 100 beats/min that is not increasing, or if the infant exhibits signs of airway obstruction after 30 seconds of positive pressure ventilation, it is recommended that tracheal intubation be considered (Fig. 37-1). In the premature infant, often a neutral head position is advantageous for intubation as opposed to a *sniffing position*. Once intubated, careful attention to breath sounds must be paid since small movements of the endotracheal tube or the patient's head may result in extubation or mainstem bronchial intubation. This is especially evident in the

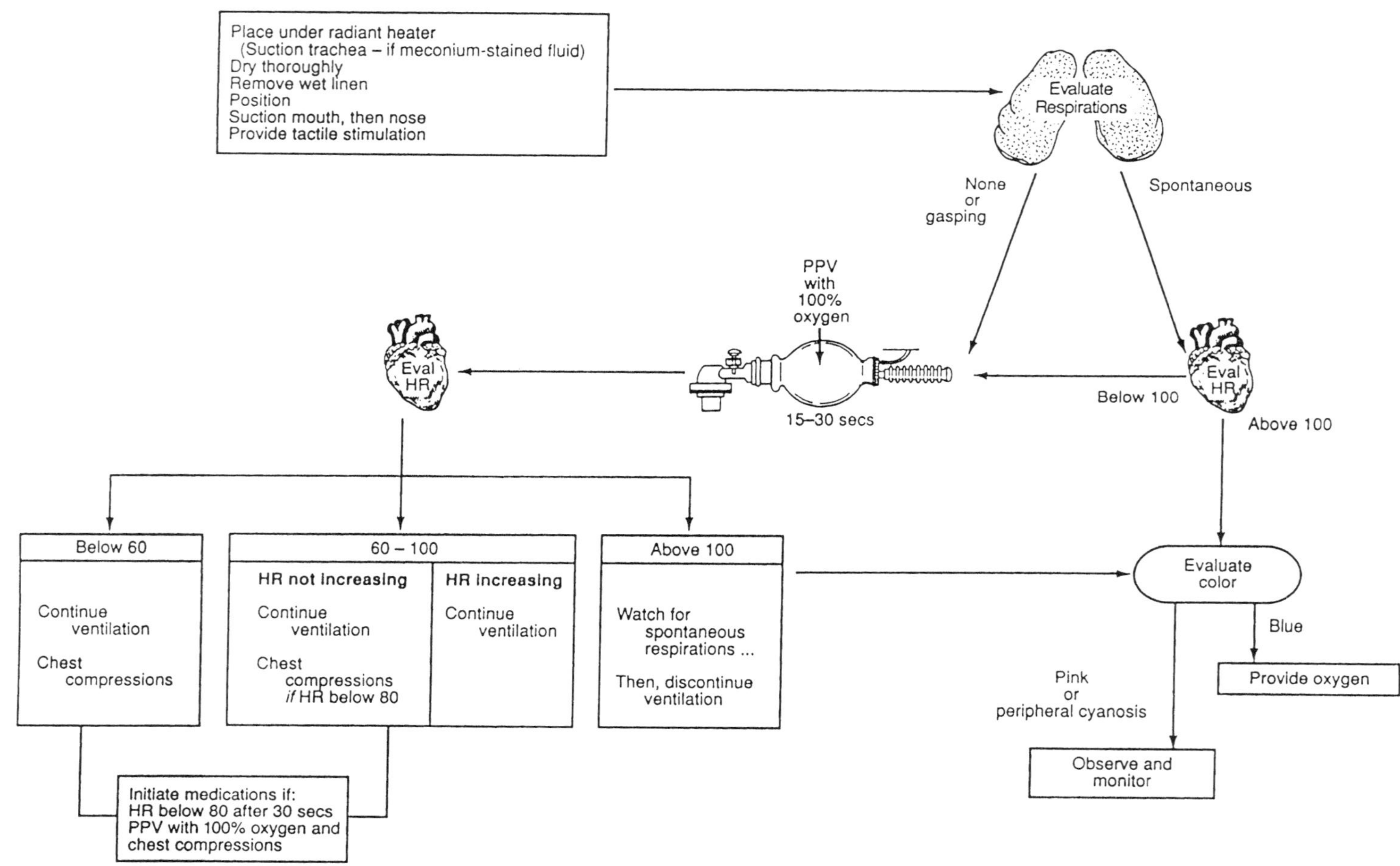

Fig. 37-1.
Overview of resuscitation in the delivery room. From *Textbook of Neonatal Resuscitation,* 1990, American Heart Association.

preterm infant whose carina-to-glottis distance may be less than 5 cm. In any infant suspected of having a diaphragmatic hernia, an endotracheal tube should be electively placed if ventilation is required, since mask ventilation can lead to air entering the bowel, thus further compromising respiration.

Meconium Aspiration: To Intubate or Not To Intubate?

The management of the newborn passed through meconium-stained fluid remains a clinical dilemma. The passage of meconium occurs in 10% to 15% of all deliveries[3] and has been thought to be a sign of fetal distress. Five percent of neonates born through meconium-stained fluid will develop meconium aspiration syndrome (MAS).[3] This syndrome causes much morbidity and mortality, with mortality estimates approaching 50%.[4] Therefore it is imperative that all safe and effective measures be employed, in the care of the newborn passed through meconium-stained fluid, to reduce the occurrence of MAS. However, on examination of the literature and clinical practice, it becomes evident that the care of the newborn passed through meconium-stained fluid is not a settled issue.

Some clinicians recommend an *aggressive* airway management strategy, suggesting tracheal suctioning to remove the meconium-stained fluid even in the vigorous infant.[4] Other clinicians recommend that airway management entail only that which permits oxygenation.[5]

A study by Murphy et al.[6] examined the pulmonary vasculature in infants with fatal MAS. In 10 of 11, the authors noted severe structural abnormal muscularization of the smallest intraacinar arteries. The authors concluded that these changes must have occurred before birth and that the persistent pulmonary hypertension associated with the fatal MAS may be a result of these changes in the pulmonary musculature and not a result of pulmonary vasospasm.

In a study by Falciglia et al.[7] examining suctioning of the neonate before and after delivery of the chest, the authors concluded that MAS is an intrauterine event not affected by the timing of suctioning. They do note that DeLee suctioning should not be abandoned, for it may decrease the severity of MAS in infants destined to develop the syndrome.

Tyson[8] has reviewed the literature on MAS. He concludes that routine delivery room intubation and suctioning may be morbidity producing, leading to airway trauma, stridor, hypoxia, and bradycardia. The author recommends against tracheal suctioning of the vigorous infant in the presence of meconium-stained fluid, but reserves the procedure for the depressed infant with meconium in the pharynx.

In a large retrospective study by Wiswell et al.[4] over 5600 liveborn neonates were examined of whom 31% had meconium-stained fluid, of whom 82% were intubated and suctioned in the delivery room. The authors emphasize that a significantly high number of neonates who were not intubated and suctioned, who then developed MAS, required longer periods of ventilation, had higher incidence of pneumothoracies, had higher morbidity, and had a higher incidence of requiring extracorporeal membrane oxygenation (ECMO) than those who developed MAS but were intubated and suctioned.

Wiswell et al[4] concluded that intubation and suctioning in the delivery room has a low incidence of complications. In fact, the authors reported no complications of hoarseness, stridor, laryngospasm, or persistent bradycardia in the 608 neonates intubated in the delivery room in their study population. They also state that a substantial number of neonates who developed MAS were not depressed at birth. A small number of the neonates, who were in the group of vigorous, normal-appearing infants passed through meconium stained fluid, went on to develop MAS. Additionally, they concluded that those who develop MAS, but were not intubated and suctioned, may be at higher risk. It is based on these and other findings that the authors believe that a selective approach should not be used in the management of the neonate passed through meconium-stained fluid.

It should be clear from the above studies and conclusions that the management of the neonate passed through meconium-stained fluid remains controversial.

The AHA[1] recommends that for the neonate exposed to thin or watery meconium (nonparticulate) probably no special management is needed. They recommend for the neonate exposed to thick (pea soup, particulate) meconium, that as soon as the baby's head is delivered, a 10-Fr catheter or larger should be used to thoroughly suction the mouth, pharynx, and nose. As soon as the infant is placed under the warmer and before drying, residual meconium in the hypopharynx should be removed by suctioning under direct vision, and the trachea then should be intubated and suctioned. They also recommend repeated intubation and suctioning until returns are nearly free of meconium.

It is essential to have a member of the newborn care team monitor the neonate's heart rate during intubation and suctioning. An oxygen source may be placed near the infants mouth during the intubation and suctioning. Gastric emptying should be done to help eliminate any meconium-containing gastric contents that could potentially be aspirated. Gastric emptying should be delayed until the infant is at least 5 minutes of age, if possible, to avoid a vagal response leading to apnea and bradycardia.[1]

High-frequency ventilation and ECMO have been used in the treatment of MAS.

In animal models, lung injury by a variety of causes has led to surfactant inactivation. Investigators have raised the issue that fatty acid injury with surfactant inactivation may play a role in MAS. This information is cited by Austen et al.[9] in their investigation of whether surfactant supplementation may be of benefit to the infant with MAS. Full-term infants having respiratory failure associated with pneumonia or MAS were treated with intratracheal calf surfactant. None of the treated infants required ECMO, had tension pneumothoracies after entry into the study, required oxygen supplementation for more than 14 days, or required oxygen at discharge, and none died. Austen et al. conclude that surfactant supplementation may be of benefit for newborns with respiratory failure due to MAS.

Circulation

The AHA[1] recommends that chest compressions be initiated if, after 15 to 30 seconds of positive-pressure ventilation with 100% oxygen, the heart rate is less than 60 or between 60 and 80 beats/min and is not increasing (Fig. 37-1). Chest compressions must always be accompanied by ventilation with 100% oxygen. The AHA recommends beginning medications if the heart rate is below 80 beats/min after 30 seconds of positive-pressure ventilation with 100% oxygen and chest compressions.

Neonatal Pharmacology

Pharmacologic resuscitation of the premature newborn gives the caregiver many unique challenges. Anatomic and physiologic differences between the neonate and older children and adults are multiple and complex. The neonate's fluid-filled lungs, propensity to revert to a transitional circulation, and drug volume of distribution play important roles in the resuscitation. These distinctions, coupled with etiologic differences for requiring resuscitation, make for a challenging resuscitation effort, especially when one bases their plan solely on adult CPR and ACLS protocols.

This section presents the AHA recommendations from their *Textbook of Neonatal Resuscitation.*[1] Focus then is placed on the recent studies and recommendations made by the Emergency Care Panel for Neonatal Pharmacology to the panel of Emergency

Care Committee, as analyzed by Burchfield et al.[10]

The AHA recommends initiating medication use under specific conditions, as depicted in Fig. 37-2. The AHA-recommended dosage schedules are seen in Table 37-1. No longer does the AHA recommend atropine or calcium in the acute phase of neonatal resuscitation. Dopamine is suggested after prolonged resuscitation with an infant in shock failing to respond to the protocol in Fig. 37-2. Naloxone may be given at any time respiratory depression is suspected from maternal narcotic administration in the resuscitative effort.

Recently much attention has been focused on the use of high-dose epinephrine administration during resuscitation.[11-18] As Burchfield et al.[10] point out, resuscitative doses for the newborn frequently have been extrapolated from adult guidelines, without scientific analysis. As is also mentioned, the terminal cardiac activity of the neonate usually is a bradydysrhythmia, as opposed to the more frequently seen ventricular fibrillation in the adult population requiring resuscitation.

Adult studies of patients in ventricular fibrillation,[11-12] have demonstrated benefit from epinephrine doses up to 0.2 mg/kg. Extending this dose to the neonatal resuscitation is of theoretical concern, since most dysrhythmias in the immediate neonatal period are bradydysrhythmias, which may not benefit from high-dose epinephrine. Additionally, concern exists of creating a hemodynamic course of hypotension followed by hypertension, since in animal neonatal models this sequence has been associated with intraventricular hemorrhage. However, Goetting et al.[19,20] demonstrated benefit in using high-dose epinephrine in children with bradydysrhythmias who did not respond adequately to smaller doses of epinephrine.

Burchfield et al.[10] note that the "epinephrine dosage was recommended to remain at 10-30 μg/kg for the first and subsequent doses administered by either the IV or endotracheal routes." This decision was partly based on the lack of scientific studies in the neonate with high-dose epinephrine and the concern with using a drug in high dose that may have a low therapeutic index in the neonate.

The majority of panelists recommended sodium bicarbonate for prolonged resuscitation when the infant does not respond adequately to other measures. This was not a unanimous recommendation, with some panelists suggesting the elimination of sodium bicarbonate due to the lack of proven scientific benefit and the fact that some animal studies showed detrimental effects.[10,21]

The panelists now recommend volume expansion "when there is strong suspicion of hypovolemia unresponsive to other resuscitative efforts." The dose of naloxone was recommended to be 0.1 mg/kg, which is in agreement with the AHA recommendations.[1] Also in agreement with the AHA is that calcium and atropine are not recommended in the delivery room resuscitation.

The authors[10] raised the issue of the effect on drug delivery via an endotracheal tube in the neonate who possibly has fluid-filled lungs, small pulmonary surface to body ratio, and right-to-left intracardiac shunting at the foramen ovale and ductus arteriosus. No definitive consensus was presented as to whether pulmonary absorption and delivery would be negatively or positively affected. The AHA[1] recommends that if medication is given via the endotracheal tube, it should be immediately followed by positive-pressure ventilation to distribute the drug

Special Considerations

Tocolytics

To prevent delivery of premature infants, tocolytic therapy has been employed. Trials of tocolytic agents have had inconsistent results. A recent study[22] showed a decrease in morbidity in the group of infants of mothers who received ritodrine. How-

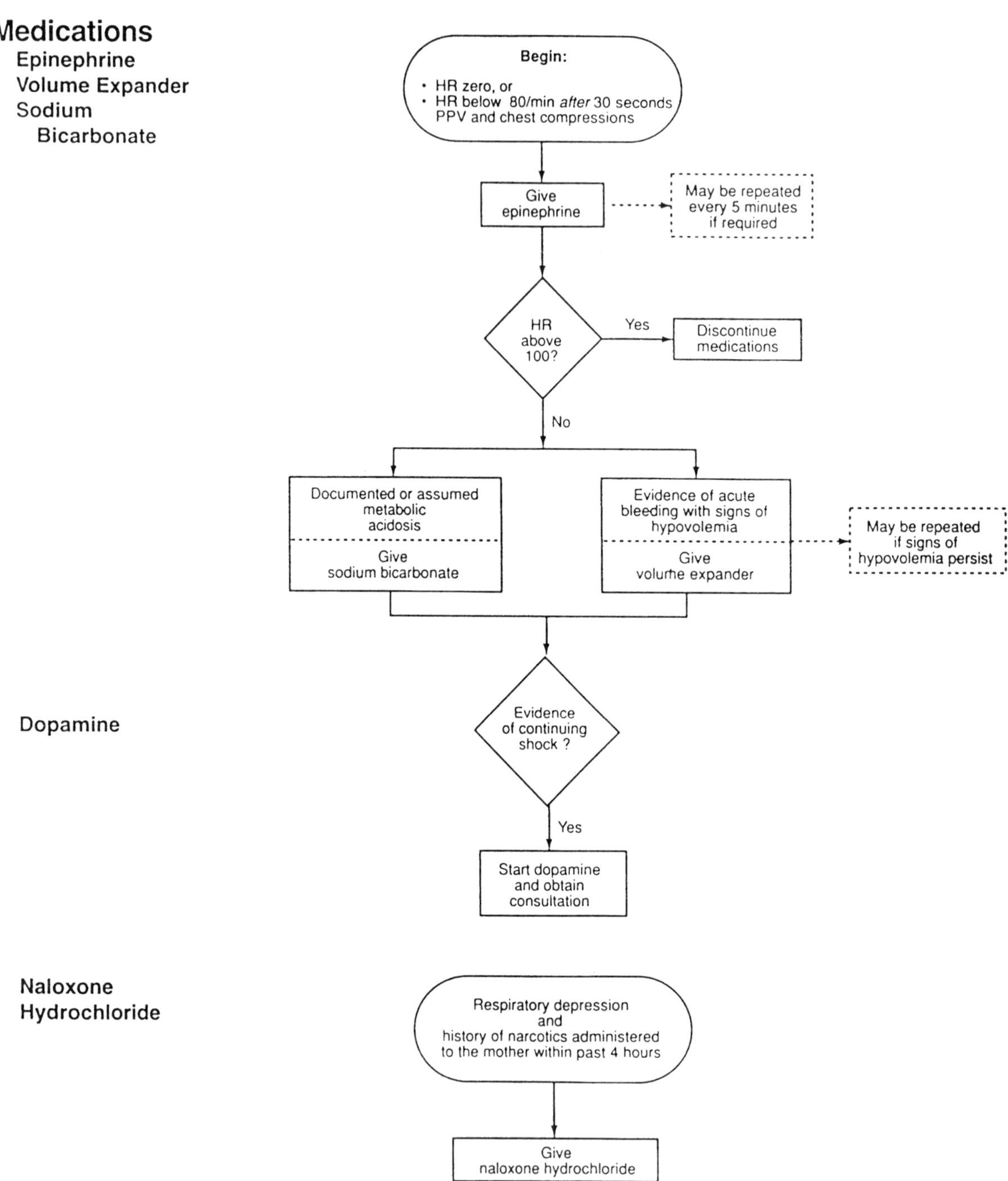

Fig. 37-2.

Key points related to the use of medications during neonatal resuscitation. *From* Textbook of Neonatal Resuscitation, *1990, American Heart Association.*

TABLE 37-1

Medications for Neonatal Resuscitation

Medication	Concentration to Administer	Preparation	Dosage/ Route	Total Dose/Infant			Rate/ Precautions
Epinephrine	1:10,000	1 ml	0.1-0.3 ml/kg IV or ET	weight		total ml	Give rapidly
				1 kg		0.1-0.3 ml	
				2 kg		0.2-0.6 ml	
				3 kg		0.3-0.9 ml	
				4 kg		0.4-1.2 ml	
Volume expanders	Whole blood 5% Albumin Normal saline Ringer's lactate	40 ml	10 ml/kg IV	weight		total ml	Give over 5-10 min
				1 kg		10 ml	
				2 kg		20 ml	
				3 kg		30 ml	
				4 kg		40 ml	
Sodium bicarbonate	0.5 mEq/ml (4.2% solution)	20 ml or two 10-ml prefilled syringes	2 mEq/kg IV	weight	total dose	total ml	Give *slowly,* over at least 2 min Give only if infant being effectively ventilated
				1 kg	2 mEq	4 ml	
				2 kg	4 mEq	8 ml	
				3 kg	6 mEq	12 ml	
				4 kg	8 mEq	16 ml	
Naloxone	0.4 mg/ml	1 ml	0.1 mg/kg (0.25 ml/kg) IV, ET IM, SQ	weight	total dose	total ml	Give rapidly IV, ET preferred IM, SQ acceptable
				1 kg	0.1 mg	0.25 ml	
				2 kg	0.2 mg	0.50 ml	
				3 kg	0.3 mg	0.75 ml	
				4 kg	0.4 mg	1.00 ml	
	1.0 mg/ml	1 ml	0.1 mg/kg (0.1 ml/kg) IV, ET IM, SQ	1 kg	0.1 mg	0.1 ml	
				2 kg	0.2 mg	0.2 ml	
				3 kg	0.3 mg	0.3 ml	
				4 kg	0.4 mg	0.4 ml	
Dopamine	$\frac{6 \times \text{weight (kg)} \times \text{desired dose } (\mu g/kg/min)}{\text{desired fluid (ml/hr)}}$ =	mg of dopamine per 100 ml of solution	Begin at 5 μg/kg/min (may increase to 20 μg/kg/min if necessary) IV	weight	total μg/min		Give as a continuous infusion using an infusion pump Monitor HR and BP closely Seek consultation
				1 kg	5-20 μg/min		
				2 kg	10-40 μg/min		
				3 kg	15-60 μg/min		
				4 kg	20-80 μg/min		

IM, Intramuscular; ET, endotracheal; IV, intravenous; SQ, subcutaneous; HR, heart rate; BP, blood pressure.
From *Textbook of Neonatal Resuscitation,* 1990, American Heart Association.

ever, tocolytic therapy may not be without risk to the developing fetus. Another recent study[23] demonstrated that antenatal indomethacin therapy for preterm labor appears to have increased the risk of necrotizing enterocolitis, intracranial hemorrhage, and patent ductus arteriosus in infants born at or before 30 weeks' gestational age.

Terbutaline was administered to the mother in our case discussion. This agent can be given intramuscularly, orally, or subcutaneously. There are numerous maternal side effects of terbutaline therapy, which include hyperglycemia, hypokalemia, lactic acidosis, hypotension, tachycardia, pulmonary edema, congestive heart failure, and dysrhythmias. The mother also may experience nausea, vomiting, headache, and nervousness. The neonatal side effects of maternally administered terbutaline include tachycardia, fetal hyperglycemia, rebound fetal hypoglycemia, hypokalemia, and hypotension. Fetal asphyxia also has been reported in response to maternally induced hypotension or increased uterine vascular resistance.

Surfactant Therapy

Fetal Surfactant Therapy and Maternal Corticosteroid Therapy

Avery and Mead reported in 1959 that in preterm infants with RDS, lung extracts did not possess the same low surface tension characteristics as that of normal lungs.[24] This was attributed to a deficiency of surfactant. Pulmonary surfactant functions by lowering surface tension, and possesses the ability of rapidly forming a monolayer in the actively respiring lung.[25] Surfactant also may possess an immune function.[26]

Numerous studies since Avery and Mead's initial work have demonstrated significant reductions in morbidity and mortality by the intratracheal administration of animal and synthetic surfactant.

Surfactant therapy initially focused on treating patients with RDS. Alternatively, surfactant therapy now can be used in the delivery room for patients at risk of developing RDS.

The parturient in our case discussion received a 3-day course of steroid therapy to mature the fetal lungs in anticipation of failed tocolysis. Maternal corticosteroid therapy has been shown to significantly decrease morbidity and RDS by about 50% in premature infants at risk of these complications.[27] Maternal corticosteroid use has been shown to also decrease the incidence of patent ductus arteriosus, intraventricular hemorrhage, and necrotizing enterocolitis. In studies of both sheep and rabbits, the effects of prenatal corticosteroid therapy and postnatal surfactant therapy were additive.[28] Jobe et al[28] evaluated the interaction of maternal corticosteroid use and neonatal surfactant therapy (beractant [Survanta]), concluding that the combined use significantly improves neonatal outcome. They note that the combined therapy results in additive benefit in mean airway pressures, inspired oxygen concentration requirements, and alveolar-to-arterial oxygen ratios. The authors state that the combined use prevented deaths during their 28-day study period. Additionally, they note that the incidence of pulmonary hemorrhage was decreased in the combined-use group. This is very interesting since pulmonary hemorrhage is the only consistently noted adverse outcome directly related with surfactant therapy.

In the Brigham and Women's Hospital, all infants are initially resuscitated in the delivery room. They are then transported to the adjoining NICU. If surfactant therapy is deemed appropriate, the first dose is given in the NICU; surfactant is not administered in the delivery room. No clear benefit has been observed in infants treated with surfactant before breathing or before receiving mechanical ventilation versus being treated in the early postdelivery period.[28] Others have expressed concern that the instillation of large volumes of surfactant during immediate resusciative efforts actually may hinder the process of newborn resuscitation.

Other Measures in the Prophylaxis of Respiratory Distress Syndrome

In an extensive review of the literature, Soll and McQueen[25] did not recommend postnatal steroids, aminophylline, or digoxin in the prophylaxis against neonatal RDS. Interestingly, although not currently recommended by Soll and McQueen, they noted that inositol supplementation may have positive effects on survival in infants with respiratory distress syndrome, showing a decreased incidence of bronchopulmonary dysplasia and death at 28 days. Inositol is a six-carbon sugar alcohol found in breast milk. It has been shown to be a precursor of the phospholipid components of membranes and also may function as a second messenger.[29] Other research[30] also has shown that inositol was effective in promoting surfactant synthesis after steroid use.

Fetal Tracheal Intubation During Delivery

The importance of the establishment of an airway is paramount to successful neonatal care. Ultrasound now enables clinicians to diagnose potentially compromised airways in utero. Head and neck masses traditionally lead to high mortality owing to their effects on airway patency and securement. Two case reports of fetal tracheal intubation with intact uteroplacental circulation are described.[31] One patient was a 36-week-old fetus with a 8-cm by 10-cm neck mass. A cesarean section was performed under general endotracheal anesthesia. After the head was delivered through the incision, the child was intubated with some difficulty. The authors noted that during the intubation the fetal heart rate was 110 beats/min and a pulse oximiter probe on the ear lobe showed saturation readings between 78% and 82%. Apgar scores were 3, 5, and 8 at 1, 5, and 10 minutes, respectively. Umbilical vein blood gas was pH 7.40, with carbon dioxide partial pressure (P_{CO_2}) of 45 mm Hg and oxygen partial pressure (P_{O_2}) of 39 mm Hg.

The other child described was a 30-week-old fetus with a large pharyngeal mass. Under general endotracheal anesthesia, a hysterotomy was performed and the fetal head was delivered. A 10-cm by 10-cm epignathus teratoma was present. The child was intubated with much difficulty in about 5 minutes. Again, intact uteroplacental circulation was maintained during intubation. The authors reported a fetal heart rate of 100 to 120 beats/min during the intubation period. Apgar scores were 2 and 4 at 1 and 5 minutes, respectively. After volume resuscitation was begun, initial postductal arterial blood gas analysis showed a pH of 7.36, P_{CO_2} of 39 mm Hg and P_{O_2} of 136 mm Hg.

The authors discussed their preference for maternal general endotracheal anesthesia with halothane, noting that this offered them uterine relaxation and tocolysis. They also noted that halothane crosses the placenta and provided them with fetal anesthesia, which had the benefit of providing fetal immobility during tracheal intubation, but possibly had the negative effect of neonatal depression. The authors stated that regional anesthesia could have provided adequate maternal anesthesia, but they believed it would not offer adequate uterine relaxation, possibly leading to premature separation of the placenta. Additionally, maternal regional anesthesia would not have provided fetal skeletal muscle relaxation.

Thus the authors described two successful intubations of fetuses with large head and neck masses while maintaining intact uteroplacental circulation in parturients under general endotracheal anesthesia.

Inhaled Nitric Oxide Therapy

Nitric oxide (NO) usually is thought of as a toxic pollutant, being a component of automobile exhaust. Not until the late 1980s was NO realized to be a significant endothelium-derived relaxing factor.[32] Recently much attention has been focused on the possible roles that NO may play in mammals in both normal and disease states in the regulation of vascular tone.[33] NO has been implicated in septic shock.[34] NO also may function as a neurotransmitter.[35] Anesthesiologists have focused much attention on inhaled NO. Inhaled NO has great appeal since it is a selective pulmonary vasodilator that acts rapidly, is reversible, and has low toxicity in clinical doses without significant systemic effects. Many animal and human studies demonstrate rapid pulmonary vasodilation with clinically significant decreases in pulmonary artery pressure, pulmonary vascular resistance, and an increase in oxygen saturation with little or no change in mean arterial pressure and systemic vascular resistance.[36-38]

An excellent review of inhaled NO addresses work on the use of this agent for the treatment of persistent pulmonary hypertension of the newborn (PPHN).[33] Kinsella et al.[39] examined the effects of 10 to 20 ppm of inhaled NO on nine infants with the diagnosis of PPHN. Their results demonstrated increase in arterial Po_2, without a change in systemic blood pressure. All of the infants showed improvement. Six of the infants were gradually weaned from the inhaled NO and recovered without the need for extracorporeal membrane oxygenation. In a similar work by Roberts et al.[40] inhaled nitric oxide was used as a "bridge" to treat hypoxemia until ECMO could be established.

Inhaled NO in the treatment of PPHN appears to offer much promise. It will be exciting to see if significant reductions in morbidity and mortality will be achieved with this therapy.

Viability

When faced with the care of an extremely premature infant, many clinical, ethical, and social questions arise. It is beyond the scope or intent of this chapter to debate these issues, but for completeness a recent study by Allen et al.[41] will be discussed briefly that addressed 6-month survival and morbidity in 142 preterm infants born at 22 to 25 weeks' gestational age, who were all treated with surfactant at birth. Results of this study demonstrated that of 29 infants born at 22 weeks, none survived; of 40 infants born at 23 weeks, 6 survived; of 34 infants born at 24 weeks, 19 survived; and of 39 infants born at 25 weeks, 34 survived. Additionally, the study showed that the greater level of immaturity was associated with a higher incidence of neonatal complications. The authors also reported that of infants born at 23 weeks' gestational age, only 2% survived without severe central nervous system abnormalities. In an excellent editorial,[42] Hack and Fanaroff comment on the difficult ethical dilemma of aggressively resuscitating or not, the very premature newborn. Hack and Fanaroff[42] noted that the authors'[40] conclusions with regard to resuscitation were in accordance with the Fetus and Newborn Committee of the Canadian Pediatric Society, which recommends for infants born at 22 weeks or less having a birth weight of less than 500 g, only comfort care be given; for infants born at 23 to 24 weeks, a decision should be made based on the infant's condition at birth and the family views; whereas an infant born at 25 to 26 weeks should receive full resuscitative efforts.

Summary

1. The American Society of Anesthesiologist's Guideline VII for Regional Anesthesia in Obstetrics states that qualified personnel, other than the anesthesiologist attending to the mother, should be immediately available to assume responsibility for resuscitation of the newborn.
2. If the Anesthesiologist becomes involved with the care of the newborn, the infant should be placed under radiant warming

lights, dried thoroughly, suctioned orally, and given gentle tactile stimulation while assessing respiration and heart rate. If respirations are spontaneous, heart rate is above 100 beats/min, and color is pink, observation and routine monitoring are indicated. If color is blue, oxygen should be administered immediately. If respirations are not present or if ineffective gasping is occurring, the infant should be given positive-pressure ventilation with 100% oxygen for 15 to 30 seconds while heart rate is evaluated. If the heart rate is greater than 100 beats/min, the resuscitator should watch for spontaneous respirations. If the heart rate is 60 to 100 beats/min, but increasing, ventilation should be continued. If the heart rate is less than 60 or is 60 to 80 beats/min, but not increasing after 15 to 30 seconds of positive-pressure ventilation with 100% oxygen, then chest compressions should be initiated. For a heart rate less than 60 beats/min, chest compressions should be begun. (Notice that chest compressions always are accompanied by 100% oxygen.)

3. Epinephrine should be given for a heart rate of 0 or a heart rate of less than 80 beats/min after 30 seconds of positive-pressure ventilation with 100% oxygen and chest compressions. A dose of 0.1 to 0.3 ml/kg of epinephrine 1:10,000 should be rapidly given via the endotracheal tube or intravenous. This dose may be repeated every 5 minutes, if required.
4. The AHA no longer recommends atropine or calcium in the acute phase of neonatal resuscitation.
5. The AHA recommends dopamine after prolonged resuscitation in the infant in shock who is failing to respond to the protocol in Fig. 37-2.
6. The AHA recommends that naloxone be given in a dose of 0.1 mg/kg intravenously or via the endotracheal tube for respiratory depression and a history of narcotics administered to the mother within the last 4 hours. Intramuscular or subcutaneous naloxone also is acceptable.
7. Maternal terbutaline therapy can lead to neonatal tachycardia, hyperglycemia, rebound hypoglycemia, hypokalemia, and hypotension.

References

1. Leon Chameides, American Heart Association, American Academy of Pediatrics, Neonatal Resuscitation Steering Committee, editors: In *Textbook of Neonatal Resuscitation,* Dallas, 1990, American Heart Association.
2. Apgar V: A proposal for a new method of evaluation of the newborn infant, *Curr Res Anesth Analg* 1953; 32:260.
3. Wiswell TE, Henley MA: Intratracheal suctioning, systemic infection and the meconium aspiration syndrome, *Pediatrics* 1992; 89:203.
4. Wiswell TE, Tussle JM, Turner BS: Meconium aspiration syndrome: have we made a difference? *Pediatrics* 1990; 85:715.
5. Katz VL, Bowers WA: Meconium aspiration syndrome: reflections on a murky subject, *Am J Obstet Gynecol* 1992; 166:171.
6. Murphy JD, Vawter GF, Reid LM: Pulmonary vascular disease in fatal meconium aspiration, *J Pediatrics* 1984; 104:758.
7. Falciglia HS, Henderschott C, Potter P, et al: Does De Lee suction at the perineum prevent meconium aspiration syndrome? *Am J Obstet Gynecol* 1992; 167:1243.
8. Tyson JE: *Immediate care of the newborn infant.* In Sinclair JC, Bracken MB, editors: *Effective care of the newborn infant,* New York, 1992, Oxford University Press.
9. Auten RL, Notter RH, Kendig JW, et al: Surfactant treatment of full-term newborns with respiratory failure, *Pediatrics* 1991; 87:101.
10. Burchfield DJ, Berkowitz ID, Berg RA, et al: Medications in neonatal resuscitation, *Ann Emerg Med* 1993; 22:435.
11. Paradis NA, Martin GB, Rosenberg J, et al: The effects of standard and high dose epinephrine on coronary perfusion

pressure during prolonged cardiopulmonary resuscitation, *JAMA* 1991; 265:1139.
12. Gonzalez ER, Ornato JP, Garnett AR, et al: Dose-dependent vasopressor response to epinephrine during CPR in human beings, *Ann Emerg Med* 1989; 18:920.
13. Callaham M, Barton CW, Kayser S: Potential complications of high-dose epinephrine therapy in patients resuscitated from cardiac arrest, *JAMA* 1991; 265:1117.
14. Ornato JP: High-dose epinephrine during resuscitation: a word of caution, *JAMA* 1991; 265:1160.
15. Stiell IG, Herbert PC, Weitzman BN: High-dose epinephrine in adult cardiac arrest, *N Engl J Med* 1992; 327:1045.
16. Brown CG, Martin DR, Pepe PE: A comparison of standard-dose and high-dose epinephrine in cardiac arrest outside the hospital, *N Engl J Med* 1992; 327:1051.
17. Polin K, Leikin JB: High-dose epinephrine in cardiopulmonary resuscitation, *JAMA* 1993; 269:1383 (letter).
18. Callaham M: High-dose epinephrine in cardiopulmonary resuscitation, *JAMA* 1992; 269:1383 (letter).
19. Goetting MG, Paradis NA: High-dose epinephrine in refractory pediatric cardiac arrest, *Crit Care Med* 1989; 17:1258.
20. Goetting MG, Paradis NA: High-dose epinephrine improves outcome from pediatric cardiac arrest, *Ann Emerg Med* 1991; 20:22.
21. Hein HA: The use of sodium bicarbonate in neonatal resuscitation: help or harm? *Pediatrics* 1993; 91:496.
22. The Canadian Preterm Labor Investigators Group: Treatment of preterm labor with the beta-adrenergic agonist ritodrine, *N Engl J Med* 1993; 329:1602.
23. Norton ME, Merrill J, Cooper BA, et al: Neonatal complications after the administration of indomethacin for preterm labor, *N Engl J Med* 1993; 329:1602.
24. Avery ME, Mead J: Surface properties in relation to atelectasis and hyaline membrane disease, *Am J Dis Child* 1959; 97:517.
25. Soll RF, McQueen MC: *Respiratory distress syndrome.* In Sinclair JC, Bracken MB, editors: *Effective care of the newborn infant,* New York, 1992, Oxford University Press.
26. Jobe AH: Pulmonary surfactant therapy, *N Engl J Med* 1993; 328:861.
27. Crowley P, Chalmers I, Keirse M: The effects of corticosteroid administration before preterm delivery: an overview of the evidence from controlled trials, *Br J Obstet Gynaecol* 1990; 97:11.
28. Jobe AH, Mitchell BR, Gunkel JH: Beneficial effects of the combined use of prenatal corticosteroids and postnatal surfactant on preterm infants, *Am J Obstet Gynecol* 1993; 168:508.
29. Michell RH: Inositol phospholipids and cell surface receptor function, *Biochim Biophys Acta* 1975; 415:81.
30. Hallman M: Effect of extracellular myoinositol on surfactant phospholipid synthesis in the fetal rabbit lung, *Biochim Biophys Acta* 1984; 795:67.
31. Schulman SR, Jones BR, Slotnick N, et al: Fetal tracheal intubation with intact uteroplacental circulation, *Anesth Analgesia* 1993; 76:197.
32. Moncada S, Palmer RMJ, Higgs EA: Nitric oxide: physiology, pathophysiology, and pharmacology, *Pharmacol Rev* 1991; 43:109.
33. Pearl, RG: Inhaled nitric oxide: the past, the present, and the future, *Anesthesiology* 1993; 78:413.
34. Kilbourn RG, Jubran A, Gross SS, et al: Reversal of endotoxin-mediated shock by NG-methyl-L-arginine, an inhibitor of nitric oxide synthesis, *Biochem Biophys Res Commun* 1990; 172:1132.
35. Snyder SH, Bredt DS: Biological roles of nitric oxide, *Sci Am* 1992; 266:62.
36. Frostell CG, Blomquist H, Hedenstierna G: Inhaled nitric oxide selectively reverses human hypoxic pulmonary vasoconstriction without causing systemic vasodilation, *Anesthesiology* 1993; 78:427.
37. Sellden H, Winberg P, Gustafsson LE, et al: Inhalation of nitric oxide-reduced pulmonary hypertension after cardiac surgery in a 3.2-kg infant, *Anesthesiology* 1993; 78:577.
38. Girard C, Lehot JJ, Pannetier JC, et al: Inhaled nitric oxide after mitral valve replacement in patients with chronic pulmonary artery hypertension, *Anesthesiology* 1992; 77:880.
39. Kinsella JP, Neish SR, Sheffer E, et al: Low-dose inhalational nitric oxide in persistent pulmonary hypertension of the newborn, *Lancet* 1992; 340:819.
40. Roberts JD, Polaner DM, Lang P, et al: Inhaled nitric oxide in persistent pulmonary hypertension of the newborn, *Lancet* 1992; 340:818.
41. Allen MC, Donohue PK, Dusman AE: The limit of viability: neonatal outcome of infants born at 22 to 25 weeks gestation, *N Engl J Med* 1993; 329:1597.
42. Hack MH, Fanaroff AA: Outcomes of extremely immature infants: a perinatal dilemma, *N Engl J Med* 1993; 329:1649.

38

Non-Obstetric Surgery during Pregnancy

A 26-year-old primigravida is admitted to the hospital with acute abdominal pain in the right lower quadrant. Exploratory laparotomy is advised. Discuss the anesthetic management as if the gestation were 6 weeks, 14 weeks, 24 weeks, and 37 weeks.

Recommendations by Norman Blass, M.D.

Normally, when one thinks of surgery in the pregnant patient, it is in the context of anesthesia for labor, delivery, and cesarean section. Acute appendicitis during gestation is relatively uncommon, but is the most performed extrauterine indication for laparotomy during pregnancy. The incidence of this disease in pregnancy is about 1 in 800 to 1 in 2000.[1]

The treatment of suspected acute appendicitis is immediate surgery. The most important component of management in the gravida is early diagnosis. Treatment must not be delayed because of the increased maternal and fetal morbidity and mortality that can occur with appendiceal perforation in the parturient.[2]

It is very important for an anesthesiologist to realize that anesthetics administered to a pregnant patient may cause special problems. Maternal safety must be assured and teratogenicity, intrauterine fetal asphyxia, and fetal wastage avoided. However, with an understanding of maternal-fetal physiology, the potential adverse effects of drugs administered, and the consequences of the surgical procedure performed, reasonable recommendations can be made for giving anesthesia to a pregnant patient at any gestational age.

Maternal Safety

Maternal safety depends a great deal on the physiologic changes that occur during pregnancy.

These changes influence anesthetic and surgical management.

Cardiovascular Alterations

Anatomically, the gradual elevation of the diaphragm causes the heart to be pushed upward and forward, yielding left-axis shift and the positioning of the apical beat to the fourth intercostal space. Usually there are no Q waves in lead AVF and it is common for the T wave to be flattened or inverted in lead III. (This is not evidence of myocardial ischemia.[3])

Murmurs are ordinarily *physiologic,* but must be distinguished from early cardiac disease. Systolic murmurs usually are *ejection murmurs* and are believed to arise from an increase in the patient's stroke volume.[4] The heart rhythm may be irregular and both atrial and ventricular premature *beats* are common.[5]

An important aspect of cardiovascular change during gestation is an increase in cardiac output. This rise is achieved early in pregnancy (first 10 weeks) and reaches 30% to 40% above the nonpregnant state by the end of the first trimester. The highest level is reached between the twentieth and twenty-fourth weeks of pregnancy. The heart rate increases by about 15 beats/min. Although the general understanding is that stroke volume increases, determined from simultaneous measurements of cardiac output and rate, the rapid rate changes that occur may alter the average stroke volume from what was previously perceived. Of note is that pregnant women with artificial pacemakers, which give a fixed rate, undergo pregnancy with no apparent problems.[6]

Relatively little change occurs in systolic blood pressure during normal gestation, but a reduction in diastolic pressure does begin about the early part of the second trimester. This pressure does not return to the prepregnancy level until the thirty-sixth week of gestation. Thus pulse pressure is highest in the midtrimester.

The position that the gravida assumes has a profound effect on her blood pressure. If a pregnant patient lies on her back during the second half of gestation, the weight of the uterus not only may compress her inferior vena cava, causing significant hypotension, but may also compress the abdominal aorta. This compression is evidenced by the femoral pressure being lower than the brachial artery pressure. The potential for aortocaval compression, plus sympathetic blockade from epidural or spinal anesthesia, may reduce maternal cardiac output and fetal perfusion very rapidly. To prevent the hypotension this situation can produce, preinduction fluid boluses, left uterine displacement, and the judicious use of ephedrine should be used.

Essentially there are no valves between the femoral veins and the heart, and when a pregnant woman lies supine there is no real difference in pressure between these veins and the right atrium. Pregnancy produces a definite increase in femoral venous pressure, whereas the atrial pressure does not change. Consequently there must be an obstruction between these veins and the heart when the patient lies down. The weight of the enlarged uterus on the inferior vena cava, the pressure of the fetal presenting part on the iliac veins, and a high-pressure venous return from the uterine veins causing *back pressure* below their inflow are all possible causes.[7]

Venous return, via the azygos and epidural veins, is increased, causing the size of the epidural space to be reduced. Consequently the volume of local anesthetic needed for a given level of anesthesia is reduced and increases the possibility of getting a *bloody tap* epidural. In addition, as it passes out intervertebral foramen, each spinal nerve root is accompanied by an epidural vein which, being engorged, will decrease the size of the opening. The decrease in the size of the epidural space and the blockage of the intervertebral foramen may explain the one-third decrease in the amount of local anesthetic required to produce a given level of epidural block in the parturient compared with the nonpregnant patient.

All clotting factors—fibrinogen, platelets, and factors V, VI, and VIII—increase throughout pregnancy. A concomitant progressive decrease in fibrinolytic activity occurs as the gestation advances. These changes increase the risk of thromboembolic phenomena during pregnancy and the puerperium.

Blood volume increases about 30% to 40% (1500 ml) by the thirtieth to thirty-fourth weeks. Both the plasma and cellular elements increase, but the hematocrit decreases because the increase in plasma volume is greater.[8]

The leucocyte count rises so that white counts of 15,000 to 16,000 are not unusual. However, there is no *shift to the left* in the normal gravida.[9]

Respiratory Alterations

The respiratory system undergoes anatomic and functional changes. Anatomically, a relatively short neck and larger breasts may make laryngoscopy and intubation difficult. Edema and congestion of the mucosa of the upper airway may cause obstruction and necessitate the use of a no. 7 or no. 7.5 endotracheal tube. The increased vascularity of the lining of the respiratory tract can cause profuse bleeding after instrumentation (especially from the nose or pharynx).

The subcostal angle can increase to more than 100° and diaphragmatic excursion increases to approximately 6 cm at term. The diaphragm is not *splinted* by the enlarging uterus; thus its resting level is 4 cm higher at the end of gestation. However, the transverse diameter of the thoracic cage compensates for this by increasing up to 2 cm. Far from being less effective, the diaphragm is the major contributor to respiration because the relaxed abdominal musculature is of lessened importance.[10]

During gestation, tidal volume rises from the prepregnancy rate of 500 ml/min to about 700 ml/min, an increase of about 40%. The respiratory rate ordinarily persists at 15 breaths/min, allowing a rise in minute volume from 7 L/min to 10 L/min, an increase of 40% at term.

As the pregnancy approaches term, the expiratory reserve volume decreases from 1300 to 1100 ml. The residual volume declines from 1500 to 1200 ml, thus reducing the functional residual capacity (FRC) about 500 ml (20%).[11] The decline in these parameters are slow and progressive. Airway closure during tidal ventilation may occur in 50% of parturients in the supine position, since FRC impinges on closing volume. FRC decreases still further in certain conditions such as obesity, general anesthesia, and the Trendelenburg position. Closing volume increases with age, smoking, and preexisting lung disease, and these factors may contribute to the development of atelectasis postoperatively.[12]

These changes in lung volumes, ventilation, and maternal hyperventilation alters the gravida's blood gases. Hyperventilation peaks by the second trimester and produces a partially compensated respiratory alkalosis (arterial oxygen pressure [Pao_2] = 100 to 105 torr, arterial carbon dioxide pressure [$Paco_2$ = 30 to 32 torr, pH = 7.45, HCO_3 = 21). This respiratory alkalosis will also move the oxygen-hemoglobin dissociation curve to the left (P50 reduced), so there is impairment of oxygen release to the tissues, including the placenta. Oxygen consumption rises significantly by midpregnancy due to the enlarging placenta, fetus, and uterus.[13]

Because of these respiratory changes, hypoxia and hypercapnia may develop very rapidly when the parturient encounters prolonged apnea subsequent to a difficult intubation or if the patient should inspire an inadequate oxygen mixture. Preoxygenation for 3 to 4 minutes should precede induction of general anesthesia and intubation should be rapid and smooth. If time does not permit preoxygenation, then four deep breaths of oxygen should be administered.

The minimum alveolar concentration (MAC) for halothane is 25% less than in the nonpregnant state and the MAC for isoflurane is about 44% less. There is less dilution of inspired gases so that induction with, and emergence from, anesthetic gases and volatile agents is more rapid.[14]

Renal Alterations

Changes in renal blood flow are similar to the alterations in cardiac output. Maximum flow is apparently reached by the end of the second trimester and is maintained until term with little alteration produced by position changes. Increases of 50% to 80% above the nonpregnant state can be expected.

The glomerular filtration rate (GFR) has a biphasic change during gestation, with an increase to 125 ml/min by 25 weeks and a subsequent slight decrease at about 38 weeks. These renal modifications are not maternal responses to fetal demand because the maximal changes occur in the first trimester when fetal metabolic requirements are minimal. In addition, the GFR does not increase at term, when the fetus is at its largest size.[15]

In the nonpregnant patient, renin acts on the substrate angiotensinogen formed in the liver to produce angiotensin I, then angiotensin II, a vasoconstricting agent. In normal gestation, the amount of circulating renin starts to rise early in the first trimester and increases progressively until term. Concentrations of angiotensinogen and angiotensin increase as the pregnancy continues, but vasoconstriction and blood pressure elevations do not occur. Parturients are resistant to angiotensin from the tenth week of gestation. There is minimal transfer of renin or angiotensin to the fetus via the placenta.

Estrogen causes an increase in renin substrate. Progesterone, a natriuretic compound, produces a relative hyponatremia, thus stimulating the renin-angiotensin system. It is paradoxical that pregnancy is characterized by high renin-angiotensin and aldosterone levels, expansion of blood volume, and increased renal blood flow. An explanation for this phenomenon is an apparent decrease in sensitivity to angiotensin during pregnancy.[16]

Because renal blood flow and the GFR increase during pregnancy, serum levels of uric acid, creatinine, and blood urea nitrogen are considerably reduced during pregnancy; what would be regarded as *normal* levels of these chemistries may indicate renal insufficiency. Renal threshold for glucose diminishes and tubular reabsorption may not keep pace with the increase in GFR, so glycosuria is common.

Gastrointestinal Alterations

Progesterone decreases gastrointestinal motility and the sphincter tone of the gastroesophageal junction. Acidity and gastric volume both are increased during pregnancy, which makes parturients more likely to have vomiting, regurgitation, and potential aspiration during general anesthesia. This phenomenon may occur as early as the twentieth week of gestation. There is also an increased incidence of hiatal hernia during pregnancy.[17]

All gravidas, from about the twentieth week of gestation, are considered to have full stomachs. It is of utmost importance in the anesthetic management of pregnant women that the airway be protected by means of a cuffed endotracheal tube inserted with rapid sequence induction and applied cricoid pressure. The acidity of the gastric secretions can be reduced satisfactorily by giving the parturient a clear antacid and an H_2-blocker before induction of anesthesia.

Endocrine Alterations

Endocrine abnormalities are difficult to detect during pregnancy since many of the normal physiologic changes mimic disease states (particularly hypothyroidism and hyperthyroidism). The parturient usually is euthyroid, although the basal metabolic rate, protein-bound iodine, and thyroid size all increase. Endorphins rise during pregnancy and may alter the pregnant patient's need for narcotic pain relief, particularly when close to term.[18]

Pregnancy is associated with hyperplasia of the β-cells of the islets of Langerhans. They secrete more insulin and are more sensitive to glucose than those of nonpregnant women. Despite this hyperinsulinemia, the disposal of glucose is impaired, resulting in higher circulating levels and contributing to the diabetogenic nature of pregnancy.[19]

Hepatic Alterations

Bilirubin is unaltered, but aspartine transferase (AST), alanine aminotransferase (ALT), alkaline phosphatase, and cholesterol are slightly elevated during pregnancy. Bromsulphthaein excretion often is reduced. Of interest to anesthesiologists, although relatively unimportant clinically, is the 28% decrease in plasma cholinesterase that occurs from early in gestation to 1 week or more after delivery.[20] As with any general anesthetic, the monitoring of neuromuscular blockade with a peripheral nerve stimulator is indicated.

Fetal Safety

It is of vital importance to the patient, obstetrician, surgeon, and anesthesiologist that there be minimal to no untoward effects of medications and anesthetics to the development or growth of the fetus.

It is estimated that 9% to 10% of birth defects are the result of maternal exposure to exogenous agents.[21] Classic teratology has been defined as the study of grossly visible congenital malformations induced during organogenesis by exogenous agents. A more modern definition is "any exogenous agent, chemical or physical, that can produce a permanent abnormality of structure or function in an organism that is exposed during embryonic or fetal life."[22] Therefore functional deficits, including behavioral difficulties, are included.

Not every pregnant woman who is exposed to even a proven teratogen faces any problems. The susceptibility to teratogens varies with the developmental stage of the fetus at the time of the exposure. Before or during early implantation, teratogenicity leads to abortion. Further along during the gestational period, malformations, growth retardation, functional deficiency, or even fetal death may occur.

Many factors must be considered to accurately determine the significance of a parturient's exposure to any potential teratogenetic agent. Factors that influence the potential for the development of abnormalities are as follows:[22]

1. Genetic factors
2. Nature of the agent
3. Dosage of the agent
4. Access to the fetus
5. Fetal development stage: the peak period of susceptibility in the human is from the fifteenth through the thirtieth days after conception, declining to the ninetieth day. This is the time of organogenesis.

Statistics concerning the teratogenetic role of anesthetics are not incontrovertible. There is no evidence of increased toxicity to the mother that can be attributed to anesthesia, and there is no evidence of such effect on the human fetus. Surveys of the number of pregnant women who undergo surgery are fraught with inaccurate figures. It is variously reported that about 70,000 pregnant women undergo nonobstetric surgery each year.[23]

In the clinical situation, separating the effects of

anesthesia from the effects of the surgery may prove difficult. It is known that reproductive malfunction, such as abortion and prematurity, is high during gestation (5.5% to 35%)[24] when surgery is performed on gravidas. There is no proof that this pertains to teratogenicity. It is likely that this wastage can be attributed to the procedure that is being performed (such as handling the peritoneum, manipulation of the uterus, etc.).

To determine the safety of anesthetics with regard to fetal development, most studies have focused on animal investigations. The applicability of animal data to humans is suspect, but cannot be ignored. It must be understood that in animal studies, the concentrations of anesthetic drugs and the duration of exposure are far in excess of those used in clinical situations.

Nitrous oxide apparently causes a decrease in the synthesis of methionine synthetase, an enzyme used in the formation of DNA. It has been postulated that this could interfere with morphologic fetal growth, especially during the time of rapid fetal growth and development, and therefore that nitrous oxide should be avoided during gestation, particularly during the first half of pregnancy. It has been shown, however, that there were no significant effects on plasma methionine after administering 60% to 70% nitrous oxide up to 4 hours in a clinical setting.[25] More research is needed in humans before a definitive statement can be made as to the use of nitrous oxide during pregnancy. Interestingly, these untoward effects can be reduced or prevented with the concomitant administration of halothane or isoflurane.

The volatile halogenated hydrocarbon anesthetics have been variously reported to produce fetal wastage and neonatal morphologic changes in several species of animals. The concentration of the anesthetic, the chronicity of application, and the time during gestation when given contribute to the deleterious effect achieved. It does appear that a single administration of a volatile agent for a surgical procedure does not compromise the fetus with regard to teratogenicity. No morphologic neonatal effects have occurred in the human that could in any way be ascribed to an anesthetic agent.[26]

Local anesthetics have not been implicated in producing morphologic defects in laboratory animals, but cytotoxic effects of certain local anesthetics on hamster lung fibroblasts have been described.[27]

Investigators have studied the effects of exposure of operating room personnel to trace levels of gases on fertility, fetal loss, and mutagenic changes, even though this is not directly related to maternal and fetal problems during surgery. When studies were done before operating room scavenging systems were used, average concentrations were found in the region of anesthetic machine popoff valves of halothane of 10 ppm and of nitrous oxide of 500 ppm. With the use of good scavenging systems and control of leakage from the anesthetic machine, these figures have been dramatically lowered.[28]

Studies concerning the relationship between anesthetic exposure while working in the operating suite and eventual reproductive outcome have been hampered by flawed design, poor controls, or problems with data collection. A frequent finding in many of these epidemiologic studies was that pregnant operating room personnel who were exposed to anesthetic gases while working in the operating suite had a rate of spontaneous abortion twice that of nonexposed women. A 1971 study from Stanford that addressed the incidence of abortions and fetal anomalies in dentists and their female aides revealed a dose-related increase in the number of abortions in the assistants and in the dentists' wives.[29]

In 1985 investigators examined six surveys and concluded that chronic exposure to trace gases in the operating suite predisposed to an increased rate of abortion. Their statement regarding congenital anomalies was much less consistent with any definitive outcome. However, a report from a Swedish survey, also done in 1985, concluded that "work in anesthesiology or operating rooms had no effect on the incidence of hospitalization for miscarriage, perinatal death, or malformations detected in the neonatal period."[30]

Appendectomy during Gestation

Appendicitis occurs most frequently during the second and third decades of life, a highly fertile period in a woman's life. A Swedish registry review[30] documented a reported incidence of acute appendicitis during gestation of one in 936 pregnancies; interestingly, misdiagnosis occurred in 36% of the cases, with an apparently higher rate of error in the latter portion of the gestation. Misdiagnosis was presumed to have occurred because of cephalad rise of the appendix as the uterus enlarges.

The diagnosis of acute appendicitis can be difficult to establish in a parturient. Signs, symptoms, and laboratory findings may be altered by the physiologic changes of pregnancy (the white blood cell count is elevated) and by the enlarging gravid uterus. While the pregnancy progresses, the appendix rises upward and outward to the flank. Frequently the classic right lower quadrant area of pain localization may be shifted to a different location. In fact, the reported accuracy of clinical judgement is as low as 58% to 68%. Nevertheless, the treatment of suspected appendicitis during pregnancy is immediate surgical intervention, irrespective of the patient's gestational status. The most important criteria for management are early diagnosis and avoidance of delay. In pregnancy, increased maternal and fetal morbidity and mortality are associated with appendiceal perforation. Consequently, immediate surgery is necessary when appendicitis is suspected in a pregnant patient.[31]

Anesthetic management of the parturient, who is presumably healthy and is to have an exploratory laparotomy for acute appendicitis, is influenced by the gestational age of the fetus. One study from University of California Los Angeles in 1990 revealed that 32% of the patients had surgery in the first trimester, 44% in the second trimester, 16% in the third trimester, and 8% in the puerperium. If the patient is 6 weeks' pregnant, it is conceivable that neither the surgeon, the patient nor the anesthesiologist may realize that an early gestation exists. All women of childbearing age should be questioned about their last menstrual period before any surgical or anesthetic procedure.[32]

There is a significant increase in spontaneous abortion in women who have exploratory surgery in the first trimester, but no evidence exists for the development of congenital abnormalities in the offspring who survive the initial surgical procedure.[33] Diagnostic procedures to reduce this incidence of fetal wastage obviously would be extremely beneficial.

Diagnostic error of about 35% to 36% is quoted as average. Sonography has been used as a diagnostic tool. In one series, 45 patients with the presumptive diagnosis of acute appendicitis underwent *graded compression scanning*. Criterion for definitive diagnosis was *visualization of an incompressible appendix*. In three late third-trimester patients, sonography could not be used because of uterine size. However, in the 42 remaining patients, sonography correctly identified 15 of 16 cases of acute appendicitis. These investigators believe that this diagnostic tool can be of great value, particularly in the first half of the gestational period, when the fetus is at great risk for either abortion or premature labor, presumably due to the surgery.[32]

To lessen fetal wastage from exploratory laparotomy, laparoscopic appendectomy has been attempted in pregnant women. It has been stated that this technique is minimally traumatic to the parturient and fetus. There has been no apparent difficulty with gas insufflation, either to the mother or to the fetus. When perforation of the appendix is discovered, exploratory laparotomy is performed.[34]

Discussion of the Three Situations Presented

Surgery and anesthesia for acute appendicitis in the first trimester can be accomplished satisfactorily if the anesthesiologist understands the various factors that may alter the patient's condition.

Several axioms are pertinent: First, *the management of the case is more important than the agents used.* The physiologic changes that occur in the parturient require changes in the anesthetic management, differing from the nonpregnant state. No anesthetic technique is truly precluded for surgery on the pregnant patient. The avoidance of maternal hypoxia, hypotension, and hypovolemia is of greater importance than the anesthetic technique selected. It is necessary to remember that hypoxia or prolonged hypotension may produce fetal abnormalities.[35]

Second, *regional anesthesia, where feasible, should be considered because local anesthetics are probably safe from teratogenetic effects.* General anesthesia is definitely acceptable for maternal and fetal well-being. Whatever the choice of anesthetic technique, the patient needs to be fully informed of the ramifications of the procedure selected. If subarachnoid block is selected, a large-bore intravenous line should be placed and sufficient fluids given to compensate for the patient's preoperative vomiting and to protect against the sympathetic blockade produced by the anesthetic. An oral nonparticulate antacid is advisable even though the gestation is in an early stage. Pain, fever, pregnancy, and peritonitis can contribute to delayed gastric emptying and increased gastric acidity.

The advantages of subarachnoid blockade include the following:

1. Minimum amount of local anesthetic (possibly increased fetal safety)
2. Rapid onset of anesthesia
3. A definite end-point to the block
4. Easy administration—a subarachnoid block is easier to administer than an epidural block, and usually produces more profound anesthesia.

The disadvantages of subarachnoid anesthesia are as follows:

1. Hypotension can be precipitous and severe
2. The dermatome level achieved is not rectifiable
3. Postdural puncture headache may occur, the incidence of which has been dramatically reduced using small-caliber pencil-point spinal needles.

If epidural anesthesia is chosen, adequate preoperative fluids and an antacid both are indicated, as with spinal anesthesia.

There are several advantages of epidural anesthesia for appendectomy if regional anesthesia is selected:

1. The propensity for hypotension that exists with spinal anesthesia is lessened, both because of the slower onset of the block and the fact that small, incremental doses of local anesthetics are administered until the desired level is achieved.
2. If an epidural catheter is used, problems with adequacy of dermatome level and duration of blockade are greatly diminished.
3. The catheter technique makes available postoperative pain relief with the administration of extradural narcotics.

The disadvantages of epidural anesthesia include the following:

1. An increased complexity of technique, with greater chance of failure

2. Slower onset of anesthesia that may preclude its use in urgent situations
3. The need for larger amounts of local anesthetic compared with spinal anesthesia.

When the clinician selects major conduction anesthesia for the management of first-trimester acute appendicitis, the patient should receive an appropriate amount of intravenous fluids to compensate for preoperative loss and the sympathetic blockade produced by the anesthetic (usually about 1500 to 2000 ml). Preferably the block should be done with the patient in the lateral position and with a narrow-gauge (25 to 27) pencil-point needle. The parturient should receive oxygen by either nasal cannula or face mask throughout the entire procedure (administered as soon as the block is in place). Hypotension must be treated immediately with a bolus of crystalloid and ephedrine given in increments of 10 mg intravenously. The duration of hypotension and subsequent altered uteroplacental perfusion directly affects neonatal outcome. The choice of local anesthetic depends on a knowledge of the advantages and disadvantages of the various types of local anesthetic available. For spinal anesthesia, the local anesthetics most frequently used are hyperbaric lidocaine, tetracaine, or hyperbaric spinal bupivacaine.

For epidural anesthesia, the local anesthetics that may be used include bupivacaine, lidocaine, etidocaine, or 2-chloroprocaine. The concomitant addition of epinephrine is controversial. Whether epinephrine causes intervillous vasoconstriction and fetal acidosis is subject to debate.

The drug 2-chloroprocaine has achieved some notoriety because of the development of persistent and painful postoperative backache, and because it apparently interferes with opioid receptors in the spinal column and thus may interfere with postoperative epidural narcotic pain relief.

If general anesthesia is selected, the patient should be placed on the operating table with the head slightly elevated. The usual monitoring equipment is applied and the patient should be preoxygenated for 3 to 5 minutes (four deep breaths would be satisfactory in an emergency situation). Induction should be performed in a manner that is thoughtful and careful. Regurgitation and aspiration in a gravida who is in pain and possibly frightened is possible, even in the first trimester. Before the start of the induction, it is advisable to give the patient a nonparticulate antacid. Rapid-sequence induction with intubation should be performed. Because gastric emptying time usually is delayed, gastric suction should be started before the surgical incision. Whether one uses nitrous oxide when the patient is in the first trimester of gestation depends on the anesthesiologist's attitude toward the potential problems with fetal DNA. No difficulty with a solitary use of nitrous oxide in a clinical situation has been reported, and recent studies apparently confirm no difficulty in the use of nitrous oxide.[26]

Since the greatest potential fetal problem in the first trimester is abortion, it behooves the surgeon to be gentle with the adjacent surrounding tissues and to disturb the pregnancy as little as possible.

If the patient is in the second trimester (about 24 weeks), it becomes necessary to alter thinking with regard to the anesthetic management. The period of organogenesis has almost been completed and the possibility of organ teratogenicity, although still present, is not the paramount factor regarding the fetus. The major problem in a patient whose pregnancy is of this gestational age is the onset of premature labor and the subsequent loss of the neonate due to lack of development. Surgical manipulation of the uterus, while attempting to delineate the appendix, may lead to irritability and contractility of the uterus and thus may cause late abortion or premature labor.

As the pregnancy grows, aortocaval compression and potential maternal hypotension become more common. The syndrome manifests itself by arterial hypotension, rapid pulse, sweating, and faintness. It occurs in about 10% of gravidas because most patients can compensate if their sympathetic system functions properly. Nevertheless, a patient in the midsecond trimester and beyond should not lie supine, and the patient should be in the lateral position when transported to the operating suite. Usually a wedge should be placed under the right hip and the table should be tilted to the left during the procedure.

Although regurgitation and aspiration are commonly linked to the third trimester of pregnancy, they may occur as early as the fourth or fifth month of gestation. To reduce the acidity and volume of stomach, the use of clear antacids, H_2-receptor blockers, and metoclopromide should be considered before anesthesia is induced.

Although theoretically applicable as the fetus approaches maturity, fetal electronic monitoring during surgery is extremely difficult, if not impossible, during intraabdominal procedures. Regional, spinal, epidural, or general anesthesia are acceptable. Some unpublished data suggest that uterine hypotonia and uterine artery vasoconstriction may occur with exposure to local anesthetics. A regional technique that results in high blood levels of local anesthetics may result in a decrease in uteroplacental perfusion. Careful attention to dosage and to the correct placement of the anesthetic should obviate this potential problem.

Different general anesthetic techniques have different effects on the uteroplacental circulation. By making an inference from combined human and animal studies, it is my opinion that thiopental–nitrous oxide anesthesia may, in certain circumstances, result in uterine hypoperfusion and fetal acidosis. Nitrous oxide is known to increase sympathetic tone. The gravid uterine artery has a low basal level of adrenergic tone, and this may explain the effects of nitrous oxide. However, inhalation agents such as halothane, isoflurane, enflurane, and desflurane reduce uterine tone and, provided blood pressure and cardiac output are maintained, sustain uterine perfusion.

Propofol may cause significant hypotension during induction in gravid women and thus produce a decrease in uteroplacental blood flow.

Ketamine, when used in doses greater than 1 mg/kg, or α-adrenergic vasopressors directly increase uterine tone and probably should be avoided.

Of major importance to the survival of the fetus at this gestational age is the necessity for the surgeon to be gentle with tissues and to try not to manipulate the uterus so as to induce uterine contractility and premature labor.

When the surgical procedure is to take place in a woman who is at 37 weeks' gestation, the pregnancy is essentially a term pregnancy. By definition, 38 weeks is term, and therefore, 37 weeks is very close to term. All of the parameters that apply to the patients who are in the first and second trimester apply to the third-trimester patient with additional major considerations. On opening the abdomen of a patient who is 37 weeks' pregnant, it is usual to find the uterus approximately the size of a watermelon and quite possibly obstructing the view and approach to the other abdominal organs, including the appendix. Furthermore, the location of the appendix is altered at this stage of gestation. As the uterus enlarges and becomes an intraabdominal organ, the cecum increasingly is lifted from its position in the cecal fossa. As a result of this displacement, the appendix may be located as high as the right upper quadrant. If the operation that is to be performed is the expected appendectomy, it might be possible to leave the uterus undisturbed and proceed with the surgery. If, however, the disease process encountered is not acute appendicitis, but a different disease process (e.g., gallbladder diseases), it may be necessary to *empty* the uterus by cesarean section, since the fetus is definitely viable. This procedure would allow adequate access to the diseased organ and permit its removal.

The technique of anesthesia for this particular patient is the same as that for the patient with a pregnancy of about 24 weeks. Regional anesthesia may be used, but a dermatome level of T-4 will be needed and hypotension must be avoided. General anesthesia requires a rapid-sequence induction, cricoid pressure, and endotracheal intubation with a no. 7 to no. 7.5 endotracheal tube. During the procedure, as long as the fetus is in situ, the fractional inspired oxygen concentration (FiO_2) should be 50%.

Fetal heart rate and uterine contraction monitoring should be started as soon as the surgery is terminated. Tocolytics may be administered by the obstetricians if necessary.

Summary

Nonobstetric surgery in a pregnant patient is potentially hazardous. The medical team must be aware of maternal physiologic changes and their significance for both mother and fetus. Maternal and fetal homeostasis must be maintained to achieve a satisfactory outcome for both mother and child. Medical acumen, based on current available knowledge, should lead to a healthy mother and neonate and give the surgeon the opportunity to satisfactorily perform the operation. There is no evidence that a single acute exposure to modern anesthetic agents endangers the pregnancy. Avoidance of hypoxia, hypotension, and hypovolemia is therefore of greater importance than is the choice of a particular anesthetic agent. No specific technique or anesthetic agent has established superiority with regard to fetal outcome.

1. When applicable, major conduction anesthesia should be employed in the first trimester to avoid teratogenetic concerns. Local anesthetic doses should be reduced by one third, even during the first trimester of pregnancy.
2. General anesthesia may prove advantageous later by allowing maximum oxygenation, the avoidance of hypotension, and by providing uterine relaxation.
3. If general anesthesia is to be used, prudence dictates the use of drugs that have been available for many years and that have a good safety record. These include thiopental, muscle relaxants, and the narcotics. The inhalational agents may be used to limit uterine activity and to try to eliminate maternal recall.
4. In most instances, optimal maternal care will provide the best outcome for both mother and neonate.

References

1. Mahmoodian S: Appendicitis complicating pregnancy, *South Med J* 1992; 85:19.
2. Tamir IL, Bongard FS, Klein SR: Acute appendicitis in the pregnant patient, *Am J Surg* 1990; 160:571.
3. Rubler S, Damani PM, Pinto ER: Cardiac size and performance during pregnancy estimated with echocardiography, *Am J Cardiol* 1977; 40:534.
4. Cutforth R, MacDonald CB: Heart sounds and murmurs in pregnancy, *Am Heart J* 1966; 71:741.
5. Metcalfe J, Ueland K: Maternal cardiovascular adjustments to pregnancy, *Prog Cardiovasc Dis* 1974; 16:363.
6. Ginns HM, Hollinrake K: Complete heart block in pregnancy treated with an internal cardiac pacemaker, *J Obstet Gynaecol Br Commonw* 1970; 70:710.
7. Kerr MG: The mechanical effects of the gravid uterus in late pregnancy, *J Obstet Gynaecol Br Commonw* 1965; 72:513.
8. Pritchard JA: Hematologic aspects of pregnancy, *Clin Obstet Gynecol* 1960; 3:378.
9. Pitkin RM, Witte DL: Platelet and leukocyte counts in pregnancy, *JAMA* 1980; 242:2696.
10. DeSwiet M: *The respiratory system.* In Hytten FE, Chamberlain G, editors: *Clinical physiology in obstetrics, ed 2,* Oxford, 1991, Blackwell.

11. Milne JA: The respiratory response to pregnancy, *Postgrad Med J* 1979; 55:318.
12. Russell IF, Chambers WA: Closing volume in normal pregnancy, *Br J Anaesth* 1981; 53:1043.
13. Andersen GJ, James GB, Mathers NP, et al: The maternal oxygen tension and acid base status during pregnancy, *J Obstet Gynaecol Br Commonw* 1969; 76:16.
14. Palahniuk RJ, Shnider SM, Eger III EI: Pregnancy decreases the requirements for inhaled anesthetic agent, *Anesthesiology* 1974; 41:82.
15. Davison JM, Dunlop W: Changes in renal hemodynamics and tubular function induced by normal human pregnancy, *Semin Nephrol* 1984; 4:198.
16. Brown MA, Sinosich MJ, Saunders DM, Gallery EDM: Potassium regulation and progesterone–aldosterone interrelationships in human pregnancy: a prospective study, *Am J Obstet Gynecol* 1986; 155:349.
17. Macfie AG, Magides AP, Richmond MN, Reilly CS: Gastric emptying in pregnancy, *Br J Anaesth* 1991; 67:54.
18. Glinoer D, DeNayer P, Bourdoux P, et al: Regulation of maternal thyroid during pregnancy, *J Clin Endocrinol Metab* 1990; 71:276.
19. Brudnell JP, Beard R: Diabetes in pregnancy, *Clin Endocrinol Metab* 1972; 1:673.
20. Combes B, Adams RH: *Pathophysiology of the liver in pregnancy.* In Assali NS, editor: *Pathophysiology of gestation, vol 1,* New York, 1971, Academic Press.
21. Mortensen ML, Sever LE, Oakley GP: *Teratology and the epidemiology of birth defects.* In Gabbe SG, Niebyl JR, Simpson JL, editors: *Obstetrics: normal and problem pregnancies.* New York, 1986, Churchill-Livingston.
22. Blass NH: *Anesthesia for surgical operations during pregnancy.* In Datta S, Ostheimer G, editors: *Common problems in obstetric anesthesia,* Chicago, 1987, Year Book Publishers.
23. Sorensen VJ, Bivens BA, Obeid FN, et al: Management of general surgical emergencies in pregnancy, *Am Surg* 1990; 56:245.
24. Brodsky JB, Cohen EN, Brown BW Jr, et al: Surgery during pregnancy and fetal outcome, *Am J Obstet Gynecol* 1980; 138:1165.
25. Nunn JF: *Nitrous oxide inactivates methionine synthetase.* In Eger EI, editor: *Nitrous oxide,* New York, 1985, Elsevier Science Publishing.
26. Mazze RI, Fujinaga M, Rice SA, et al: Reproductive and teratogenic effects of nitrous oxide, halothane, isoflurane and enflurane in Sprague-Dawley rats, *Anesthesiology* 1985; 64:334.
27. Sturrock JE, Nunn JF: Cytotoxic effects of procaine, lignocaine, and bupivacaine, *Br J Anaesth* 1979; 51:273.
28. Eger EI II: Fetal injury and abortion associated with occupational exposure to inhaled anesthetics, *J Am Assoc Nurse Anesth* 1991; 59:309.
29. Cohen EN, Bellville JW, Brown BW Jr: Anesthesia, pregnancy and miscarriage: a study of operating room nurses and anesthetists, *Anesthesiology* 1971; 35:343.
30. Ericson HA, Kallen AJB: Hospitalization for miscarriage and delivery outcome among Swedish nurses working in operating rooms 1973-1975, *Anesth Analg* 1985; 64:981.
31. Richards C, Daya S: Diagnosis of acute appendicitis in pregnancy, *Can J Surg* 1989; 32:358.
32. Lim HK, Sang Hoon Bae, Gwy Suk Sec: Diagnosis of acute appendicitis in pregnant women: value of sonography, *Am J Roentgenol* 1992; 159:539.
33. Snider SM, Webster GM, Maternal and fetal hazards of surgery during pregnancy, *Am J Obstet Gynecol* 1963; 92:891.
34. Schreiber JH: Laparoscopic appendectomy in pregnancy, *Surg Endosc* 1990; 4:100.
35. Smith BF: Teratology in anesthesia, *Clin Obstet Gynecol* 1974; 17:145.

39

Postpartum Tubal Ligation

A 35-year-old multigravida has an uneventful vaginal delivery without any anesthetic. The patient has previously requested a postpartum tubal ligation. How soon should this be performed after delivery? Outline the anesthetic management of the patient requesting postpartum tubal ligation. Discuss the choices of anesthesia.

Recommendations by Amr E. Abouleish, M.D.
Ezzat I. Abouleish, M.D.

Postpartum tubal ligation (PPTL) is a simpler and safer method of sterilization than interval laparoscopic tubal coagulation. With PPTL, certain factors should be considered:

1. Possibility of gastric aspiration
2. Local anesthetic drug requirement
3. Cholinesterase level
4. Maternal general condition
5. Neonatal general condition
6. Anesthetic techniques.

Possibility of Gastric Aspiration

Gastric Emptying

Obstetric patients are at increased risk of aspiration of gastric contents secondary to pain, stress, and narcotics, as well as mechanical and hormonal factors. Many of the factors contributing to vomiting, regurgitation, and aspiration are alleviated by delivery. For example, pain and stress, which are the main causes of delayed gastric emptying, usually end by delivery.[1] By the time the patient is ready for PPTL, the effects of narcotics administered early in labor have terminated. After delivery the size of uterus decreases; hence the mechanical

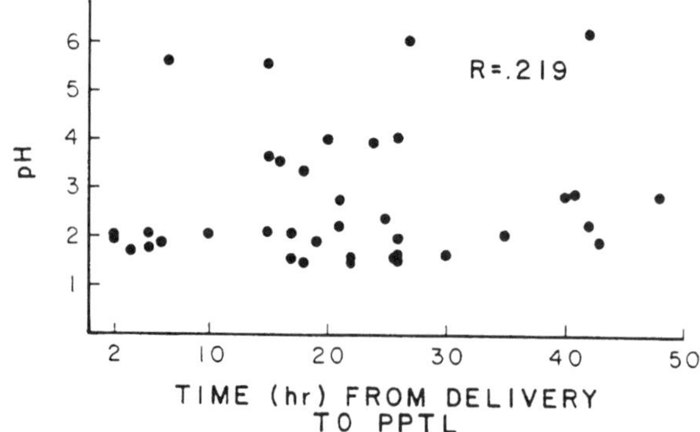

Fig. 39-1.
Correlation between time (hours) from delivery to PPTL and gastric pH. *(From Uram M, Abouleish E, McKenzie R, et al: The risk of aspiration pneumonitis with postpartum tubal ligation,* Soc Obstet Anesth Perinatol *1982:[abstr].)*

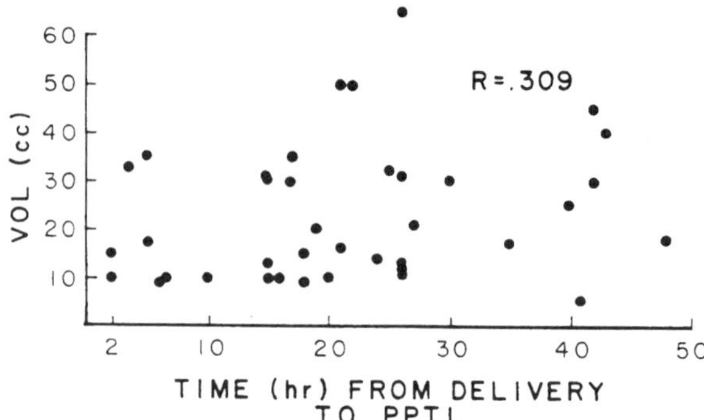

Fig. 39-2.
Correlation between time (hours) from delivery to PPTL and gastric volume *(From Uram, et al: The risk of aspiration pneumonitis with postpartum tubal ligation,* Soc Obstet Anesth Perinatol *1982;2 [abstr].)*

changes due to the increased intraabdominal pressure also are decreased. Progesterone, which originally causes relaxation of ligaments, for example, gastroesophageal ligaments, dramatically decreases. Desphande et al. found that during labor, the already elevated plasma progesterone level either stayed elevated or increased further, being 13 to 20 μg/dl.[2] However, within 10 to 20 minutes after delivery, progesterone levels decrease by 25% to 50% of the intrapartum level. It is important to remember that the exact time that gastric emptying returns to the nonpregnant state is still not clear.

Gastric Volume and pH

Patients with a gastric volume more than 25 ml and a pH less than 2.5 are arbitrarily considered at risk of pneumonitis should aspiration occur. Blouw et al. compared the gastric volume and pH of 21 patients undergoing PPTL at least 8 hours after delivery with those of 11 patients of the same age group who had not recently been pregnant and were undergoing elective tubal ligation.[3] They found 33% of the postpartum patients and 64% of the control patients to be at high risk of aspiration. They concluded that gastric emptying must have occurred sometime between delivery and 8 hours thereafter. To explore this interval, we examined the gastric volume and pH of 40 patients in whom PPTL was performed between 2 and 48 hours after delivery.[4] We found that 28% of the postpartum patients were at high risk, an incidence comparable with that of Blouw et al. No correlation existed between the risk factors and the delivery-to-surgery time, the duration of the first stage of labor, the duration of the second stage of labor, or the interval from the last meal to the onset of labor (Figs. 39-1 and 39-2). With these data, we concluded that, regarding the risk of aspiration, the patient's safety was not enhanced by delaying general anesthesia to more than 2 hours after delivery. James et al.[5] further extended the search to explore the risk in this 8-hour period by examining gastric pH and volume in three groups, divided according to the delivery-to-PPTL interval, and comparing them with a control group of female surgical patients of the same age and weight. They found no significant difference in gastric pH or volume among early (1 to 8 hours), intermediate (9 to 23 hours), or late (24 to 25 hours) postpartum groups. Neither were they able to demonstrate a difference between postpartum and elective surgical patients: 60% of all their patients were at risk. They warned about aspiration pneumonitis, however, and recommended sodium citrate administration and cricoid pressure in all PPTL patients.

Interval Between Delivery and Surgery

Despite the reports described in the previous section, the safe interval between delivery and surgery still is controversial. A March 1992 statement from the Committee on Obstetrics, Maternal and Fetal Medicine, of the American College of Obstetricians and Gynecologists indicates that there are no contraindications to proceeding with a tubal sterilization in the immediate postpartum period if a woman has had a major anesthetic for her delivery and the anesthetic can be continued safely. Nonetheless, a major anesthetic (conduction, regional, or general inhalation) to accomplish a tubal sterilization should be continued only after careful evaluation by the anesthesia service. Because the parturient may have an increased risk of regurgitation and aspiration of acidic gastric contents, many anesthesiologists prefer to wait for a period of time after delivery to allow for increased gastric emptying. Postpartum sterilization is an elective procedure, and one should not proceed unless conditions are safe. Therefore, the Committee did not specify any specific time interval, leaving it to the discretion of the anesthesiologist. The American Society of Anesthesiologists does not have a stand on this particular issue.

In our hospitals at the University of Texas Medical Branch (Galveston) and the University of Texas Medical School (Houston), the delivery-to-PPTL interval is not the only factor determining the timing of PPTL. Such operations are performed in the labor and delivery suite only when anesthesia, obstetric, and nursing staff are free to provide the service without compromising the care of the women in labor. Assuming that this criterion is met, how soon after delivery can the operation be performed? If a major anesthetic is to be initiated, we wait at least 8 hours, preferably until the next morning when more manpower is readily available. (In the editor's hospitals, if manpower is not a problem, PPTL is done if necessary under spinal anesthesia immediately after delivery.)

The problem of the risk of aspiration and the timing of surgery can be resolved to a great extent if PPTL has been anticipated. In a patient in whom PPTL is expected, continuous epidural analgesia or spinal anesthesia may be used for parturition. Not only does the patient benefit from the relief of pain offered by the anesthetic technique during parturition, but there is also sufficient time to test the safety and efficacy of that technique before the tubal ligation. It is also more economical and safer to use one anesthetic than two. When epidural anesthesia is chosen for vaginal delivery and tubal ligation, after the delivery, the epidural is reinstated to reach a T-4 level, the dermatomal level required for any intraabdominal operation, including tubal ligation.[6] With a lower dermatomal level, for example, T-10, skin incision may be tolerable but intraabdominal manipulations and pulling on the fallopian tubes cause pain. In a patient with cardiovascular disease in whom a relatively high block to T-4 is risky, a lower level is acceptable and anesthesia is supplemented by intraperitoneal instillation of 80 ml of 0.5% lidocaine 5 minutes earlier.[7] With this technique the blood level of lidocaine in a puerperal woman was found to be safe (about 2 μg/ml) and well below the toxic level (9 to 10 μg/ml). When subarachnoid block for both delivery and tubal ligation is chosen, the drug used is bupivacaine to cover both delivery and the tubal ligation. The dose should be adequate to reach the T-4 level, that is, if cesarean section is to be performed. Combined spinal and epidural or continuous spinal anesthesia for both delivery and tubal ligation are excellent alternatives. The analgesia for early labor can be conducted using intrathecal (IT) 10 μg sufentanil with or without 2.5 mg bupivacaine (1 ml 0.25%).[8-10] The analgesia after IT injection of sufentanil begins almost instantaneously. Although the addition of a small dose of bupivacaine (2.5mg) does not have any significant effect on the motor power, it does prolong the duration of analgesia when added with sufentanil and allows the use of episiotomy and repair if required.[11] The introduction of IT sufentanil has been well received by patients, obstetricians, and nursing staff because of its intense, rapid analgesia with minimal motor, sensory, or vasomotor paralysis. The main side effect is itching. After delivery, epidural anesthesia can be used for tubal ligation as described earlier. With continuous spinal anesthesia, analgesia for labor can be obtained by the use of IT narcotic with or without local anesthetic. After delivery, the level and intensity of the block can be achieved by titrating hyperbaric bupivacaine dosage (0.75% in 8.25% dextrose) to achieve a T-4 dermatomal level. Unfortunately, because of a dozen cases in two reports of development of cauda equina syndrome after the use of continuous spinal technique with 5% hyperbaric lidocaine,[12,13] the Food and Drug Administration rescinded its approval of the use of the technique using catheters smaller than 27-gauge until further studies prove its safety. Five percent hyperbaric lidocaine has been used for spinal anesthesia for more than 25 years. Moreover, a multicenter prospective study of more than 10,000 spinal anesthetics has shown that 5% hyperbaric lidocaine is both safe and effective.[14] However, recent reports have clouded lidocaine's record.[15-17] Obviously, more studies of the safety of continuous spinal catheter technique with microcatheters and 5% hyperbaric lidocaine are required.

Local Anesthetic Drug Requirements

Datta and associates found that bupivacaine caused a more rapid onset and a more profound degree of conduction block in isolated vagus nerve from pregnant rabbits compared with that from nonpregnant animals.[18,19] Moreover, they found that when progesterone had been administered intramuscularly for 4 days to nonpregnant rabbits that underwent ovariectomy, susceptibility of the vagus nerve to bupivacaine block increased and the recovery period was prolonged.[20] This action could have resulted from alterations in local anesthetic diffusion through the nerve sheath or actual change in membrane sensitivity to local anesthetics.

With pregnancy, the hormonal effect, by increasing the susceptibility of these nerves, and the mechanical effect, by causing engorgement of the vertebral veins and reducing cerebrospinal fluid volume, explain the fact that the local anesthetic requirement for each spinal segment block after spinal anesthesia is less in cesarean section than in gynecologic operation, the ratio being 1:1.5. During the postpartum period, both the progesterone level and the mechanical compression of the inferior vena cava are reduced, but are still above the nonpregnant state. Therefore the correspondence doses of local anesthetic for PPTL lies between that for cesarean section and gynecologic operation. For example, with spinal or epidural anesthesia the dose requirement of the local anesthetic per segment with cesarean section compared with PPTL is 1:1.3.[21,22] With epidural anesthesia, the dose requirement during the postpartum increased gradually over the cesarean section requirement to reach that of gynecologic level after 36 hours.

Cholinesterase Level

The reduction by 30% in cholinesterase level during pregnancy continues during the postpartum period.[23-25] This decrease results largely from an increase in blood volume (30%). After the injection of succinylcholine in puerperal patients, the recovery time (time from 25% to 75% recovery) and the maximal recovery of muscular paralysis (time from complete paralysis to 90% recovery) were increased by 30 seconds and 3 minutes, respectively, compared with those who were not pregnant.[25] This prolongation of action may be statistically, but not clinically, significant. The net result is that there is no clinically significant prolongation of the duration of succinylcholine action in the postpartum period.[26] Although the duration of action may be increased, the intubating dose of succinylcholine (1.5 mg/kg) is unchanged and should not be reduced in a pregnant or puerperal woman. Any reduction of the intubating dose leads only to inadequate relaxation, difficult intubation, and possible aspiration. Whenever a muscle relaxant is administered, a nerve stimulator should be used to guide the timing of intubation and regulate subsequent doses. After the intubating dose, subsequent doses are tailored to the patient's need, guided by the response to nerve stimulation. Any prolonged apnea after the administration of succinylcholine in a pregnant or puerperal patient should not be blamed on the physiologic reduction of cholinesterase level, because the level must be reduced by at least 50% before prolonged apnea occurs after succinylcholine administration. Therefore, when such a problem arises, abnormal cholinesterase should be suspected. Further investigations of the genotype of the patient, her husband, their children, and her close relatives may prevent such a complication in other members of her family.

Maternal General Condition

The patient's condition should be evaluated before the decision to undertake PPTL. If the patient is cardiovascularly unstable or has a life-threatening disease, surgery should be postponed, to be done electively when the condition is resolved, or other methods of contraception should be used.

Sometimes PPTL is postponed because of a low hemoglobin (Hb) level. The magic values of 10 g/dl Hb and hematocrit of 30% should not be the rule. With pregnancy, hemodilution occurs, and Hb values between 10 and 12 g/dl and hematocrits between 29% and 39% are normal.[27] After delivery, there can be further dilution caused by intravenous administration of fluids during labor, the antidiuretic effect of oxytocin, and the shift of fluid from the extravascular to the intravascular compartment in preparation for postpartum diuresis. Postponing surgery based on a Hb value of less than 10 g/dl may lead to unwanted pregnancy and more risk in terminating it. If the postpartum patient is not bleeding, has a stable cardiovascular system and a Hb value of 7.5 g/dl or higher, we do not hesitate to administer anesthesia, whether spinal, epidural, or general.

Neonatal General Condition

Usually the patient contemplates PPTL during pregnancy on the assumption that her baby is going to be normal. However, this may not be the case. Therefore, the condition of the neonate should be considered before the final decision to perform PPTL.

Anesthetic Techniques

The types of anesthesia available for PPTL are spinal, epidural, general, or local.

Spinal Anesthesia

Spinal anesthesia is the simplest and safest technique. The dangers of general anesthesia, namely, difficulty in intubation and the problem of aspiration pneumonitis, are almost absent with spinal anesthesia. The cardiotoxicity and neurotoxicity of local anesthetic drugs arising from inadvertent intravascular or subarachnoid injection associated with epidural anesthesia are eliminated with spinal anesthesia. Moreover, with a spinal block, the onset of action is fast, the analgesia is superb, and the recovery is smooth. The incidence and severity of hypotension and the occurrence of nausea and vomiting are much less with PPTL than with cesarean section because of the decreased size of the uterus leading to reduced incidence of supine hypotension syndrome.[21] The main objection to spinal anesthesia by lay people, as well as some physicians, is the incidence of postdural puncture headache (PDPH). With the advent of pencil-tip spinal needles, for example, Whitacre or Sprotte, the incidence and severity of PDPH have been greatly reduced. In more than 1000 patients the incidence of PDPH with a 25-gauge Whitacre needle was 1%, with very few of these patients requiring epidural blood patch.[28] In addition, after a 24-gauge Sprotte needle was used, the incidence rate of PDPH was less than 20% of the rate when a 26-gauge Quincke needle was used.[29] By using a 27-gauge Whitacre needle, this complication, if indeed it ever occurs, should be extremely rare. The flow rate through a 27-gauge Whitacre needle is the same as through a 25-gauge Whitacre or a 26-gauge Quincke needle.[30,31] Therefore, anesthesiologists used to the latter needles should not hesitate to use a 27-gauge Whitacre needle. Moreover, by using a pencil-tip needle, identification of the subarachnoid space is easy, as the "give" of the ligamentum flavum and dura is better felt than with Quincke needles. Details of spinal anesthesia follow.

Epidural Anesthesia

Epidural anesthesia offers no advantages over spinal anesthesia and should not be considered for a short procedure like PPTL unless an epidural catheter is already in place after its use for delivery. With respect to the patient's safety for an operation less than 2 hours in duration, the price of epidural anesthesia is too high. This price with respect to spinal anesthesia includes the danger of inadvertent intravascular or intrathecal injection, a more complicated procedure, and less adequate analgesia. However, if the patient has had epidural anesthesia for labor, the use of this anesthetic technique for PPTL is warranted. When epidural anesthesia is reinstated many hours after the delivery, certain precautions should be taken:

1. A history of the reliability of epidural analgesia for labor should be confirmed.
2. The patient's back should be examined to ensure that an appropriate length of the catheter is still present. The catheter may be displaced from the epidural space by too much movement of the patient, inadequate taping, and perspiring by the patient.
3. The first 10 ml of the local anesthetic should be injected with the patient on her side to exclude leakage of the catheter or superficial position of its tip, which can lead to subcutaneous crepitus or swelling.
4. If epidural injection of an adequate dose of a local anesthetic (e.g., 20 to 30 ml of 3% chloroprocaine) cannot achieve an adequate bilateral level of block (i.e., at least T-6 dermatomal level), spinal anesthesia should be considered rather than struggling with an inadequate block and exposing the patient to its dangers. The administration of spinal anesthesia immediately after verification of inadequate epidural anesthesia and after the administration of a large dose of a local an-

esthetic sometimes leads to a more excessive level of block than anticipated. The mechanism of this occurrence is unclear: cerebrospinal fluid volume may have decreased owing to its compression by the epidurally injected large volume of local anesthetic, both techniques may have had an additive effect, or accessing of the epidural may have injected local anesthetic into the subarachnoid space through the created hole in the dura. It may therefore be safer to let the epidural block wear off before administering a spinal anesthetic.

General Anesthesia

General anesthesia is indicated in situations such as the patient's refusal to have regional anesthesia, the anesthesiologist's inability to perform a block, or a contraindication to regional exists. The conduct of general anesthesia here should not differ from that for other intraabdominal surgical procedures, with the exception of certain points discussed below.

Thirty milliliters of 0.3 M sodium bicitrate is given orally about 5 minutes before surgery, and cricoid pressure is applied with the onset of unconsciousness. H_2-receptor antagonists (e.g., cimetidine, ranitidine) or upper gastrointestinal stimulants (e.g., metoclopramide) usually are not required and may have undesirable side effects. For example, cimetidine may cause cardiovascular collapse if given intravenously and can interfere with the metabolism of other drugs such as lidocaine or diazepam. Metoclopramide may cause extrapyramidal symptoms or agitation as well as inhibition of pseudocholinesterase.[32] Moreover, the use of metoclopramide is not a guarantee to empty the stomach in the peripartum period,[33] and its action is nullified by the prior use of atropine, glycopyrrolate, or opioids.[34] Therefore, the administration of metoclopramide or cimetidine alone without antacids is not advisable. Rapid-sequence induction using either thiopental (4 mg/kg) or propofol (2 mg) plus succinylcholine (1.5 mg) and cricoid pressure should be used. Because the operation usually is short, muscular relaxation can be maintained by a succinylcholine infusion guided by the use of a nerve stimulator. Anesthesia can be maintained by nitrous oxide:oxygen, supplemented by an inhalation anesthetic such as isoflurane.

Local Anesthesia

In certain cases and countries, local anesthesia can be the only safe or available method to use. Moreover, the instillation of a local anesthetic intraperitoneally can supplement a borderline spinal or epidural block and is safer than adding general anesthesia. Local anesthesia has been successfully used for both PPTL and internal laparoscopic tubal ligation.[7,35-37] After adequate intravenous sedation of the patient, the umbilical region is infiltrated with 0.5% lidocaine. After the abdominal incision is performed, 80 ml of the local anesthetic solution is administered by the surgeon under direct vision. After intraperitoneal administration of 100 ml of 0.5% lidocaine, the blood lidocaine level was only 2.2 μg/ml, a figure well below the toxic level of 10 μg/ml.[7] After a 5- to 10-minute waiting period, surgery can be resumed to perform the tubal ligation.

Preferred Technique: Spinal

Because our technique of choice for this patient is spinal anesthesia, we will describe it in more detail. Surgery is delayed for 8 hours, preferably performed the next morning when personnel are more readily available. No oral intake is allowed for 8 hours before surgery. Although water may have a better pH than other common liquids[38] and the administration of water up to 2 hours after surgery is recommended,[39] water's buffering capacity is limited.[40] Thus, the safest method is to abstain from

TABLE 39-1

DOSES (IN MG) OF LOCAL ANESTHETICS REQUIRED FOR SPINAL ANESTHESIA IN THE LATERAL HORIZONTAL POSITION AT L2-3 INTERSPACE*

Procedure and Anesthetic	Height			
	150 cm (5ft)	157.5 cm (5ft 3in)	165 cm (5ft 6in)	172.5 cm (5ft 9in)
Cesarean section†				
Lidocaine	50	60	70	80
Bupivacaine	8	9	10	11
Tetracaine	8	9	10	11
Postpartum tubal ligation				
Lidocaine	65	75	85	100
Bupivacaine	10	10	12.5	13.5
Tetracaine	10	11	12.5	13.5

*Add more local anesthetic with sitting position or the use of L3-4 interspace (e.g., 1.5 mg bupivacaine or equivalent for either situation).

†Add 0.2 mg morphine and 0.2 mg epinephrine.

drinking or eating for 8 hours. For fluid and energy supply during this 8-hour period, intravenous infusion of an electrolyte solution containing 5% dextrose is safer than oral intake. Although spinal anesthesia is planned and the patient will be awake and can control her airway, the possibility that the patient will require general anesthesia cannot be excluded in case unforeseen surgical complications lead to an extensive intraabdominal operation. Moreover, the spinal block may extend unintentionally to a too-high level, requiring control of the airway and ventilation. Under these two circumstances, intubation will be necessary and the possibility of aspiration should be considered. Oral intake of antacid, as described earlier, can be an added safety procedure.

Intravenous infusion of lactated Ringer's solution, 15 ml/kg, is administered within 20 minutes of the spinal block. While monitors are being applied, intravenous sedation of the patient is performed. The authors prefer L2-3 over L3-4 because of a more predictable level associated with the former interspace. Because L3-4 is at the hub of the lumbar lordosis, an unpredictable amount of the local anesthetic can move toward the caudal area, and is thus lost from spreading cephalad to achieve an adequate level. The dose of the local anesthetic should be higher than for cesarean section and less than that for a gynecologic operation such as abdominal hysterectomy. We found the ratio of the doses to achieve the same dermatomal level, T-4 in cesarean section to PPTL, to be 1:1.30.[21] The doses of local anesthetic required to achieve a T-4 dermatome may[41-43] or may not[44-46] correlate with patient height. One of us (E. I. A.) chooses the dose of local anesthetic based on patient height (Table 39-1), whereas the other (A. E. A.) uses a fixed dose of local anesthetic for patients 5 ft to 6 ft tall: either 12 mg hyperbaric 0.75% bupivacaine or 60 mg hyperbaric 5% lidocaine. The addition of 0.2 mg epinephrine intensifies the block and prolongs its duration of action.[47] However, the addition of epinephrine in a short procedure with minimal intraabdominal manipulation, like PPTL, usually is not required. The addition of 0.2 mg morphine to hyperbaric bupivacaine also intensifies the spinal block and prolongs the postoperative analgesia.[48] Ten micrograms of fentanyl also can intensify the block, however, with shorter duration of postoperative pain relief. The combination of adrenaline and bupivacaine provides better analgesia than the addition of either one alone.[49] Although the addition of both adrenaline and morphine to bupivacaine is valuable in cesarean section, the use of hyperbaric bupivacaine alone in the above-mentioned dosage is adequate for PPTL.

After the injection of the local anesthetic, the patient is turned on her back and monitored closely. Displacing the uterus to the left is not required during PPTL because the incidence of supine hypotension syndromes was significantly less than with cesarean section, 7% versus 83%,[21] and the dosage of ephedrine required to correct hypotension was significantly smaller, 1.6 ± 5.2 mg versus 19.2 ± 14.2 mg. Therefore, despite the fact that ephedrine is an effective prophylactic measure in cesarean section under spinal anesthesia[50] and is recommended for use with PPTL,[51] we prefer intravenous administration of 10-mg increments of ephedrine when required. Also, the incidence of nausea and vomiting was less with PPTL than with cesarean section, 1% and 0% compared with 19% and 10%, respectively, because of the greater stability of the cardiovascular system with tubal ligation.

Summary

1. With PPTL, aspiration pneumonitis is a serious problem. Although the factors that predispose to aspiration during parturition are reduced, they are not totally eliminated. Despite our recommendation of a waiting period of 8 hours, the time at which the puerperal patient can be considered to return to normal *nonpregnant* gastrointestional physiology is still unknown. Therefore, keeping the patient awake by using regional anesthesia is safer than general anesthesia. If general anesthesia is indicated, precautions should be taken to avoid aspiration, mainly by using preanesthetic antacid, rapid-sequence induction, and cricoid pressure.
2. Spinal anesthesia is the preferred technique. The reasons are as follows:
   (1) *safety*—it is safer than general anesthesia and epidural anesthesia; by using a pencil-tip needle of a small gauge (e.g., 27-gauge Whitacre needle), the incidence and severity of PDPH should be of no great concern; (2) *simplicity;* (3) *rapid onset of action;* and (4) *reliable and intense analgesia.*
3. The dose of spinal anesthesia is higher than that for cesarean section and less than that for gynecologic operations; the ratio of cesarean section to PPTL is 1:1.30.

References

1. Whitehead BEM, Smith M, O'Sullivan G: An evaluation of gastric emptying times in pregnancy and parturim. In *Abstracts of Scientific Papers, Society of Obstetric Anesthesia and Perinatology,* Annual Meeting, 1990.
2. Desphande GN, Turner AK, Sommerville IF: Plasma progesterone and pregnanediol in human pregnancy, during labour and postpartum, *J Obstet Gynaecol Br Empire* 1960; 67:954.
3. Blouw R, Scatliff J, Craig DB, et al: Gastric volume and pH in postpartum patients, *Anesthesiology* 1976; 45:456.
4. Uram M, Abouleish E, McKenzie R, et al: The risk of aspiration pneumonitis with postpartum tubal ligation. In *Abstracts of Scientific Papers, Society for Obstetric Anesthesia and Perinatology,* Annual Meeting, 1982.
5. James CF, Gibbs CP, Banner T: Postpartum perioperative risk of aspiration pneumonia, *Anesthesiology* 1984; 61:756.
6. Abouleish E: *Subarachnoid block:* In Abouleish E, editor: *Pain Control in Obstetrics,* Philadelphia, 1977, JB Lippincott.
7. Cruikshank DP, Laube DW, DeBaker LF: Intraperitoneal li-

docaine anesthesia for postpartum tubal ligation, *Obstet Gynecol* 1973; 42:127.

8. Abouleish A: Intrathecal sufentanil: a therapeutic option in managing obstetric pain, *Obstet Pain Manag* 1933; 1:1.
9. Camman WR, Minzter BH, Denney RA, Datta S: Intrathecal sufentanil for labor analgesia, *Anesthesiology* 1993; 78: 870.
10. Cammann W, Abouleish A: Spinal epidural analgesia throughout labour, *Lancet* 1993; 341:1095.
11. Collis RE, Baxandall MC, Srikantharajah ID, et al: Combined spinal epidural analgesia with ability to walk throughout labour, *Lancet* 1993; 341:767.
12. Rigler ML, Drasner K, Krejcie TC, et al: Cauda equina syndrome after continuous spinal anesthesia, *Anesth Analg* 1991; 72:275.
13. Schell RM, Brauer FS, Cole DJ, Applegate RL: Persistent sacral root deficits after continuous spinal anaesthesia, *Can J Anaesth* 1991; 38:908.
14. Phillips OC, Ebner H, Nelson AT, Black MH: Neurologic complications following spinal anesthesia with lidocaine: a prospective review of 10,440 cases, *Anesthesiology* 1969; 30:284.
15. Drasner K, Rogler ML, Sessler DI, Stolelr ML: Cauda equina syndrome following intended epidural anesthesia, *Anesthesiology* 1992; 77:582.
16. Schneider M, Ettlin T, Kaufmann M, et al: Transient neurologic toxicity after hyperbaric subarachnoid anesthesia with 5% lidocaine, *Anesth Analg* 1993; 76:1154.
17. deJong RH: Last round for a "heavyweight"? *Anesth Analg* 1994; 78:3.
18. Datta S, Lambert DH, Gregus J, et al: Differential sensitivities of mammalian nerve fibers during pregnancy, *Anesth Analg* 1983; 62:1070.
19. Flanagan HL, Datta S, Lambert DH, et al: Effect of pregnancy on bupivacaine-induced conduction blockade in the isolated rabbit vagus nerve, *Anesth Analg* 1987; 66:123.
20. Flanagan HL, Datta S, Moller RA, Covino BG: Effect of exogenously administered progesterone on susceptibility of rabbit vagus nerves to bupivacaine, *Anesthesiology* 1988; 39:A676.
21. Abouleish EI: Postpartum tubal ligation requires more bupivacaine for spinal anesthesia than does cesarean section, *Anesth Analg* 1986; 65:897.
22. Brooks GZ, Mandel ALZ: The early postpartum dermatomal spread of epidural 2-chloroprocaine. In *Abstracts of Scientific Papers, Society for Obstetric Anesthesia and Perinatology,* Annual Meeting, San Antonio, Texas, 1984.
23. Shnider SM: Serum cholinesterase activity during pregnancy, labor, and puerperium, *Anesthesiology* 1965; 26:335.
24. Evans RJ, Wroe JM: Plasma cholinesterase changes during pregnancy, *Anaesthesia* 1980; 35:651.
25. Ganga CC, Heyduk JV, Marx GF, Sklar GS: A comparison of the response to suxamethonium in postpartum and gynaecological patients, *Anaesthesia* 1982; 37:903.
26. Blitt CD, Petty WC, Alberternst EE, et al: Correlation of plasma cholinesterase activity and duration of action of succinylcholine during pregnancy, *Anesth Analg* 1977; 56:78.
27. Garn SM, Redella SA, Petzold AS, Falkner F: Maternal hematologic levels and pregnancy outcome, *Semin Perinatol* 1981; 5:155.
28. Hurley RJ, Lambert D, Hertwig L, Datta S: Postdural puncture headache in the obstetric patient: spinal vs. epidural anesthesia, *Anesthesiology* 1992; 77:A1018.
29. Ross BK, Chadwick HS, Mancuso JJ, et al: Sprotte needle for obstetric anesthesia: decreased incidence of post-dural puncture headache, *Reg Anesth* 1992; 17:29.
30. Abouleish E, Mitchell M, Miller H, et al: Comparative flow rates of saline in commonly used spinal needles including pencil tip needles, *Reg Anesth* 1994; 1934.
31. Abouleish E, Mitchell M, Warters D: In search of the optimal spinal needle, *Anesthesiology* 1992; 77:A1016.
32. Kao YJ, Tellez J, Turner DR: Dose-dependent effect of metoclopramide on cholinesterases and suxamethonium metabolism, *Br J Anaesth* 1990; 65:220.
33. Cohen SE, Barrier G: Does metoclopramide decrease gastric volume in cesarean section patients? *Anesthesiology* 1983; 59:A403.
34. Barash PG, Cullen BF, Stoelting RK, editors: *Clinical anesthesia,* Philadelphia, 1989, JB Lippincott.
35. Munson AK, Scott JR: Postpartum tubal ligation under local anesthesia, *Obstet Gynecol* 1972; 39:756.
36. Peterson HB, Hulka JF, Spielman FJ, et al: Local versus general anesthesia for laparoscopic sterilization: a randomized study, *Obstet Gynecol* 1987; 70:903.
37. Deep R, Vicchnicki MB: Laparoscopic tubal ligation under peritoneal lavage, *Reg Anesth* 1985; 10:24.
38. Abouleish E, Merriman T: In obstetrics: keep the water colorless and clear, *Anesth Analg* 1991; 73:674.
39. Lam KK, So HY, Gin T: Gastric pH and volume after oral fluids in the postpartum patient, *Can J Anaesth* 1993; 40:218.

40. Abouleish E, Meisenheimer B, Lin J Rashad N: pH of stomach contents, *Anesth Analg* 1992; 74:930.

41. Moore DC: Factors influencing spinal anesthesia, *Reg Anesth* 1982; 7:20.

42. Greene NM: Distribution of local anesthetic solution within the subarachnoid space, *Anesth Analg* 1985; 64:715.

43. Santos A, Pederson H, Finster M, Edstrom H: Hyperbaric bupivacaine for spinal anesthesia in cesarean section, *Anesth Analg* 1984; 63:1009.

44. Norris MC: Height, weight, and the spread of subarachnoid hyperbaric bupivacaine in the term parturient, *Anesth Analg* 1988; 67:555.

45. Norris MC: Patient variables and the subarachnoid spread of hyperbaric bupivacaine in the term parturient, *Anesthesiology* 1990; 72:478.

46. Hartwell BL, Aglio LS, Hauch MA, Datta S: Vertebral column length and spread of hyperbaric subarachnoid bupivacaine in the term parturient, *Reg Anesth* 1991; 16:17.

47. Abouleish E: Epinephrine improves the quality of spinal hyperbaric bupivacaine for cesarean section, *Anesth Analg* 1987; 66:395.

48. Abouleish E, Rawal N, Fallon K, Hernandez D: Combined intrathecal morphine and bupivacaine for cesarean section, *Anesth Analg* 1988; 67:370.

49. Abouleish E, Rawal N, Tobon-Randal B, et al: A clinical and laboratory study to compare the addition of 0.2 mg morphine, 0.2 epinephrine or their combination to hyperbaric bupivacaine for spinal anesthesia in cesarean section, *Anesth Analg* 1993; 77:457.

50. Kang YG, Abouleish E, Caritis S: Prophylactic intravenous ephedrine infusion during spinal anesthesia for cesarean section, *Anesth Analg* 1982; 61:839.

51. Gajraj NM, Victory RA, Pace NA, et al: Comparison of an ephedrine infusion with crystalloid administration for prevention of hypotension during spinal anesthesia, *Anesth Analg* 1993; 76:1023.

40

Maternal Infection

A 25-year-old primigravida is admitted to the labor floor with a history of spontaneous rupture of membrane. Her temperature is 101° F and her pulse is 120 beats/min. On vaginal examination, she is 5-cm dilated and in active labor. The obstetrician requests epidural analgesia for her pain relief.

Recommendations by Harvey Carp, Ph. D., M.D.
David H. Chesnut, M.D.

Infection in the parturient is a common clinical problem encountered by obstetric anesthesiologists and has important fetal, maternal, and anesthetic implications. This chapter briefly reviews the more common causes of fever in the parturient, including chorioamnionitis and urinary tract infections. Furthermore, the potential risks and benefits of regional anesthesia in the febrile parturient are discussed. Finally, recommendations for the anesthetic management of the febrile parturient are formulated.

Common Etiologies of Fever

Chorioamnionitis

Chorioamnionitis is one of the most common infections occurring in the parturient and is present in about 1% of all pregnancies.[1-6] The diagnosis of chorioamnionitis is based on clinical signs and consists of a syndrome of fever higher than 38° C plus maternal or fetal tachycardia, uterine tenderness, or foul-smelling amniotic fluid.

In most cases, bacteria gain access to the amniotic cavity and the fetus by ascending through ruptured membranes; chorioamnionitis develops in a significant number of parturients with premature rupture of the membranes.[1] Bacteroides, group B streptococci, and *Escherichia coli* are common organisms isolated from the amniotic fluid of parturients with chorioamnionitis. Importantly, maternal bacteremia has been reported to occur in about 10% of parturients with the clinical diagnosis of chorioamnionitis.[1-6]

Neonatal complications of this infection include

sepsis, meningitis, pneumonia, and increased perinatal death. Maternal complications include postpartum infection, postpartum hemorrhage, sepsis, and even death. In addition, several studies report an increased incidence of cesarean deliveries in pregnancies complicated by chorioamnionitis.

Clearly the patient with chorioamnionitis represents a high-risk patient and obstetric management of these complex cases, continues to evolve. Most investigators agree that there is a need for timely delivery of the fetus. In recent studies excellent maternal and neonatal results have been reported without the use of arbitrary time limits, and when cesarean delivery was performed for standard obstetric indications and not for the diagnosis of chorioamnionitis alone.

Perinatologists agree that antibiotics are indicated in patients with chorioamnionitis. However, there is not complete agreement regarding the type and timing of antibiotic therapy. For many years pediatricians requested that maternal antibiotic therapy be delayed until after delivery to avoid the possibility that intrapartum therapy might effect the results of neonatal blood cultures. However intrapartum antibiotic therapy is becoming more common as a result of recent reports, suggesting a decrease in neonatal and morbidity when antibiotic treatment is begun during rather than after delivery.[7,8]

Urologic Infections

Urinary tract infections are common infectious complications of pregnancy. Urinary stasis and decreased ureteric tone caused by the gravid uterus, as well as by the smooth muscle relaxant effects of progesterone, probably predispose parturients to urinary infections and also make it more likely that infection in the bladder may ascend into the kidneys to produce pyelonephritis.[1,9,10]

Symptoms of acute pyelonephritis usually are dramatic and this infection is a serious threat to fetal and maternal well-being.

About 10% of parturients with pyelonephritis will develop transient bacteremia during the course of this infection.[1,9,10] The most common organisms are *E. coli, Klebsiella,* and *Proteus* species. Interestingly, a recent report suggested that acute pyelonephritis during pregnancy may be associated with development of the adult respiratory distress syndrome.[11]

In addition to maternal complications, pyelonephritis has important fetal implications. This infection has been associated with a significantly increased risk of premature delivery as well as fetal infectious complications.

Regional Anesthesia in the Febrile Parturient

Clinical Studies

Clinicians have long suspected that an association exists between the performance of a dural puncture during a period of bacteremia and the subsequent development of meningitis. Similar concerns apply to the performance of epidural block and the development of epidural abscess. However, these concerns are based largely on anecdotal reports of central nervous system infection after regional anesthesia, and are not readily supported by clinical studies.[12-17]

Early medical researchers feared that diagnostic lumbar puncture actually might cause meningitis rather than aid in its diagnosis.[18-23] They reasoned that the rich venous plexus surrounding the spinal cord could be disrupted by lumbar puncture and allow the direct introduction of bacteria into the central nervous system by the spinal needle. Alternatively, disruption of the dural barrier could permit hematogenous spread of infection into the central nervous system. Epidural block involves the introduction of a foreign body and frequently involves blood vessel disruption. As such, this technique could produce a nidus for subsequent infection.

To validate this hypothesis six separate, retrospective clinical studies have been performed to evaluate the risk of diagnostic lumbar puncture.[18-23] These studies did not involve the administration of regional anesthesia. However, these reports have provided differing conclusions regarding the association between dural puncture performed during a period of bacteremia and meningitis. Four of these studies clearly do not support an association between dural puncture and meningitis.[18-21] In fact, one of these studies concluded that, "The development of bacterial meningitis in children with occult bacteremia is stongly associated with the species of bacteria that causes the infection, but not with a lumbar puncture."[21] Whereas two studies did provide some evidence for an association between dural puncture and meningitis,[22,23] both of them have serious methodologic flaws. One study was performed during an epidemic of meningitis.[23] Although the authors found high rates of meningitis after lumbar puncture, they did not compare these values to a control group not undergoing lumbar puncture. The second study reported an association between lumbar puncture and meningitis only in infants younger than 1 year of age.[22] However, these investigators could not exclude the possibility that pediatricians participating in this unblinded retrospective study performed more lumbar punctures in sicker appearing children already at a higher risk for meningitis.

In summary, each of the epidemiologic studies performed to date have serious methodologic flaws and do not provide a clear-cut answer to the question of whether dural puncture performed during a period of bacteremia is a significant risk factor for the development of meningitis. Part of the uncertainty surrounding the risk of dural puncture may be due to the fact that the development of meningitis is a complex process requiring many steps, only one of which involves the integrity of the meninges.

Some anesthesiologists have cited anecdotal reports of meningitis after spinal anesthesia during a presumed period of bacteremia as evidence that dural puncture may cause meningitis.[12-17] However, many of these patients were debilitated or immunosuppressed, and already at risk for the development of meningitis in the absence of spinal anesthesia. Adding to the confusion are two recent cases of meningitis reported to occur after epidural block for labor.[17] Both patients in this study were afebrile and without clinical signs of infection at the time of epidural placement. In fact, the epidural was in place for less than 1 hour in one of the patients. Similarly, two cases of epidural abscess have been reported several days after epidural catheter removal in parturients without signs of infection at the time of the anesthetic.[16]

In view of the fact that the development of central nervous system infection is a complex process, it is not surprising that epidemiologic studies of spinal and epidural anesthesia involving thousands of patients find the incidence of infectious complications related to anesthesia to be extraordinarily rare. Dripps and Vandam prospectively studied patients receiving 10,098 spinal anesthetics between 1948 and 1951 and reported no cases of central nervous system (CNS) infection.[24] Similarly, three reviews of over 500,000 obstetric patients who received regional anesthesia reported no cases of meningitis and only two cases of epidural space infection (not associated with maternal infection).[25-27] Surely some of these parturients were bacteremic at the time of the regional anesthetic, given the frequency with which parturients develop fever and infection during labor. A study by Blanco et al. found a 1% incidence rate of bacteremia in a random sample of patients in the labor ward, and most studies report an 8% to 10% incidence rate of bacteremia in parturients with chorioamnionitis.[2-5] Furthermore, most studies have reported that the level of fever was a poor predictive indicator of bacteremia in these patients. Blanco et al. reported that almost half of the bacteremic patients with choriomanionitis had temperatures below 38.8° C.[5] Furthermore, Bader et al. reported no difference in the mean temperatures between bacteremic and nonbacteremic patients with chorioamnionitis.[28]

Unfortunately, there are no good predictive factors to identify the subgroup of febrile patients with chorioamnionitis who are bacteremic at the time of an anesthetic. Therefore, two groups of investigators evaluated the risk of CNS infection after regional anesthesia administered to febrile patients with chorioamnionitis. Bader et al. retrospectively studied 279 parturients with chorioamnionitis and found no evidence of CNS infection after epidural or spinal block for labor and cesarean delivery.[28] Eight percent of the subjects had blood cultures for diagnosis of type of infection and nearly two thirds of the patients were not treated with antibiotics before the regional block. Similarly, Ramanathan et al. studied 139 parturients with chorioamnionitis and also found no evidence of meningitis or epidural abscess after regional anesthesia.[29] These investigators treated almost all of the subjects with antibiotics before the anesthetic.

Taken together, the bulk of clinical evidence does not support an association between regional anesthesia and the development of CNS infection. However, some degree of uncertainty does remain because of the relatively small numbers of patients who have been studied, the retrospective design of most studies, and the possibility of bias in patient selection.

Experimental Studies

To better define the risk of dural puncture performed during bacteremia, this author performed animal experiments under more closely controlled conditions than is possible during clinical studies.[30] In brief, rats were rendered bacteremic by producing a flank abscess using *E. coli*. Next, cisternal dural puncture was performed on the bacteremic animals, 24 hours after which the cisterna magna was surgically drained and the spinal fluid was cultured for evidence of meningitis. As shown in Table 40-1, 12 of the 40 animals undergoing dural puncture during *E. coli* bacteremia developed meningitis. Bacteremic animals not undergoing dural puncture did not develop meningitis, and dural puncture in the absence of bacteremia did not result in infection. Importantly, none of the bacteremic animals given a dose of gentamicin 15 minutes before the dural puncture developed meningitis.

Although animal models of disease permit careful control of experimental variables, clinical conditions cannot be duplicated exactly. Applying this experimental study to clinical practice has several limitations. The level of bacteremia produced in the rats exceeded the transient, low-grade bacteremia produced in most obstetric patients. In fact, the animals most likely had hemodynamic and metabolic changes characteristic of early sepsis. In addition, although *E. coli* is a common cause of bacteremia in surgical and obstetric patients, it is an uncommon cause of meningitis. Furthermore, the relative size of the dural tear produced by the 26-gauge needle used in this study is larger in rats compared with that in humans. In addition, the cisternal site of dural puncture is not normally used in clinical anesthesia. Lastly, spinal anesthesia involves the injection of a local anesthetic, and these drugs have been reported to be bacteriostatic.[31]

These experimental differences render the clinical relevance of the animal data in the current study

TABLE 40-1

ASSOCIATION BETWEEN BACTEREMIA AND THE RECOVERY OF ESCHERICHIA COLI FROM CEREBROSPINAL FLUID AFTER DURAL PUNCTURE

No.	Bacteremia* CFU/ml	Gentamicin†	Dural Puncture	Cerebrospinal Fluid *E. coli*‡
40	40 ± 22 (5-100)	No	Yes	12/40§
40	48 ± 25‖ (2-100)	No	No	0/40
30	0 (0)	No	Yes	0/30
30	49 ± 35 (5-110)	Yes	Yes	0/30

No., No. of rats in each group; CFU, colony-forming units.

*Data expressed as mean ± SD (range in parentheses).

†Gentamicin administered before dural puncture.

‡Data expressed as the no. of animals with *E. coli* cultured from spinal fluid per total no. of animals in that group.

§ $P < 0.05$ compared with other groups.

‖Not statistically different compared with the bacteremic group undergoing cisternal puncture.

From Carp H, Bailey S: The association between meningitis and dural puncture in bacteremic rats, *Anesthesiology* 1992;76:739.

difficult to interpret. However, these experimental data and the results of previous animal studies suggest that dural puncture during bacteremia may be a risk factor for the development of meningitis. However, antibiotic treatment before the dural puncture appears to eliminate this risk.

Human Immunovirus Infection

Human immunovirus (HIV) infection is increasingly common in parturients, and obstetric anesthesiologists will be called on to administer regional anesthesia to these women for labor or cesarean delivery. In view of the high incidence of neurologic dysfunction associated with HIV infection, many clinicians avoid regional anesthesia in these patients. Neurologic dysfunction may be the result of the increased incidence of tuberculous, and fungal and viral infections of the CNS secondary to HIV-induced immunsupression.[32] In addition, the direct action of HIV itself within the CNS may result in aseptic meningitis, myelopathy, and neuropathy.[33] In fact, about 40% of individuals with HIV infection show clinical evidence of serious neurologic disease with progression of their infection to acquired immunodeficiency syndrome (AIDS).[33]

The HIV infection produces several unique medical problems that may affect the choice of regional anesthesia in these patients. For example, what is the risk to the HIV-positive parturient of direct introduction of HIV virus–containing blood into the CNS as a result of dural puncture? Most studies suggest that HIV infects the CNS early in the natural course of HIV infection, before symptoms appear, and it seems that dural puncture would be unlikely to introduce HIV into an uninfected CNS.[33,34] An additional concern would be the introduction of other viruses, fungi, or mycobacteria into the CNS of a parturient, with the subsequent development of meningitis as a result of HIV-related immunosupression. In particular, *Mycobacterium tuberculosis* is emerging as one of the most frequent causative agents of meningeal infections in HIV-positive patients.[32] In contrast to the recommendation for the use of prophylactic antibiotics in bacteremeic patients (vida supra), such prophylaxis may not be effective in the case of individuals infected with *M. tuberculosis* as a result of the high frequency of drug-resistant organisms.[32]

In spite of these theoretical concerns, no reports of meningitis as a result of diagnostic lumbar puncture in an HIV-positive patient appear to have been made. In fact, the results of two preliminary studies involving a small number of HIV-positive parturients reported no neurologic or infectious complications after epidural or spinal anesthesia.[35,36] Furthermore, epidural blood patch did not produce complications in six HIV-positive patients.[37] However, further studies will be required to confirm these preliminary results, suggesting that regional anesthesia is safe in the HIV-positive parturient.

Anesthetic Management: Recommendations

In my opinion, the bulk of clinical and experimental evidence suggests that regional anesthesia can be safely administered to healthy patients at risk for bacteremia. Regional anesthesia does not need to be avoided in patients at risk for transient, low-grade bacteremia, including the parturient with the presumptive diagnosis of chorioamnionitis. Furthermore, appropriate antibiotic therapy initiated before the anesthetic should lessen the risk of meningitis or epidural abscess in patients with evidence of systemic infection. In my practice I do not hesitate to administer spinal or epidural block to patients with evidence of systemic infection, provided appropriate antibiotic therapy has begun. This recommendation applies to case of the febrile parturient with the presumptive diagnosis of chorioamnionitis described at the beginning of the chapter. Although the choice of anesthesia needs to be individualized, it is prudent to avoid regional anesthesia in untreated patients with overt clinical signs of sepsis.

Finally, "We do not give regional anesthesia in the absence of other relevant information. Rather, we provide care for febrile patients who require anesthesia for labor, delivery or emergency surgery. When one considers the risks of infection with regional anesthesia one should ask: What are the alternatives? What are the consequences of witholding regional anesthesia in a febrile patient? For example, what is the greater risk in a febrile parturient: meningitis or epidural abscess after spinal or epidural anesthesia, or failed intubation and aspiration during general anesthesia?"[38]

Summary

1. Fever is a common clinical finding in parturients and usually is the result of maternal infection.
2. Chorioamnionitis and pyelonephritis are the most common antepartum infections and may produce serious maternal or perinatal morbidity.
3. The bulk of clinical and experimental evidence suggests that regional anesthesia may be safely performed in parturients at risk for transient bacteremia as well as patients with established infection, provided there is no evidence of overt sepsis.
4. Treatment of maternal infections with antibiotics, before regional block, is appropriate and prudent in cases of maternal infection, before the administration of regional block.

References

1. Gibbs RS, Sweet RL: *Maternal and fetal infections.* In Creasy RK, Resnik R, editors: *Maternal-fetal medicine: principles and practice,* Philadelphia, 1989, WB Saunders.
2. Gibbs RS, Castillo MS, Rogers PJ: Management of acute chorioamnionitis, *Am J Obstet Gynecol* 1980; 136:709.
3. Duff P, Sanders R, Gibbs RS: The course of labor in term

patients wtih chorioamnionitis, *Am J Obstet Gynecol* 1983; 147:391.

4. Yoder PR, Gibbs RS, Blanco JD, et al: A prospective, controlled study of maternal and perinatal outcome after intraamniotic infection at term, *Am J Obstet Gynecol* 1983; 45:695.
5. Blanco JD, Gibbs RS, Casteneda YS: Bacteremia in obstetrics: clinical course, *Obstet Gynecol* 1981; 58:621.
6. Satin AJ, Mayberry MC, Leveno KJ, et al: Chorioamnionitis: a harbinger of dystocia, *Obstet Gynecol* 1992; 79:913.
7. Gibbs RS, Djinsmoor MJ, Newton ER, Ramamurthy RS: A randomized trial of intrapartum versus immediate postpartum treatment of women with intra-amniotic infection, *Obstet Gynecol* 1988; 72:823.
8. Gilstrap LC, Leveno KJ, Cox SM, et al: Intrapartum treatment of acute chorioamnionitis: impact on neonatal sepsis, *Am J Obstet Gynecol* 1988; 159:579.
9. Gilstrap LC, Cunningham FG, Whalley PJ: Acute pyelonephritis in pregnancy: an anterospective study, *Obstet Gynecol* 1974; 57:409.
10. Kass EH: Bacturia and pyelonephritis of pregnancy, *Arch Intern Med* 1960; 205:194.
11. Cunningham FG, Lucas MJ, Hankins GDV: Pulmonary injury complicating antepartum pyelonephritis, *Am J Obstet Gynecol* 1987; 156:797.
12. Berman RS, Eisele JH: Bacteremia, spinal anesthesia, and development of meningitis, *Anesthesiology* 1978; 48:376.
13. Roberts SP, Petts HV: Meningitis after obstetric spinal anesthesia, *Anaesthesia* 1990; 45:376.
14. Barrie HJ: Meningitis following spinal anesthesia, *Lancet* 1941; i:242.
15. Loarie DJ, Fairley HB: Epidural abscess following spinal anesthesia, *Anesth Analg* 1978; 57:351.
16. Ngan Koo WD, Jones MR, Thomas P, Worth RJ: Extradural abscess complicating extradural anesthesia for caesarean section, *Br J Anaesth* 1992; 69:647.
17. Ready LB, Helfer D: Bacterial meningitis in parturients after epidural anesthesia, *Anesthesiology* 1989; 71:988.
18. Pray LG: Lumbar puncture as a factor in the pathogenesis of meningitis, *Am J Dis Child* 1941; 295:62.
19. Eng RHK, Seligman SJ: Lumbar puncture-induced meningitis, *JAMA* 1981; 245:1456.
20. Smith KM, Deddish RB, Ogata ES: Meningitis associated with serial lumbar punctures and post-hemmorrhagic hydrocephalus, *J Pediatrics* 1986; 109:1057.
21. Shapiro ED, Aaron NH, Wald ER, Chiponis D: Risk factor for the development of bacterial meningitis among children with occult bacteremia, *J Pediatrics* 1986; 109:15.
22. Teele DW, Dashefsky B, Rakusan T, Klein JO: Meningitis after lumbar puncture in children with bacteremia, *N Engl J Med* 1981; 305:1079.
23. Wegeforth P, Latham JR: Lumbar puncture as a factor in the causation of meningitis, *Am J Med Sci* 1919; 158:183.
24. Dripps RD, Vandam LD: Long-term follow-up of patients who received 10,098 spinal anesthetics, *JAMA* 1954; 156: 1486.
25. Scott DB, Hibbard B: Serious non-fatal complications associated with extradural block in obstetric practice, *Br J Anaesth* 1990; 64:537.
26. Crawford JS: Some maternal complications of epidural analgesia for labour, *Anaesthesia* 1985; 40:1219.
27. Hellmann K: Epidural anesthesia in obstetrics: a second look at 26,127 cases, *Can Anaesth Soc J* 1965; 12:398.
28. Bader AM, Gilbertson L, Kirz L, Datta S: Regional anesthesia in women with chorioamnionitis, 1992; 17:84.
29. Ramanathan J, Vaddadi A, Mercer BM, et al: Epidural anesthesia in women with chorioamnionitis, *Anesth Rev* 1992; 19:35.
30. Carp H, Bailey S: The association between meningitis and dural puncture in bacteremic rats, *Anesthesiology* 1992; 76:739.
31. James FM, George RH, Naiem H, White GJ: Bacteriologic aspects of epidural analgesia, *Anesth Analg* 1976; 55:187.
32. Berenguer J, Moreno S, Laguna F, et al: Tuberculous meningitis in patients infected with the human immunodeficiency virus, *N Engl J Med* 1992; 326:668.
33. Elder GA, Sever JL: AIDS and neurological disorders: an overview, *Ann Neurol* 1988; 23(suppl):S4.
34. Resnick L, Berger JR, Shapshak P, Tourtelotte WW: Early penetration of the blood-brain barrier by HIV, *Neurology* 1988; 38:9.
35. Hughes SC, Dailey PA, Landers D, et al: The HIV + parturient and regional anesthesia: clinical and immunologic response, *Anesthesiology* 1992; 77:A1036.
36. Gershon RY, Williams DM, Berry AJ, et al: The effect of anesthesia on the HIV infected parturient, *Anesthesiology* 1992; 77:A1037.
37. Tom DJ, Gulevich SJ, Shapiro HM, et al: Epidural blood patch in the HIV-positive patient: review of clinical experience, *Anesthesiology* 1992; 76:943.
38. Chestnut DH: Spinal anesthesia in the febrile patient, *Anesthesiology* 1992; 76:667.

41

Latex Allergy

A 32-year-old primigravida, at 28 weeks' gestation, comes to the hospital for an anesthesia consultation because of latex allergy. How will you approach this case?

Recommendations by Dana A. Vildus, M.D.

Latex, the milky sap obtained from *Hevea brasiliensis,* has been used in the manufacture of various medical products for many years; however, only recently, contact urticaria and anaphylaxis due to its use have been described. The first case of contact urticaria was described in 1979[1] and in 1984 it was confirmed by skin prick testing as an IgE-mediated anaphylaxis.[2] Cases of intraoperative anaphylaxis were first reported in 1989.[3,4] Latex sensitivity and anaphylaxis has been reported in the obstetric population after vaginal examination,[5] after vaginal delivery,[6] and after cesarean section.[7,8] With this growing number of reports of severe reactions to latex and the prevalence of latex products in the health care environment, the prevention and management of latex anaphylaxis in the obstetric population merits attention.

High-Risk Population

Two populations are known to be at increased risk for the development of latex sensitivity. The first group is health care professionals, especially operating room personnel who routinely use latex gloves. In one study, 7.4% of physicians and 5.4% of nurses were sensitive to latex, a much higher incidence than either the other hospital employees (1.3%) or the general population (0.8%).[9] Sixty-seven percent of these latex-allergic patients had a history of atopy and in fact, latex gloves used on eczematous hands may predispose to latex allergy.

Another high-risk group includes patients with prolonged or frequent exposure to latex from multiple surgical procedures or from the routine care of a dysfunctional bladder or colon. This includes patients with myelodysplasia and congenital urologic abnormalities.[10,11] In fact, one study found 34% of children with spina bifida had antibodies to latex antigens.[12]

Preoperative Assessment

A thorough history is essential in the initial evaluation of the patient. The first step is to identify high-risk patients, particularly those with multiple allergies, atopy, and eczema. Patients should be questioned about itching, erythema, swelling, or wheezing after using latex medical or household gloves, during dental or medical examinations where latex products were used, while using condoms, or even while inflating balloons. In addition, patients with a history of intraoperative anaphylaxis for unknown reasons should be suspected of latex sensitivity.

Patients in whom latex sensitivity is suspected should be referred to an allergist for appropriate testing. The most common tests for latex allergy are the skin-prick test (SPT), the intradermal test (IDT), and the radioallergosorbent test (RAST).

The SPT involves incubating extracts of latex in saline, then placing a drop of the solution (1:10 wt/vol) on the forearm. A skin prick then is made and a wheal and flare response is measured after 10 minutes. At the same time, positive and negative controls with histamine and saline are placed.[13] The IDT is more sensitive but carries more of a risk for a systemic reaction. The solution is diluted 100- to 1000-fold less than for SPT and is injected intradermally.[14] These reactions are graded 1+ to 4+, with 2+ being a weak positive reaction (the reaction to latex is half as strong as the reaction to histamine) and 4+ being strong positive (the reaction to latex is greater than is the histamine test reaction).[13] Since anaphylaxis may be induced with skin testing, it is necessary to have epinephrine and resuscitative equipment available.

The RAST test is an in vitro test that measures latex-specific IgE antibodies by exposing the antigen to the patient's antibody-containing serum. This complex then is incubated with radiolabeled anti-human IgE, and the radioactivity then is measured. The activity is proportional to the quantity of IgE antibody bound during the initial phase of the test.[14] RAST is not yet a substitute for skin testing since false-negative results do occur, especially in people with milder allergies.[13] Direct skin testing is more sensitive, less expensive, and less time consuming, but carries the risk of anaphylaxis. Because of this risk, direct skin testing probably should be avoided in the pregnant patient. Since the RAST test is relatively insensitive, if one suspects latex allergy by clinical history, then one should treat the patient as though she were allergic to latex.

Recommendations for Management

If a patient is suspected to be allergic to latex, the only known effective treatment is avoidance of latex products. Pharmacologic prophylaxis, such as combined administration of H_2-blockers, corticosteroids, and diphenhydramine have been cited in case reports[15,16]; it is unclear that these measures prevent or decrease the severity of anaphylaxis, should it occur.

Foremost is the necessity to avoid exposure to latex, especially in the form of gloves. Repeated mucosal exposure to latex gloves during surgery or vaginal examination favors absorption of antigen. Synthetic gloves, such as those made of neoprene (Neolon) or sytrene butadiene (Tactylon) are available alternatives. Any rubber ports in intravenous tubing should not be punctured; instead, drugs should be administered through stopcocks. All drugs need to be drawn up from glass ampules, or multiple-dose vials with rubber tops need to be removed before withdrawing the drug. Medications given via glass syringes can be used. If freshly drawn, drugs administered through rubber-tip plunger syringe systems have been reported as not presenting any problems, since the contact time is insufficient for any significant quantity of antigen to become dissolved.[14] The blood pressure cuff is rubber based and may cause a contact dermatitis. This can be avoided by wrapping the area underneath with soft cotton or cast padding. Epidural catheters have been used safely. The catheter adapter may contain a small amount of latex, but soaking it in saline will elute the responsible proteins.

If a general anesthetic is needed, it is necessary to avoid old-style endotracheal tubes and certain airways. It is necessary to use plastic endotracheal tubes, circuits, and face masks, and a prewashed or nonlatex reservoir bag. Once washed multiple times, the latex antigen is reduced to safe levels. It is not feasible to change some components in the anesthesia machine itself, such as the ventilator bellows, but one can decrease the amount of airborne antigens by placing a passive humidifier in the circuit.

Avoidance of latex is of paramount importance. Communication between obstetricians, nurses, and anesthesiologists must be maintained so that everyone is prepared to avoid and treat latex allergy. At Bringham and Womens's Hospital (Boston) a *latex allergy kit* is available that contains alternatives to latex-containing products. A checklist is helpful (Table 41-1), but companies often do not list components found in patient care products. It may be necessary to contact the manufacturers directly to determine if their products contain latex or if a latex-free alternative is available.

Should latex anaphylaxis occur in the pregnant patient, treatment should be aimed at maintaining both maternal and fetal oxygenation. Bronchospasm and hypotension should be treated with supplemental oxygen, left uterine displacement, fluids, and vasopressors. In extreme cases, intubation of the trachea may be necessary. Epinephrine is the drug of choice in anaphylaxis; however, doses needed to treat anaphylaxis are not the same as those needed for cardiac arrest. Since epinephrine is a potent

TABLE 41-1
CHECKLIST FOR LATEX-ALLERGIC PATIENTS

Preoperative

- Patients with a history of chronic care with latex-based products, e.g., spina bifida patients
- History of intolerance to latex-based products: balloons, rubber gloves, condoms, dental dams, rubber urethral catheters
- History of intraoperative anaphylaxis of uncertain etiology
- Careful coordination of surgical/anesthesia/nursing teams
- Check with central supply for availability of alternatives

Intraoperative

Anesthesia Equipment

- Gloves
- Airways/endotracheal tubes
- Masks
- Rebreathing bags
- Ventilator bellows
- Circuit
- Multidose vials
- Intravenous equipment/tourniquet/rubber bands
- Blood pressure cuffs
- Syringe plungers

Surgical Equipment

- Drains (e.g., penrose)
- Urinary catheters
- Instrument mats
- Surgical gloves
- Rubber-shod clamps
- Vascular tags
- Bulb syringes for irrigation
- Rubber bands

Postoperative

- Medic alert tag
- Warnings posted on chart
- Warnings posted on bed

uterine artery vasoconstrictor, the minimum effective dose to correct hypotension and bronchospasm should be used. The dose can range from 0.1 μg/kg[14] to 5 μg/kg,[17] depending on the severity of symptoms.

Second-line drugs are bronchdilators, such as β-2-agonists and aminophylline, antihistamines, and corticosteroids. Epinephrine and other bronchodilators can cause uterine relaxation and may increase bleeding if delivery occurs. Diphenhydramine (0.5 to 1 mg/kg) should be administered to reduce the likelihood that circulating histamine will subsequently attach to unoccupied histamine receptors. All antihistamines cross the placenta, but diphenhydramine has minimal adverse effects in the neonate.[18] Corticosteroids also are administered for the treatment of an allergic reaction, and may in fact be helpful in ameliorating protracted reactions, especially those associated with bronchospasm.[19]

Summary

1. A patient should have a prior consult with an anesthesiologist before her admission and obtain a Medic Alert bracelet.
2. On the day of delivery, a *latex allergy kit* should be kept in the delivery area. All personnel must be aware of patient's allergy, and avoiding latex products is imperative.
3. A patient may deliver either vaginally or by cesarean section. For labor and delivery, regional analgesia using an epidural technique is a safe choice. For cesarean section, regional anesthesia, or if indicated, general anesthesia can be provided, safely using the nonlatex alternatives recommended.
4. One should be prepared to treat anaphylaxis with appropriate resuscitative drugs and equipment readily available.

References

1. Nutter AF: Contact urticaria to rubber, *Br J Dermatol* 1979; 101:597.
2. Turjanmao K, Reunala T, Tuimala R, Karkkainea T: Severe IgE-mediated allergy to surgical gloves: proceedings from the XV Nordic Congress of Allergology, Turku, Finland, *Allergy* 1984; (suppl 2):35 (abstract).
3. Gerber AC, Jong W, Zbinden S, et al: Severe intraoperative anaphylaxis to surgical gloves: latex allergy, an unfamiliar condition, *Anesthesiology* 1989; 71:800.
4. Slater JE: Rubber anaphylaxis, *N Engl J Med* 1989;820:1126.
5. Axelsson JGK, Johansson SGO, Wrangsjo K: IgE-mediated anaphylactoid reactions to rubber, *Allergy* 1987; 42:46.
6. Laurent J, Malet R, Smiejan JM, et al: Latex hypersensitivity after natural delivery, *J Allergy Clin Immunol* 1992; 89:779.
7. Turjanmaa K, Reunela T, Tuimala R, Karkkainen T: Allergy to latex gloves: unusual complication during delivery, *Br Med J* 1988; 297:1029.
8. Leynadier R, Pecquet C, Dry J: Anaphylaxis to latex during surgery, *Anaesthesia* 1989; 44:547.
9. Turjanmaa K: Incidence of immediate allergy to latex gloves in hospital personnel, *Contact Dermatitis* 1987; 17:270.
10. Sethna NF, Sockin SM, Holzman RS, Slaten JE: Latex anaphylaxis in a child with a history of multiple anesthetic drug allergies, *Anesthesiology* 1992; 77:372.
11. Moneret-Vantrin DA, Laxenaire MC, Bavoux F: Allergic shock to latex and ethylene oxide during surgery for spina bifida, *Anesthesiology* 1990; 73:556.
12. Slater JE, Mastello LA, Shaer C: Rubber specific IgE in children with spina bifida, *J Urol* 1991; 146:578.
13. Turjanmaa K, Reunda T, Rasanen L: Comparison of diagnostic methods in latex surgical glove contact urticaria, *Contact Dermatitis* 1988; 19:241.
14. Holzman RS: Latex allergy: an emerging operation room problem, *Anesth Analg* 1993; 76:635.
15. Sockin SM, Young MC: Preoperative prophylaxis of latex anaphylaxis, *J Allergy Clin Immunol* 1991; 87:269.
16. Swartz JO, Braude BM, Gilmour RF, et al: Intraoperative anaphylaxis to latex, *Can J Anaesth* 1990; 37:589.
17. Stoelting RK: Allergic reactions during anesthesia, *Anesth Analg* 1983; 62:341.
18. Halpern S: *Anesthesia for pregnant patient with immunologic disorders.* In: Shnider SM, Levinson G, editors: *Anesthesia for obstetrics,* ed 3, Baltimore, 1993, Williams and Wilkins.
19. Bochner BS, Lichtenstein LM: Anaphylaxis, *N Engl J Med* 1991; 324:1785.

42

Drug Addiction

A 28-year-old primigravida, at 29 weeks' gestation, is admitted to the labor floor with a blood pressure of 220/120 mm Hg and a heart rate of 130 beats/min. She gives a history of smoking crack *before admission to the hospital. Discuss the anesthetic management of this patient for labor, delivery, and cesarean section.*

Recommendations by David J. Birnbach, M.D.

Substance abuse continues to be a major problem facing our society. Obstetricians, pediatricians, and anesthesiologists are encountering an increasing number of pregnant women who use illicit substances, whether recreationally or as addicts.[1] Perinatal substance abuse has been linked to many maternal and neonatal complications that may have a profound effect on the patient's response to the administration of anesthesia. The use of cocaine, for example, is associated with a high morbidity and mortality, especially in the patient undergoing anesthesia. This chapter emphasizes the detection, anesthetic management, and treatment of the cocaine-abusing parturient, and also discusses the anesthetic implications of amphetamine, narcotic, and alcohol abuse in pregnancy.

Cocaine Abuse

Cocaine use has been described by the Director of the National Institute on Drug Abuse as a "major public health threat."[2] Whereas the use of most illicit substances in the U.S. has remained stable or has even declined over the last decade, the use of cocaine has increased dramatically.[3] It has been suggested that cocaine use in U.S. actually has reached epidemic proportions, with greater than 5 million Americans using this drug regularly.[3,4]

Cocaine use, although it has increased over the last decade, is not a new phenomenon. Archeologic findings suggest that pre-Incans in Peru and Bolivia were the first to discover the stimulant effect of the coca plant. Cocaine was used predominantly by the natives of South America until it was isolated by

Niemann in 1859.[5] In the nineteenth century cocaine was brought to prominence by the descriptions by prominent physicians and authors of its benefits in treating many ailments. Sigmund Freud was one of the most famous proponents of cocaine, stating that it could cure depression, alleviate disorders of the stomach, treat asthma, and cure drug addiction.[6] The medical use of cocaine was described by Koller,[7] who documented its local anesthetic properties, and Halstead, the father of modern surgery, who first used cocaine to perform nerve blocks and ultimately became cocaine dependent himself.[8]

By the early 1900s the adverse effects of cocaine were being reported, and in 1906 the Food and Drug Act began to regulate its use. Although Coca Cola originally used cocaine as an additive ingredient, due to this Act the beverage company began using decocainized coca leaves.[9] The present U.S. epidemic of cocaine abuse is considered to be the third, the first two being in the 1890s and 1920s.[10]

Evidence of recent increased cocaine use can be seen in the increases in cocaine-related emergency visits and cocaine-related overdose deaths. In the 10-year period from 1976 to 1986, there was a more than fifteenfold increase in emergency department visits attributed to cocaine abuse.[11] The recent increase in cocaine-related mortalities most likely is due to the higher purity and lower cost of cocaine. The price of cocaine has steadily decreased over the last decade, to the point where prices for cocaine are similar to marijuana, removing a barrier to its widespread use.

Recent studies show that the rate of cocaine use by pregnant women in the U.S. also is growing, and that an increasing number of infants are being born to cocaine-abusing mothers.[12] More than 5 million American women of childbearing age use illicit drugs, with almost 1 million of these women using cocaine.[13] Because many cocaine-abusing patients deny drug use,[14,15] the exact extent of prenatal cocaine use is not known. It has been estimated, however, that as many as 45% of women cared for at urban teaching hospitals may be using cocaine during their pregnancies.[16] Although unregistered patients tend to have high rates of cocaine use, perhaps as high as 50% or greater,[17] registered pregnant patients also have been found to be using cocaine[18,19] In 1988 10% of women delivering at a New York City hospital were found to have positive results for cocaine on urine toxicology testing.[20] Likewise, studies from Chicago, Detroit, and California also have reported cocaine-positive results in about 10% of their parturients.[21,22] When the rates of cocaine use were compared between a high-risk center and a private hospital, 11% of patients in the public hospital versus 1% of patients in the private hospital reported cocaine use.[19] Cocaine use is not restricted to inner city patients, however, and evidence now suggests that it is occurring in all parts of this country and across cultural and economic boundaries.[23,24] Pregnant cocaine users are significantly more likely to have had no or inadequate prenatal care.[25] Other characteristics that may be associated with cocaine abuse include use of other illicit substances, cigarette smoking, positive serology testing for sexually transmitted diseases, and acquired immunodeficiency syndrome (AIDS).

Cocaine (benzoylmethylecgonine, C17H21NO4) is an alkaloid derived from the Erythroxylon coca.[26] This drug affects all major organ systems and may cause life-threatening complications such as myocardial ischemia and infarction, even in the absence of preexisting cardiac disease. Mortality from cocaine may occur even after the ingestion of small doses. Potential mechanisms to explain myocardial ischemia in young, healthy cocaine-abusing patients without a history of cardiac disease include coronary artery vasospasm, thrombus, cardiomyopathy, and myocardial depression.[27-29] Although the lethal dose of orally administered cocaine has been reported to be as high as 1200 mg, death has been reported after the administration of as little as 20 mg of cocaine.[30] Several teams of investigators have demonstrated that pregnancy enhances the cardiovascular toxicity of cocaine.[31,32] Table 42-1 reviews the maternal manifestations of cocaine abuse. Fig. 42-1 summarizes the mechanisms of cocaine-induced myocardial depression and dysfunction.

Administration of cocaine may occur via the oral, intranasal, and intravenous routes. Additionally, cocaine hydrochloride can be prepared to yield free-base cocaine, which can be smoked. This alkalinized, smokable form of cocaine is known as *crack* and currently is the most widely used form of cocaine. Crack has become popular because it provides the abuser with advantages of intense euphoria and almost instant onset, along with a low price. This free-base form of cocaine (crack) is manufactured by mixing the hydrochloride salt with an alkali. Crack is more stable on heating, vaporizes readily, and has a high bioavailability when smoked.[26] Pharmacologic effects of cocaine are mediated by alterations of norepinephrine, dopamine,

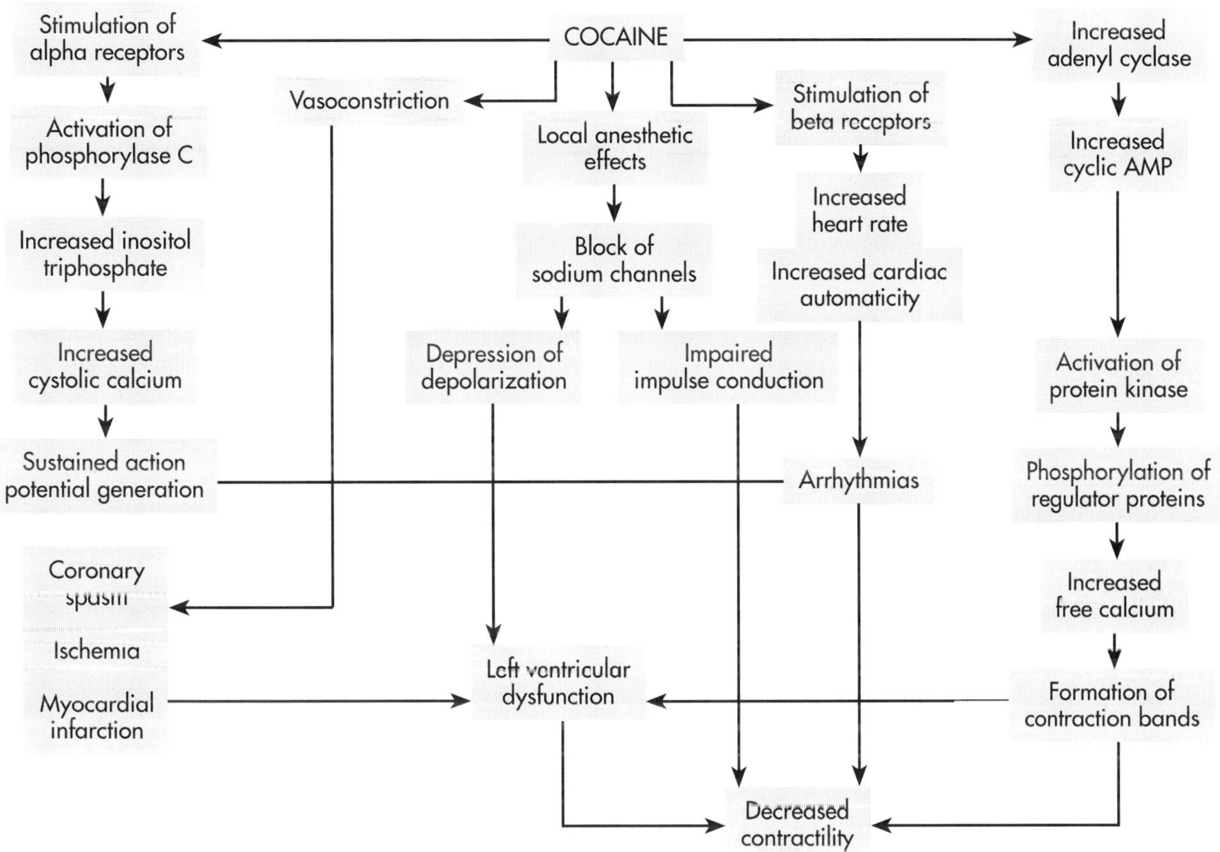

Fig. 42-1.

Mechanisms of cocaine-induced myocardial depression and dysfunction. *(From Birnbach DJ:* Substance abuse. *In Chestnut DH, editor:* Obstetric anesthesia, *ed 1, St. Louis, 1994, Mosby-Year Book.)*

TABLE 42-1
LIFE-THREATENING COMPLICATIONS OF COCAINE ABUSE

Cardiovascular[27-29,33-36]	Myocardial infarction, arrhythmias, asystole, aortic rupture
Central nervous system[36-39]	Convulsions, stroke, hemorrhage
Gastrointestinal[40-43]	Ischemia, elevation of liver enzymes, hepatotoxicity, hepatic failure
Hematologic[44,45]	Thrombocytopenia, DIC
Pulmonary[46,47]	Aspiration bronchospasm, pneumothorax, pneumomediastinum
Renal[48]	Renal failure
Infectious[49,50]	HIV infection

DIC, Disseminated intravascular coagulation; HIV, human immunovirus.

and serotonin.[26,51] The intense euphoria associated with cocaine is thought to be due to accumulation of dopamine in the synaptic cleft.[26] The harmful effects of cocaine, such as vasoconstriction and hypertension, occur as a result of an accumulation of catecholamines. Cocaine is metabolized principally by plasma and hepatic cholinesterases with about 5% excreted unchanged in the urine.[26] The volume of distribution of cocaine is 1.2 to 1.9 l/kg.[52] Cocaine metabolism may differ in mother and fetus, and also may differ in pregnant versus nonpregnant women.[53,54] Breakdown of cocaine is reviewed in Fig. 42-2.

Cocaine plasma levels remain detectable for 4 to 6 hours. The half-life of cocaine varies significantly between individuals. Since the mean elimination half-life for cocaine is less than 1 hour, cocaine detection generally is performed on urinary metabolites of cocaine rather than on cocaine itself. Urine testing for cocaine metabolites will continue to give positive results for 24 to 72 hours after cocaine use, depending on the degree of use. Because of differences in metabolism, infant toxicology tests may give positive results for a period after the maternal urine test results become negative.[55] Preliminary data in rats show that the fetal liver can metabolize cocaine to norcocaine, but not to cocaine methyl ester. This altered metabolism may be due to lower fetal levels of plasma cholinesterases and an immature fetal liver. Failure to efficiently break down cocaine may contribute to increased fetal cocaine toxicity.[56]

A difficult aspect of medical care for the parturient who is abusing cocaine is recognition of her addiction. A majority of pregnant cocaine addicts deny drug use when interviewed by their physicians.[14,15] Physical examination may lead to the suspicion of cocaine abuse when there is unexpected hypertension and tachycardia. It has been suggested that physicians should consider the possibility of cocaine abuse in every hypertensive pregnant woman.[57] The American Academy of Pediatrics recommends a thorough maternal history, obtained in a nonthreatening, organized manner, as the key to diagnosis of drug exposure in infants.[58] Based on clinical examination, it may be difficult to differentiate between cocaine intoxication and preeclampsia since both can present with hypertension, proteinuria, and edema. Cocaine abuse may be mistakenly diagnosed as severe preeclampsia since cocaine may cause excessive excretion of protein as well as edema, blurred vision, and

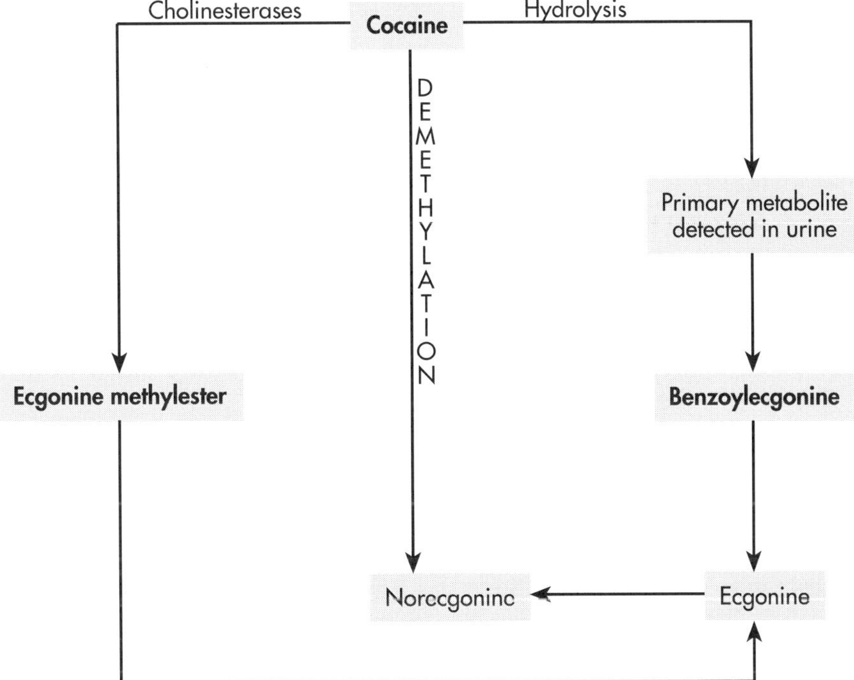

Fig. 42-2.
Metabolism of cocaine.

headache.[57] Table 42-2 reviews the signs and symptoms of cocaine abuse.

Lack of prenatal care and cigarette smoking are of predictive value in the recognition of the cocaine abuser.[15,25,59] Parturients who present to the labor and delivery floor with no prenatal care are four times more likely to have positive toxicology results for cocaine. Table 42-2 reviews the risk factors for patients who should be considered to be at high risk of antenatal cocaine abuse.

Most often the diagnosis of cocaine abuse is confirmed with urine toxicology testing. Current laboratory screening methods for cocaine metabolites include gas chromatography, mass spectrometry, and radioimmunoassay. Gas-liquid chromatographic techniques can identify low cocaine levels, but both radioimmunoassay and enzyme immunoassay techniques have been successfully used to detect urinary benzoylecgonine. The problem with laboratory-performed assays is the inevitable lag time. For an anesthesiologist being confronted with an acute situation such as fetal distress, the knowledge of cocaine use that the lab will provide in 48

TABLE 42-2
Signs and Symptoms of Cocaine Abuse

Hypertension
Tachycardia
Convulsions
Hyperreflexia
Tremors
Hyperpyrexia
Acidosis

hours is of very little benefit. A newly developed method for detection of urinary benzoylecgonine that allows physicians to test the urine instantly is the OnTrak Abuscreen TM assay (Roche Diagnostics, Branchburg, NJ). The OnTrak assay, which is a latex agglutination inhibition test for benzoylecgonine, provides a result within 4 minutes; this allows the perinatal team to make appropriate clinical decisions regarding the care of the patient. Recently this test was evaluated on 100 women at risk for cocaine abuse at St. Luke's–Roosevelt Hospital Center in New York City. It was observed that the OnTrak test had a 100% sensitivity and specificity when compared with the standard hospital laboratory test.[17]

Although the data on the pharmacology of cocaine during pregnancy in humans are somewhat limited, there are adequate animal and human data to demonstrate that cocaine use in pregnancy is dangerous to both mother and fetus. This danger is exaggerated by the popular misconception that cocaine does not cross the placenta and is a safe way to achieve easier and faster childbirth.

Cocaine is poorly ionized at physiologic pH, is lipophilic, and has a low molecular weight. Therefore it is no surprise that investigators find that cocaine easily crosses the placenta. The administration of cocaine to pregnant ewes has been shown to result in the rapid appearance of cocaine in the fetal circulation.[60,61] It has been demonstrated by several investigators that cocaine freely crosses the placenta and produces direct effects on the fetus.[62] Investigators have observed dose-dependent increases in maternal blood pressure and uterine vascular resistance.[31] Indirect effects also occur in the pregnant cocaine-abusing patient. Maternal vasoconstriction causes decreased uteroplacental blood flow, uteroplacental insufficiency, and decreased fetal oxygenation.[61] Because pretreatment of gravid ewes with phentolamine has not been found to alter the uterine vascular response to cocaine, it has been suggested that the vasoconstrictive effect of cocaine may be due to both adrenergic and nonadrenergic mechanisms.

In addition to the neonatal risk associated with cocaine use in pregnancy, there is also an added maternal risk compared with the nonpregnant cocaine user. Woods and Plessinger compared the hemodynamic sequelae of cocaine in the pregnant and nonpregnant ewe and found that although both groups exhibited increases in heart rate and blood pressure, the pregnant animals had a twofold increase in cardiovascular changes.[31] Cocaine also has been shown to produce cardiac arrhythmias at substantially lower doses in pregnant compared with nonpregnant ewes.[63]

The effects of maternal cocaine use are incremental and cumulative.[64] It has been reported that first-trimester maternal cocaine abuse may result in spontaneous abortion and may cause neurologic abnormalities as well as congenital abnormalities.[65,66] Although there have been some conflicting reports, many authors believe that cocaine may have teratogenic effects including urogenital, skeletal, ophthalmologic, and cardiac abnormalities.[62,67-70] Explanation for fetal abnormalities due to maternal cocaine ingestion included the following:

- Vasoconstriction secondary to cocaine may cause hypoxia, which may disrupt morphogenesis
- Cocaine may cause a local ischemic effect, which may interfere with peristalsis
- Abnormalities of ionized calcium secondary to cocaine may interfere with ureteral peristalsis, leading to hydronephrosis.[71,72]

Other fetal abnormalities that have been reported after maternal cocaine abuse include irritability, seizures, abnormalities of motor function, hypotonia, electroencephalographic abnormalities, renal dysfunction, and prune-belly syndrome.[73,74] Women who abuse cocaine during pregnancy are at a greater risk of delivering infants who are low birth weight, premature, small for gestational age, shorter, and who have smaller head circumferences when compared with women who are not using drugs in pregnancy.[75] Adverse developmental effects secondary to perinatal cocaine use will have an increasing impact on the medical, educational, social welfare, and justice systems in our society.[24] A report by the U.S. Senate Finance Committee states that the government will spend $15 billion dollars annually to prepare cocaine-affected children to enter kindergarten.[76]

Maternal cocaine use has been implicated in multiple obstetric complications including an increased incidence of spontaneous abortion, preterm labor, abruptio placenta, and fetal distress.[65,77,78] Recently there has been a report of uterine rupture and extensive bladder laceration after cocaine use.[79] Maternal and fetal hormonal and electrolyte abnormalities also have been noted. The abnormalities of fetal glucose that may be seen are not insulin induced. The increased levels of corticotropin (ACTH) may be a result of pituitary stimulation or possibly due to changes in ACTH releasing factor.[80]

The American College of Obstetrics and Gynecology recently has made several recommendations regarding the management of pregnant patients who use cocaine:[81]

1. The obstetrician should obtain a drug history at the first prenatal visit and the patient should be warned about the dangers of drug use during pregnancy
2. A woman who acknowledges use of cocaine should be counseled and offered support to aid in her abstinence.
3. The obstetrician should consider periodic urine testing *to encourage and reinforce continual abstinence.*
4. The obstetrician should consider testing of the mother or the neonate (or both) in cases of unexpected fetal growth restriction or in women with abruptio placentae and no history of chronic hypertension.
5. Some states consider in utero drug exposure to be a form of child abuse or neglect under the law, and require that physicians report positive results of drug tests in pregnant women or their newborn infants.
6. When a maternal test gives positive results for cocaine metabolites, the neonatologist or pediatrician should be advised of the infant's exposure in utero.

Anesthesia in the Cocaine-Abusing Parturient

When requested to provide an anesthetic for a cocaine-abusing parturient, the anesthesiologist must weigh the risks and benefits of regional versus general anesthesia in each case. At St. Luke's–Roosevelt Hospital Center in New York City, where a large population of pregnant women who abuse cocaine is treated, it has been observed that life-threatening events are more common during general anesthesia than during regional anesthesia in the cocaine-abusing parturient for cesarean section.[82] The most frequently encountered problems in this cocaine-abusing population undergoing general anesthesia are severe hypertension and arrhythmias after laryngoscopy and intubation.

Although regional anesthesia may be associated with fewer life-threatening events, it still places the patient at considerable risk. In another study at this institution, it was found that these patients are at increased risk for hypotension during regional anesthesia, and ephedrine may not be an effective vasopressor in these patients.[82] Because of these findings, it is the practice of our anesthesiology staff to prepare a dilute solution of phenylephrine so that it is readily available should the patient develop ephedrine-resistant hypotension. Additionally, cocaine abuse may place patients at risk for platelet abnormalities. Several cases of cocaine-induced thrombocytopenia have been reported in the literature.[44,45,83] Therefore in our high-risk patient population, any cocaine-positive patient, or any patient at high risk for cocaine abuse (Table 42-3) has a platelet count performed before placement of an epidural anesthetic.

If regional anesthesia is selected for the cocaine-abusing parturient, these patients often require opioid supplementation during surgery. Possible explanations for this include an abnormal affect in these cocaine abusers, a bias on the part of the anesthesiologist to sedate patients who abuse drugs, or perhaps a neurophysiologic alteration in the central nervous system of cocaine abusers, which changes not only their perception of pleasure, but also their perception of pain.[84,85]

If general anesthesia is indicated, the patient is vulnerable to hypertension, arrhythmias, and myocardial ischemia. At this hospital, as at many others, severe hypertension secondary to cocaine abuse is treated with labetalol.[86] Vertommen and coworkers[87] evaluated the use of hydralazine in the treatment of cocaine-induced hypertension in gravid ewes. They found that although hydralazine restored mean arterial systemic pressure (MAP) to baseline, it also resulted in profound maternal tachycardia. Labetalol, unlike hydralazine, decreased both MAP and heart rate. These authors concluded that "labetalol may be preferable to hydralazine for treatment of the acutely cocaine-intoxicated parturient."[88] Cocaine abuse represents a relative contraindication to the use of propranolol, since β-blockade may cause unopposed α-adrenergic receptor stimulation and worsened hypertension.[89]

Because of the risk of arrhythmias in these patients, halothane administration should be avoided. This volatile agent places the patient at risk of sensitization of the myocardium to the elevated catecholamines and therefore to the development of malignant arrhythmias.[26] Ketamine also may potentiate the cardiac effects of cocaine by further increasing catecholamine levels. The exact opposite may occur however, since in the case of the patient who is a chronic cocaine abuser with depleted catecholamine levels, there is a risk of hypotension after administration of ketamine.

TABLE 42-3
PARTURIENTS AT HIGH-RISK FOR COCAINE ABUSE

Unregistered patients (no prenatal care)
Preterm labor
Hypertensive
Abruptio placenta
Positive serology for sexually transmitted diseases
Cigarette smoking

Legal and Ethical Issues

In June 1988 District of Columbia Superior Court Judge Wolf ordered Brenda A. Vaughn to serve a sentence in jail because she was pregnant and had tested positive for cocaine. The U.S. Attorney's Office had agreed to probation instead of jail time; however, Judge Wolf issues the sentence stating that "I'm going to keep her locked up until the baby is born because she tested positive for cocaine when she came before me."[90] In July 1989 Florida Judge Eaton found Ms. Jennifer Johnson guilty of two felony counts for delivering a drug to a minor. Judge Eaton concluded that Ms. Johnson had passed cocaine to her children through the umbilical cord as they were being born.[91] Some of the legal protection for the unborn child is subject to challenge based on the U.S. Supreme Court decision in Roe v. Wade, where the court held that the word *person* as used in the fourteenth amendment does not include the unborn.[92] Despite the conclusion that a fetus is not a *person,* the court did state that individual states had an important and legitimate interest in *protecting the potentiality of human life*. Other courts, however, have ruled that pregnant women who abuse drugs are not guilty of criminal charges.[93] At stake when creating rules to protect the fetus from the mother's addiction is an infringement on the mother's right to privacy. A particular area of concern is the mother's right to refuse toxicology testing. The courts have indirectly addressed this sensitive issue in several cases, where they have concluded that in certain circumstances it is reasonable to test without *individualized suspicion*.[94] Other courts have also held that the *right to privacy* was an issue in a patient's refusal to allow testing or therapy. Recently several courts have found that a patient even has the right to refuse to undergo a cesarean section under the right to privacy inherent in the Constitution.[95]

The federal Child Abuse Prevention and Treatment Act prevents a state from receiving federal funds unless the state has a statute providing for the reporting of known and suspected instances of child abuse and neglect. Although all states have such reporting requirements, each state differs in specifics. A majority of states impose both civil and criminal penalties on health care practitioners who are required to make child abuse reports and fail to do so. In New York, for example, a physician who knows of child abuse and fails to report it can be found guilty of a class A misdemeanor. Although one New York court has held that a newborn baby who is having withdrawal symptoms is a prima facie neglected baby,[96] another has stated that there is no evidence that the state legislature intended to "regulate a pregnant woman's body or to control her diet, medication, exercise, or smoking habits on behalf of a fetus."[97]

These cases illustrate some of the difficult legal issues and present confusion surrounding the illicit use of drugs by women during pregnancy. These and other ethical and legal issues have been dealt with at the legislative level only recently. Until it is clearly defined, the best alternative is to inform all high-risk patients that they will be tested for toxicology and obtain informed consent. Additional legal protection is afforded by testing all patients, so that no case can be made for discrimination.

Cocaine addicts often abuse other drugs. Alcohol, amphetamines, heroin, phencyclidine, LSD, and marijuana all have been reported as additives to cocaine.[98,99]

Amphetamine Abuse

The amphetamine drugs are sympathomimetics that cause profound central nervous system stimulation. These drugs may be abused individually or in conjunction with other drugs such as cocaine and heroin. Acute ingestion of amphetamines causes signs and symptoms which resemble those of cocaine ingestion and include hypertension, tachycardia, agitation confusion, arrhythmias, hyperreflexia, and fever.[100] These symptoms in a parturient can be mistaken for preeclampsia or eclampsia.[101] Although there was some controversy regarding the association between the use of amphetamines and congenital abnormalities in the 1970s,[102] it is now widely believed that the illicit use of amphetamines in pregnancy is associated with intrauterine growth retardation, preterm labor and delivery, abruptio placenta, fetal distress, and an increased risk of perinatal mortality.[103]

Amphetamine abuse may cause fetal distress and thus necessitate emergency cesarean section. The acute ingestion of amphetamines increases the dose requirements for general anesthetic agents, whereas the chronic ingestion of amphetamines decreases the minimum alveolar concentration of volatile anesthetics.[104] Since it is often difficult to differentiate between acute and chronic abusers, it is prudent to gradually titrate doses to effect in these patients. As with cocaine abusers, agents which sensitize the myocardium to catecholamines, such as halothane, should be avoided. Ephedrine may not function to increase blood pressure in the presence of baseline tachycardia and may be relatively contraindicated if the baseline heart rate is too fast. Therefore, if choosing a regional anesthetic for cesarean section in the amphetamine-abusing patient with a baseline tachycardia, phenylephrine should be available to treat hypotension. Cases of cardiac arrest during cesarean section in women who chronically abuse amphetamines have been reported in patients undergoing both general and epidural anesthesia.

Narcotic Abuse

The opioids that are abused in pregnancy include heroin, morphine, demerol, methadone, and fentanyl. Although a decrease is being seen at the St. Luke's–Roosevelt Hospital Center in the incidence of patients who present to the labor floor who are intravenously abusing narcotics, it has been estimated that 250,000 women in the U.S. are intravenous drug abusers, with 90% of these being of childbearing age.[105] Heroin is the most commonly intravenously abused narcotic in our patient population. Heroin, being a diacetyl morphine has a reduced polarity and thus an even faster placental passage than morphine. Heroin is rapidly hydrolyzed to 6-monoacetylmorphine and excreted in the urine.

Perinatal abuse of opioids may be associated with AIDS, hepatitis, endocarditis, pulmonary, renal, and cardiac disease.[105,106] Other associated problems in the opioid-abusing parturient include medical complications of adulterants mixed with opioids, such as talcosis when talc is mixed with heroin.[107] Additionally, when sclerosis of veins occurs, injection of opioids into central veins has been reported as a cause of pneumothorax, hemothorax, pneumomediastinum, and embolism.[108]

Acute withdrawal syndrome may be recognized by tremors, anxiety, muscle pains, nausea, vomiting, anorexia, gastrointestinal pain, dehydration, tachycardia, hypertension, and mydriasis. These symptoms peak at 48 to 72 hours after the last narcotic intake and may be treated with the administration of narcotic or clonidine.[109] The use of opioid antagonists or mixed agonist/antagonist drugs may precipitate acute withdrawal, and therefore should not be used in these patients.[110] To prevent withdrawal in a hospitalized patient, she must receive her usual daily baseline narcotic dose, irrespective of additional considerations of acute pain relief.[111]

Narcotic overdose is characterized by coma miosis and respiratory depression. When treating the patient with narcotic overdose, the most important factor is securing the airway, since these patients are not able to protect their airway and need *full stomach* precautions.

Despite use of large doses of local anesthetics, regional techniques may provide inadequate pain relief in some opioid abusers.[112] This apparent decrease in pain tolerance in the opioid abuser may be due to a decreased production of endogenous opioid peptides. General anesthesia may be safely used in the opioid-addicted parturient; however, these patients may have abnormal liver function and therefore, when possible, should receive drugs that are not hepatically detoxified. Postoperative pain management can be achieved using patient-controlled analgesia, even in the opioid abuser.[113] In the rehabilitated opiate abuser, narcotics can be avoided, if so desired, by use of regional anesthesia and postoperative administration of parenterally administered nonsteroidal antiinflammatory drugs such as ketorolac.[114]

Alcohol Abuse

The alcoholic parturient poses many problems to the anesthesiologist. Table 42-4 reviews the sequelae and anesthetic implications of alcohol abuse. Alcohol is a known teratogen and its use in pregnancy is associated with the fetal alcohol syndrome.[115] Signs and symptoms of this syndrome include cra-

TABLE 42-4
Sequelae of Alcohol Abuse and Anesthetic Implications

Sequelae	Anesthetic Implications
Cardiomyopathy	Increased risk of myocardial depression during general anesthesia
Increased gastric acid	Increased risk of pulmonary aspiration of gastric contents
Cross tolerance with barbiturates	Increased induction dose of sodium thiopental required except when the patient is acutely intoxicated
Decreased albumin concentration	Increased sensitivity to many drugs as a result of decreased protein binding
Coagulopathy	Possible contraindication to the administration of regional anesthesia
Esophageal varices	Increased risk of bleeding with passage of a nasogastric tube, esophageal stethoscope, temperature probe, and suction catheter
Ascites	Abnormalities of intravascular volume and electrolytes
Liver disease	Decreased pseudocholinesterase activity and abnormal response to drugs that undergo hepatic metabolism
Electrolyte abnormalities	Prolonged activity of muscle relaxants

From Birnbach DJ: Substance abuse. In Chestnut DH, editor: *Obstetric anesthesia*, ed 1, St Louis, 1994, Mosby Year Book.

niofacial, cardiac, renal, and musculocutaneous abnormalities. Because a safe level of alcohol intake in pregnancy has never been established, abstinence is the safest course during pregnancy or in women who plan to become pregnant.[116]

When an acutely ethanol-intoxicated parturient is admitted to our labor and delivery suite, she is immediately seen by an anesthesiologist and tested not only for alcohol but for cocaine, since patients who abuse alcohol often abuse other drugs. Recently Kurth et al. demonstrated that ethylcocaine, which is formed by the mixture of ethanol and cocaine, is a very potent cerebral vasoconstrictor.[117] This suggests that the combination of alcohol and cocaine may be especially hazardous.

In the absence of coagulopathy or neuropathy, the practice at this hospital is to anesthetize alcohol-abusing parturients with regional anesthesia. Occasionally, we are unsuccessful in our regional anesthesia attempts with these patients because of psychosis or combative behavior. Alcoholic patients may have cardiomyopathies and have exaggerated response to myocardial depressants. If acutely intoxicated, decreased amounts of anesthetic will be needed intraoperatively, since the patient is "preanesthetized."[118] All alcohol-abusing patients are referred on admission for detoxification workup and delirium tremens prophylaxis.

Summary and Discussion of the Management of the Illustrated Case

This case involves the management of a cocaine-abusing patient who is hypertensive, tachycardiac, and in preterm labor. The following is a review of the proposed anesthetic management:

1. *Identification of drug abuse*—history and physical examination; urine for toxicology testing; and instant evaluation with OnTrak.
2. *Prepare for immediate cesarean section* (these patients have a higher risk of fetal distress)—history and physical examination, and an airway evaluation; have the operating room ready, type and crossmatch blood; the pediatrician should be present; intravenous hydration with lactated Ringer's; aspiration prophylaxis (Bicitra [sodium citrate dihydrate]).
3. *Treatment of hypertension*—monitoring should include electrocardiogram (ECG) and pulse

oximeter, arterial line; with a normal ECG, give intravenous labetalol; with the ECG showing ischemia, give intravenous nitroglycerine.

4. *Treatment of angina and/or hypertension*—labetalol if ECG is normal; nitroglycerine if ECG shows ischemia.
5. *Treatment of arrhythmias*—hypertension should be treated (as above); ventricular fibrillation with verapamil; ventricular tachycardia with lidocaine.
6. *Tocolysis*—hydration (as above); material heart rate less than 100 beats/min, give terbutaline with or without magnesium sulphate; heart rate more than 120 beats/min, give magnesium (one should avoid terbutaline).

References

1. Knisely JS, Spear ER, Green DJ, et al: Substance abuse patterns in pregnant women, *NIDA Res Monogr* 1991; 108:280.
2. Jaffe JH: *Cocaine use in America: epidemiologic and clinical perspectives, NIDA Res Monogr* 1985; 61:1-226.
3. Abelson HI, Miller JD: A decade of trends in cocaine in the household population, *NIDA Res Monogr* 1985; 61:35.
4. Adams EH, Kozel NJ: Cocaine use in America: introduction and overview, *NIDA Res Monogr* 1985; 61:1.
5. Fleming JA, Byck R, Barash PG: Pharmacology and therapeutic applications of cocaine, *Anesthesiology* 1990; 73:518.
6. Byck R: *Cocaine papers: Sigmund Freud,* New York, 1975, Stonehill Publishing.
7. Altman AJ, Albert DM, Fournier GA: Cocaine's use in ophthalmology: our 100 year heritage, *Surv Ophthalmol* 1985; 29:300.
8. Petersen RC, Stillman RE, editors: Cocaine, 1977. NIDA Res Monograph 13. National Institute on Drug Abuse. Washington, D.C., 1977, U.S. Government Printing Office.
9. Beattie GF: Soft drink flavours: their history and characteristics, *Perfumery Essential Oil Rec* 1956; 47:437.
10. Byck R: *Cocaine use and research: three histories.* In: Fisher S, Rashkin A, Uhlenhuth EH, editors: *Cocaine: clinical and behavioral aspects,* New York, 1986, Oxford University Press.
11. Colliver J: *A decade of DAWN: cocaine-related cases, 1976-1985,* Washington DC, 1987, National Institute on Drug Abuse, Division of Epidemiological and Statistical Publication.
12. Vega WA, Bohdan K, Hwang J, Noble A: Prevalence and magnitude of perinatal substance exposures in California, *N Engl J Med* 1993; 329:850.
13. Select Committee on Children, Youth, and Families, United States House of Representatives: *Women, addiction, and perinatal substances abuse,* Washington, D.C., 1990, U.S. Government Printing Office.
14. Knisely JS, Spear ER, Green DJ, et al: Substance abuse patterns in pregnant women, *NIDA Res Monogr* 1991; 108:280.
15. Birnbach DJ, Weiss W, Grunebaum A: Epidural anesthesia for cesarean section in cocaine abusing patients, *Soc Obstet Anesth Perinatol* 1989; F-6 (abstract).
16. Volpe JJ: Effect of cocaine use on the fetus, *N Engl J Med* 1992; 327:399.
17. Birnbach DJ, Stein DJ, Thomas K, et al: Instant recognition of the cocaine abusing parturient: evaluation of a new technique, *Anesthesiology* 1993; 79:A987 (abstract).
18. Schutzman DL, Frankenfield-Chernicoff M, Clatterbaugh HE, Singer J: Incidence of intrauterine cocaine exposure in a suburban setting, *Pediatrics* 1991; 88:825.
19. Streissguth AP, Grant TM, Barr HM, et al: Cocaine and the use of alcohol and other drugs during pregnancy, *Am J Obstet Gynecol* 1991; 164:1239.
20. Matera C, Warren WB, Moomjy M, et al: Prevalence of use of cocaine and other substances in an obstetric population, *Am J Obstet Gynecol* 1990; 163:797.
21. McCalla S, Minkoff HL, Feldman J, et al: The biologic and social consequences of perinatal cocaine use in an inner city population, *Am J Obstet Gynecol* 1991; 164:625.
22. Gillogley KM, Evans AT, Hansen RL, et al: The perinatal impact of cocaine, amphetamine, and opiate use detected by universal intrapartum screening, *Am J Obstet Gynecol* 1990; 163:1535.
23. Vega WA, Kolody B, Hwang J, Noble A: Prevalence and magnitude of perinatal substance exposures in California, *N Engl J Med* 1993; 329:850.
24. Nair BS, Watson RR: Cocaine and the pregnant woman, *J Reprod Med* 1991; 36:862.
25. McCalla S, Minkoff HL, Feldman J, et al: Predictors of cocaine use in pregnancy, *Obstet Gynecol* 1992; 79:641.

26. Fleming JA, Byck R, Barash PG: Pharmacology and therapeutic applications of cocaine, *Anesthesiology* 1990; 73:518.
27. Kloner RA, Hale S, Alker K, Rozkalla S: The effects of acute and chronic cocaine use on the heart, *Circulation* 1992; 85:407.
28. Nahas GG, Trouve R, Manger WM: Cocaine, catcholamines and cardiac toxicity, *Acta Anesthesiol Scand* 1990; 34:77.
29. Billman GE: Mechanisms responsible for the cardiotoxic effects of cocaine, *FASEB J* 1990; 4:2469.
30. Price KR: Fatal cocaine poisoning, *J Forensic Sci Soc* 1974; 14:329.
31. Woods JR Jr, Plessinger MA: Pregnancy increases cardiovascular toxicity to cocaine, *Am J Obstet Gynecol* 1990; 162:529.
32. Plessinger MA, Woods JR Jr: Progesterone increases cardiovascular toxicity to cocaine in nonpregnant ewes, *Am J Obstet Gynecol* 1990; 163:1059.
33. Liu SS, Forrester RM, Murphy GS, et al: Anaesthetic management of a parturient with myocardial infarction related to cocaine use, *Can J Anaesth* 1992; 39:858.
34. Fraker TD, Temesy-Armos PN, Brewster PS, Wilkerson RD: Mechanism of cocaine induced myocardial depression in dogs, *Circulation* 1990; 81:1012.
35. Mendelson MA, Chandler J: Postpartum cardiomyopathy associated with maternal cocaine abuse, *Am J Cardiol* 1992; 70:1092.
36. Levine SR, Brust JCM, Futrell N, et al: Cerebrovascular complications of the use of the "crack" form of alkaloidal cocaine, *N Engl J Med* 1990; 323:699.
37. Merriam AE, Medalia A, Levine B: Partial complex status epilepticus associated with cocaine abuse, *Biol Psychiatry* 1988; 23:515.
38. Spivey WH, Eurle B: Neurologic complications of cocaine abuse, *Ann Emerg Med* 1990, 19:1422.
39. Lichtenfeld PJ, Rubin DB, Feldman RS: Subarachnoid hemorrhage precipitated by cocaine snorting, *Arch Neurol* 1984; 41:223.
40. Nalbandian H, Sheth N, Dietrich R, Georgiou J: Intestinal ischemia caused by cocaine ingestion: report of two cases, *Surgery* 1988; 97:374.
41. Mallat A, Dhumeaux D: Cocaine and the liver, *J Hepatol* 1991; 12:275.
42. Kothur R, Marsh F, Posner J: Liver function tests in non parenteral cocaine users, *Arch Intern Med* 1991; 151:1126.
43. Kloss MW, Rosen GM, Raukman EJ: Cocaine-mediated hepatotoxicity: a critical review, *Biochem Pharmacol* 1984; 33:169.
44. Orser B: Thrombocytopenia and cocaine abuse, *Anesthesiology* 1991; 74:195.
45. Burday MJ, Martin ES: Cocaine induced thrombocytopenia, *Am J Med* 1991; 91:656.
46. Forrester JM, Steele AW, Waldron JA, Parsons PE: Crack lung: an acute pulmonary syndrome with a spectrum of clinical and histopathologic findings, *Am Rev Respir Dis* 1990; 142:462.
47. Ettinger NA, Albin RJ: A review of the respiratory effects of smoking cocaine, *Am J Med* 1989; 87:664.
48. Merigan KS, Roberts JR: Cocaine intoxication: hyperpyrexia, rhabdomyolysis and acute renal failure, *Clin Toxicol* 1987; 25:135.
49. Minkoff HL, McCalla S, Delke I, et al: The relationship of cocaine use to syphilis and human immunodeficiency virus infections among inner city parturient women, *Am J Obstet Gynecol* 1990; 163:521.
50. Chiasson MA, Stoneburner RL, Hildebrandt DS, et al: Heterosexual transmission of HIV-1 associated with the use of smokable free base cocaine, *AIDS* 1991; 5:1121.
51. Gold MS, Washton AM, Dackis CA: Cocaine abuse: neurochemistry, phenomenology, and treatment, *Natl Inst Drug Abuse Res Monogr Ser* 1985; 61:130.
52. Chow MJ, Ambre JJ, Ruo TI, et al: Kinetics of cocaine distribution, elimination, and chronotropic effects, *Clin Pharmacol Ther* 1985; 38:318.
53. Sandberg JA, Olsen GD: Cocaine pharmacokinetics in the pregnant guinea pig, *J Pharmacol Ther* 1991; 258:477.
54. Sandberg JA, Olsen GD: Cocaine and metabolite concentrations in the fetal guinea pig after chronic maternal cocaine administration, *J Pharmacol Exp Ther* 1992; 260:587.
55. Chasnoff IJ, Lewis DE, Griffith DR, Willey S: Cocaine and pregnancy: clinical and toxicological implications for the neonate, *Clin Chem* 1989; 35:1276.
56. Stettler RW, Bohman VR, Standard DI, et al: Cocaine metabolism during pregnancy in maternal, placental, and fetal compartments: an in-vivo animal model, *Am J Obstet Gynecol* 1992; 166:361A.
57. Towers CV, Pircon RA, Nageotte MP, et al: Cocaine intoxication presenting as preeclampsia and eclampsia. Obstet Gynecol 1993; 81:545.

58. American Academy of Pediatrics, Committee on Substance Abuse, *Pediatrics* 1990; 86:639.
59. Spence MR, Williams R, Digregorio JG, et al: The relationship between recent cocaine use and pregnancy outcome, *Obstet Gynecol* 1991; 78:326.
60. DeVane CL, Burchfield DJ, Abrams RM, et al: Disposition of cocaine in pregnant sheep, *Dev Pharmacol Ther* 1991; 16:123.
61. Moore TR, Sorg J, Miller L, et al: Hemodynamic effects of intravenous cocaine on the pregnant ewe and fetus, *Am J Obstet Gynecol* 1986; 155:883.
62. Bingol N, Fuchs M, Diaz V, et al: Teratogenicity of cocaine in humans, *J Pediatr* 1987;110:93.
63. Woods JR, Plessinger MA, Scott K, Miller RK: Perinatal cocaine exposure to the fetus: a sheep model for cardiovascular evaluation, *Ann NY Acad Sci* 1989; 562:267.
64. Nair BS, Watson RR: Cocaine and the pregnant woman, *J Reprod Med* 1991; 36:862.
65. Chasnoff IJ, Burns WJ, Schnoll SH, et al: Cocaine use in pregnancy, *N Engl J Med* 1985; 313:666.
66. Chasnoff IJ, Griffith DR, MacGregor S, et al: Temporal patterns of cocaine use in pregnancy, *JAMA* 1989; 261:1741.
67. Fantel AG, Macphail BJ: The teratogenicity of cocaine, *Teratology* 1982; 26:17.
68. Webster WS, Brown-Woodman PD: Cocaine as a cause of congenital malformations of vascular origin: experimental evidence in the rat, *Teratology* 1990; 41:689.
69. Chavez GF, Mulinare J, Cordero JF: Maternal cocaine use during early pregnancy as a risk factor for congenital urogenital anomalies, *JAMA* 1989; 262:795.
70. Viscarello RR, Ferguson DD, Nores J, Hobbins JC: Limb-body wall complex associated with cocaine abuse: further evidence of cocaine's teratogenicity, *Obstet Gynecol* 1992; 80:523.
71. Chasnoff IJ, Chisum GM, Kaplan WE: Maternal cocaine use and genitourinary tract malformation, *Teratology* 1988; 37:201.
72. Van Allen MI: Fetal vascular disruption: mechanisms and some resulting birth defects, *Pediatr Ann* 1981; 10:219.
73. Oro AS, Dixon SD: Perinatal cocaine and methamphetamine exposure: maternal and neonatal correlates, *J Pediatr* 1987; 111:571.
74. Doberczak TM, Shanzer S, Senie RT, Kandall SR: Neonatal neurologic and electroencephalographic effect of intrauterine cocaine exposure, *J Pediatr* 1988; 113:354.
75. Handler A, Kistin N, Davis F, Ferro C: Cocaine use during pregnancy: perinatal outcomes, *Am J Epidemiol* 1991; 133:818.
76. Associated Press: *Enormous cost of addicted babies,* December 1, 1989.
77. MacGregor SN, Keith LG, Chasnoff IJ, et al: Cocaine use during pregnancy: adverse perinatal outcome, *Am J Obstet Gynecol* 1987; 157:686.
78. Mastrogiannis DS, Decavalas GO, Verma UMA, Tejani N: Perinatal outcome after recent cocaine use, *Obstet Gynecol* 1990; 76:8.
79. Hsu CD, Chen S, Feng TI, Johnson TRB: Rupture of uterine scar with extensive maternal bladder laceration after cocaine abuse, *Am J Obstet Gynecol* 1992; 167:129.
80. Owiny JR, Jones MT, Sadowsky D, et al: Cocaine in pregnancy: the effect of maternal administration of cocaine on the maternal and fetal pituitary-adrenal axes, *Am J Obstet Gynecol* 1991; 164:658.
81. American College of Obstetrics and Gynecology, Committee on Obstetrics: Maternal and Fetal Medicine: *Cocaine in pregnancy,* Committee Opinion no. 114, September 1992.
82. Birnbach DJ, Stein DJ, Thomas K, et al: Cocaine abuse in the parturient: what are the anesthetic implications? *Anesthesiology* 1993; 79:A988.
83. Leissinger CA: Severe thrombocytopenia associated with cocaine use, *Ann Intern Med* 1990; 112:708.
84. Birnbach DJ, Grunebaum A, Collins E, Cohen A: The effect of cocaine on regional anesthesia, *Am J Obstet Gynecol* 1991; 164:A557.
85. Gawin FH: Cocaine addiction: psychology and neurophysiology, *Science* 1991; 251:1580.
86. Gay GR, Loper KA: The use of labetalol in the management of cocaine crisis, *Ann Emerg Med* 1988; 17:282.
87. Vertommen JD, Hughes SC, Rosen MA, et al: Hydralazine does not restore uterine blood flow during cocaine-induced hypertension in the pregnant ewe, *Anesthesiology* 1992; 76:580.
88. Hughes SC, Vertommen JD, Rosen MA, et al: Cocaine induced hypertension in the ewe and response to treatment with labetalol, *Anesthesiology* 1991; A1075.
89. Ramoska E, Sacchetti A: Propranolol induced hypertension

in the treatment of cocaine intoxication, *Ann Emerg Med* 1985; 14:1112.

90. Washington Post, July 23, 1988, p. 41.
91. *State of Florida v. Jennifer Johnson,* no. 89-890-CFA, Circuit court, Seminole County, Fla., 1989.
92. 410 U.S. 113, 158, 162-164 (1973).
93. *People of California v. Pamela Rae Stewart* no. M-508197, Municipal Court of the State of California, San Diego Judicial District, 1987.
94. *Skinner v. Railway Labor Executives Association* 489 U.S. 602, 109 S.Ct. 1402, 103 L.Ed.2d 639 (1989).
95. District of Columbia Court of Appeals no. 87-609 (1990).
96. 76 Misc.2d 617, 351 NYS 2d 337 (1974).
97. 533 NYS 2d 241, NY Family Court, (1988).
98. Samuels J, Schwalbe SS, Marx GF: Speedballs: a new cause of intraoperative tachycardia and hypertension, *Anesth Analg* 1991; 72:397.
99. Slutsker L, Smith R, Higginson G, Fleming D: Recognizing illicit drug use by pregnant women: reports from Oregon birth attendants, *Am J Public Health* 1993; 83:61.
100. Ong BH: Hazards to health: dextroamphetamine poisoning, *N Engl J Med* 1962; 266:1321.
101. Elliot RH, Rees GB: Amphetamine ingestion presenting as eclampsia, *Can J Anaesth* 1990; 37;130.
102. Nora JJ, McNamara DG, Fraser FC: Dextroamphetamine sulphate and human malformations, *Lancet* 1967; 1:570.
103. Little BB, Snell LM, Gilstrap LC: Methamphetamine abuse during pregnancy. outcome and fetal effects, *Obstet Gynecol* 1988; 72:541.
104. Johnston RR, Way WL, Miller RD: Alteration of anesthetic requirement by amphetamine, *Anesthesiology* 1972; 36:357.
105. Hoegerman G, Schnoll S: Narcotic use in pregnancy, *Clin Perinatol* 1991; 18:51.
106. Kliman L: Drug dependence and pregnancy: antenatal and intrapartum problems, *Anaesth Intensive Care* 1990; 18:358.
107. Gross EM: Autopsy findings in drug addicts, *Pathol Annu* 1978; 13:35.
108. Lewis JW, Groux N, Eliet JP, et al: Complications of attempted central venous injections performed by drug abusers, *Chest* 1980; 4:613.
109. Gold MS, Pottash AL, Extein I, Kleiber HD: Clonidine in acute opiate withdrawal, *N Engl J Med* 1980; 302:1421.
110. Weintraub SJ, Naulty JS: Acute abstinence syndrome after epidural injection of butorphanol, *Anesth Analg* 1985; 64:452.
111. Wood PR, Soni N: Anaesthesia and substance abuse, *Anaesthesia* 1989; 44:672.
112. Scheutz F: Drug addicts and local anesthesia: effectivity and general side effects, *Scand J Dental Res* 1982; 90:99.
113. Boyle RK: Intra- and postoperative anaesthetic management of an opioid addict undergoing cesarean section, *Anaesth Intensive Care* 1991; 19:276.
114. Litvak KM, McEvoy GK: Ketorolac: an injectable nonnarcotic analgesic, *Clin Pharm* 1990; 9:921.
115. Lemoine P, Harroussean H, Borteyrn JP: Les enfants deparents alcoolques: anomalies observees. A propos de 127 cas, *Quest Med* 1968; 25:477.
116. Council on Scientific Affairs, American Medical Association: Fetal effects of maternal alcohol use, *JAMA* 1983; 249:2517.
117. Kurth CD, Monitto CL, Albuquerque ML, et al: Effect of cocaine and cocaine metabolites on the cerebral microvasculature in piglets, *Anesthesiology* 1992; 77:A1039.
118. Bruce DL: Alcoholism and anesthesia, *Anesth Analg* 1983; 62:84.

43

Cardiopulmonary Resuscitation in Parturients

A 29-year-old primigrada, 32 weeks' gestation, is admitted to the labor floor with a history of dyspnea. She complains of pain in her left leg. While being examined by the obstetrician, the patient complains of severe pains in her chest and becomes unconscious and cyanotic. Discuss the management.

Recommendations by Deborah M. Barron, M.D.
Lesley I. Gilbertson, M.D.

Cardiopulmonary arrest in the pregnant patient is a rare medical emergency estimated to occur once in every 30,000 patients.[1] At Brigham and Women's Hospital, Boston, in the last decade there have been eight arrests in over 90,000 deliveries. Proper management requires immediate knowledgeable intervention of the entire medical team to provide the optimal outcome for both mother and fetus. Cardiopulmonary resuscitation in pregnancy is unique because there are in fact two patients, one of whom is totally dependent of the other. However, the treatment priorities for the pregnant patient are the same as for the nonpregnant patient. The primary responsibility of an obstetric anesthesiologist always is first to the life of the mother, but the optimal medical care of the mother also is the best care for the fetus.

Causes of Cardiopulmonary Arrest

The causes of cardiopulmonary arrest include conditions which predate the pregnancy and conditions that are exacerbated by or develop due to the pregnancy (Table 43-1). Women with a preexisting medical condition such as hypertension, cardiac disease, endocrine, pulmonary and collagen vascular disease have an increased risk of having a cardiac arrest during pregnancy.[2] Pregnant women without significant medical problems also have arrested from myriad causes. Causes of these arrests include cerebrovascular accidents; acquired valvular disease; maternal arrhythmia; myocardial infarctions; anesthesia complications; thromboembolism, amniotic fluid and air embolisms; hypermagnesemia; trauma; septicemia; preeclampsia; pregnancy-associated cardiomyopathy; hypovolemia secondary to hemorrhage; and drug overdose. Of all these causes, the most common cause of arrest is hypovolemia secondary to hemorrhage.[3] Of drug intoxication, cocaine has become a more prevalent problem in the obstetric population.[4] Cocaine toxicity can manifest as ischemia, infarctions, arrhythmias, myocarditis, aortic rupture, congestive heart failure, dilated cardiomyopathy, and sudden death.[5,6]

TABLE 43-1

Causes of Cardiopulmonary Arrest During Pregnancy

Preexisting heart disease
Congenital heart disease
Acquired heart disease
Coronary artery disease
Myocardial infarction
Arrhythmia
Acute heart disease
Drug-induced arrhythmia: iatrogenic
Drug-induced arrhythmia: illicit drugs, especially cocaine
Pericardial tamponade: iatrogenic after perforation of the heart by central catheters
Pericardial tamponade
Pregnancy-associated cardiomyopathy
Pregnancy-induced hypertension; toxemia
Angioedema of larynx/anaphylaxis
Envenomation
Lightning
Cerebral vascular accident
Asthma
Pulmonary embolus/amniotic fluid embolism
Aspiration pneumonia
Overwhelming infection/septicemia
Trauma
Poisoning and drug overdose
Iatrogenic (e.g., hypermagnesemia)
Hemorrhage/hypovolemia

Physiologic Changes in Pregnancy

Many physiologic changes of pregnancy can influence resuscitation of the pregnant patient. Physical changes of pregnancy include the change of body habitus, laryngeal edema, enlargement of the mammary glands, and increased vascularity of the mucosa. Changes in the pulmonary system include an increased tidal volume, respiratory rate, and minute ventilation to meet the increased oxygen requirements of the pregnancy. These changes, combined with the decreased functional residual capacity, contribute to the rapid decreases in arterial and venous oxygen tensions of pregnant women compared with nonpregnant women when apneic.[7] The cephalad displacement of the diaphragm 4 to 6 cm by the gravid uterus[8] and the enlargement of the breasts can contribute to a decreased compliance in artificial ventilation.[9,10] The cardiovascular state of pregnancy is a high-flow, low-resistance system because of increased plasma and blood volume, cardiac output, and increased maternal heart rate associated with decreased systemic vascular resistance. A special concern in a supine pregnant patient is the effect the gravid uterus has both on the arterial and venous system. The obstruction of the inferior vena cava and pelvic veins by the gravid uterus can sequester as much as 30% of the circulated blood volume.[11,12] This decrease in venous return to the heart results in a lower cardiac output and lower blood pressure. The uterine compression also compromises the aortoiliac vessels and affects both the renal and uterine blood supply. The displacement of the abdominal contents upward by the uterus also can cause the thorax to be less compressible, thus affecting external chest compression effectiveness (Table 43-4).

TABLE 43-2
Difficult Airway Cart

Bronchoscope
Bronchoscopy cart
Bronchoscope suction adapter
5% Lidocaine ointment: lollipop
2% Viscous lidocaine: gargle
4% Lidocaine solution: atomizer
Atomizer
Lubricant: bronchoscope lubricant
Tongue blade: 5% lollipop
Nasal swabs: cocaine
Nasal trumpets: small and large (for application 5% lidocaine and nasal dilator)
Blue towels, cotton gauze
ETT: nasal—uncut, oral—cut (place in warm bottle of normal saline)
Ovassapian airway
Non-Luer-lock 10-ml syringe with 4% lidocaine or normal saline irrigation
Light source
Suctions (one for bronchoscope and one with Yankauer for oral suction)
Transtracheal kit
4% Lidocaine: 3 ml in 5-ml syringe with 21-gauge needle
Alcohol patches
Medications
Cocaine
Glycopyrolate
Droperidol
Lidocaine
Phenylephrine
Fentanyl
Midazolam

ETT, Endotracheal tube.

Equipment

Emergency resuscitative equipment must always be both readily available and accessible. All medical staff should know the location of the equipment and be familiar with the type of equipment available. All emergency equipment must include basic airway management equipment, resuscitative drugs, a tank of oxygen, intravascular catheters, resuscitation fluids, and a defibrillator or pacemaker. Since difficult intubations are estimated to be encountered in 5% of obstetric patients given general anesthetics,[13] a separate *difficult airway cart* should be created to include both nonsurgical and surgical airway equipment (Table 43-2). Cardiopulmonary arrest can occur anywhere, which necessitates equipment being preassembled in a portable kit. This portable emergency kit should include all primary airway equipment and drugs, yet remain light enough to be mobile (Table 43-3).

Management

Management of the pregnant patient in cardiopulmonary arrest begins with the fundamentals of any resuscitation situation. These include securing

TABLE 43-3
Portable Emergency Equipment

Rigid laryngoscope blades (Macintosh nos. 3 and 4, Miller nos. 2 and 3) of different types and sizes
Short-handled laryngoscope handle (Datta Briwa handle)
Endotracheal tubes of various sizes (5,6,7,8)
Endotracheal guides: stylets, light wands
Forceps to allow manipulation of tip of tube (McGill forceps) or tube which allows tip manipulation
Emergency nonsurgical airway of preference (mask, laryngeal mask airway, esophageal-tracheal device)
Equipment for cricothyroidotomy
Exhaled carbon dioxide detector
Emergency drugs
Tape and ties to secure airway

TABLE 43-4

ANATOMIC AND PHYSIOLOGIC EFFECTS OF PREGNANCY AFFECTING CLOSED-CHEST CARDIOPULMONARY RESUSCITATION

Increased heart rate
Increased blood and plasma volume
Increased cardiac output
Decreased arterial blood pressure
Decreased systemic vasculature resistance, except in toxemic syndromes
Increased respiratory rate and tidal volume
Increased minute ventilation
Decreased functional residual capacity
Increased oxygen consumption
Decreased arterial P_{CO_2}
Decreased serum bicarbonate
Enlarging uterus and supine position
Decreased compliance for artificial ventilation
Decreased compliance for thoracic compression
Uterine compression of aorta and inferior vena cava
Decreased venous return
Aortoiliac occlusion with decreased renal and uterine arterial flow
Increased rate of acid metabolite production
Decreased gastric motility
Relaxed gastroesophageal sphincter

P_{CO_2}, Carbon dioxide pressure.

an airway, ventilating with oxygen, and establishing hemodynamic stability. The airway must be secured with prompt endotracheal intubation if possible, but mask ventilation with cricoid pressure is better than no ventilation at all. Because of the increased mucosal vascularity, which can cause easy bleeding, nasal intubation is not recommended. Endotracheal intubation addresses three concerns of the arresting parturient. First, a properly placed endotracheal tube enables patients to be ventilated with 100% oxygen. Second, since all pregnant patients past 12 weeks of gestation are deemed *full stomachs,* endotracheal intubation allows for airway protection against aspiration. Finally, endotracheal intubation secures a route for administration of emergency drugs, specifically atropine, lidocaine, naloxone, and epinephrine. If this route is used, one should remember that the dose administered should be two and one half times the recommended intravenous dose. The delivered endotracheal dose should be diluted to a 10 ml dose and followed by two positive-pressure breaths. Equipment for oral intubation should include rigid laryngoscope of choice, short-handled laryngoscope handle, a styletted endotracheal tube one size smaller than would normally be used, oxygen supply, bag-valve device, and suction apparatus. Proper placement should be confirmed by auscultation and a portable carbon dioxide detector. If a detector is used, remember that the tube may be in the correct position without a change in the detector because there is no cardiac output and hence no carbon dioxide delivery to the lungs. Other means to confirm placement can include a fiberoptic bronchoscope or esophageal detector device bulb.[14] Since parturients are more likely to be difficult to intubate compared with nonpregnant patients,[15] familiarity and knowledge with both surgical and nonsurgical airways is imperative.[16] Nonsurgical airways include face mask, laryngeal mask, transtracheal jet ventilation, and esophageal-tracheal devices. These devices can be used by themselves, as an adjunct to securing endotracheal intubation, or as a bridge until a definite surgical airway can be secured. Comparison of the laryngeal mask airway and esophageal-tracheal device in an obstetric population suggests that the esophageal-tracheal device may have an advantage.[17] This benefit is due to the ability to provide positive-pressure ventilation and a decreased aspiration risk, since the esophageal cuff prevents gastric contents from entering the trachea. After establishing an airway, ventilation should be accomplished with a bag-valve device attached to a high concentration of oxygen at a rate of one ventilation for each 5 chest compressions in a two-person rescue, or two ventilations to 15 compressions for a one-person rescue.[18] Because both arterial and venous systems are compressed by the uterus,[11,12,19] left uterine displacement is critical. This displacement relieves this compression, and is accomplished by either having a medical care provider manually displace the uterus to the left, or by placing a wedge or folded towel under the patient's right hip, which produces a 15° angle. This key maneuver decompresses the vasculature and still allows for the upper torso to remain flat and available for adequate chest compressions.

When pulselessness has been established, external chest compressions should be initiated. Proper hand position is the key for properly performed chest compressions. Compressions must be performed on the lower half of the sternum, with the heel of both hands delivering a 60-lb force.[18] The compression depth should be one and one half to two inches at a rate of 80 to 100 beats/min. Each compression should be smooth and regular with equal compression:relaxation ratio. Complications of improperly performed chest compressions include sternal fracture, pneumothorax, hemothorax, lung contusion, and lacerations of the spleen and liver. Consideration can be given to simultaneous ventilation and chest compression, which in dogs has been shown to produce both higher blood pressures and improved carotid flow.[20] Next, two large-bore intravenous catheters (no. 14 or 16) must be placed by whatever means necessary. Antecubitals are an excellent site since their placement will not be impeded by the chest compressions. Other sites include internal and external jugular veins or subclavian veins. When emergency access is required, both the subclavian and internal jugular veins remain patent when peripheral veins collapse. But with these access sites are inherent risks, such as subclavian or carotid artery punctures and pneumothorax. Venous cutdowns are an alternative means of access. Fluid resuscitation should use either normal saline or Ringer's lactate solution, not 5 percent dextrose in water (D_5W). These fluids should be administered as rapidly as possible, preferably warmed.

Monitors

Cardiac monitors should be attached to the patient as soon as possible, but not if it would delay the initiation of the proper cardiopulmonary resuscitation. One should remember the axiom, *treat the patient not the monitors.* An electrocardiogram (ECG) should not be necessary to establish pulselessness, but this is necessary to differentiate between ventricular fibrillation and pulseless electrical activity (formerly called electromechanical dissociation [EMD]). An arterial blood gas reading, a complete chemistry profile, complete blood count, and a coagulation profile should be obtained. One should remember to assess for tracheal deviation, and to observe for bilateral chest wall excursion and auscultation of both lungs, which assures both correct tube placement and eliminates the possibility of a pneumothorax. Muffled heart sounds may indicate the possibility of cardiac tamponade. If the clinical picture improves, an arterial line, central venous pressure, or pulmonary artery line can be placed as indicated.

Guidelines

With an ECG and pulse check, both the electrical and mechanical activity of the heart can be assessed, which enables the clinician to apply the correct algorithm[21] (Figs. 43-1 through 43-4 and Table 43-5, p. 488). The treatment priorities for a pregnant patient are the same as for a nonpregnant patient. Pregnancy is not a contraindication to external defibrillation.[22] If defibrillation is required, the left breast may need to be displaced for placement of the pads or paddles to the apex of the heart. For patients in ventricular fibrillation from bupivacaine

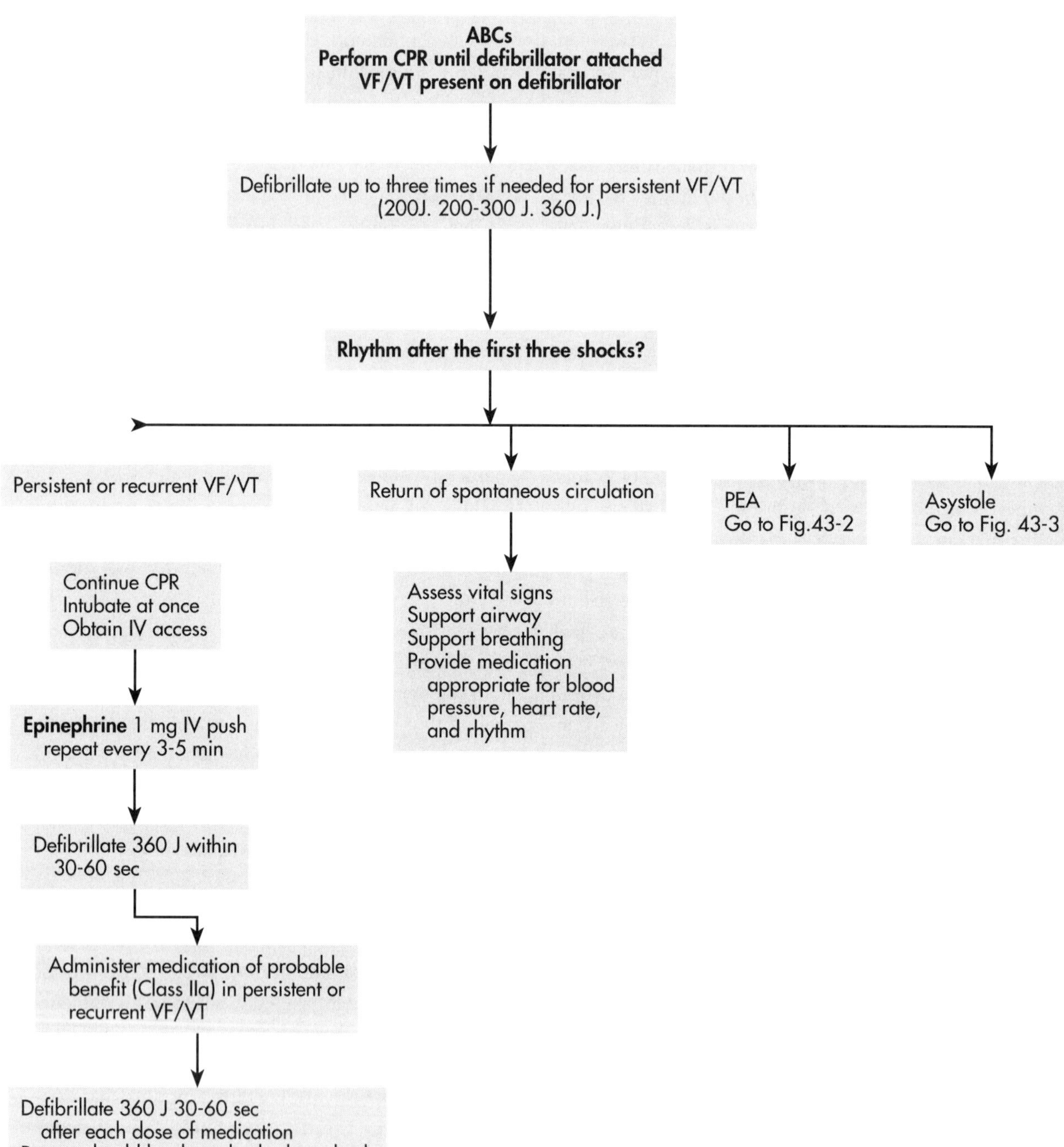

Fig. 43-1.
Ventricular fibrillation/pulse ventricular tachycardia algorithm (VF/VT).[21] PEA, pulseless electrical activity.

Includes: Electromechanical dissociation (EMD)
Pseudo- EMD
Idioventricular rhythms
Ventricular escape rhythms
Bradyasystolic rhythms
Postdefibrillation idioventricular rhythms

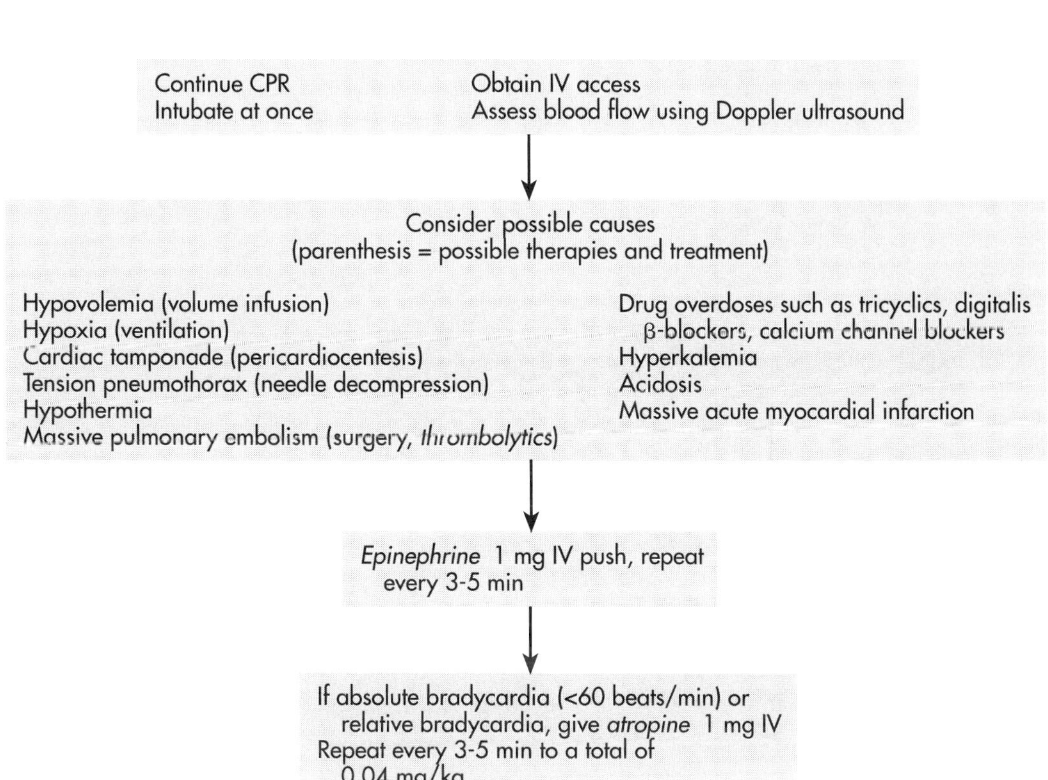

Fig. 43-2.
Pulseless electrical activity (PEA) algorithm.[21]

toxicity, lidocaine must be avoided and the first-line drug should be bretylium. Lidocaine, atropine, procainamide, and bretylium all have been used in pregnant patients. Concern regarding epinephrine in pregnancy is based on its α-agonist properties, which could contribute to decreased uterine perfusion; however, in a code situation, its therapeutic effects greatly outweigh this potential risk. If the standard dose of a resuscitation drug does not elicit the normal response, consideration should be given to increasing the dose to correct for the increased blood volume of pregnancy.

Protocol

Protocols for the medical management of the mother and delivery of her fetus vary from institution to institution, and familiarity with one's own institutional protocol is of great importance. If the

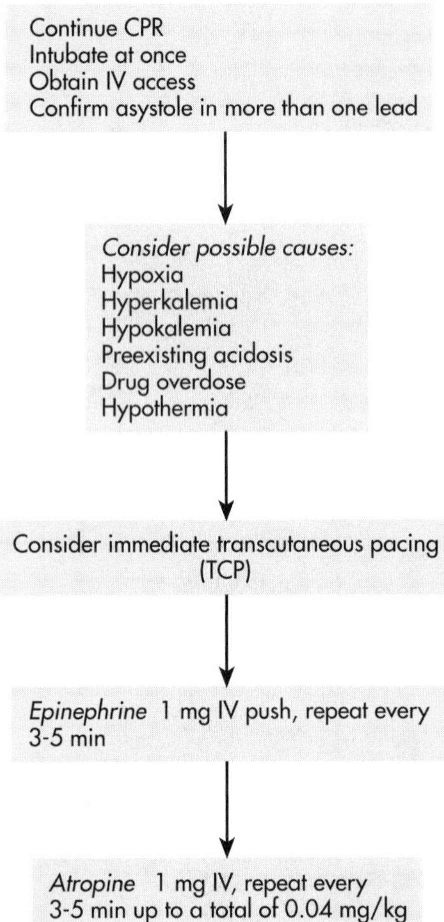

Fig. 43-3.
Asystole treatment algorithm.[21]

mother has not been resuscitated by 4 minutes of CPR, the chance of a successful outcome is reduced. At our institution, our protocol states that any pregnant woman with a uterine size greater than 20-weeks will have an immediate cesarean section performed at 4 minutes of resuscitation with the goal of delivery of the fetus by 5 minutes. Uterine size does not always correlate with gestational age in the case of macrosomia, multiple gestation, and other special conditions. On physical examination, a 20-week uterine size is easy to determine because this is when the fundal height is palpated at the level of the umbilicus. The dichotomy in the resuscitation protocol based on uterine size rather than gestational age presumes that once the uterus is of a 20-week size, it then causes significant arterial and venous compromise. With the delivery of the fetus, the occlusion of the great vessels is eliminated and the vena cava is returned to normal.[23]

The rationale for this approach is based on the improved outcome for both the mothers and their babies. Irreversible brain damage is known to occur from anoxia within 4 to 6 minutes without ad-

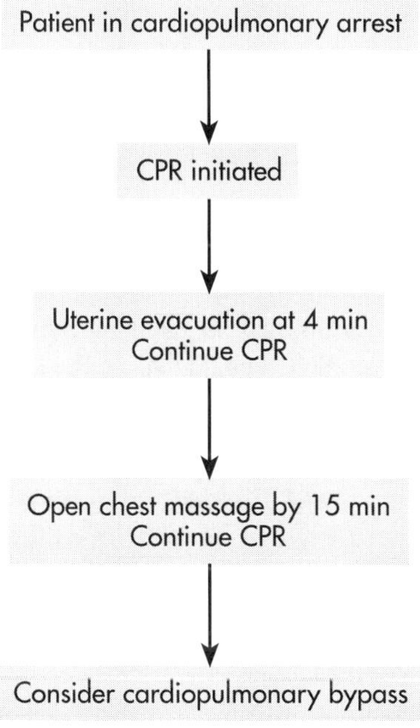

Fig. 43-4.
Management plan for pregnant patient in cardiopulmonary arrest.

equate cerebral perfusion.[18] Pregnant patients become anoxic more quickly from apnea than nonpregnant patients.[13] In a series of five cardiac arrests, the three women who underwent immediate cesarean section recovered and did well, in contrast to the two women whose operation was started after 6 minutes who had irreversible brain damage.[24] In one case, a late-term pregnant woman had a respiratory arrest; although her heart showed electrical activity, there was no measurable blood pressure despite active resuscitation. On evacuation of her uterus, her blood pressure immediately rose to 80 torr.[25] Based on cases and investigations, there is speculation that delivery of the fetus is possibly the most important intervention in the resuscitation of the mother.

Although improvement in maternal outcome would be enough to justify early delivery of the fetus, it is clear that is also improves fetal outcome. It has been estimated that the oxygen reserve of the fetus is only 2 minutes.[26] In pregnant animal models, brain damage was noted as early as 6 minutes after fetal asphyxia.[27] The literature presents impressive support that the shorter the interval from maternal arrest to the delivery of the fetus, the better the fetal outcome. Most healthy survivors were delivered within 5 minutes, with only a few healthy infants being delivered more than 10 minutes after arrest[28] (Table 43-6). During a code, fetal monitoring is not advisable or practical because of the noise during the resuscitative efforts. Secondly, it will not give information that will affect clinical management. If the mother is successfully resuscitated within 4 minutes, then the fetal status will be evaluated. If not successful at 4 minutes, our protocol requires cesarean section, regardless of the fetal status. For best maternal and fetal outcome, strict adherence to the *4-minute* rule is strongly advocated. During the evacuation of the uterus, external chest compressions should be continued with immediate preparations begun to perform a thora-

TABLE 43-5
Drug Therapy

Class I: definitely helpful
Class IIa: acceptable, probably helpful
Class IIb: acceptable, possibly helpful
Class III: not indicated, may be harmful
The recommended dose of epinephrine is 1 mg IV push every 3-5 min; if this approach fails, several class IIb dosing regimens can be considered
Intermediate: epinephrine 2-5 mg IV push, every 3-5 min
Escalating: epinephrine 1-mg, 3-mg, or 5-mg IV push, 3 min apart
High: epinephrine 0.1 mg/kg IV push, every 5 min
Sodium bicarbonate
Class I: 1 mEq/kg if patient has known preexisting hyperkalemia
Class IIa
If known preexisting bicarbonate-responsiveness acidosis
If overdose with tricyclic antidepressants
To alkalinize the urine in drug overdoses
Class IIb
If intubated and long arrest interval
On return of spontaneous circulation after long arrest interval
Class III
Hypoxic lactic acidosis
Medications for VF
Lidocaine 1.5 mg/kg IV push; repeat in 3-5 min to total loading dose of 3 mg/kg; then use
Bretylium 5 mg/kg IV push; repeat in 5 min at 10 mg/kg
Magnesium sulfate 1-2 g IV in torsades de pointes or suspected hypomagnesemic state or severe refractory VF
Procainamide 30 mg/min in refractory VF (maximum total 17 mg/kg)
Atropine
Class IIb: shorter dosing intervals in pulseless electrical activity and asystolic arrest

IV, Intravenous; VF, ventricular fibrillation

cotomy for the start of open-chest massage[29] (Table 43-7).

Although no studies specifically address open versus closed chest massage in the pregnant population, for patients with chest trauma, massive pulmonary embolism, and profound hypovolemia, thoracotomy and open-chest massage can be effective interventions.[30] Studies in both humans and animals have shown superior hemodynamic parameters from open-chest massage.[31-33] In experimental studies with dogs, open-chest massage improved cardiac output, arterial pressures, and blood flow to the carotid and coronary arteries. However, the survival advantage of open-chest massage compared with closed massage declined with increasing the interval from arrest to initiation of the opening of the thorax.[32] When beginning open-chest massage and all other medical interventions, consideration should be given to placing the patient on cardiopulmonary bypass if possible. Every therapeutic option must be considered for these patients since they are a healthy population who will do well if they survive the arrest. The four main indications for bypass are profound hypothermia, bupivacaine toxicity, hemorrhage secondary to hypovolemia, and pulmonary embolism.

Obstetric Code Team

Clearly the management of an obstetric arrest requires the integral cooperation of all the medical care providers. At Brigham and Women's Hospital, a separate obstetric code team has been established that includes participants from a variety of services. This unique team includes anesthesiologists, thoracic surgeons, obstetricians, pediatricians-neonatologists, and obstetric-critical care nurses. At all times, the anesthesiologist is the code leader with a primary responsibility to the mother. Each member of the team has clearly delineated roles to be performed. The anesthesi-

TABLE 43-6

Postmortem Cesarean Delivery with Surviving Infants with Reports of Time from Death of the Mother to Delivery

Time from Maternal Death to Delivery (Min)	Surviving Infants	
	No.	Percent (of Births Reported)
0-5	42 Normal infants	70
6-10	7 Normal infants	13
	1 With mild neurologic sequelae	
11-15	6 Normal infants	12
	1 With severe neurologic sequelae	
16-20	1 With severe neurologic sequelae	1.7
21+	2 With severe neurologic sequelae	3.3
	1 Normal infant	

From Katz VL, Dotters DJ, Droegemueller W: Perimortem cesarean delivery, *Contempt Obstet Gynecol* 1986; 68:571.

ologist secures an airway, ventilates with oxygen, ascertains the cardiac rhythm, directs chest compressions, and establishes intravascular access. The thoracic surgeon assists in obtaining vascular access and prepares to perform a left thoracotomy when instructed. The obstetrician prepares to perform an emergency cesarean section. The pediatrician awaits the delivery of the fetus, prepared to perform a full neonatal resuscitation. The obstetric nurses obtain needed equipment and drugs, and record events in code. Our protocol advocates early aggressive intervention, which includes cesarean section at 4 minutes with delivery of the fetus by 5 minutes, and a low threshold for converting to open-chest massage and consideration of cardiopulmonary bypass. For medical care providers to work cohesively in a code situation, it is not enough that they know their roles; they should actually practice their tasks. Impromptu *mock codes* can benefit the entire medical team. The medical care providers should actually bring the crash cart to a room, prepare drugs, and open a cesarean section kit. For example, the obstetrician's responsibility is not to help in resuscitation, but to immediately gown and glove and prepare for a expeditious cesarean section. These simulated codes reinforce the knowledge base and clarify each person's role as a member of the code team.

Summary

Cardiopulmonary arrest in the pregnant patient is a rare medical emergency which requires a clear, organized, timely medical intervention for successful outcome.

1. As in any resuscitation situation securing an airway, ventilating with oxygen, and establishing hemodynamic stability with left uterine displacement are the priorities. For the parturient in cardiopulmonary arrest, remember that the anatomic and physiologic affects of pregnancy will affect resuscitation.
2. If resuscitation is not successful by 4 minutes, a perimortem cesarean section should be performed since it is associated with im-

TABLE 43-7
Technique of Open-Chest Cardiac Massage

1. Open the chest and pericardium with an incision through the left fifth intercostal space
2. One hand: the ventricles are cupped by the fingers and palm of the right hand and the heart is compressed against the sternum and squeezed by the fingers
3. Two hands: if there is sufficient exposure the heart is enclosed, one hand below, the other hand above the heart; compression is produced by squeezing the hands together and squeezing the fingers
4. One-handed massage without a firm opposing force, either the sternum or the other hand, is less effective
5. Sixty compressions per minute is adequate if good filling and emptying of the ventricles are achieved
6. Endotracheal intubation is essential to maintain adequate ventilation
7. Broad-spectrum antibiotic coverage should be initiated immediately
8. Open-chest massage can be a bloody business; today, precautions for hepatitis B virus and human immunodeficiency virus must be observed

From Lee RV, Rodgers BD, White LM, et al: Cardiopulmonary resuscitation of pregnant women, *Am J Med* 1986; 81:311.

proved maternal and fetal outcome.

3. A team approach with each member clearly understanding their role ensures the best possible outcome for mother and baby.

References

1. Department of Health and Social Security: *Report on confidential inquiries into maternal deaths in England and Wales 1976-78, 1979-81,* London, 1982, 1986, HMSO.
2. Hibbard LT: Maternal mortality due to cardiac disease, *Clin Obstet Gynecol* 1975; 18:27.
3. Pritchard JA, MacDonald PC, Gant NF: *Obstetrics in broad perspective.* In Pritchard JA, MacDonald PC, Gant NF, et al: editors: *Williams obstetrics, ed 17,* New York, 1985, Appleton-Century-Crofts.
4. Streissguth AP, Grant TM, Barr HM, et al: Cocaine and the use of alcohol and other drugs during pregnancy, *Am J Obstet Gynecol* 1991; 164:1239.
5. Kloner RA, Hale S, Alker K, et al: The effect of acute and chronic cocaine use on the heart, *Circulation* 1992; 85: 407.
6. Rezkalla SH, Hale S, Loner RA: Cocaine induced heart disease, *Am Heart J* 1990; 120:403.
7. Archer GW, Marx GF: Arterial oxygen tension during apnoea in parturient women, *Br J Anaesth* 1974; 46:358.
8. Rubin A, Russo N, Goucher D: The effect of pregnancy upon pulmonary function in normal women, *Am J Obstet Gynecol* 1956; 72:963.
9. Weinberger SE, Weiss ST, Cohen WR, et al: Pregnancy and the lung, *Am Rev Respir Dis* 1980; 121:559.
10. Gee JBL, Packer BS, Millen JE, et al: Pulmonary mechanics during pregnancy, *J Clin Invest* 1967; 46:945.
11. Kerr MG, Scott DB, Samuel E: Studies of the inferior vena cava in late pregnancy, *Br Med J* 1964; 1:532.
12. Bieniarz J, Crottogini JJ, Curucher E, et al: Aortocaval compression by the uterus in late human pregnancy, *Am J Obstet Gynecol* 1968; 100:203.
13. Gibbs CP: Gastric aspiration: prevention and treatment, *Clin Anesthesiol* 1986; 4:47.
14. Zaleski L, Abello D, Gold MI: The esophageal dector device, *Anesthesiology* 1993; 79:244.
15. Samsson GL, Young JR: Difficult tracheal intubation: a retrospective study, *Anesthesia* 1987; 42:487.
16. Lawlor M, Johnson C, Weiner M: Airway management in obstetric anesthesia, *Int J Obstet Anesth* 1993; 3:225.
17. Wissler RN: The esophageal-tracheal combitube, *Anesth Rev* 1993; 20:147.
18. Albaran-Sotelo R, Flint LS, Kelly K, editors: *Basic life support.* Dallas, 1990, American Heart Association.
19. Ureland K, Novy MG, Perterson EN, et al: Maternal cardiovascular dynamics, *Am J Obstet Gynecol* 1969; 104:856.
20. Chandra N, Snyder LD, Weisfeldt ML: Abdominal binding during cardiopulmonary resuscitation in man, *JAMA* 1981; 246:351.
21. Albarran-Sotelo R, Flint LS, Kelly K, et al, editors: *Textbook of advanced cardiac life support, ed 2,* Dallas, 1990, American Heart Association.
22. Curry JJ, Quintana FJ: Myocardial infarction with ventricular fibrillation during pregnancy treated by direct current defibrillation with fetal survival, *Chest* 1970; 58:82.
23. Kerr MG: The mechanical effects of the gravid uterus in later pregnancy, *J Obstet Gynecol Br Commonw* 1965; 72:513.
24. Marx GF: Cardiopulmonary resuscitation of late-pregnancy women, *Anesthesiology* 1982; 56:156.

25. DePace NL, Betesh JS, Kotler MN: Postmortem cesarean section with recovery of both mother and offspring, *JAMA* 1982; 248:971.
26. Longo LD, Hill EP, Power GC: *Factors affecting placental oxygen transfer.* In Longo LD, Bartels H, editors: *Respiratory gas exchange and blood flow in the placenta,* Bethesda, Md, 1972, Public Health Service 345-91k (DHEW (NIH) 73-361) as quoted in Greenberger PA, Patterson R: Management of asthma during pregnancy, *N Engl J Med* 1985; 312:897.
27. Windle WF: Brain damage at birth, *JAMA* 1968; 206:1967.
28. Katz VL, Dotters DJ, Droegemueller W: Perimortem cesarean delivery, *Contempt Obstet Gynecol* 1986; 68:571.
29. Lee RV, Rodgers BD, White LM, et al: Cardiopulmonary resuscitation of pregnant women, *Am J Med* 1986; 81:311.
30. Stephenson HE Jr: Pathophysiological considerations that warrant open-chest cardiac resuscitation, *Crit Care Med* 1980; 8:185.
31. DelGuerico LRM, Feins NR, Cohn JD, et al: Comparison of blood flow during external and internal cardiac massage in man, *Circulation* 1965; 32(suppl):171 (abstract).
32. Sanders AB, Kern KB, Ewy GA: Improved survival from cardiac arrest with open chest massage, *Ann Emerg Med* 1983; 12:138 (abstract).
33. Jacobsen S: Current status of open chest procedures, *Clin Emerg Med* 1983; 2:121.

44

Morbid Obesity

A 30-year-old primigravida with 39 weeks' gestation comes for preoperative consultation for cesarean section. She is morbidly obese with a blood pressure of 160/95 mm Hg. She is being treated with hypotensive medications. Discuss the anesthetic management.

Recommendations by Donald H. Wallace, M.D.

Obesity is common, affecting about 25% of the population, as determined by insurance height and weight tables.[1] Obesity usually results from excessive calorie intake and reduced energy expenditure or production. Increased numbers of adipocytes may be present in the first year, and hereditary, socioeconomic, and psychological factors contribute to the obese state. The adipocyte has increased stores of triglycerides because of outlined changes in intermediary metabolism (Fig. 44-1). About 5% of the obese are defined as the morbidly obese (MO), having a body weight double the height/weight tables' ideal body weight, or 100 lb more than ideal weight. Regional distribution of adipose tissue, as in truncal or abdominal obesity, is measured at the bedside by waist/hip circumference ratio, which is accepted as associated with increased morbidity. The severity of obesity also is assessed by several other indices[2,3]; however, recently the body mass index (BMI) has been selected[4] as a parameter in the study of excessive maternal weight and pregnancy outcome (BMI = weight [kg]/height [m^2], 25 is normal, and > 30 is frank obesity).

The MO pregnant woman is considered to be *high risk,* and challenges the anesthesiologist when the obstetrician schedules cesarean section (Tables 44-1 and 44-2). It is reported[5] that 88% of obese pregnant women have increased gastric volumes greater than 25 ml and a gastric pH less than 2.5; also, a reduced rate of gastric emptying increases the risk of aspiration. In addition, obese patients have a higher incidence of hiatal hernia. A study of

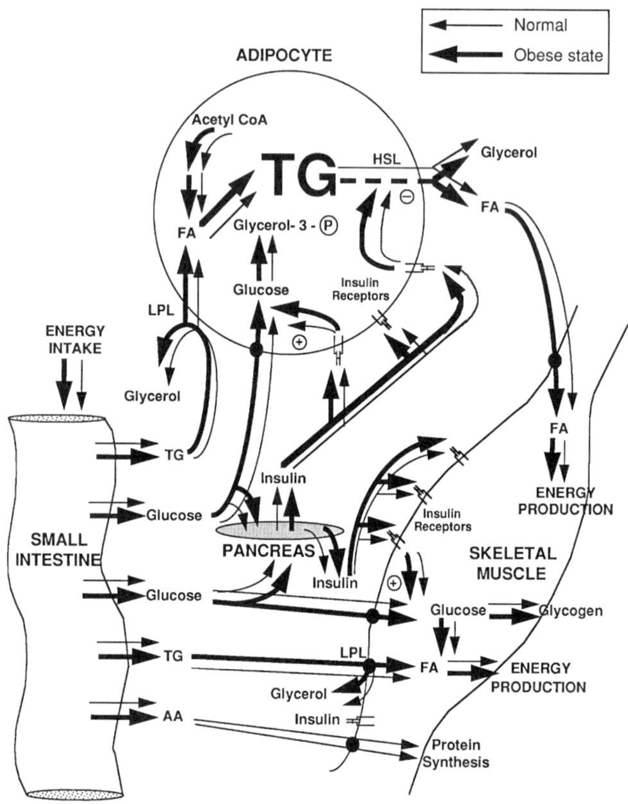

Fig. 44-1.

Intermediary metabolism of obesity. In a normal person, during steady state, energy intake is equal to the energy production or expenditure. Obesity results from an excessive energy intake and reduced energy expenditure or production. Excessive energy intake presents a load of triglyceride, glucose, and amino acids in the circulation for disposal. Storage of fat in adipocytes occurs after glycogen stores in liver and skeletal muscles are repleted. Excessive stimulation of β-cells of the pancreas by glucose causes increased secretion of insulin, which in turn leads to accumulation of triglyceride in adipocytes. In severe obesity, insulin receptor expression may be down-regulated in skeletal muscles as well as in adipocytes, thus leading to insulin resistance. Digestion of food releases triglycerides, glucose, and amino acids from the intestines into the circulation. Glucose can be used to produce energy by body tissues, especially skeletal muscles, or can be stored as glycogen in liver or skeletal muscles. Triglycerides in circulation are hydrolyzed by lipoprotein lipase (LPL), which is present on capillary endothelium, to fatty acids and glycerol. Fatty acids in turn can be used for energy production by skeletal muscles, or may be stored after reesterification in adipocytes. The process of reesterification of fatty acids in adipocytes needs insulin-stimulated glucose transport and production of glycerol-3-phosphate. Triglycerides stored in adipocytes can be released after lipolysis, which is under the control of hormone-sensitive lipase (HSL). Insulin suppresses HSL activity and stimulates LPL activity as well as endogenous fatty acid synthesis and esterification of fatty acids; and therefore, excess insulin action results in a net accumulation of triglycerides in the adipocytes. How insulin affects these activities after interaction with insulin receptors is not clear.

TABLE 44-1

Obstetric Complications in Obese Patients

Perinatal mortality
Prolonged gestation
Dysfunctional labor
Failed induction
Prolonged 2nd stage of labor
Chorioamnionitis
Difficult intubation
Increased risk of blood loss $>$ 1000 ml at C-section
Prolonged surgery
Postpartum hemorrhage
Thrombophlebitis
Wound infection
Wound dehiscence

TABLE 44-2

Increased Risk to the Fetus in Obese Mothers

Macrosomia
Twin gestation
Malpresentation
Birth asphyxia
Birth trauma
Shoulder dystocia
Neonatal hypoglycemia
Cord accidents
Meconium staining

lower esophageal sphincter tone[6] in the obese has demonstrated normal mean lower esophageal sphincter pressure in most. Drugs that affect the lower esophageal sphincter pressure are shown in Table 44-3.

Maternal adaptations to pregnancy in the MO include even greater oxygen demands because of fat cell metabolism. Oxygen consumption increases by

TABLE 44-3

Effect of Selected Drugs on the Lower Esophageal Sphincter Pressure

Increase	Decrease	No Change
Metoclopramide	Atropine	Propranolol
Prochlorperazine	Glycopyrrolate	Oxprenolol
Neostigmine	Dopamine	Cimetidine
Suxamethonium	Sodium nitroprusside	Ranitidine
Metoprolol	Ganglion blockers	Atracurium
Antacids	Thiopental	
Halothane		
Enflurane		
Opioids		

TABLE 44-4

Respiratory Changes

Respiratory compromise is caused by
Increased lumbar lordosis: abdominal volume
Thoracic kyphosis: decreased volume thorax
Abdominal fat: displaces diaphragm upward
Thoracic fat: decreased chest wall compliance
In morbid obesity
Decreased IRV
Decreased vital capacity
Decreased total lung capacity
Decreased inspiratory capacity
Decreased MVV
Decreased ERV and FRC, FRC $<$ CC
Closure of dependent alveoli
Increased V/Q mismatch
Arterial hypoxemia

100% as weight increase doubles. The work of breathing is increased by excess layers of fat over the chest and abdomen, which mechanically splint the chest wall and diaphragm. Increased thoracic kyphosis and thoracolumbar lordosis limit rib movement (Table 44-4). The supine position reduces ventilation and respiratory reserves, and may not be tolerated. Obese hypoventilation syndrome,[7] with its characteristic hypercarbia, hypoxemia, somnolence, edema, polycythemia, and cardiomegaly, occurs in 5% to 10% of the MO population.

Chronic hypertension is more common in the nonpregnant and pregnant obese populations, with an increase in pregnancy-induced hypertension (PIH). Blood volume and cardiac output are increased by 35% to 45% during pregnancy; blood volume in the obese increases in proportion to their body mass. There is considerable enlargement of the vascular bed[8] in the MO, and there is a significant increase in cardiac work and output. An excess weight of 100 kg may increase cardiac output by 200% with marked increase in stroke volume (Table 44-5).

Circulatory changes also are significant with changes in position.[9] Changing the MO from the sitting to the supine position has elevated oxygen consumption by 11%, and pulmonary capillary wedge pressure (PCWP) by up to 30%. Respiratory obstruction relieved by tracheal intubation has reduced PCWP from 38 to 5 mm Hg in an obese patient.[10] Cardiac arrest has occurred after placing MO patients in the supine position for surgery.[11]

Abnormal glucose tolerance tests, gestational diabetes, insulin-resistant diabetes, diabetic neuropathy, and retinopathy are more common in the obese. Fatty accumulation in the liver and abnormalities in insulin and triglyceride metabolism occur, and there might be associated coagulopathy with hepatic failure. Biotransformation of volatile agents[12-14] such as halothane and enflurane results in elevated serum bromide and inorganic fluoride levels (Table 44-6).

Psychological problems are common in the MO pregnant woman.[15] It is important to explain the reasons for careful history and physical examination, and to discuss risks and benefits of alternative methods of anesthesia. Making special preparations for transport, and discussing activities within the labor and delivery suite and while transferring to the delivery bed will help to obtain the cooperation and assistance of an anxious and sometimes depressed woman. All members of the health care team should

TABLE 44-5
CARDIOVASCULAR CHANGES

Increased cardiac output
Pregnancy: 35%-45%
Obesity: up to 200% with blood flow to fat at 2-3 ml/100 g may require CO increase by 2000 ml/min
LVEDV at upper range of normal
Cardiac work and myocardial oxygen consumption
Increased 45% during labor
Increased 80% immediately after delivery
Increased BP
Normal SVR
Increased mean PA and PCWPs

TABLE 44-6
THE RISK FOR ASSOCIATED ANTENATAL DISEASE IS 5 TO 10 TIMES THE RATE SEEN IN THE NORMAL POPULATION

Gestational diabetes mellitus
Hypertension (chronic or PIH)
Urinary tract infections
Coronary artery disease
Cirrhosis
Cholelithiasis
Polycythemia
Cardiomegaly
Edema
Hypercarbia

avoid disparaging remarks about the patient's size or appearance.

The preanesthetic evaluation determines the degree of reduction in respiratory reserves. Facial and oropharyngeal edema, and increased tongue size can result in difficult laryngoscopy in the hypertensive woman at term. Rolls of cervical fat and greatly enlarged breasts restrict range of movement of the neck, and add to the difficulty of laryngoscopy and tracheal intubation (Table 44-7). Response to anesthetic drugs in the obese is determined by altered biotransformation, hepatic and renal clearance, drug binding, and volumes of distribution.

Pharmacokinetics of the administered drugs are changed in MO parturients (Table 44-8). In the MO woman,[16] the optimal induction dose of sodium pentothal which has a longer elimination half-life because of increased volume of distribution, is unclear. I limit the dose to 500 mg or less despite body weight exceeding 150 kg, although 4 mg/kg is the usual induction dose to limit potential for awareness and stress-caused reductions in uterine blood flow. Succinylcholine requirements are not based on lean body weight, since pseudocholine esterase activity is increased in the obese, and duration of action remains normal with doses calculated on a milligram per kilogram basis. Excellent relaxation for tracheal intubation is obtained with doses up to 200 mg, and I monitor relaxation with a peripheral nerve stimulator. There is normal response to nondepolarizing muscle relaxants. Recovery usually is rapid after nitrous oxide–fentanyl and low-dose (0.3 to 0.4 minimum alveolar concentration [MAC]) isoflurane anesthesia, an agent with minimal biotransformation that ensures amnesia.

TABLE 44-7

Predictors of a Difficult Airway

- Short, thick neck
- Mandibular length/posterior depth < 3.6
- Thyromental distance < 6 cm
- Limited extension of atlantooccipital joint
- Limited opening of mouth < 6 cm
- Long incisors with overbite increase
- High, arched palate
- Mallampati class 3

TABLE 44-8

Pharmacokinetics in Obesity

- Drug biotransformation may be altered due to
  - Hepatic dysfunction
  - Diabetes
  - Changes in splanchnic blood flow
  - Prolonged biotransformation in fatty tissue
- Renal clearance and excretion decreased due to decrease in
  - Glomerular filtration
- Biliary excretion hampered by
  - Gallstones
  - Pancreatitis
- Hyperlipoproteinemia may affect drug binding
  - Benzodiazepines & thiopental
    - Increased V_d
    - Increased elimination half-life
  - Volatile agents
    - Elimination time increases due to fat solubility
  - Fentanyl and sufentanyl
    - Normal V_d
    - Normal elimination half-life
    - Normal clearance
  - Vecuronium
    - Prolonged recovery with decreased hepatic blood flow and hepatic elimination
  - Succinylcholine
    - Increased requirements due to increased pseudocholinesterase
    - Increased V_d

V_d, Volume of distribution.

Anesthesia for Cesarean Section

Reviews in the literature confirm problems with both general anesthesia and regional anesthesia.[17-23] Anesthetic and obstetric outcome[24] in a series of MO parturients confirmed the high incidence of antepartum disease and emergency cesarean section. Epidural anesthesia was feasible; however, a high initial failure rate also confirmed the need for early catheter placement and critical assessment of the segmental blockade with catheter replacement, if indicated.[24] However, epidural anesthesia is favored for nonemergent deliveries.[25] Furthermore, difficult tracheal intubation occurred in 6 of 17 of the MO women, in contrast to 0 of 8 control women.[24] It is well established that the cesarean section rate is increased in the MO, and maternal death is reported as 5 to 13 times more likely with emergency than with elective cesarean section. Maternal death directly attributed to cesarean section is five to six times more likely during emergency cesarean section than death attributed to vaginal delivery. Pregnancy increases the potential for difficult intubation. In the obstetric population, 1 in 300 to 1 in 750 attempted tracheal intubations fail.[26-29] It is hard to prospectively identify which airway would be especially difficult for intubation.[24]

Whether the woman consents to general anesthesia or epidural anesthesia, anesthetic management requires[30] prophylaxis against aspiration, safety in management of the airway, adequate ventilation, and the minimization of additional cardiovascular stress. Careful transportation to the operating delivery room and positioning of the woman to avoid discomfort, respiratory stress, and aortocaval compression (by providing adequate uterine tilt) are essential throughout preparation for anesthesia and surgery. Immediately after positioning on the operating bed of appropriate size, continuous electronic monitoring of the fetal heart rate is routine practice at Parkland Memorial Hospital.

General Anesthesia

Preparation for the induction of general anesthesia and maintenance before and after delivery are summarized in Table 44-9. Inserting a radial arterial cannula allows sampling for arterial blood gas analysis and gives the advantage of continuous blood pressure monitoring. I monitor end-tidal concentrations of physiologic gases and anesthetic gases. Acute oxygenation with 100% oxygen starts[31-34] during the final preparations for the abdomen for surgery and placement of the Foley catheter and urinometer. I use the short-handled laryngoscope[35] when performing rapid-sequence induction with cricoesophageal compression. A *difficult airways* cart

TABLE 44-9

Steps for General Anesthesia in the Obese Parturient

1. Insert two large intravenous catheters (16 gauge); warm Ringer's lactate solution for infusion
2. Sodium citrate 0.3 mol/L orally 30 ml within 30 min of induction
3. Tilt uterus to left, ECG, BP cuff, pulse oximeter
4. Clear face mask, administer 100% oxygen
5. Thiopental 4 mg/kg, succinylcholine 1.0-1.5 mg/kg
6. Cricoesophageal compression from loss of consciousness until tracheal placement and cuff inflation, capnograph, and chest evenly ventilated by auscultation
7. Administer $N_2O:O_2$ (50%:50%), isoflurane 0.6-0.7 MAC
8. Monitor NMB by peripheral nerve stimulator: atracurium 0.2-0.3 mg/kg
9. Reduce isoflurane to 0.3-0.4 MAC after delivery; intravenous fentanyl 100 μg repeated as necessary
10. Oxytocin infusion (20 U/L of Ringer's lactate)
11. Empty stomach with a large-bore suction catheter
12. Extubate when parturient is awake, following commands, and satisfies usual criteria for extubation

kept within our delivery suite contains all necessary equipment and local anesthetic agents for the alternative of awake intubation under topical anesthesia. If history or evaluation of the airways predicts difficult tracheal intubation, I perform oral fiberoptic intubation through an intubating airway. It is best to avoid blind nasal intubation because there is a risk of serious epistaxis in the obstetric population.

In the elective cesarean section, time to complete planning with the obstetrician and the MO woman adds safety to the delivery of a high-risk pregnancy (Table 44-10). If intubation fails after rapid-sequence induction, a failed intubation drill[36] is immediately instituted to restore maternal oxygenation. Failure to stop trying to intubate the trachea is associated with maternal death.[37] With expert assistance, mask ventilation is started with cricoid pressure maintained if oxygenation is being restored in the unconscious, paralyzed patient. If the face mask does not fit during maintenance of jaw thrust to open the posterior pharyngeal space and allow ventilation, a laryngeal mask airway[38] may be lifesaving. Although this device does not protect against aspiration, it does facilitate restoration of ventilation. Anesthesiologists are becoming increasingly familiar with this new device, and it is clinically useful in other surgical populations. It is kept available in our difficult airways cart for emergency use. Transtracheal jet ventilation and cricothyrotomy are other emergency procedures that may prove lifesaving.

TABLE 44-10
STEPS TO MINIMIZE RISKS OF DIFFICULT AND FAILED INTUBATION

Shoulder roll
Helps get breasts and abdominal fat out of way
Elevate occiput
Sniffing position helps align airway
Helps lessen anteriorly displaced larynx
Consider awake intubation (oral)
Acute oxygenation 100% O_2 denitrogenate for 3-5 min
Superior to four MVVs
Expert assistance immediately available
Follow failed intubation drill
Restore maternal oxygenation
Use of LMA
Cricothyrotomy/jet ventilation
Tracheostomy

In the labor and delivery suite, PIH is managed by magnesium sulphate and hydralazine protocols.[39] Blood pressure is then controlled for maternal and fetal safety. Continuous electronic fetal heart rate monitoring confirms continued fetal well-being. Obstetrician and anesthesiologist are aware of possible drug interactions when pharmacotherapy has continued during pregnancy for control of chronic hypertension. In the delivery operating room, monitoring of continuous radial arterial blood pressure allows additional hydralazine to be administered to attenuate the stress response that occurs at laryngoscopy and tracheal intubation. Labetolol (serial doses up to 1 mg/kg) also is effective in modifying a serious increase in systolic and diastolic blood pressures, which will occur if blood pressure is inadequately controlled. In the absence of deliberate volume expansion, I have found that serial doses (50 μg) of nitroglycerin (total 150 to 200 μg) effectively controls blood pressure immediately before rapid-sequence induction, and blunts the pressor response to tracheal intubation.

Maintenance of neuromuscular blockade is monitored by peripheral nerve stimulator throughout surgery. The intermediate-acting agent atracurium establishes nondepolarizing neuromuscular blockade, and is preferred especially in the presence of hepatic or renal impairment. I avoid succinylcholine infusion in the MO because large volumes may be administered during surgery of longer duration, with risk of type II block. This would be undesirable postoperatively when absence of neuromuscular blockade is essential to allow extubation, especially with the known high risk of respiratory failure and arrest in the MO after delivery.[40-42]

After delivery I maintain balanced anesthesia with nitrous oxide/isoflurane (0.3 to 0.4 MAC). Fentanyl is administered after clamping the cord for intraoperative and postoperative analgesia. These low end-tidal concentrations are effective for amnesia and do not prevent the contraction of the uterus in response to oxytocin.[43,44]

Regional Anesthesia

Epidural Anesthesia

Technical difficulty is anticipated because of anatomic considerations when the anesthesiologist plans regional anesthesia in the MO parturient. Epidural anesthesia for elective cesarean section is accepted for the many advantages it offers, and would be the anesthetic of choice in this case. It is important that bleeding and coagulation abnormalities are excluded before intraspinal methods are selected. A platelet count of 100,000 mm^3 or more also is desirable, and has been a useful guideline during evaluation for regional anesthesia. Bleeding time tests are not always clinically useful in predicting safety when the platelet count is less than 100,000 mm^3. The thromboelastogram allows diagnosis of bleeding or coagulation abnormalities in other surgical populations at the bedside or in the operating room, but this device remains under investigation in the obstetric population.

Obesity and edema increase the percutaneous distance between the skin and the epidural space.[45] For successful epidural anesthesia the needle and catheter insertion should be close to the midline. If the needle is advanced increasingly laterad, lateral placement of the catheter will ensue.[46] A high incidence of unsatisfactory blocks has been reported when the point of the needle is greater than 6 to 9 cm from the skin puncture site.[47-49] I recommend positioning the MO woman sitting; evaluation of the entire back at the time of the preanesthetic interview is recommended. The lumbar spinous processes are sometimes found to be palpable because of the distribution of body fat. If not, the midline can be approximated from the occiput, vertebra prominens, dorsolumbar spinous processes, intercrestal line, and lumbosacral region. In the delivery, preparation of a wide skin area is advantageous, and use of a fine needle and local infiltration is recommended to identify the spinous processes and midlumbar interspace. Exploration with a fine needle through the interspace allows identification of the ligamentum flavum. The needle may then be removed or left as a guide along which to slide the epidural needle. It has been helpful in my practice to use the method of indirect sonographic guidance in obese pregnant patients, a method that is available at the bedside in most labor and delivery suites.[45]

The advantages of continuous epidural anesthesia over spinal anesthesia include the ability to inject incremental boluses of local anesthetic, less hypotension, and ability to limit cephalad extension of the segmental blockade. Less motor block accompanies the high sensory levels required for cesarean section, and the risk of impaired ventilation in the MO woman is less with peak cephalad spread to a T-6 level. Furthermore, the sitting position during onset of epidural anesthesia in the MO woman limits cephalad spread of the segmental block.[50,51] Like Dewan,[16] I have maintained a slightly flexed, partly sitting position in women who could not be positioned supine, without obscuring the surgical field. Choice of abdominal incision[23] varies; obstetricians in this center prefer an extended midline incision above the panniculus.[52] This choice improves surgical access.

I test my catheters using incremental doses of lidocaine with the woman in the sitting and semi-sitting positions. This is followed by incremental doses of 0.5% bupivacaine until a T-6 level is obtained. Addition of fentanyl (100 μg) to the 0.5% bupivacaine to maximize intraoperative and postoperative analgesia is recommended.

Spinal Anesthesia

Subarachnoid block is now a frequent choice for cesarean section because the technologic advances with finer needles reduces the incidence and severity of postdural puncture headache. In this case, however, a rapid onset of conduction block and spread cephalad may result in hypotension and impairment of respiratory muscle activity. The increased dose of hyperbaric agent necessary to increase duration of spinal anesthesia also increases the risk of a high spinal block. This would seriously impair respiratory muscle activity and further complicate anesthetic management. In this case, continuous spinal anesthesia, which allows incremental injections of hyperbaric agent through an intrathecal catheter, should be considered. I have found continuous spinal anesthesia a satisfactory alternative to epidural anesthesia for intraoperative management. Incremental injections of hyperbaric bupivacaine or tetracaine allow the gradual spread of the block to a T-6 level.

Postpartum Management and Pain Control

Epidural analgesia should be continued in the extended care unit (ECU) after delivery. The many preoperative risk factors in the MO caution the health care team to monitor pain control and oxygenation continuously. The advantageous effects of epidural analgesia[22] have been demonstrated in surgical populations. Comparison of intramuscular and epidural morphine[53] revealed reduced morphine requirement, earlier ambulation, fewer pulmonary complications, and absence of clinically observed respiratory depression when the epidural route was used. Epidural morphine[54] caused less depression of the ventilatory response to carbon dioxide than parenteral narcotics. Use of epidural morphine in the high-risk MO should be restricted to the ECU. The partly sitting, head-up position[16] is recommended.

After general anesthesia, if extubation criteria are not satisfied, then controlled ventilation should be continued in the ECU until this can be safely accomplished with the woman fully awake, well oxygenated, and capable of continuing adequate spontaneous ventilation.

Acknowledgement

With thanks to Abhimanyu Garg, M.D., Center for Human Nutrition, University of Texas Southwestern Medical Center at Dallas; Brenda Jackman for assistance with art work; and Janet Miller for secretarial assistance.

References

1. Metropolitan Life Insurance Company: New weight standards for men and women, *Stat Bull* 1959; 40:3.
2. Billewicz WZ, Kemsley WFF, Thomson AM: Indices of obesity, *Br J Prev Soc Med* 1962; 16:183.
3. Keys A, Fidanza F, Karvonen MJ, et al: Indices of relative weight and obesity, *J Chronic Dis* 1972; 25:329.
4. Johnson JWC, Longmake JA, Frentzen B: Excessive maternal weight and pregnancy outcome, *Am J Obstet Gynecol* 1992; 167:2:353.
5. Vaughan RW, Bauer S, Wise L: Volume and pH of gastric juice in obese patients, *Anesthesiology* 1975; 43:686.
6. O'Brien TF: Lower esophageal sphincter pressure (LESP) and esophageal function in obese humans, *J Clin Gastroenterol* 1980; 3:145.
7. Burwell CS, Robin ED, Whaley RD, Bickelmann AG: Extreme

obesity associated with alveolar hypoventilation: a Pickwickian syndrome, *Am J Med* 1956; 21:811.

8. Smart GA: *Diseases of metabolism: obesity.* In Hunter D, editor: *Price's textbook of the practice of medicine, ed 9,* London, 1956, Oxford Medical Publications.
9. Paul D, Hoyt J, Boutros A: Cardiovascular respiratory changes in response to changes of posture in the very obese, *Anesthesiology* 1976; 45:73.
10. Teeple E, Ghia J: An elevated pulmonary wedge pressure resulting from an upper respiratory obstruction in an obese patient, *Anesthesiology* 1983; 59:66.
11. Tseuda K, et al: Obesity supine death syndrome: reports of two morbidly obese patients, *Anesthesiology* 1975; 43:686.
12. Young SR, Stoelting RK, Peterson C, Madura JA: Anesthetic biotransformation and renal function in obese patients during and after methoxyflurane or halothane anesthesia, *Anesthesiology* 1975; 42:451.
13. Bentley JB, Vaughan RW, Miller MS, et al: Serum inorganic fluoride levels in obese patients during and after enflurane anesthesia, *Anesth Analg* 1979; 58:409.
14. Bentley JB, Vaughan RW, Gandolfi AF, Cork RC: Halothane biotransformation in obese and nonobese patients, *Anesthesiology* 1982; 57:94.
15. Blass NH: *The morbidly obese pregnant patient.* In Datta S, editor: *Anesthetic and obstetric management of high risk pregnancy,* St. Louis, 1991, Mosby–Year Book.
16. Dewan DM: *The obese parturient.* In James FM, Wheeler AS, Dewan DM, editors: *Obstetric anesthesia: Pre complicated patient, ed 2,* Philadelphia, 1988, FA Davis Co.
17. Catenacci AJ, Anderson JD, Boersma D: Anesthetic hazards of obesity, *JAMA* 1973; 175:657.
18. Fox GS: Anesthesia for intestinal short circuiting in the morbidly obese with reference to the pathophysiology of gross obesity, *Can Anaesth Soc J* 1975; 22:307.
19. Gould AB: Effect of obesity on respiratory complications following general anesthesia, *Anesth Analg* 1962; 41:448.
20. Buckley FP, Robinson NB, Simonowitz DA, Dellinger EP: Anaesthesia in the morbidly obese, *Anaesthesia* 1983; 38:840.
21. Bromage PR, Fox GS: Obesity: its relation to anesthesia, *Anaesthesia* 1976; 31:557.
22. Gelman S, Laws HL, Potzick J, et al: Thoracic epidural vs. balanced anesthesia in morbid obesity: an intraoperative and postoperative hemodynamic study, *Anesth Analg* 1980; 59:902.
23. Hodgkinson R. Husain FJ: Caesarean section associated with gross obesity, *Br J Anaesth* 1980; 52:919.
24. Hood DD, Dewan DM: Anesthetic and obstetric outcome in morbidly obese parturients, *Anesthesiology* 1993; 79:1210.
25. Kliegman RM, Gross T: Perinatal problems of the obese mother and her infant, *Obstet Gynecol* 1985; 66:299.
26. Lee JJ, Larson RH, Buckley JJ, Roberts RB: Airway maintenance in the morbidly obese, *Anesth Rev* 1980; 7:33.
27. Turnbull AC, Tindall VR, Beard RW, et al: *Report on confidential enquiries into maternal deaths in England and Wales 1982-1984,* London, 1989, Department of Health and Social Security, Reports on Health and Social Subjects.
28. Rocke DA, Murray WB, Rout CC, Gouws E: Relative risk analysis of factors associated with difficult intubation in obstetric anesthesia, *Anesthesiology* 1992; 77:67.
29. Lyons G: Failed intubation, *Anaesthesia* 1985; 40:759.
30. Cohen SE: *Anesthesia for the morbidly obese pregnant patient.* In Shnider SM, Levinson G, editor: *Anesthesia for obstetrics ed 3* Baltimore, 1993, Williams & Wilkins.
31. Norris M, Dewan D: Preoxygenation for cesarean section: a comparison of two techniques, *Anesthesiology* 1985; 62:827.
32. Gambee A, Hertzka R, Fisher D: Preoxygenation techniques: comparison of three minutes and four breaths, *Anesth Analg* 1981; 60:691.
33. Vaughan RW, Wise L: Intraoperative arterial oxygenation in obese patients, *Ann Surg* 1976; 84:35.
34. Wyner J, Brodsky J, Merrell R: Massive obesity and arterial oxygenation, *Anesth Analg* 1981; 60:691.
35. Datta S, Briwa J: Modified laryngoscope for endotracheal intubation of obese patients, *Anesth Analg* 1981; 60:120.
36. Tunstall ME, Sheik A: Failed intubation protocol: Oxygenation without aspiration, *Clin Anesthesiol* 1986; 4:171.
37. Scott DB: Endotracheal intubation: friend or foe? *Br Med J* 1986; 292:157.
38. McLune S, Regan M, Moore J: Laryngeal mask airway for cesarean section, *Anaesthesia* 1990; 45:227.
39. Cunningham FG, McDonald PC, Gant NF: *Hypertensive disorders in pregnancy.* In *Williams obstetrics, ed 18,* East Norwalk, Conn, 1989, Appleton and Lange.
40. Vaughan RW, Engelhardt RC, Wise L: Postoperative hypoxemia in obese patients, *Ann Surg* 1974; 180:877.
41. Vaughan RW, Wise L: Choice of abdominal operative incision in the obese patient: a study using blood gas measurements, *Ann Surg* 1975; 181:829.
42. Vaughan RW, Wise L: Postoperative arterial blood gas measurements in obese patients: effect of position on gas exchange, *Ann Surg* 1975; 182:705.

43. Wallace DH, Cosentino SL, Shearer VE, et al: The effect of isoflurane 1% or low-dose and regional anesthesia on uterine tone at cesarean section, *Anesthesiology* 1989; 7:A874.
44. Andrews W, Ramin S, Wallace DH, et al: Effect of type of anesthesia on blood loss at elective repeat cesarean section, *Am J Perinatol* 1992; 9(3):197.
45. Wallace DH, Currie JM, Gilstrap LC, Santos R: Indirect sonographic guidance for epidural anesthesia in obese pregnant patients, *Reg Anesth* 1992; 17:233.
46. Bromage PR: *Epidural analgesia,* Philadelphia, 1978, WB Saunders.
47. Narang VPS, Lintner SPK: Failure of extradural block in obstetrics: a new hypothesis, *Br J Anaesth* 1988; 60:402.
48. Usubiaga JE, Reis A, Usubiaga LE: Epidural misplacement of catheters and mechanisms of unilateral blockade, *Anesthesiology* 1970; 32:158.
49. Hehre FW, Sayig JM, Lowman RM: Etiologic aspects of failure of continuous lumbar peridural anesthesia, *Anesth Analg* 1960; 39:511.
50. Hodgkinson R, Husain F: Obesity and the cephalad spread of analgesia following epidural administration of bupivacaine for cesarean section, *Anesth Analg* 1980; 59:89.
51. Hodgkinson R, Husain F: Obesity, gravity, and spread of epidural anesthesia, *Anesth Analg* 1981; 60:421.
52. Rawal N, Sjostrand U, Christoffersson E, et al: Comparison of intramuscular and epidural morphine for postoperative analgesia in the grossly obese: influence on postoperative ambulation and pulmonary function, *Anesth Analg* 1984; 63:583.
53. Doblar D, et al: Epidural morphine following epidural local anesthesia: effect on ventilatory and airway occlusion pressure responses to CO_2, *Anesthesiology* 1981; 55:423.

45

Autoimmune Disease

A 29-year-old primigravida at 36 weeks' gestation comes for an anesthesia consult. She has systemic lupus erythematosus with involvement of multiple organs. Discuss the anesthetic management for labor, delivery, and cesarean delivery.

Recommendations by Martha A. Hauch, M.D.

The patient with an autoimmune disease has a condition in which endogenous antibodies are produced to react with that patient's own host tissues. As a result of this *internal war,* various end-organ damage may occur. Systemic lupus erythematosus (SLE) often is considered a prototype for the autoimmune diseases and is discussed first.

Systemic Lupus Erythematosus

Characteristics of SLE include the presence of autoantibodies and circulating immune complexes, complement level depression, and the deposition of complement-fixed immune complexes within tissues and vessel walls. It is a multisystem disease that most frequently affects female patients, especially during their reproductive years. It is believed that SLE complicates about 1 in 1600 to 5000 pregnancies.[1] However, prospective case-controlled studies have shown no significant increase in exacerbation of SLE with pregnancy.[2,3] The disease is notable for the presence of a host of various autoantibodies, some of which appear to be diagnostic for the disease itself and others which are believed to produce or contribute to its many clinical manifestations. Also notice that certain drugs such as procainamide hydrochloride, hydralazine hydrochloride, and anticonvulsants can produce SLE, albeit in a milder form, since there is no associated renal or central nervous system disease. The various end-organ manifestations of the disease are listed in Table 45-1. As demonstrated in the table, SLE has the ability to damage every major organ in the

TABLE 45-1
End-Organ Involvement in SLE

Skin	Malar (butterfly) rash, discoid rash, photosensitivity, oral and nasopharyngeal ulcerations, subcutaneous nodules, alopecia
Neuromuscular	Seizures, psychosis, depression, nonerosive arthritis, myalgias, myositis, peripheral neuropathy, ascending polyneuritis
Hematologic	Hemolytic anemia, leukopenia, thrombocytopenia, lymphopenia
Renal	Proteinuria, glomerulonephritis, hypoalbuminemia
Pulmonary	Pleuritis, interstitial disease, sterile infiltrates
Cardiac	Pericarditis, myocarditis, endocarditis, cardiomyopathy, coronary artery disease
Immune	Positive lupus erythematosus cell Prep; abnormal titer of anti-DNA antibody, anti-Smith antibody; false-positive syphilis serologic results; abnormal titer of antinuclear antibody (ANA), lupus anticoagulant antibody (LAC), anticardiolipin antibody (ACA)
Hepatic	Hepatomegaly, lupoid hepatitis
Spleen	Splenomegaly
Constitutional	Fever, fatigue, malaise, anorexia, weight loss

SLE, Systemic lupus erythematosus; Prep, preparation.

body, and the effects of special concern to the anesthesiologist are now discussed in detail.

Cardiopulmonary Effects

Some of the most serious consequences of SLE involve the cardiorespiratory system. Cardiomyopathy may stem from direct involvement of the cardiac muscle tissue, resulting in myocarditis or possibly congestive heart failure. Chronic hypertension also may lead to cardiomyopathy. Coronary artery vasculitis, endocarditis, or pericarditis also may occur. The most common cardiac manifestation of SLE is pericarditis with or without a significant pericardial effusion. On physical examination, the anesthesiologist should listen for the presence of a friction rub (evidence of pericarditis), murmur (suggestive of possible endocarditis, also known as Libman-Sachs disease), or an S3 (evidence of congestive heart failure). The electrocardiogram (ECG) findings most commonly reveal nonspecific t wave changes or elevated S-T segments suggestive of pericarditis.[4] An echocardiogram also may be useful to evaluate valvular function or the presence of a pericardial effusion.

Pulmonary system review may reveal a history of hemoptysis or dyspnea, which may indicate the presence of pleural effusions, pulmonary infarcts, or pulmonary vasculitis causing interstitial disease. On physical examination, one should be alerted to the presence of rales (suggestive of congestive failure) or a pleural rub (indicative of an effusion or pneumonitis). Pulse oximetry or arterial blood gas sampling from a patient with severe lung involvement may reveal severe hypoxemia. Pulmonary function testing may demonstrate a restrictive pattern with decreased vital capacity or a diffusion abnormality.

Renal Involvement

Since one of the leading causes of death in these patients is renal failure, the anesthesiologist should look for the presence of mild to severe hypertension with or without abnormalities in blood urea nitrogen (BUN), creatinine, or albumin values. Complicating this problem is the suggestion in the literature that patients with cardiac involvement may be more prone to the development of preeclampsia. Findings such as hypertension and proteinuria may be due to preeclampsia rather than a lupus flare. It is difficult to differentiate between a lupus flare and preeclampsia, but the diagnosis often is crucial since the management is drastically different. A lupus flare is managed medically with steroids and possibly immunosuppressive agents, whereas severe preeclampsia is an indication for urgent delivery. If a determination is unable to be made, renal biopsy should be considered. In the majority of patients, evidence of lupus nephritis antedates pregnancy.[3,5] Most studies indicate a relatively uncomplicated course during pregnancy if the nephritis is in remission before conception. The most severe exacerbations occur in patients with active disease at conception, manifesting as hypertension, proteinuria, and declining creatinine clearance.[6]

Immunologic Abnormalities

Various immunologic abnormalities have been identified in SLE patients, including the presence of antiphospholipid antibody (which may also be known as anticardiolipin antibody [ACA] or lupus anticoagulant (LAC). About 80% of patients with LAC have enzyme-linked immunosorbent assay (ELISA) antiphospholipid antibody, but only 10% to 50% of patients with ELISA antiphospholipid antibody have LAC.[7] The presence of both does not necessarily worsen one's prognosis or condition. Interestingly, these antibodies also have been reported in a substantial number of patients *without* known autoimmune disease. The presence of these antibodies results in a prolongation of the partial thromboplastin time (PTT) and rarely, the prothrombin time (PT) secondary to their reaction with phospholipid antigens used in the test.[8] However, there is no correlation between the prolonged coagulation test values and clinical bleeding. More often than not, the presence of LAC and ACA usually is associated with a thrombotic picture.[9] Thromboses of the deep veins, peripheral arteries, and retinal vessels have been reported, as well as pulmonary embolism and cerebrovascular events.[10] Placental thromboses and infarctions also have been reported.[11] The presence of these antibodies also has been associated with maternal thrombocytopenia. Antiphospholipid antibody syndrome (APS) is defined by the presence of antiphospholipid antibody and/or LAC and any or all of the following: recurrent thromboses, recurrent fetal losses, and thrombocytopenia.[12] Because of the increased frequency of fetal losses in patients with these antibodies, current data favor prophylaxis with low-dose aspirin or heparin over prednisone.[7] Since most authorities treat thrombotic episodes in these patients with anticoagulant drugs, regional anesthesia is contraindicated unless this therapy is reversed.[13]

In addition to these antibodies, additional antibodies to red blood cells, neutrophils, lymphocytes, and platelets also may be present in patients with SLE. These may result in hemolytic anemia, leukopenia, lymphocytopenia, and thrombocytopenia as well. Because of the presence of these antibodies, cross-matching blood for these patients may be difficult and should be anticipated.

Anti-Ro (also known as SSA) is an antibody directed toward nonnuclear histone antigens and is found in 25% to 30% of patients with SLE.[6] The presence of this antibody in SLE mothers has been associated strongly with the rare occurrence of isolated complete congenital heart block (CHB) in their infants. Women without SLE also may carry this antibody; however, CHB is a permanent disorder and, in the absence of other cardiac anomalies, is associated with a 5% mortality rate.[3]

Neurologic Involvement

Another common organ to be involved in a variety of ways is the central nervous system. Patients may present with peripheral sensory neuropathies, transverse myelitis, seizures, or a Guillain-Barre picture. Behavioral changes including depression, paranoia, mania, and schizophrenia have been frequently reported. Movement disorders such as chorea, athetosis, and hemiballismus also may be present. One of the more common causes of death in these patients is as a result of cerebrovascular hemorrhage. The anesthesiologist should carefully document the type and location of any existing neuropathies and look for signs and symptoms suggestive of increased intracranial pressure before performing an anesthetic.

Joints

The presence of arthritis in the proximal joints of the hands, wrists, and knees, occasionally along with Raynaud's phenomenon, may pose problems in obtaining intravenous access or in positioning the patient for a regional anesthetic. In addition, long-term steroid therapy may result in a vascular necrosis of the major joints.

Hepatic Involvement

Lastly, lupoid hepatitis has been reported in patients presenting as jaundice, hepatomegaly, and hyperglobulinemia. In some cases of SLE, hypersplenism from the autoimmune destruction of blood cells is an important cause of thrombocytopenia.[14]

Medications

When taking a medication history, the anesthesiologist should realize that corticosteroids usually are the mainstay of drug therapy in patients who are not in remission from their disease. Stress doses should be used during labor and delivery as well as in the immediate puerperium. The use of steroids in pregnancy may be associated with glucose intolerance. Infants born to mothers receiving chronic steroids should be monitored for adrenal suppression, although this is rare.[6] The use of immunosuppressive agents such as azathioprine (Imuran) occasionally is necessary and may antagonize neuromuscular blocking agents used for muscle relaxation. Antimalarials, such as chloroquine, also are used occasionally. Although infrequent, serious toxic effects of these drugs include visual disturbances, retinopathy, peripheral myopathy and neuropathy, thrombocytopenia, aplastic anemia, and cardiomyopathy.

Anesthetic Management

The management of the SLE patient during labor and delivery is best accomplished by a team approach involving rheumatologists, obstetricians, anesthesiologists, and pediatricians, As has been mentioned, obtaining a thorough review of systems and medication history is essential in the SLE patient since the medical history often is complex and may carry major anesthetic implications. If not already obtained, initial laboratory evaluation on the patient's arrival to the labor floor should include ANA and complement levels as well as a baseline evaluation of renal function (BUN, creatinine, 24-hour urine for total protein and creatinine clearance).[6] The presence of ACA and/or LAC also should be determined. Because of the increased risk of stillbirth, regular assessment of fetal well-being on a weekly basis should begin by 28 weeks' gestation, usually in the form of a nonstress test followed by a contraction stress test or biophysical profile if fetal well-being cannot be documented. Ideally, a vaginal delivery at term is aimed for unless there is some other obstetrical indication for early or abdominal delivery. Premature labor and delivery has been documented to occur more frequently in patients with SLE.[2,3]

Literature on the anesthetic management of the pregnant SLE patient is scarce. Minimal monitoring should include pulse oximetry. The presence of severe cardiopulmonary decompensation (e.g., cardiomyopathy with congestive heart failure [CHF], restrictive lung disease with hypoxemia and/or limited reserves) or renal failure (worsening proteinuria, rising creatinine values) may warrant the placement of invasive monitors. Care should be taken to optimize maternal-fetal well-being through the use of left uterine displacement position throughout labor, supplemental oxygen therapy, and strict maintenance of normal maternal blood pressure and heart rate.

Improved placental perfusion may occur with the

use of epidural analgesia as a result of its ability to lower maternal catecholamine blood levels and improve uterine blood flow. Obviously, before the technique is performed, coagulation studies should be obtained. As discussed earlier, some of these patients may have thrombocytopenia and the occasional patients may even have clinical bleeding secondary to a truly positive prolongation of their PT and PTT. Patients with either ACA or LAC antibodies, however, may have falsely elevated PTs and PTTs, and may require a bleeding time to rule out a true coagulopathy if the platelet count is borderline (between 90,000 and 150,000/mm^3). Patients with platelet counts below 90,000 to 100,000/mm^3, regardless of PTs and PTTs, are perhaps at too great a risk for epidural hematoma to consider the elective use of epidural analgesia. Patients on heparin should have a normalization of their coagulation profile before regional analgesia is considered.

If cesarean delivery is needed, regional anesthesia also may be administered, provided there is no clinical coagulopathy present, as evidenced by a normal platelet count with or without a bleeding time. The patient with severe hypertension or renal compromise who may not handle sudden intravascular volume shifts well may better tolerate the slower onset of epidural, as opposed to spinal, anesthesia. Given the possibility of the presence of cardiac or restrictive lung disease in some of these patients, care should be taken to avoid great swings in blood pressure, heart rate, and oxygen saturation if general anesthesia is needed. In addition, patients with hepatic or renal decompensation may not be able to normally metabolize and excrete medications eliminated via these routes.

Rheumatoid Arthritis

Rheumatoid arthritis is the most common systemic rheumatic disease and affects female patients three times more often than male patients. The etiology of the disease appears to be determined by a combination of genetic, hormonal, and psychosomatic factors.[15] The disease is most typically characterized by symmetrical inflammation of the synovial joints, the most commonly affected being the metacarpophalangeal, proximal interphalangeal, and wrist joints.

Pregnancy appears to induce remission in most patients with this disease.[16,17] However, many of these patients go on to have an exacerbation of their symptoms after delivery.

Of particular concern to the anesthesiologist, in addition to the joint pathologic manifestations, should be the extraarticular manifestations of the disease, some of which can be life-threatening. In addition to taking a careful history (including medications, previous complications and operations), a thorough physical examination concentrating on the areas listed below are mandatory.

Airway Involvement

Inflammation of the synovial joints of the airway is a common area of involvement in this disease. In particular, the temporomandibular joint may have undergone ankylosis, leaving it difficult to open the patient's mouth for intubation. Involvement of the cricoarytenoid joint may result in edematous constriction of the glottis, perhaps even necessitating emergency tracheostomy.[18] Rheumatoid nodules in the vocal cords also have been known to arise. To make the situation worse, cervical spine disease is reported in 35% to 50% of patients and may result in severe flexion deformity of the neck along with atlantoaxial instability. This may result in spinal cord damage, especially with neck extension.[19]

A recent onset of hoarseness or change in voice quality may indicate, albeit in an insidious fashion, laryngeal involvement of the disease. The anesthesiologist can avoid potential problems with endotracheal intubation by having the patient open her mouth and then look for visualization of the uvula and tonsillar pillars in addition to evaluating her ability to asymptomatically extend her neck. The patient with poor visualization of these oral structures and severe, painful neck extension should be considered for elective, fiberoptic intubation if general anesthesia is deemed necessary.

Cardiopulmonary Involvement

Thorough examination of the patient's heart and lungs may detect arthritic involvement of these organs. Restrictive lung disease created by degenerative kyphosis of the spine, inflammatory fixation of the ribs, rheumatoid pleural effusions, and pulmonary fibrosis is made more severe by the presence of a large, gravid uterus. This added restriction may result in a markedly reduced functional residual capacity and thus a diminished ability of the patient to push during the second stage of labor, secondary to decreased oxygen reserves. The presence of severe restrictive disease also may contraindicate a high level of sensory anesthesia with the use of regional anesthesia, since this may further compromise respiratory effort. Elective pulmonary function testing, along with baseline pulse oximetry, in the third trimester may alert the obstetric care team to these possible problems. Also notice that the most common extraarticular feature of this disease, rheumatoid nodules, may occur in the lungs leading, on occasion, to pneumothorax or bronchopleural fistulas if cavitation and rupture occur.

Cardiac involvement may take the form of pericarditis, valvular disease, conduction defects, or cardiomyopathy. Care should be taken to listen for a friction rub or distant heart sounds (suggestive of an effusion), murmurs, or a third heart sound. Visceral granulomas have been known to commonly occur in the myocardium, valvular rings, coronary arteries, and aortic root. Suspicious findings on routine exam require additional evaluation with an ECG with or without an echocardiogram. In the occasional patient with constrictive pericarditis during pregnancy, successful management has been described using restriction of activity, avoidance of diuretics and β-blockers, and use of epidural anesthesia for labor.[20]

Joints

In addition to involvement of airway joints, inflammation also may affect the hip, knee, and lumbar intervertebral joints. Deformities in these areas therefore will limit spine and hip flexion and abduction. If these limitations are present, the anesthesiologist should warn the patient that proper positioning for a regional anesthetic may be difficult or even impossible. Severe hip disease may warrant vaginal delivery with special stirrups, no stirrups, or at times even necessitate cesarean delivery.[21]

Neurologic Effects

Because of occasional peripheral nerve involvement, especially in those patients with Felty's (rheumatoid arthritis, splenomegaly, leukopenia) and Sjogren's (rheumatoid arthritis, keratoconjunctivitis sicca, xerostomia) syndromes, a thorough examination should be performed to detect the presence of sensory deficits. These deficits should be documented, since these patients may later receive a regional anesthetic.

Vascular Manifestations

Of all the extraarticular manifestations of this disease, vasculitis is potentially the most life-threatening. Immune complexes are deposited in vascular walls of capillaries, arterioles, arteries, venules, and veins. This vasculitis has been known to present in the form of microinfarcts (commonly seen in the nailbed), mesenteric infarction, and gangrene.[22]

Medications

Certain medications taken by the patient may dictate choice of anesthetic technique for delivery.

Ingestion of aspirin results in interference with platelet function, so recent heavy ingestion may warrant a bleeding time if a regional anesthetic is contemplated. However, the *postaspirin* bleeding time is not always thought to be a reliable indicator of platelet function or hemostatic capability.[23] Although the bleeding time may normalize 2 to 3 days after cessation of aspirin ingestion, platelet function may take up to 7 days to return to normal.[24] Likewise, an abnormal bleeding time is not always correlated with inadequate hemostatic function.[25] A retrospective analysis of 805 patients receiving 1013 spinal or epidural anesthetics, of whom 26% were taking aspirin, revealed no postoperative neurologic dysfunction.[24] However, patients receiving aspirin and/or other antiplatelet therapy did have a significantly higher incidence of minor hemorrhagic complications such as blood-tinged cerebrospinal fluid or bloody aspiration from the spinal or epidural needle or catheter. Rather than letting a bleeding time from patients on antiplatelet therapy dictate whether a regional technique may be used, the authors suggest that expert, atraumatic regional technique be performed on an individualized basis, along with scrupulous monitoring for early signs of cord compression (prompt neuroradiologic evaluation of pain in the back or legs) in the perioperative as well as the postoperative period.

Nonsteroidal antiinflammatory drugs (NSAIDs) have been associated with hepatic toxicity, so baseline serum glutamic oxaloacetic transaminase and serum glutamic pyruvic transaminase levels should be documented. These drugs generally are not used during pregnancy, however.

Steroid use may result in adrenal suppression, and recent steroid ingestion (within 6 months) dictates giving the patient maximum supplementation (300 mg of hydrocortisone over 24 hours) to cover her possibly inadequate adrenal function. In addition, osteoporosis secondary to chronic corticosteroid treatment dictates careful positioning of these patients at all times during labor and delivery to avoid fractures.

Adverse drug reactions to gold therapy include extensive skin eruptions, oral ulcers, membranous glomerulonephropathy, agranulocytosis, and aplastic anemia. These patients need thorough evaluation of dermal integrity, complete blood cell count with differential, BUN levels, creatinine levels, and urinalysis.

Anesthetic Management

Management of the parturient with rheumatoid arthritis thus greatly depends on the type and degree of multiorgan involvement and, in part, the medications that the patient is currently taking. As mentioned earlier, peripheral neuropathies may exist and, although they do not contraindicate the use of regional anesthesia, they should be documented before initiation of conduction blockade. In addition, if only for medical and legal reasons, normal clotting studies should be verified before placement of a regional anesthetic. Performing regional anesthesia may be technically difficult, however, in the patient with severe joint contractures and restricted range of motion.

The patient with severe airway abnormalities warrants special care. A large intravascular or subarachnoid injection of local anesthetic intended for the epidural space may result in seizures or a total spinal blockade with loss of the glottic reflex. Needless to say, this would be catastrophic in the full-stomach patient (as all pregnant patients are regardless of the status of nothing by mouth) who may be impossible to ventilate or intubate in the usual manner because of rheumatoid involvement of her airway. Because of rapid, and at times unpredictable, spread of anesthesia, spinal anesthesia for cesarean delivery in the patient with severe airway disease is not advised. However, it can also be argued that the laboring "nonepiduralized" patient with severe airway abnormalities is at tremendous risk of airway complications if a fetal distress situation should arrive necessitating urgent cesarean delivery. Thus, for laboring patients, I advise cautious use of epidural analgesia. The level of sensory anesthesia must be raised cautiously with no more than 3 ml of local anesthetic at a time with continuous watch for signs and symptoms of subarachnoid (especially with sudden, dramatic relief of contraction pain) or intravascular injection. It is no doubt safest to secure the airway of the patient with severe involvement before cesarean delivery (most easily done via awake oral fiberoptic intubation). However, this may not always be practical or easily done, especially if the anesthesiologist is not skilled at difficult fiberoptic intubation in the relatively minimally sedated patient with a full stomach. Under no circumstances should a patient with a full stomach or with a compromised airway be delivered by cesarean delivery using a "Hail Mary" emergent rapid sequence induction, since this may likely result in both fetal *and* maternal death. An abdominal wall field block with local infiltration is a much safer alternative should this situation arise. Obviously, the use of early epidural analgesia is the best way to avoid this potentially disastrous scenario.

Regardless of anesthetic technique, a large-bore intravenous catheter should be placed early on in labor, since these patients may experience increased blood loss secondary to aspirin therapy on top of their baseline anemia of pregnancy. Patients with extensive cardiopulmonary disease may require invasive monitoring, especially those with constrictive pericarditis, valvular lesions, or exercise-limiting restrictive lung disease. Pericardiectomy during pregnancy has been reported to be successful in the patient with severe constrictive pericarditis.[26]

Depending on the degree of spine and cardiopulmonary involvement, postpartum pain relief after operative delivery may be achieved via a variety of methods. If an epidural or subarachnoid catheter was placed preoperatively, it may be used postoperatively to deliver epidural or intrathecal narcotics with or without a dilute concentration of local anesthetics. The patient whose hematologic or anatomic problems contraindicated regional anesthesia may be managed with a patient-controlled analgesia (PCA) device to deliver intravenous pain relief. In addition, use of the NSAID, ketorolac, may potentiate the analgesia of either technique.

Immune Thrombocytopenic Purpura

Immune thrombocytopenic purpura (ITP) is characterized by a reduced platelet count, increased peripheral destruction of platelets by platelet-reactive antibodies via the reticuloendothelial system, and augmented platelet production as evidenced by increased circulating megathrombocytes.[27] The disease is thought to complicate at least 1 to 2 of every 10,000 pregnancies and is the most common cause of thrombocytopenia in the first and second trimesters.[28,29] The etiology of thrombocytopenia in the pregnant patient also may be due to other disease processes, however, such as preeclampsia and the hemolysis–elevated liver enzymes—low platelet count (HELLP) syndrome, thrombocytopenic purpura, hemolytic uremic syndrome, SLE, type II von Willebrand disease, and disseminated intravascular coagulation. Thus, a thorough history and physical examination (in addition to hematologic evaluation of the patient's peripheral blood film) is essential to rule out other causes of thrombocytopenia and treat the patient with true ITP appropriately.

Early involvement of the anesthesiologist is of value, since these patients may come for splenectomy before delivery, or certainly may require anesthesia for delivery, whether vaginal or cesarean. The main issues for the anesthesiologist concern (1) medications the patient is taking to manage the ITP, and (2) the maternal and fetal platelet counts, either of which may dictate route of delivery and choice of anesthetic technique.

Medications

Prednisone remains the mainstay of drug therapy in the pregnant patient who begins to run platelet counts of less than 30,000/mm^3 or who begins to clinically manifest signs of hemostatic decompensation (petechiae, purpura, epistaxis, etc.). Sixty percent to 70% of patients will respond to this approach.[30] These patients will need to be treated with full-dose peripartum steroid coverage.

Patients who are unresponsive to steroid therapy may be tried on a regimen of intravenous gamma globulin with or without concomitant steroid administration. After intravenous IgG therapy, platelet counts usually begin to rise by 48 hours and are maximal after 6 days of therapy.[31] This effect has been reported to last 1 to 4 weeks.

The patient who fails these approaches is then considered for splenectomy. Removing the spleen removes a large source of antibody production, as well as a reservoir of macrophages. Splenectomy ideally is performed in the second trimester.[32] General anesthesia via rapid-sequence induction usually is needed for this procedure.

Platelet Count

In this disease process, one needs to be concerned not only about the maternal platelet count but the fetal count as well. This is because maternal platelet-reactive IgG is able to cross into the fetal circulation and bind to fetal platelets, thereby marking them for destruction via the fetal reticuloendothelial system. The most disastrous consequence of neonatal thrombocytopenia is intracranial hemorrhage with resultant neurologic damage. Although argued by some, passage of the fetal head through the birth canal is thought to be the major factor responsible for this complication. Unfortunately a reliable method has not yet developed for predicting the degree of fetal thrombocytopenia, since no correlation exists between maternal and fetal platelet counts or with the level of maternal platelet-associated IgG and the neonatal platelet count.[33,34]

Patients with apparent incidental thrombocytopenia (which may represent new-onset ITP during pregnancy, or simply an acceleration of the normal physiologic process of gestationally increased platelet destruction) and platelet counts above 75,000/mm^3 are thought to be able to undergo vaginal delivery. The recognition and diagnosis of this *incidental thrombocytopenia* syndrome is important, because infants born to these women appear to have a markedly reduced risk of developing thrombocytopenia compared with infants born to women who manifest the disease before pregnancy.[35] This conclusion came from a series of 1357 women who had platelet counts ranging from 97,000 to 150,000/mm^3. Women with apparent incidental thrombocytopenia and platelet counts less than 75,000/mm^3 are recommended to undergo percutaneous umbilical cord blood sampling (PUBS) for determination of the fetal platelet count.[35,36] Women with fetal platelet counts greater than 50,000/mm^3 may have a vaginal delivery. It has been suggested, partly because of conflicting and insufficient data in the literature, that women with fetal platelet counts less than this undergo cesarean delivery.[37]

Fetal scalp sampling as a means of ascertaining the fetal platelet count has been advocated by some experts over the more technically difficult, and potentially riskier, PUBS technique. However, this procedure requires fetal membranes to be ruptured and a fairly dilated cervix with an engaged fetal head to be present.

Anesthetic Management

Once a route of delivery has been determined, the anesthesiologist may then ponder the issue of technique of choice. Certainly the patient manifesting clinical signs of bleeding (as discussed earlier) should not be considered a safe candidate for regional anesthesia. However, there is much controversy as to the acceptable minimal platelet count in the asymptomatic thrombocytopenic patient.

The bleeding time has been demonstrated by Harker and Slichter to remain normal until platelet concentrations fall to less than 100,000/mm^3 in the average patient, hence the common teaching that levels greater than this probably are safe for regional anesthesia.[38] They also demonstrated that platelet recovery after transfusion averages 65% of the amount infused in both normal patients *and* patients with ITP. However, platelet survival, as determined by peripheral platelet counts, was reduced to 48 to 230 minutes in ITP patients.[39]

Ideally, if platelet transfusion is deemed necessary, single-donor plateletpheresis should be done and the platelet count should be expected to peak 1 hour after transfusion.

In terms of neurologic sequelae with the use of regional anesthesia in ITP patients, Rolbin et al. recently reported a series of 61 pregnant patients, of whom 3 had platelet counts less than 100,000/mm^3, who had no neurologic sequelae after epidural anesthesia.[40] In a follow-up retrospective review of 2929 parturients, of whom 24 had platelet counts less than 100,000/mm^3, Rasmus et al. did not find that peripartum thrombocytopenia, with platelet counts as low as 18,000/mm^3, increased the risk of neurologic complications after a regional anesthetic.[41] In that study, 12 of those patients had lumbar epidural anesthetics (platelet counts from 18,000 to 90,000/mm^3) and 2 had spinal anesthetics (platelet counts 24,000 and 35,000/mm^3, respectively) without neurologic complaints. Interestingly, of the 24 patients with platelet counts less than 100,000/mm^3, 2 were diagnosed with ITP, but not until into the postpartum period since there was no suspicion of thrombocytopenia before delivery. Thus it is beginning to appear that even patients with mild thrombocytopenia may safely receive regional anesthesia. However, as always, the risk of epidural or spinal hematoma (with the potentially catastrophic complication of paraplegia) must be weighed against the complications resulting from a failed intubation with the use of general anesthesia (aspiration, hypoxemia, possible maternal death).

Finally, one should always remember that other analgesic options do exist if regional anesthesia is contraindicated. Kleiman and co-workers reported excellent results with the use of PCA using fentanyl in a parturient with a platelet function abnormality.[42] In that case, the patient received a 50-μg loading dose of fentanyl, after which 20-μg boluses of the drug were self-administered every 3 minutes as needed. A total of 400 μg over 3.5 hours were used without maternal or neonatal respiratory sequelae. However, observation of the baby in an *intensive care* setting for at least 6 hours was recommended since the neonatal half-life of fentanyl can vary from 75 to 440 minutes.[43] Narcotic-induced decreases in beat-to-beat variability also should be anticipated.

Polymyositis and Dermatomyositis

These two diseases are characterized by damage to skeletal muscle by a lymphocyte inflammatory process resulting in symmetrical proximal muscle weakness. When the muscular findings are associated with dermatologic changes, the disease is termed *dermatomyositis*. An infectious origin is suggested by epidemiologic studies in the childhood form of the disease and in adults by the occurrence of polymyositis in human immunovirus–infected individuals.[44] Although rare, there is a female preponderance of 2 : 1 with this disease, along with a bimodal age of onset occurring either in the late childhood-teen years or around 50 years of age. There have been only limited reviews in the literature concerning pregnancy and these disease entities, with the outcome of pregnancy varying with the age of onset and the degree of disease activity at the time of conception.[45,46] There seems to be a high incidence of fetal losses with the adult-onset form and strict antepartum surveillance usually is the norm.

Although the disease is fairly uncommon, the anesthesiologist should be aware of certain problems inherent to this disease process that carry significant anesthetic implications.

Cardiopulmonary Effects

Myocardial fibrosis may lead to conduction defects and/or an inflammatory cardiomyopathy. At the very least, an ECG should be obtained and a good history and physical examination should be done to rule out cardiac decompensation.

Pulmonary fibrosis or pneumonitis may be present with this disease as well. The patient should be questioned for a history of shortness of breath, dyspnea, or decreased exercise tolerance. The patient in whom pulmonary involvement is suspected should have a baseline pulse oximetry value and arterial blood gas sampling. Pulmonary function tests may shed light on the degree of pulmonary decompensation.

Airway Involvement

Dysphagia due to weakness of the striated muscles of the pharynx may render the patient more susceptible to aspiration of secretions and gastric contents. Thus, the pregnant patient with this disease is considered to have even a *fuller* stomach than an otherwise healthy patient. In addition, patients may have joint involvement typical of rheumatoid arthritis or SLE that may render endotracheal intubation difficult.

Neuromuscular Effects

Proximal muscle weakness usually first occurs in the lower extremities. A thorough examination of muscle strength should be carried out before initiation of any anesthetic so as not to confuse the cause of postpartum muscle weakness.

Although there is no evidence that the disease affects the neuromuscular junction, Wylie and Churchill-Davidson reported subjective improvement in peripheral weakness in these patients after administration of anticholinesterases and, therefore, cautioned use of muscle relaxants.[47] Flusche et al. reported significantly delayed recovery from vecuronium in a patient with polymyositis in addition to multiple other medical problems.[48] However, Brown et al. recently reported normal onset, peak effect, and recovery with both succinylcholine and atracurium in a patient with active dermatomyositis.[49]

Medications

Corticosteroids are the treatment of choice to restore strength and normalize the creatine phosphokinase level. Therefore these patients should receive stress-steroid doses when coming to labor and delivery. When the patient is on cyclosporin therapy, there may be sensitization to vecuronium-induced neuromuscular blockade.[50]

Ankylosing Spondylitis

Ankylosing spondylitis is a rheumatic disease characterized by inflammation of the apophyseal, sacroiliac, and costovertebral joints of the spine. It most commonly arises in the childbearing years, and the primary sites of involvement are the cervical spine and pubic symphysis in pregnant patients. A retrospective review found that with pregnancy, symptoms worsened in 30% of patients, improved in 30%, and were unchanged in 40%.[51] In addition, it was noted that most patients will experience a temporary flare in the first 6 postpartum months. In terms of the disease's effect on pregnancy, most women have completely normal pregnancies, and vaginal delivery usually is indicated. However, the disease does dictate several anesthetic considerations for patient management during labor and delivery.

Cardiopulmonary Involvement

A small percentage of patients with ankylosing spondylitis may develop proximal aortitis. Fibrotic degeneration may lead to the development of aortic insufficiency or destruction of the atrioventricular bundle with subsequent heart block.[52] Mitral valve involvement may occur as well. Fortunately, most of these cardiac complications are seen in patients who have had the disease more than 15 to 30 years and thus do not often present in pregnancy. However, this should not dissuade the anesthesiologist from eliciting a thorough cardiac history along with performing cardiac auscultation and obtaining a baseline ECG.

Respiratory complications result from progressive ankylosis, causing limitations in thoracic and cervical extension, and thus preventing chest expansion by producing fixation of the thoracic cage. Diffuse pulmonary fibrosis, cyst formations, and secondary amyloidosis also may occur.[53] In addition, the pregnant patient's gravid uterus will create further diminution in lung volumes, causing a severe restrictive process. Pulmonary function testing (which can even be done at the bedside) and baseline oximetry readings should be obtained if any symptoms of dyspnea or shortness of breath are elicited. Patients with severe restrictive disease may not be candidates for high levels of regional anesthesia because of their already compromised lung volumes.

Airway Abnormalities

Perhaps of most concern to the obstetric anesthesiologist is the presence of airway abnormalities in these patients. If the duration of the disease is 16 years or more, 75% of patients develop cervical ankylosis and have a high risk of cervical fractures.[54] Cervical spine involvement may range from slightly decreased limitation of neck movement to complete neck fusion, usually in the flexed position. Loss of normal flexibility with increasing osteoporosis predisposes the spine to fracture, usually at the C-5-6 and C-6-7 levels, even after relatively minor trauma.[52] Because of the danger of undiagnosed fractures, some experts advise that every patient having ankylosing spondylitis have preoperative spine radiographs, even though visualization of low cervical fractures may be difficult if not impossible.[53,54] Cervical spinal injuries in ankylosing spondylitis are reported to be accompanied by transection of, or extensive injuries to, the spinal cord in 50% of cases.[55] Therefore it is suggested in the literature that fiberoptic transnasal (since orotracheal intubation may push the cranial fragment of the cervical spine ventrally) or retrograde tracheal intubation of the patient with long-standing ankylosing spondylitis be performed while the patient is awake. This is no doubt made much more difficult in the pregnant patient considering the hypertrophy of the nasal mucosa.

In addition to cervical spine involvement, the disease process also may affect mobility of both the temporomandibular joint (thus adequate oral opening should be checked) and the cricoarytenoid joint (inquiries into hoarseness, dysphagia, or dyspnea should be made). Cricoarytenoid involvement may make the vocal cords more susceptible to trauma or may result in fixation of the cords.[54]

Neuromuscular Effects

In addition to the aforementioned cervical problems, additional disease may result from spinal fractures elsewhere or by development of a cauda equina syndrome. Pain, numbness, or weakness in the lower limbs and difficulty with micturation or defecation often are presenting complaints, and the syndrome appears to occur when the disease is inactive.[55] Focal epilepsy and peripheral nerve lesions also have been described with the disease.[53] Restriction in lumbar flexion and calcification of interspinous ligaments may make regional anesthesia difficult or impossible. Obviously, all of these patients should be questioned and examined for any limitations in spine movement or presence of existing neurologic impairment before initiation of an anesthetic.

Progressive Systemic Sclerosis

Progressive systemic sclerosis (PSS), also known as *scleroderma,* is a multisystem disease characterized by the excessive production of connective tissue along with intimal proliferation and adventitial fibrosis of small vessels. The disease has a 3 : 1 female-to-male ratio with a 10 : 1 preponderance in the reproductive age groups.[56] However, since the peak age of onset is in the third to fifth decade, the disease is uncommon in pregnancy. When it does occur in the pregnant patient though, about 50% will notice an acceleration in the disease process.[57] In addition, the incidence of spontaneous abortion, stillbirth, premature labor, and perinatal mortality is high.[58]

In terms of pathogenesis, studies suggest that both the immune and connective tissue systems are abnormal in this disorder. A primary defect in the immune system has been suggested to result in the production of lymphokines, which then stimulate connective tissue synthesis and cause the typical connective tissue changes seen in scleroderma.[59] The spectrum of disease varies from isolated peripheral cutaneous symptoms to widespread multisystem involvement. The organ involvements of special significance to the anesthesiologist need to be discussed in detail to appreciate their implications for anesthetic management.

Cardiopulmonary Implications

Over the years there has been some controversy over the frequency, cause, and clinical implications of the myocardial involvement seen in this disease. However, autopsy studies in affected patients have demonstrated that myocardial progressive systemic sclerosis is a distinct entity with relatively frequent occurrence that may lead to arrhythmias, CHF, angina pectoris with normal coronary arteries, and sudden death.[60] Intermittent vascular spasm, resulting in *contraction band necrosis,* similar to what is seen in the digits, is thought to play a role in the damage. In addition, chronic pericardial effusion with CHF also may be present and is thought to be a harbinger of renal failure.[59] Systemic hypertension is a result of renal arteriolar intimal proliferation with vascular obstruction and subsequent impairment in renal perfusion. A baseline ECG should be obtained in addition to performing a thorough history and physical. Any question of cardiac decompensation should be followed through with additional studies such as echocardiography.

In terms of simply obtaining vital signs, Korotkoff sounds have been reported to be difficult to auscultate and may not accurately reflect central pressures.[61] Arterial catheterization may be needed to monitor blood pressure, although this may precipitate spasm and necrosis in smaller arteries.

Pulmonary hypertension is a major cause of death in this disease.[62] It appears more often in patients with the CREST syndrome than the other variants of the disease. This acronym stands for *c*alcinosis, *R*aynaud's phenomenon, *e*sophageal motility disorder, *s*clerodactyly and *t*elangiectasia. Pulmonary fibrosis from the sclerodermatous involvement of the lungs causes decreased inspiratory capacity, decreased compliance, decreased diffusion capacity, and increased residual volume.[63] Hypoxemia may result from decreases in diffusion capacity. Warm ambient temperatures have been shown to produce an improvement in diffusion capacity.[64] Pulmonary function testing should be performed along with pulse oximetry to obtain a baseline assessment of prelabor respiratory reserve.

Renal Involvement

Patients who have renal involvement may have either fulminant, hypertensive, oliguric renal failure, or acute renal failure with normal blood pressure.[65] Renal disease may occur at any time during pregnancy, but usually occurs in the third trimester and may appear abruptly in patients with previously documented normal renal function. In patients with known renal disease who do not wish to terminate their pregnancy, baseline assessment of renal function (including a 24-hour urine collection) should be performed. Careful attention to blood pressure and renal status must be maintained throughout pregnancy, while also monitoring fetal growth and well-being, given the higher incidence of stillbirths and premature labor.

Because renal blood flow has been shown to significantly fall with the exacerbation of Raynaud's from cold temperatures, keeping the patient with renal involvement warm is mandatory.[66] Although there is no specific treatment for the renal lesion, it is generally thought advisable to control systemic hypertension to prevent renal vasoconstriction.[59] Hemodialysis or renal transplantation have been used in appropriate patients.

Airway Abnormalities

Sclerodermatous skin contractures, along with temporomandibular joint dysfunction, can severely limit opening of the mouth, making conventional intubation difficult or impossible.[61] Telangiectasias, present orally or nasally, may on rare occasions bleed profusely if traumatized with airway equipment. The already higher risk of aspiration with pregnancy is made worse by the presence of gastroesophageal sphincter incompetence and esophageala dysmotility in these patients. Metoclopramide may be helpful in increasing gastroesophageal sphincter tone in this situation. In addition, anatomic deformities (described characteristically as a fish-mouth appearance) in patients with scleroderma may make even simple mask oxygenation difficult. Laryngeal involvement, presenting as edema, also has been reported.[67]

Therefore if endotracheal intubation is needed, most experts recommend awake fiberoptic intubation. Limited oral opening, perhaps preventing placement of an Ovassapian-type airway for the fiberscope, must be weighed against traumatizing nasal telangiectasias in the pregnant patient. Preparations for tracheostomy should always be made in the event that the airway is lost during intubation attempts. For these reasons, regional anesthesia has been strongly encouraged by some for cesarean delivery whenever possible.[61] However, one must keep in mind that, if the regional route is chosen, the possibility for general anesthesia may then arise on an urgent basis. This scenario has prompted some experts to advocate always securing the airway via elective intubation followed by general anesthesia over regional anesthesia in patients with severe airway manifestations of scleroderma. Obviously, this decision has to be made on an individual basis only after a thorough examination of the patient's airway and regional landmarks (because there can be severe changes in ligament and spine flexibility) has been performed.

Neuromuscular Effects

In addition to the aforementioned ligament and joint changes of the back and spine, atrophy of the vasa nervorum leading to mononeuritis multiplex has been noted. Thus, a thorough examination of the patient's peripheral sensory function should be made before performing any regional anesthetic. Prolonged anesthesia with the use of both lidocaine and chloroprocaine has been described.[61,68]

Skin

In addition to the aforementioned integumentary problems, one should expect difficulty in obtaining intravenous access secondary to thickened, fibrotic skin and vasospasm. A warm room and warm intravenous fluids are essential in maximizing success at venous, and arterial if needed, cannulation.

Gastrointestinal Abnormalities

Esophageal reflux, with esophagitis and stricture, may occur with this disease. Decreased intestinal motility may lead to bacterial overgrowth and secondary malabsorption because of deconjugation of bile salts. Malabsorption of vitamin K then may lead to a blood clotting abnormality with a prolongation of the PT.[62]

Autoimmune Hemolytic Anemia

In this disease process, the patient develops autoantibodies to the antigens on her red blood cells. These antibodies are primarily divided into two classes: the warm reacting antibodies and the cold antibodies. Warm antibodies are primarily of the IgG type and may cross the placenta. Warm antibodies are associated with hematologic malignancies, SLE, viral infections, and drug ingestion (such as methyldopa). Cold antibodies are associated with mycoplasma infections and mononucleosis, and are typically of the IgM type. A positive direct Coomb's test is the most commonly used method for diagnosis.

Autoimmune hemolytic anemia usually worsens during pregnancy. Clinical features include the signs and symptoms due to anemia and splenomegaly. Laboratory findings demonstrate low hematocrit levels and hyperbilirubinemia, and occasionally leukopenia and thrombocytopenia.

The anesthesiologist should be aware that transfusion therapy may be complicated in these patients because the autoantibody is directed to a component of the Rh locus that is present on the erythrocytes of essentially all potential donors.[69] In emergencies, the least incompatible cells available should be used for transfusion. In cold agglutinin disease, all intravenous solutions (including blood) should be warmed before administration so as not to aggravate the hemolysis. Treatment for warm antibody hemolytic anemia consists of corticosteroids, which need to be given in stress doses at the time of labor and delivery. They are not effective in the cold antibody anemias, however. In difficult cases of either type, immunosuppressive therapy has been used.

Summary

Of all the diseases which have been discussed, SLE is one of the most common autoimmune diseases occurring in the parturient. To summarize the anesthetic management of the case presented:

1. Multiple systems may be involved involving cardiopulmonary, renal, neuromuscular, hepatic, and immune functions.
2. Depending on the severity of the disease and extent of organ involvement, invasive monitors may be necessary.
3. Patients with hepatic or renal dysfunction may not be able to normally metabolize and excrete medications eliminated via these routes.
4. The presence of ACA and/or LAC may result in a prolongation of the PTT and, rarely, the PT secondary to their reaction with phospholipid antigens used in the tests. Although the presence of these antibodies has most commonly been associated with thrombocytopenia and thrombotic complications, an occasional patient may manifest a coagulopathy Therefore, before considering regional anesthesia, it should be determined that the platelet count and bleeding time are within normal limits.

References

1. Hollingsworth JW, Resnick R: *Rheumatologic and connective tissue disorders.* In Creasy RK, Resnick R, editors: *Maternal Fetal medicine: principles and practice,* Philadelphia, 1989, WB Saunders.
2. Lockshin MD, Reinitz E, Druzin ML, et al: Lupus pregnancy case control prospective study demonstrating absence of lu-

pus exacerbation during or after pregnancy, *Am J Med* 1984; 77:893.

3. Mintz G, Rodriguez-Alvarez E: Systemic lupus erythematosus, *Rheum Dis Clin North Am* 1989; 15:255.
4. Steinberg AD: *Systemic lupus erythematosus.* In Wyngaarden JB, Smith LH, Lloyd H Jr, editors: *Cecil textbook of medicine,* Philadelphia, 1988, WB Saunders/Harcourt Brace Jovanovich.
5. Hayslett JP, Reece EA: Systemic lupus erythematosus in pregnancy, *Clin Perinatol* 1985; 12:539.
6. Hauch MA, Bromley B: *Autoimmune diseases.* In Datta S, editor: *Anesthetic and obstetric management of high-risk pregnancy,* St. Louis, 1991, Mosby–Year Book.
7. Lockshin MD: Antiphospholipid antibody syndrome, *JAMA* 1992; 268:1451.
8. Malinow AM, Rickford WJK, Mokriski BLK, et al: Lupus anticoagulant: implications for obstetric anaesthetists, *Anaesthesia* 1987; 42:1291.
9. Espinoza LR, Hartmann RC: Significance of the lupus anticoagulant, *Am J Hematol* 1986; 22:331.
10. Lubbe WF, Liggins GC: Lupus anticoagulant and pregnancy, *Am J Obstet Gynecol* 1985; 153:322.
11. Hanly JG, Gladman DD, Rose TH, et al: Lupus pregnancy: a prospective study of placental changes, *Arthritis Rheum* 1988; 31:358.
12. Sammaritano LR, Gharavi AE, Lockshin MD: Antiphospholipid antibody syndrome: immunologic and clinical aspects, *Semin Arthritis Rheum* 1990; 20:81.
13. Lowson SM: Lupus anticoagulant: implications for the obstetric anaesthesiologist, *Anaesthesia* 1987; 43:508.
14. Abouleish E: Obstetric anesthesia and systemic lupus erythematosus, *M E J Anesth* 1988; 9:435.
15. Condemi JJ: The autoimmune diseases, *JAMA* 1992; 268: 2882.
16. Ostensen M, Husby G: A prospective clinical study of the effect of pregnancy on rheumatoid arthritis and ankylosing spondylitis, *Arthritis Rheum* 1983; 12:69.
17. Ostensen M, Aune B, Husby G: Effect of pregnancy and hormonal changes on the activity of rheumatoid arthritis, *Scand J Rheumatol* 1983; 12:69.
18. Person D: Juvenile rheumatoid arthritis: anesthetic and surgical considerations, *AORN J* 1986; 44:439, 442, 446.
19. Keenan MA, Stiles CM, Kaufman RL: Acquired laryngeal deviation associated with cervical spine disease in erosive polyarticular arthritis: use of the fiberoptic bronchoscope in rheumatoid disease, *Anesthesiology* 1983; 58:441.
20. Sachs BP, Lorell BH, Mehrez M, et al: Constrictive pericarditis and pregnancy, *Am J Obstet Gynecol* 1986; 154:156.
21. Thurnau GR: Rheumatoid arthritis, *Clin Obstet Gynecol* 1983; 26:558.
22. Mongan ES, Coss RM, Jacox RF, et al: A study of the relation of seronegative and seropositive rheumatoid arthritis to each other and to necrotizing vasculitis, *Am J Med* 1969; 47:23.
23. Hindman BJ: Usefulness of the post-aspirin bleeding time, *Anesthesiology* 1986; 64:368.
24. Horlocker TT, Wedel DJ, Offord KP: Does preoperative antiplatelet therapy increase the risk of hemorrhagic complications associated with regional anesthesia? *Anesth Analg* 1990; 790:631.
25. Mayumi T, Dohi S: Spinal subarachnoid hematoma after lumbar puncture in a patient receiving antiplatelet therapy, *Anesth Analg* 1983; 62:777.
26. Das PB, Gupta RP, Sukumar IP, et al: Pericardiectomy: indications and results, *J Thorac Cardiovasc Surg* 1973; 66:58.
27. Burstein SA, Harker LA: *Quantitative platelet disorders.* In Bloome AL, Thomas DP, editors: *Haemostasis and thrombosis,* Edinburgh, 1981, Churchill-Livingstone.
28. Kessler I, Lancet M, Borenstein R, et al: The obstetrical management of patients with immunologic thrombocytopenic purpura, *J Obstet Gynecol* 1982; 20:33.
29. Kelton JG: Management of the pregnant patient with idiopathic thrombocytopenic purpura, *Ann Intern Med* 1983; 99:796.
30. Berchtold P, McMillan R: Therapy of chronic idiopathic thrombocytopenic purpura in adults, *Blood* 1989; 74:2309.
31. Tchernia G, Dreyfus M, Lauriaan Y, et al: Management of autoimmune thrombocytopenia in pregnancy: response to infusion of immunoglobulins, *Am J Obstet Gynecol* 1984; 148:225.
32. Pizzuto J, Ambriz R: Therapeutic experience on 934 adults with idiopathic thrombocytopenic purpura: multicentric trial of the Cooperative Latin American Group on Hemostasis and Thrombosis, *Blood* 1984; 64:1179.
33. Cines DB, Schreiber AD: Immune thrombocytopenia: use of a Coombs antiglobulin test to detect IgG and C3 on platelets, *N Engl J Med* 1979; 300:106.
34. Samuels P, Bussel JB, Braitman LE, et al: Estimation of the risk of thrombocytopenia in the offspring of pregnant women with presumed immune thrombocytopenia purpura, *N Engl J Med* 1990; 323:229.

35. Moise KJ Jr, Carpenter RJ Jr, Cotton DB, et al: Percutaneous umbilical cord blood sampling in the evaluation of fetal platelet counts in pregnant patients with autoimmune thrombocytopenic purpura, *Obstet Gynecol* 1988; 72:346.

36. Scioscia AL, Grannum PA, Copel JA, et al: The use of percutaneous umbilical blood sampling in immune thrombocytopenic purpura, *Am J Obstet Gynecol* 1988; 159:1066.

37. McCrae KR, Samuels P, Schreiber AD: Pregnancy-associated thrombocytopenia: pathogenesis and management, *Blood* 1992; 80:2697.

38. Harker LA, Slichter SJ: The bleeding time as a screening test for evaluation of platelet function, *N Engl J Med* 1972; 287:155.

39. Harker LA, Finch CA: Thrombokinetics in man, *J Clin Invest* 1969; 48:963.

40. Rolbin SH, Abbol D, Musclow E, et al: Epidural anesthesia in pregnant patients with low platelet counts, *Obstet Gynecol* 1988; 71:918.

41. Rasmus KT, Rottman RL, Kotelko DM, et al: Unrecognized thrombocytopenia and regional anesthesia in parturients: a retrospective review, *Obstet Gynecol* 1989; 73:943.

42. Kleiman SJ, Wiesel S, Tessler MJ: Patient-controlled analgesia (PCA) using fentanyl in a parturient with a platelet function abnormality, *Can J Anaesth* 1991; 38:489.

43. Koehntop DE, Rodman JH, Brundage DM, et al: Pharmacokinetics of fentanyl in neonates, *Anesth Analg* 1986;65:227.

44. Condemi JJ: The Autoimmune Diseases, *JAMA* 1992; 268:2882.

45. Rosenzweig BA, Rotmensch S, Binette SP, et al: Primary idiopathic polymyositis and dermatomyositis complicating pregnancy: diagnosis and management, *Obstet Gynecol Surv* 1989; 44:162.

46. Gutierrez G, Dagnino R, Mintz G: Polymyositis/dermatomyositis and pregnancy, *Arthritis Rheum* 1984; 27:291.

47. Wylie WD, Churchill Davidson HC. *Neurologic conditions and anaesthesia*. In Churchill-Davidson HC, editor: *A practice of anaesthesia,* Philadelphia, 1984, WB Saunders.

48. Flusche G, Unger-Sargon J, Lambert DH: Prolonged neuromuscular paralysis with vecuronium in a patient with polymyositis, *Anesth Analg* 1987; 66:188.

49. Brown S, Shuypak RC, Chandrakant P, et al: Neuromuscular blockade in a patient with active dermatomyositis, *Anesthesiology* 1992; 77:1031.

50. Wood GG: Cyclosporine-vecuronium interaction, *Can J Anaesth* 1989; 36:358.

51. Ostensen M, Husby G: Ankylosing spondylitis and pregnancy, *Rheum Dis Clin North Am* 1989; 15:241.

52. Pirlo AF, Herren AL: Ankylosing spondylitis: case report and review of literature, *Anesthesiol Rev* 1978; 5:13.

53. Sinclair JR, Mason RA: Ankylosing spondylitis: the case for awake intubation, *Anaesthesia* 1984; 39:3.

54. Salathe M, Johr M: Unsuspected cervical fractures: a common problem in ankylosing spondylitis, *Anesthesiology* 1989; 70:869.

55. Hassan I: Cauda equina syndrome in ankylosing spondylitis: a report of six cases, *J Neurol Neurosurg Psychiatry* 1976; 39:1172.

56. Black CM, Steven WM: Scleroderma, *Rheum Dis Clin North Am* 1989; 15:193.

57. Kitzmiller JL: Autoimmune disorders: maternal, fetal and neonatal risks, *Clin Obstet Gynecol* 1978; 21:385.

58. Slate WG, Graham AR: Scleroderma and pregnancy, *Am J Obstet Gynecol* 1968; 101:335.

59. Siegel RC: Scleroderma, *Med Clin North Am* 1977; 61:283.

60. Bulkey BH, Ridolfi RL, Slayer WR, et al: Myocardial lesions of progressive systemic sclerosis: a cause of cardiac dysfunction, *Circulation* 1976; 53:483.

61. Thompson J, Conklin KA: Anesthetic management of a pregnant patient with scleroderma, *Anesthesiology* 1983; 59:69.

62. Ritchie B: Pulmonary function in scleroderma, *Thorax* 1964; 19:28.

63. Sacker MA, Akgun N, Kimbel P, et al: The pathophysiology of scleroderma involving the heart and respiratory system, *Ann Intern Med* 1964; 60:611.

64. Emmannel G, Saroja D, Gopinathan K: Environmental factors and the diffusing capacity of the lungs in progressive systemic sclerosis, *Chest* 1976; 69(suppl):304.

65. D'Angelo, Fries WA, Masi AT, et al: Pathologic observations in systemic sclerosis, *Am J Med* 1969; 46:428.

66. Cannon PJ, Hassar M, Case DB, et al: The relationship of hypertension and renal failure in scleroderma (progressive systemic sclerosis) to structural and functional abnormalities of the renal cortical circulation, *Medicine* 1974; 53:1.

67. Weisman RA, Calcaterra TC: Head and neck manifestations of scleroderma, *Ann Otol* 1978; 87:332.

68. Eisele JH, Reitan JA: Scleroderma, Raynaud's phenomenon, and local anesthetics, *Anesthesiology* 1971; 34:386.

69. Schreiber AD: *Autoimmune hemolytic anemia.* In Lichtenstein LM, Fauci AD, editors: *Current therapy in allergy, immunology, and rheumatology,* Toronto, BC, 1988, Decker.

46

Anesthesia for Pregnant Patients with Increased Intracranial Pressure

A 21-year-old primigravida with 38 weeks' gestation is transferred from a peripheral hospital. The patient gives a history of severe intermittent bifrontal headaches, blurring of vision, numbness of the fingers, and unsteady gait. Neurologic examination and investigation suggest a neoplasm of the posterior fossa with increased intracranial pressure. The obstetrician decides to perform a cesarean section. Discuss the anesthetic management.

Recommendations by Gordon L. Mandell, M.D. and Sivam Ramanathan, M.D.

Maternal malignancy complicates about 1 in 1000 pregnancies.[1] These malignancies most commonly arise in the breast, cervix, or hematopoietic system.[2] Intracerebral tumors during pregnancy are rare. Roelvink et al.[3] reported 4 cases of intracerebral tumors diagnosed during pregnancy and reviewed 223 additional cases. They reported that 38% of intracerebral tumors diagnosed during pregnancy were gliomas and 28% were meningiomas. Other tumors included acoustic neuromas and cerebellar astrocytomas.

Intracranial tumors do not occur more often during pregnancy.[4] However, pregnancy may precipitate or exacerbate the symptoms of the tumor secondary to an increase in the size of the tumor. Increased tumor size may be produced by increased edema or vascularity of the tumor.

Diagnosis of Intracranial Tumors

Intracranial tumors can appear as a change in mental status, seizures, or with signs and symptoms of increased intracranial pressure (headaches, vomiting, visual disturbances, mental status changes, papilledema, hypertension, and bradycardia). During pregnancy, the accurate diagnosis of increased intracranial pressure (ICP) may be delayed because of the similarity of presentation with preeclampsia. Signs such as hemiparesis and hemisensory deficits usually are not present with preeclampsia. A high index of suspicion and a thorough neurologic examination are key to making the correct diagnosis. In cases where an intracerebral tumor is suspected, an ophthalmologic examination should be performed and a neurologist should be consulted. With computerized axial tomography and magnetic resonance imaging, the accuracy of diagnosis is significantly improved. Once the diagnosis of an intracerebral tumor is made, neurosurgeons, anesthesiologist, and neonatologists must be consulted.

Obstetric Management

No specific guidelines exist for the management of patients with intracranial tumors during pregnancy. Although neurosurgical procedures can be successfully carried out during pregnancy, it is best if delivery precedes neurosurgical intervention. In patients with stable clinical courses, neurosurgery may be postponed until after delivery. The mode of delivery is controversial. Marx et al.[5] showed that uterine contractions alone do not increase cerebrospinal fluid pressure, but that skeletal muscle contractions, which occur in response to pain, do increase pressure. In addition, maternal expulsive efforts during the second stage increase cerebrospinal fluid pressure. Therefore it is possible to induce labor in selected cases, shortening the second stage with forceps delivery. When forceps delivery is not possible, cesarean delivery should be done. Patients with normal ICP are successfully managed with epidural anesthesia.[6] Epidural anesthesia abolishes the pain associated with labor, eliminates the maternal urge to bear down during the second stage of labor, and aids in a forceps delivery. However, patients with highly malignant tumors or those that deteriorate neurologically because of increasing ICP may require immediate intervention. If the fetus is mature, immediate cesarean delivery should be performed. If the fetus is immature, neurosurgical intervention is recommended.

Conduction Anesthesia and Increased Intracranial Pressure

In the parturient with increased ICP, the use of major conduction anesthesia is highly controversial. Lumbar puncture increases the risk of a tentorial or cerebellar herniation secondary to cerebrospinal fluid leakage.[7] Therefore spinal anesthesia is contraindicated in the patient with increased ICP. The risk of an unintentional dural puncture also exists with lumbar epidural and caudal anesthesia. In addition, lumbar epidural injection increases ICP. Hilt et al.[8] demonstrated that ICP increased in response to the injection of epidural bupivacaine and normal saline in two patients with severe head injuries with continuous ICP monitors in place. They attributed this to cranial bulk displacement of cerebrospinal fluid. Caudal injection is not without risk. Abouleish[9] reported two cases of apnea after the injection of caudal lidocaine in parturients with brain tumors, presumably the result of increased ICP. For cesarean delivery, most anesthesiologists choose general anesthesia for the parturient with increased ICP. But regardless of the anesthetic technique used, prevention of further neurologic damage is essential and management must be directed at preventing normal cerebral function.

Cerebral Blood Flow and Intracranial Pressure

The safe conduct of anesthesia requires a basic understanding of the pressure-volume relationship of the intracranial contents. Normal cerebral function is dependent on both cerebral metabolism and cerebral perfusion. Should cerebral oxygen demand exceed oxygen delivery, cerebral hypoxia and possibly irreversible nerve cell damage can occur. Cerebral hypoxia usually results from decreased oxygen delivery rather than increased oxygen demand.[10] Decreased oxygen delivery may be due to hypoxemia or ischemia. Because of inadequate stores of oxygen, neural tissue is highly dependent upon vascular perfusion to function normally.

Cerebral blood flow is described by the following formula:

$$\text{CBF} = \frac{(\text{MAP} - \text{ICP})}{\text{CVR}}$$

where CBF is cerebral blood flow, MAP is mean arterial blood pressure, ICP is intracranial pressure, and CVR is cerebrovascular resistance.

An increase in ICP reduces CBF and produces ischemia leading to cerebral hypoxia and neuronal damage. In addition to neuronal damage, increased ICP produces arterial hypertension, bradycardia and other arrhythmias, abnormal breathing patterns, apnea, and pulmonary edema.

Intracranial pressure is directly related to intracranial volume (brain tissue, cerebrospinal fluid, and intracranial blood). An increase in the volume of one of these components increases ICP unless the volume of one or the other component decreases proportionately. In the patient with an intracranial neoplasm, as tumor volume increases, cerebrospinal fluid and blood are expelled from the intracranial space. Once this mechanism is exhausted, intracranial compliance decreases. Even small changes in intracranial volume will dramatically increase ICP, thus seriously affecting CBF.

Cerebrovascular Resistance and Intracranial Pressure

Cerebrovasodilation increases CBF, intracranial blood volume, and ICP in patients with intracranial tumors, and is detrimental to the patient's recovery. In contrast, cerebrovasoconstriction can reduce elevated ICP and improve the patient's condition. Cerebrovascular resistance is affected by the following: arterial carbon dioxide tension ($Paco_2$), arterial oxygen tension (Pao_2), cerebral metabolic rate for oxygen ($CMRo_2$), and anesthetic drugs. Anesthetic management is primarily directed at producing cerebrovasoconstriction and reducing intracranial blood volume. This includes proper positioning of the head and neck to promote cerebral venous outflow, preventing increases in intrathoracic and intraabdominal pressure, controlling the airway and decreasing $Paco_2$ with hyperventilation, and selecting proper anesthetic agents that decrease CBF and $CMRo_2$.

Cerebral Blood Flow, Cerebral Metabolic Rate, and Anesthetic Agents

With the exception of ketamine, most intravenous agents used to induce general anesthesia reduce CBF and $CMRo_2$.[11] Barbiturates produce a dose-dependent reduction in CBF and $CMRo_2$, whereas in the absence of significant changes in $Paco_2$, narcotics either decrease CBF and $CMRo_2$ slightly or have no effect.[11] All volatile anesthetics decrease $CMRo_2$ but increase CBF and consequently ICP.[11] The effects of nitrous oxide on CBF and $CMRo_2$ is less than that of the volatile agents, suggesting that its use after hyperventilation is safe.[11]

Anesthetic Management

The anesthetic management of the parturient with an intracerebral tumor and increased ICP for cesarean delivery begins with the preanesthetic visit. The anesthesiologist obtains a history and physical examination, and reviews laboratory values and the recommendations from other medical consultants. Special attention is paid to the patient's current neurologic status. Because these patients may be receiving diuretics to decrease cerebral edema, the patient's intravascular volume status and electrolyte balance must be evaluated. Two types of diuretics are used to decrease brain edema: osmotic diuretics (e.g., mannitol) and loop diuretics (e.g., furosemide). In experimental animals, the intravenous administration of mannitol to the mother produces decreased total body water and increased plasma sodium and potassium concentration in the fetus.[12] Furosemide may be the diuretic of choice in the pregnant patient to decrease cerebral edema. Preoperative medication that produces excessive sedation or hypoventilation usually is avoided since an increase in $Paco_2$ can increase CBF and ICP. Because of the risk of pulmonary aspiration, the patient should receive 30 ml of sodium citrate by mouth 15 to 20 minutes before induction of anesthesia.

The patient is positioned on the operating table supine with left uterine displacement and her head slightly elevated. In addition to the standard monitors, continuous arterial pressure and end-tidal carbon dioxide monitoring is advised. Central venous pressure monitoring is used when indicated. Patients with evidence of neurogenic pulmonary edema will benefit from pulmonary artery catheter placement.

The patient is preoxygenated while the obstetrician prepares the surgical site. To protect the pregnant patient from pulmonary aspiration, induction of general anesthesia requires a rapid-sequence technique using cricoid pressure and a cuffed endotracheal tube. This technique is acceptable for the parturient with increased ICP if the patient is adequately anesthetized before laryngoscopy and intubation of the trachea. Intravenous lidocaine (1.5 mg/kg) before induction of anesthesia blunts the detrimental effects of laryngoscopy and tracheal intubation on ICP.[13] Thiopental (6 mg/kg) produces unconsciousness rapidly, lowers ICP, and is considered safe for elective cesarean delivery at this dose.[14] Although succinylcholine may increase ICP due to skeletal muscle fasciculations, 1.5 mg/kg of succinylcholine after pretreatment with a nondepolarizing muscle relaxant and a thiopental induction may be acceptable.[11] As an alternative, vecuronium may be used in a priming sequence (0.01 mg/kg) 4 minutes before thiopental administration followed by (0.1 mg/kg) to facilitate tracheal intubation. The patient can be asked to voluntarily hyperventilate before induction of anesthesia to decrease $Paco_2$.

After intubation of the trachea, ventilation is controlled to maintain $Paco_2$ between 25 and 30 mm Hg. Appropriate ventilation is key in managing the patient with increased ICP. Hyperventilation not only produces a reduction in ICP, but prevents an increase in ICP caused by cerebrovasodilating drugs such as isoflurane. However, $Paco_2$ values lower than 25 mm Hg should be avoided because of the adverse effects of hyperventilation on uterine blood flow and fetal oxygenation.

Anesthesia is maintained with 50% nitrous oxide and 0.75% isoflurane before delivery of the baby. Low-dose isoflurane (less than 1.0 minimum alveolar concentration) produces minimal effects on CBF and ICP, and is useful in preventing maternal awareness and elevations in maternal blood pressure caused by surgical stimulation.[15] After the umbilical cord is clamped, the anesthetic is supplemented with intravenous fentanyl (3 to 5 μg/kg). The inspired isoflurane concentration is decreased to 0.25%. Muscle relaxation is maintained with intravenous vecuronium. Fluid administration should be minimized to avoid increasing cerebral water content and ICP. Glucose-containing solutions should be avoided in the neurosurgical patient because they can increase cerebral edema.[11]

At the conclusion of surgery, coughing or straining should be minimized. Also, extubation of the patient's trachea should not be performed until she is awake and capable of protecting her airway. To provide a smooth emergence, it is helpful to administer 1.5 mg/kg of lidocaine intravenously. After extubation the patient should be positioned with her head elevated and given supplemental oxygen by face mask. In the postanesthesia care unit a neurologic examination should be performed, since neurologic deterioration during the postoperative period requires immediate evaluation.

Summary

1. Intracerebral tumors are rare during pregnancy and the diagnosis of increased ICP may be delayed because of the similarity of presentation with preeclampsia. However, once the correct diagnosis is made, neurosurgeons, anesthesiologists, and neonatologists should be consulted.
2. If possible, delivery should precede neurosurgical intervention. Patients with stable courses may deliver vaginally with epidural anesthesia; however, those with rapid neurologic deterioration and increased ICP may require immediate cesarean delivery under general anesthesia.
3. When ICP is elevated, using conduction anesthesia is highly controversial. Epidural anesthesia increases ICP and may cause herniation if an unintentional dural puncture occurs.
4. Increased ICP reduces CBF and produces ischemia, leading to cerebral hypoxia and neuronal damage. Anesthetic management is directed at reducing intracranial volume. This includes the following: proper positioning of the head to promote cerebral venous outflow, preventing increases in intrathoracic and intraabdominal pressure, controlling the airway and decreasing $Paco_2$ with hyperventilation, and selecting anesthetic agents that decrease CBF and $CMRo_2$.

References

1. Pollack RN, Pollack M, Rochon L: Pregnancy complicated by medulloblastoma with metastases to the placenta, *Obstet Gynecol* 1983; 81:858.
2. Koren G, Weiner L, Lishner M, et al: Cancer in pregnancy: identification of unanswered questions on maternal and fetal risks, *Obstet Gynecol Surv* 1990; 45:509.
3. Roelvink NCA, Kamphorst W, van Alphen HAM, et al: Pregnancy-related primary brain and spinal tumors, *Arch Neurol* 1987; 44:209.
4. Haas JF, Janisch W, Stanczek W: Newly diagnosed primary intracranial neoplasms in pregnant women: A population-based assessment, *J Neurol Neurosurg Psychiatry* 1986; 49:874.
5. Marx GF, Zemaitis MT, Orkin LR: Cerebrospinal fluid pressures during labor and obstetrical anesthesia, *Anesthesiology* 1961; 22:348.
6. Finfer SR: Management of labour and delivery in patients with intracranial neoplasms, *Br J Anaesth* 1991; 67:784.
7. Duffy GP: Lumbar puncture in the presence of raised intracranial pressure, *Br Med J* 1969; 1:407.
8. Hilt H, Gramm H-J, Link J: Changes in intracranial pressure associated with extradural anaesthesia, *Br J Anaesth* 1986; 58:676.
9. Abouleish E: Intracranial hypertension and caudal anaesthesia, *Br J Anaesth* 1987; 59:1478 (letter).
10. Michenfelder JD: Brain hypoxia: Current status of experimental and clinical therapy, *Semin Anesth* 1983; 2:81.
11. Messick JM, Newberg LA, Nugent M, et al: Principles of neuroanesthesia for the nonneurosurgical patient with CNS pathophysiology, *Anesth Analg* 1985; 64:143.
12. Bruns PD, Linder RO, Drose VE, et al: The placental transfer of water from fetus to mother following the intravenous infusion of hypertonic mannitol to the maternal rabbit, *Am J Obstet Gynecol* 1963; 86:160
13. Hamill JF, Bedford RF, Weaver DC, et al: Lidocaine before endotracheal intubation: intravenous or laryngotracheal? *Anesthesiology* 1981; 55:578.
14. Kosaka Y, Takahashi T, Mark LC: Intravenous thiobarbiturate anesthesia for cesarean section, *Anesthesiology* 1969; 31:489.
15. Eger EI: Isoflurane: a review, *Anesthesiology* 1981; 55:559.

Index

B

C

H

K

L

M

Q

R

S

T

U

V

W